VIRAL INFECTIONS OF THE RESPIRATORY TRACT

LUNG BIOLOGY IN HEALTH AND DISEASE

Executive Editor

Claude Lenfant
*Director, National Heart, Lung and Blood Institute
National Institutes of Health
Bethesda, Maryland*

1. Immunologic and Infectious Reactions in the Lung, *edited by Charles H. Kirkpatrick and Herbert Y. Reynolds*
2. The Biochemical Basis of Pulmonary Function, *edited by Ronald G. Crystal*
3. Bioengineering Aspects of the Lung, *edited by John B. West*
4. Metabolic Functions of the Lung, *edited by Y. S. Bakhle and John R. Vane*
5. Respiratory Defense Mechanisms (in two parts), *edited by Joseph D. Brain, Donald F. Proctor, and Lynne M. Reid*
6. Development of the Lung, *edited by W. Alan Hodson*
7. Lung Water and Solute Exchange, *edited by Norman C. Staub*
8. Extrapulmonary Manifestations of Respiratory Disease, *edited by Eugene Debs Robin*
9. Chronic Obstructive Pulmonary Disease, *edited by Thomas L. Petty*
10. Pathogenesis and Therapy of Lung Cancer, *edited by Curtis C. Harris*
11. Genetic Determinants of Pulmonary Disease, *edited by Stephen D. Litwin*
12. The Lung in the Transition Between Health and Disease, *edited by Peter T. Macklem and Solbert Permutt*
13. Evolution of Respiratory Processes: A Comparative Approach, *edited by Stephen C. Wood and Claude Lenfant*
14. Pulmonary Vascular Diseases, *edited by Kenneth M. Moser*
15. Physiology and Pharmacology of the Airways, *edited by Jay A. Nadel*
16. Diagnostic Techniques in Pulmonary Disease (in two parts), *edited by Marvin A. Sackner*
17. Regulation of Breathing (in two parts), *edited by Thomas F. Hornbein*
18. Occupational Lung Diseases: Research Approaches and Methods, *edited by Hans Weill and Margaret Turner-Warwick*
19. Immunopharmacology of the Lung, *edited by Harold H. Newball*
20. Sarcoidosis and Other Granulomatous Diseases of the Lung, *edited by Barry L. Fanburg*

21. Sleep and Breathing, *edited by Nicholas A. Saunders and Colin E. Sullivan*
22. *Pneumocystis carinii* Pneumonia: Pathogenesis, Diagnosis, and Treatment, *edited by Lowell S. Young*
23. Pulmonary Nuclear Medicine: Techniques in Diagnosis of Lung Disease, *edited by Harold L. Atkins*
24. Acute Respiratory Failure, *edited by Warren M. Zapol and Konrad J. Falke*
25. Gas Mixing and Distribution in the Lung, *edited by Ludwig A. Engel and Manuel Paiva*
26. High-Frequency Ventilation in Intensive Care and During Surgery, *edited by Graziano Carlon and William S. Howland*
27. Pulmonary Development: Transition from Intrauterine to Extrauterine Life, *edited by George H. Nelson*
28. Chronic Obstructive Pulmonary Disease: Second Edition, Revised and Expanded, *edited by Thomas L. Petty*
29. The Thorax (in two parts), *edited by Charis Roussos and Peter T. Macklem*
30. The Pleura in Health and Disease, *edited by Jacques Chrétien, Jean Bignon, and Albert Hirsch*
31. Drug Therapy for Asthma: Research and Clinical Practice, *edited by John W. Jenne and Shirley Murphy*
32. Pulmonary Endothelium in Health and Disease, *edited by Una S. Ryan*
33. The Airways: Neural Control in Health and Disease, *edited by Michael A. Kaliner and Peter J. Barnes*
34. Pathophysiology and Treatment of Inhalation Injuries, *edited by Jacob Loke*
35. Respiratory Function of the Upper Airway, *edited by Oommen P. Mathew and Giuseppe Sant'Ambrogio*
36. Chronic Obstructive Pulmonary Disease: A Behavioral Perspective, *edited by A. John McSweeny and Igor Grant*
37. Biology of Lung Cancer: Diagnosis and Treatment, *edited by Steven T. Rosen, James L. Mulshine, Frank Cuttitta, and Paul G. Abrams*
38. Pulmonary Vascular Physiology and Pathophysiology, *edited by E. Kenneth Weir and John T. Reeves*
39. Comparative Pulmonary Physiology: Current Concepts, *edited by Stephen C. Wood*
40. Respiratory Physiology: an Analytical Approach, *edited by H. K. Chang and Manuel Paiva*
41. Lung Cell Biology, *edited by Donald Massaro*
42. Heart–Lung Interactions in Health and Disease, *edited by Steven M. Scharf and Sharon S. Cassidy*
43. Clinical Epidemiology of Chronic Obstructive Pulmonary Disease, *edited by Michael J. Hensley and Nicholas A. Saunders*
44. Surgical Pathology of Lung Neoplasms, *edited by Alberto M. Marchevsky*
45. The Lung in Rheumatic Diseases, *edited by Grant W. Cannon and Guy A. Zimmerman*

46. Diagnostic Imaging of the Lung, *edited by Charles E. Putman*
47. Models of Lung Disease: Microscopy and Structural Methods, *edited by Joan Gil*
48. Electron Microscopy of the Lung, *edited by Dean E. Schraufnagel*
49. Asthma: Its Pathology and Treatment, *edited by Michael A. Kaliner, Peter J. Barnes, and Carl G. A. Persson*
50. Acute Respiratory Failure: Second Edition, *edited by Warren M. Zapol and Francois Lemaire*
51. Lung Disease in the Tropics, *edited by Om P. Sharma*
52. Exercise: Pulmonary Physiology and Pathophysiology, *edited by Brian J. Whipp and Karlman Wasserman*
53. Developmental Neurobiology of Breathing, *edited by Gabriel G. Haddad and Jay P. Farber*
54. Mediators of Pulmonary Inflammation, *edited by Michael A. Bray and Wayne H. Anderson*
55. The Airway Epithelium, *edited by Stephen G. Farmer and Douglas Hay*
56. Physiological Adaptations in Vertebrates: Respiration, Circulation, and Metabolism, *edited by Stephen C. Wood, Roy E. Weber, Alan R. Hargens, and Ronald W. Millard*
57. The Bronchial Circulation, *edited by John Butler*
58. Lung Cancer Differentiation: Implications for Diagnosis and Treatment, *edited by Samuel D. Bernal and Paul J. Hesketh*
59. Pulmonary Complications of Systemic Disease, *edited by John F. Murray*
60. Lung Vascular Injury: Molecular and Cellular Response, *edited by Arnold Johnson and Thomas J. Ferro*
61. Cytokines of the Lung, *edited by Jason Kelley*
62. The Mast Cell in Health and Disease, *edited by Michael A. Kaliner and Dean D. Metcalfe*
63. Pulmonary Disease in the Elderly Patient, *edited by Donald A. Mahler*
64. Cystic Fibrosis, *edited by Pamela B. Davis*
65. Signal Transduction in Lung Cells, *edited by Jerome S. Brody, David M. Center, and Vsevolod A. Tkachuk*
66. Tuberculosis: A Comprehensive International Approach, *edited by Lee B. Reichman and Earl S. Hershfield*
67. Pharmacology of the Respiratory Tract: Experimental and Clinical Research, *edited by K. Fan Chung and Peter J. Barnes*
68. Prevention of Respiratory Diseases, *edited by Albert Hirsch, Marcel Goldberg, Jean-Pierre Martin, and Roland Masse*
69. *Pneumocystis carinii* Pneumonia: Second Edition, Revised and Expanded, *edited by Peter D. Walzer*
70. Fluid and Solute Transport in the Airspaces of the Lungs, *edited by Richard M. Effros and H. K. Chang*
71. Sleep and Breathing: Second Edition, Revised and Expanded, *edited by Nicholas A. Saunders and Colin E. Sullivan*
72. Airway Secretion: Physiological Bases for the Control of Mucous Hypersecretion, *edited by Tamotsu Takishima and Sanae Shimura*

73. Sarcoidosis and Other Granulomatous Disorders, *edited by D. Geraint James*
74. Epidemiology of Lung Cancer, *edited by Jonathan M. Samet*
75. Pulmonary Embolism, *edited by Mario Morpurgo*
76. Sports and Exercise Medicine, *edited by Stephen C. Wood and Robert C. Roach*
77. Endotoxin and the Lungs, *edited by Kenneth L. Brigham*
78. The Mesothelial Cell and Mesothelioma, *edited by Marie-Claude Jaurand and Jean Bignon*
79. Regulation of Breathing: Second Edition, Revised and Expanded, *edited by Jerome A. Dempsey and Allan I. Pack*
80. Pulmonary Fibrosis, *edited by Sem Hin Phan and Roger S. Thrall*
81. Long-Term Oxygen Therapy: Scientific Basis and Clinical Application, *edited by Walter J. O'Donohue, Jr.*
82. Ventral Brainstem Mechanisms and Control of Respiration and Blood Pressure, *edited by C. Ovid Trouth, Richard M. Millis, Heidrun F. Kiwull-Schöne, and Marianne E. Schläfke*
83. A History of Breathing Physiology, *edited by Donald F. Proctor*
84. Surfactant Therapy for Lung Disease, *edited by Bengt Robertson and H. William Taeusch*
85. The Thorax: Second Edition, Revised and Expanded (in three parts), *edited by Charis Roussos*
86. Severe Asthma: Pathogenesis and Clinical Management, *edited by Stanley J. Szefler and Donald Y. M. Leung*
87. *Mycobacterium avium*–Complex Infection: Progress in Research and Treatment, *edited by Joyce A. Korvick and Constance A. Benson*
88. Alpha 1–Antitrypsin Deficiency: Biology • Pathogenesis • Clinical Manifestations • Therapy, *edited by Ronald G. Crystal*
89. Adhesion Molecules and the Lung, *edited by Peter A. Ward and Joseph C. Fantone*
90. Respiratory Sensation, *edited by Lewis Adams and Abraham Guz*
91. Pulmonary Rehabilitation, *edited by Alfred P. Fishman*
92. Acute Respiratory Failure in Chronic Obstructive Pulmonary Disease, *edited by Jean-Philippe Derenne, William A. Whitelaw, and Thomas Similowski*
93. Environmental Impact on the Airways: From Injury to Repair, *edited by Jacques Chrétien and Daniel Dusser*
94. Inhalation Aerosols: Physical and Biological Basis for Therapy, *edited by Anthony J. Hickey*
95. Tissue Oxygen Deprivation: From Molecular to Integrated Function, *edited by Gabriel G. Haddad and George Lister*
96. The Genetics of Asthma, *edited by Stephen B. Liggett and Deborah A. Meyers*
97. Inhaled Glucocorticoids in Asthma: Mechanisms and Clinical Actions, *edited by Robert P. Schleimer, William W. Busse, and Paul M. O'Byrne*
98. Nitric Oxide and the Lung, *edited by Warren M. Zapol and Kenneth D. Bloch*

99. Primary Pulmonary Hypertension, *edited by Lewis J. Rubin and Stuart Rich*
100. Lung Growth and Development, *edited by John A. McDonald*
101. Parasitic Lung Diseases, *edited by Adel A. F. Mahmoud*
102. Lung Macrophages and Dendritic Cells in Health and Disease, *edited by Mary F. Lipscomb and Stephen W. Russell*
103. Pulmonary and Cardiac Imaging, *edited by Caroline Chiles and Charles E. Putman*
104. Gene Therapy for Diseases of the Lung, *edited by Kenneth L. Brigham*
105. Oxygen, Gene Expression, and Cellular Function, *edited by Linda Biadasz Clerch and Donald J. Massaro*
106. Beta$_2$-Agonists in Asthma Treatment, *edited by Romain Pauwels and Paul M. O'Byrne*
107. Inhalation Delivery of Therapeutic Peptides and Proteins, *edited by Akwete Lex Adjei and Pramod K. Gupta*
108. Asthma in the Elderly, *edited by Robert A. Barbee and John W. Bloom*
109. Treatment of the Hospitalized Cystic Fibrosis Patient, *edited by David M. Orenstein and Robert C. Stern*
110. Asthma and Immunological Diseases in Pregnancy and Early Infancy, *edited by Michael Schatz, Robert S. Zeiger, and Henry N. Claman*
111. Dyspnea, *edited by Donald A. Mahler*
112. Proinflammatory and Antiinflammatory Peptides, *edited by Sami I. Said*
113. Self-Management of Asthma, *edited by Harry Kotses and Andrew Harver*
114. Eicosanoids, Aspirin, and Asthma, *edited by Andrew Szczeklik, Ryszard J. Gryglewski, and John R. Vane*
115. Fatal Asthma, *edited by Albert L. Sheffer*
116. Pulmonary Edema, *edited by Michael A. Matthay and David H. Ingbar*
117. Inflammatory Mechanisms in Asthma, *edited by Stephen T. Holgate and William W. Busse*
118. Physiological Basis of Ventilatory Support, *edited by John J. Marini and Arthur S. Slutsky*
119. Human Immunodeficiency Virus and the Lung, *edited by Mark J. Rosen and James M. Beck*
120. Five-Lipoxygenase Products in Asthma, *edited by Jeffrey M. Drazen, Sven-Erik Dahlén, and Tak H. Lee*
121. Complexity in Structure and Function of the Lung, *edited by Michael P. Hlastala and H. Thomas Robertson*
122. Biology of Lung Cancer, *edited by Madeleine A. Kane and Paul A. Bunn, Jr.*
123. Rhinitis: Mechanisms and Management, *edited by Robert M. Naclerio, Stephen R. Durham, and Niels Mygind*
124. Lung Tumors: Fundamental Biology and Clinical Management, *edited by Christian Brambilla and Elisabeth Brambilla*
125. Interleukin-5: From Molecule to Drug Target for Asthma, *edited by Colin J. Sanderson*
126. Pediatric Asthma, *edited by Shirley Murphy and H. William Kelly*

127. Viral Infections of the Respiratory Tract, *edited by Raphael Dolin and Peter F. Wright*

ADDITIONAL VOLUMES IN PREPARATION

Air Pollutants and the Respiratory Tract, *edited by David L. Swift and W. Michael Foster*

Exercise-Induced Asthma, *edited by E. R. McFadden, Jr.*

Gastroesophageal Reflux Disease and Airway Disease, *edited by Mark R. Stein*

LAM and Other Diseases Characterized by Smooth Muscle Proliferation, *edited by Joel Moss*

The Lung at Depth, *edited by Claes Lundgren and John N. Miller*

Diagnostic Pulmonary Pathology, *edited by Philip T. Cagle*

Immunotherapy in Asthma, *edited by Jean Bousquet and Hans Yssel*

Neurobiology of Sleep and Circadian Rhythms, *edited by Fred Turek and Phyllis Zee*

Multimodality Treatment of Lung Cancer, *edited by Arthur T. Skarin*

Cytokines in Pulmonary Infectious Disease, *edited by Steven Nelson and Thomas Martin*

Asthma's Impact on Society: the Social and Economic Burden, *edited by Kevin B. Weiss, A. Sonia Buist, and Sean D. Sullivan*

Anticholinergic Agents in the Upper and Lower Airways, *edited by Sheldon L. Spector*

Control of Breathing in Health and Disease, *edited by Murray D. Altose and Yoshikazu Kawakami*

Chronic Lung Disease of Early Infancy, *edited by Richard D. Bland and Jacqueline J. Coalson*

Lung Growth and Development, *edited by John A. McDonald*

Parasitic Lung Diseases, *edited by Adel A. F. Mahmoud*

Particle–Lung Interactions, *edited by Peter Gehr and Joachim Heyder*

The opinions expressed in these volumes do not necessarily represent the views of the National Institutes of Health.

VIRAL INFECTIONS OF THE RESPIRATORY TRACT

Edited by

Raphael Dolin
*Harvard Medical School
Boston, Massachusetts*

Peter F. Wright
*Vanderbilt University School of Medicine
Nashville, Tennessee*

MARCEL DEKKER, INC.   NEW YORK · BASEL

ISBN: 0-8247-0195-X

The publisher offers discounts on this book when ordered in bulk quantities. For more information, write to Special Sales/Professional Marketing at the address below.

This book is printed on acid-free paper.

Copyright © 1999 by MARCEL DEKKER, INC. All Rights Reserved.

Neither this book nor any part may be reproduced or transmitted in any form or by any means, electronic or mechanical, including photocopying, microfilming, and recording, or by any information storage and retrieval system, without permission in writing from the publisher.

MARCEL DEKKER, INC.
270 Madison Avenue, New York, New York 10016
http://www.dekker.com

Current printing (last digit):
10 9 8 7 6 5 4 3 2 1

PRINTED IN THE UNITED STATES OF AMERICA

INTRODUCTION

When the series of monographs Lung Biology in Health and Disease was conceived in 1973, the intent was to publish volumes that would bring together basic and clinical research, and to translate these research outcomes into information that would benefit patients. At that time, it was thought that a dozen or so volumes would do it!

Today, it is clear that the publisher and I grossly underestimated the vitality of research in pulmonary medicine. Nevertheless, in his introduction to this volume, *Viral Infections of the Respiratory Tract*, one of the editors, Dr. Peter F. Wright, points out that none of the many volumes already published addresses viral infections.

Although viral diseases have plagued humans for millennia, it appears that the field of virology did not open up until the 1898 report by Loeffer and Frosch indicating that there were some pathogens so small that they could go through the finest of filters. In the book titled *A History of the Life Sciences* (Marcel Dekker, Inc., 1994), Lois N. Magner refers to viruses as "the invisible microbes" and mentions that much earlier write-ups used the term *virus* with a very different meaning from that used today: "The first and most common meaning of '*virus*' was '*slime*,' presumably unpleasant, but not necessarily dangerous."

Unfortunately, the occurrence of devastating viral epidemics, such as the outbreak of HIV in the 1980s or, more recently, the 1995 Ebola outbreak, has underscored the critical importance of the viral pathogens. Furthermore, the risk of new epidemics is constantly before us. For example, the global warming threat may result in the increased incidence of hantavirus infection. Thus we believe this volume is significant and timely, and we hope that it will reinforce the interest of the pulmonary research and clinical communities in viral infections. I have no doubt that, among experts in the field and pulmonary medicine practitioners, this volume will be a landmark.

I am, indeed, very grateful to the editors, Drs. Raphael Dolin and Peter F. Wright, for undertaking this project. They and the authors have produced a unique volume and a major contribution to the field of pulmonary medicine. As the overall editor of this series of monographs, I want to express my gratitude to them all, and to thank them for the opportunity to include this monograph.

Claude Lenfant, M.D.
Bethesda, Maryland

PREFACE

Virology is one of the most rapidly evolving fields in clinical medicine. It has been the direct beneficiary of the molecular revolution, in which many of the early advances in understanding structure, genetics, and replicative strategy have been the result of work with microbes—especially viruses. The discipline of virology has focused on understanding the pathogenesis of infection. This focus has been rewarded by success in the development of viral vaccines and has perhaps been influenced by the lack of easy therapeutic interventions that antibiotics provide in bacterial infections.

The rapid progress in virology must make it difficult for those outside the field to assess current trends. There are excellent textbooks in virology and viral pathogenesis from which to build a framework in fundamental virology. Strong clinical textbooks exist in adult infectious diseases and pediatric infectious disease which thoroughly cover many of the clinical aspects of virology. The goal of this volume in the Lung Biology in Health and Disease series is to direct attention more specifically to viral aspects of respiratory disease in a way that will be useful to those without formal training in infectious disease, and to emphasize the many ways in which viral infections influence respiratory physiology and pathology. The organization of the volume is more completely articulated in the introductory chapter. We appreciate the opportunity to contribute to this distinguished series and to have the chance to acknowledge the hard work of the authors of individual chapters.

Peter F. Wright
Raphael Dolin

CONTRIBUTORS

Mark R. Denison, M.D.   Associate Professor, Department of Pediatrics, Vanderbilt University School of Medicine, Nashville, Tennessee

Floyd W. Denny, Jr., M.D.   Professor, Department of Pediatrics, University of North Carolina School of Medicine at Chapel Hill, Chapel Hill, North Carolina

Raphael Dolin, M.D.   Professor, Department of Medicine, and Faculty Dean for Clinical Programs, Harvard Medical School, Boston, Massachusetts

Ann R. Falsey, M.D.   Associate Professor, Department of Medicine, University of Rochester School of Medicine and Dentistry, and Rochester General Hospital, Rochester, New York

Barney S. Graham, M.D., Ph.D.   Professor, Department of Pediatrics, Vanderbilt University School of Medicine, Nashville, Tennessee

Stephen B. Greenberg, M.D.   Professor and Vice-Chair, Department of Medicine, Baylor College of Medicine, and Ben Taub General Hospital, Houston, Texas

Peter A. Gross, M.D.   Professor and Vice-Chairman, Department of Medicine, New Jersey Medical School, Newark, and Chairman, Department of Internal Medicine, Hackensack University Medical Center, Hackensack, New Jersey

William C. Gruber, M.D. Associate Professor, Division of Infectious Diseases, Department of Pediatrics, Vanderbilt University School of Medicine, Nashville, Tennessee

Shaw-Guang Lee, Ph.D. Principal Investigator, Department of Viral Vaccine Research, Wyeth–Lederle Vaccines and Pediatrics, Pearl River, New York

Howard Levy, M.D., Ph.D., F.C.C.M. Director, Medical Intensive Care Unit, Department of Internal Medicine, University of New Mexico Health Sciences Center, Albuquerque, New Mexico

Marilyn A. Menegus, Ph.D. Professor, Department of Microbiology and Immunology, University of Rochester School of Medicine and Dentistry, Rochester, New York

Arnold S. Monto, M.D. Professor, Department of Epidemiology, School of Public Health, University of Michigan, Ann Arbor, Michigan

Steven Q. Simpson, M.D., F.C.C.P. Associate Professor, Division of Pulmonary and Critical Care Medicine, University of Kansas Medical Center, Kansas City, Kansas

John J. Treanor, M.D. Associate Professor of Medicine, Infectious Diseases Unit, University of Rochester School of Medicine and Dentistry, Rochester, New York

Edward E. Walsh, M.D. Professor, Department of Medicine, University of Rochester School of Medicine and Dentistry, and Department of Infectious Diseases, Rochester General Hospital, Rochester, New York

Peter F. Wright, M.D. Professor and Head, Division of Pediatric Infectious Diseases, Department of Pediatrics, and Director, Center for International Health, Vanderbilt University School of Medicine, Nashville, Tennessee

CONTENTS

Introduction	Claude Lenfant	*iii*
Preface		*v*
Contributors		*vii*

1. **Introduction**   1
   Peter F. Wright

Part One   VIRAL RESPIRATORY INFECTIONS IN DIFFERENT POPULATIONS

2. **Acute Lower Respiratory Infections in Children**   5
   Floyd W. Denny, Jr.

I.	Introduction	5
II.	Classification of Acute Lower Respiratory Infections	6
III.	Etiology of Acute Lower Respiratory Tract Infections	6
IV.	Role of Respiratory Viruses as Causes of Acute Lower Respiratory Infections in Children	9
V.	Role of Various Risk Factors in the Occurrence of Acute Respiratory Infections	13
VI.	Role of Acute Respiratory Infections in Developing Countries	17
VIII.	Summary and Conclusions	20
	References	21

3. **Viral Pneumonia in Adults**   25
   Stephen B. Greenberg

I.	Introduction	25
II.	Pathogenesis	26

	III.	Comparison of Viral Pneumonia in Children and Adults	27
	IV.	Community-Acquired Viral Pneumonia	27
	V.	Diagnosis	35
	VI.	Treatment and Prevention	35
	VII.	Summary	38
		References	38

4. Viral Pulmonary Infections in Older Persons   53
Ann R. Falsey

	I.	Introduction	53
	II.	Epidemiology	54
	III.	Influenza Virus	55
	IV.	Respiratory Syncytial Virus	63
	V.	Parainfluenza Viruses	67
	VI.	Rhinoviruses	69
	VII.	Coronaviruses	71
	VIII.	Summary	72
		References	73

5. Respiratory Viral Infections in Immunocompromised Patients   83
Raphael Dolin

	I.	Introduction	83
	II.	Cancer and Leukemia	84
	III.	Bone Marrow Transplantation	85
	IV.	Solid Organ Transplantation	88
	V.	Human Immunodeficiency Virus Infection	89
	VI.	Prevention	91
	VII.	Treatment	94
	VIII.	Cytomegaloviral and Other Herpes Viral Infections	95
	IX.	Summary	96
		References	97

Part Two   VIRUSES CAUSING RESPIRATORY INFECTIONS

6. Influenza A and B Viruses   105
John J. Treanor

	I.	Introduction	105
	II.	Viral Replication	106
	III.	Pathogenesis and Host Response	109

	IV.	Epidemiology	117
	V.	Clinical Features	123
	VI.	Complications	124
	VII.	Diagnosis	125
	VIII.	Prevention and Therapy	126
	IX.	Summary	137
		References	138

7. Respiratory Syncytial Viruses — **161**
Edward E. Walsh and Barney S. Graham

	I.	Introduction and History	161
	II.	Viral Structure and Replication	162
	III.	Epidemiology	164
	IV.	Nonadaptive Immune Response to Infection	167
	V.	Adaptive Immune Response to Infection	168
	VI.	Disease Pathogenesis	171
	VII.	Clinical Manifestations	175
	VIII.	Diagnosis	178
	IX.	Therapy	180
	X.	Prevention	182
		References	184

8. Parainfluenza Viruses — **205**
Peter F. Wright

	I.	Introduction	205
	II.	Similarity to Other Respiratory Viruses	206
	III.	Replicative Strategy	207
	IV.	Pathogenesis of Parainfluenza Virus Infections	208
	V.	Epidemiology	212
	VI.	Infections in Immunocompromised Hosts	213
	VII.	Viral Diagnosis	214
	VIII.	Therapy	214
	IX	Prevention	215
	X.	Summary	216
		References	216

9. Adenoviruses — **223**
Shaw-Guang Lee and William C. Gruber

	I.	Introduction	223
	II.	Classification and Morphology of Adenoviruses	224

	III.	Life Cycle and Replication	226
	IV.	Unique Role of Specific Viral Proteins	229
	V.	Viral Pathogenesis	232
	VI.	Epidemiology	236
	VII.	Clinical Manifestations	237
	VIII.	Therapy: Antivirals and Passive Immunoglobulin Treatment	240
	IX.	Prevention: Current and Potential Vaccine Strategies	240
	X.	Adenoviruses as Gene-Delivery Vectors	242
	XI.	Summary	243
		References	244

10. The Common Cold: Rhinoviruses and Coronaviruses — **253**
Mark R. Denison

	I.	Introduction	253
	II.	Rhinoviruses	254
	III.	Coronaviruses	265
	IV.	Summary	273
		References	273

11. Hantaviruses — **281**
Steven Q. Simpson and Howard Levy

	I.	Introduction	281
	II.	Viral Replication	284
	III.	Epidemiology	286
	IV.	Clinical Manifestations	288
	V.	Pathology	294
	VI.	Viral Pathogenesis	295
	VII.	Therapy	298
	VIII.	Prevention	300
		References	300

Part Three   DIAGNOSIS

12. Laboratory Diagnosis of Infection with Respiratory Viruses — **307**
Marilyn A. Menegus

	I.	Introduction	307
	II.	Specimen Collection	308
	III.	Isolation of Viruses in Cell Culture	309
	IV.	Antigen Detection	309

V.	Immunofluorescent Antibody Staining	310
VI.	Enzyme-Linked Immunosorbent Assays	310
VII.	Polymerase Chain Reaction	311
VIII.	Serology	312
IX.	Rhinoviruses	313
X.	Respiratory Syncytial Virus	314
XI.	Influenza Viruses	314
XII.	Parainfluenza Viruses	316
XIII.	Adenoviruses	317
XIV.	Coronaviruses	318
XV.	Cytomegalovirus	319
XVI.	Herpes Simplex	321
XVII.	Conclusion	322
	References	322

Part Four TREATMENT

13. Therapy of Viral Respiratory Infections — 327
Arnold S. Monto

I.	Introduction	327
II.	Amantadine and Rimantadine	327
III.	Ribavirin	338
IV.	Other Antivirals for Treatment of Infections of the Lung	345
V.	Conclusions	345
	References	346

Part Five PREVENTION

14. Prevention of Viral Respiratory Infections — 355
Peter A. Gross

I.	Influenza Virus Vaccines	355
II.	Measles	365
III.	Varicella-Zoster Virus	367
IV.	Respiratory Syncytial Virus	368
V.	Parainfluenza Virus	369
VI.	Summary	369
	References	370

Author Index   375
Subject Index 429

1

Introduction

PETER F. WRIGHT

Vanderbilt University School of Medicine
Nashville, Tennessee

In over 100 volumes published so far, the Lung Biology in Health and Disease series has not addressed viral infections of the respiratory tract. The editors undertook the task of putting this book together because they felt this was a significant oversight! In part, the efforts of the editors and chapter authors of this monograph have been directed toward presentation of the clinical manifestations and management of illness caused by common respiratory viruses. We hope that this will allow practitioners of pulmonary medicine to become more familiar with respiratory viral illness; to recognize that newer diagnostic (Chap. 12), therapeutic (Chap. 13), and preventive (Chap. 14) measures give them many more options to modify the incidence and course of illness; and, thus, make the integration of viral diagnosis into the management of acute respiratory illness an essential component of clinical care.

There is a long-established base of knowledge in these areas of viral respiratory illness. Over the past 30 years, the etiology and epidemiology of viral respiratory pathogens have been well described, particularly in children (Chap. 2). Influenza's role in mortality and morbidity in the elderly has long been recognized (Chap. 4). More recently, the importance of other viral respiratory pathogens in disease in the immunosuppressed patient has become appreciated (Chap. 5). *Viral Infections of the Lung* will review these issues, particularly from the perspective of community acquired illness (Chap. 3).

In addition, the chapters in this monograph are intended to explore our emerging understanding of the pathogenesis of viral respiratory disease. This understanding is creating bridges of research interest between molecular virology, mucosal immunology, and pulmonary physiology. The task is to translate the symptomatology of virus-induced colds, bronchitis, pneumonia, and asthma into a physiological understanding of the underlying events and to integrate the role that viruses play either through direct interactions with the respiratory tract epithelium or through the induction of immunopathology.

The upper respiratory tract shares with the gastrointestinal tract unrelenting exposure to viruses. It is a major highway for microbes into the human host. Immune tolerance and clearance of antigens must be important components at this site to avoid a continuous state of immune activation. The exposure of the lower respiratory tract to viruses and antigens through direct inhalation is much less than that of the upper respiratory tract because of the limited size of particles that will enter the lower respiratory tract (normally less than $10 \mu m$). Once infection is established in the upper respiratory tract, it may be easier for viruses to enter the lung by inhalation because of the high titers of virus in secretions, which are typically one million per milliliter of nasal secretions, or by aspiration of the copious secretions characteristic of most viral infections. Some viruses are much more likely to cause lower respiratory tract disease, which suggests that there may be barriers to viral growth in the lung or other factors that limit progression to lower respiratory tract disease that remain to be defined.

Viruses have three patterns of replication in the respiratory tract: (1) acute infection with growth confined to the respiratory mucosal surface, of which there are many examples such as rhinoviruses (Chap. 10), influenza (Chap. 6), parainfluenza viruses (Chap. 8), and respiratory syncytial virus (Chap. 7); (2) persistent replication or latency on the respiratory mucosal surface such as adenoviruses (Chap. 9); and (3) primary replication on the respiratory mucosa as a preamble to systemic spread such as measles, varicella-zoster virus, or hantavirus (Chap. 11).

Although the replicative cycle and molecular structure of many viruses is well understood and the broad temporal picture of illness is painted, the interaction of viruses with the epithelial surface and with the mucosal immune system are not well understood at a cellular level or within the microenvironment of the respiratory tract.

Introduction

Many of the viruses discussed in this book grow exclusively on the respiratory epithelium with no evidence of invasion or extension beyond this layer. Very little is known about nonspecific barriers to viral attachment to cells, the initiation of virus replication in the epithelial cell, and mechanisms of cell death. It is not known whether viruses are selective in growth among the many different epithelial cell types. The information that is beginning to emerge about receptors for respiratory viruses such as sialic acid for influenza and the intracellular adhesion molecule, ICAM-1, for the majority of rhinoviruses, suggests that receptors are often ubiquitous proteins on which the virus has "hitchhiked" for cell entry. As these two cases exemplify, the cell receptors themselves often do not account for the specificity of viruses for mucosal surfaces.

Many viruses exit from polarized cells, such as those of the respiratory epithelium, only at the apical or conversely at the basilar surface. For viruses such as influenza, this phenomenon of exit back into the respiratory lumen from the apical surface of respiratory epithelial cells raises questions as to how viruses are seen by the immune system and what role specialized antigen-presenting cells such as interdigitating dendritic cells and microfold cells may play in antigen recognition.

Immunity to respiratory viruses appears to be a complex interaction between IgA-mediated mucosal immunity, cytotoxic T cells, and humoral antibody. IgA transcytosis across epithelial cells makes it the one arm of the immune system clearly available in the extracellular milieu. In addition, some respiratory viruses, such as influenza viruses, have evolved antigenic mutability or wholesale antigenic shift by reassortment. Other viruses, such as respiratory syncytial virus, can spread intracellularly from cell to cell by fusion, making them inaccessible to classic virus neutralization. These factors combined with the short interval between infection and disease, which allows little time for recall of memory responses, make natural or induced immunity to these agents a biological challenge.

Other areas at this interface of microbiology and physiology include (1) the interaction of viruses with pulmonary mediators of bronchoconstriction and inflammation. Respiratory syncytial virus infections have a unique causation of bronchiolitis in the newborn period and a predilection to cause a wheezing-like illness in adults; (2) the role that virally stimulated cytokines play in the induction of immunity and in the cause of symptoms associated with viral illness; and (3) the interactions between viruses and bacteria in the potentiation of disease. For example, *Staphylococcus aureus* strains can produce a protease which cleaves the influenza hemagglutinin and increases the severity of influenza in the murine model. In exchange, epithelial cell damage from influenza allows bacterial invasion; and finally (4) viruses have the promise to provide means for therapeutic intervention as vectors for the introduction of genes into cells in the respiratory tract.

We hope that in raising the above questions this book will stimulate interest in and contribute to a better understanding of respiratory viral disease, and to the promise that viruses have as important experimental tools in defining the interaction of infection with pulmonary function.

Part One

VIRAL RESPIRATORY INFECTIONS IN DIFFERENT POPULATIONS

2

Acute Viral Lower Respiratory Infections in Children

FLOYD W. DENNY, JR.

University of North Carolina School of Medicine at Chapel Hill
Chapel Hill, North Carolina

I. Introduction

Acute lower respiratory tract infections (ALRI) are a common affliction of the human host. In developed or industrialized countries, ALRI are important causes of disability and days lost from work or school, but the case fatality rate is small except in certain patients at high risk. In developing countries, ALRI are also a leading cause of death. It is the purpose of this chapter to paint a picture of the clinical impact of viruses on the lower respiratory tracts of children. All classes of microorganisms, including viruses, bacteria, parasites, and protozoa, are capable of infecting the respiratory tract, but only viruses and bacteria are common causes of infections. Since these microorganisms are inextricably involved in some respiratory infections, both will be addressed when appropriate. No effort will be made to make this chapter a review of more unusual causes of ALRI. Detailed descriptions of the pathogenesis of many of these viruses appear in subsequent chapters.

Because of the complexity of ALRI, an effort will be made to simplify the presentation by first presenting a classification of these infections. This will be followed by a review of the common infectious agents and the clinical dis-

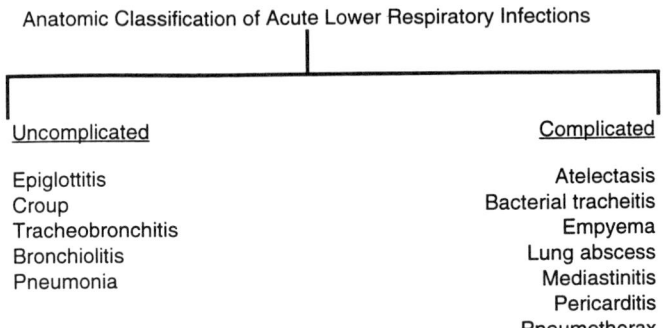

Figure 1 Classification of acute lower respiratory infections.

eases they cause, including the interaction of viruses and bacteria in causing infections, and risk factors associated with severe and fatal ALRI. As ALRI present very different problems in the populations of both developing and developed countries, this will be addressed in some detail below.

II. Classification of Acute Lower Respiratory Infections

Acute respiratory infections can be conveniently classified by separating the upper from the lower tracts at the epiglottis. The majority of ALRI can be classified by the anatomical area of the respiratory tract that is primarily affected (Fig. 1). Most infections are not accompanied by any of the listed complications. Infection may involve more than one site of the lower tract, but most infected children have a single site of major involvement. This classification of lower respiratory tract infection syndromes has been especially useful, because there is close association between the anatomical site in the clinical syndrome and other associated factors, including causative agents.

III. Etiology of Acute Lower Respiratory Tract Infections

The causative agents associated with acute respiratory infections are relatively well understood and are similar everywhere that studies have been done. Certain viruses and bacteria are causes of ALRI. These are listed in Table 1, where they are classified as common and less common. Table 1 is representative of

Table 1 Viruses and Bacteria Causing Acute Lower Respiratory Infections

Agent	Common	Less common
Viruses	Adenoviruses	Coronaviruses
	Influenza viruses	Enteroviruses
	Parainfluenza viruses	Herpes simplex viruses
	Respiratory syncytial viruses	Rhinoviruses
Bacteria	*Mycoplasma pneumoniae*	*Chlamydia pneumoniae*
	Streptococcus pneumoniae	*Haemophilus influenzae*

several reported studies (1–5). All of the listed viruses most commonly cause acute upper respiratory infections alone. In particular, coronaviruses, enteroviruses, herpes simplex virus, and rhinoviruses are primarily causes of upper respiratory infections. Viruses that are more frequently involved in ALRI are adenoviruses, influenza viruses, parainfluenza viruses, and respiratory syncytial viruses. All of the listed bacteria are widely accepted as causative agents of ALRI. *Mycoplasma pneumoniae* is an important cause of tracheobronchitis and pneumonia in older children and young adults, but it is an infrequent cause of illness in young children, when viruses are much more common (6). *Chlamydia pneumoniae* has been recognized as a cause of similar illnesses but much less frequently than *M. pneumoniae* (7).

The roles of *Streptococcus pneumoniae* and *Haemophilus influenzae* cannot be defined so easily. Both of these agents are recognized causes of ALRI but pose special problems in diagnosis. Although type b *H. influenzae* is associated commonly with acute epiglottitis and *S. pneumoniae* with lobar pneumonia in the older child, these two bacteria have not been associated closely with any of the other syndromes listed in Figure 1. They are not recognized causes of uncomplicated upper respiratory tract infections. This makes the clinical diagnosis of ALRI caused by these agents difficult. This problem is compounded by upper respiratory tract carriage of *H. influenzae* and *S. pneumoniae* in a high percentage (up to 20 and 50%, respectively) of normal children at certain ages and during certain seasons (8–9). The failure of anticapsular polysaccharide antibodies to develop in young children has also hampered etiological studies based on serological responses. At the present time, in the absence of epiglottitis or lobar pneumonia in the older child, the only way to associate *H. influenzae* or *S. pneumoniae* with lower respiratory tract infection is to isolate the bacterium from the blood or pleural space or directly from the lung by percutaneous aspiration. Because of these problems, the roles of these two bacteria as causes of ALRI in patients are largely unknown. Although studies suggest that the organisms are infrequent causes of ALRI in the United States, especially when compared with viruses and *M. pneumoniae*, there is widespread belief, and some evidence, that they play a major role in the increased morbidity and mortality associated with ALRI in developing countries (10,11).

Although it is clear that viruses are far more frequent causes of ALRI than are bacteria, precise data regarding their relative roles are not available. It is a common assumption by both nonmedical and medical personnel alike that patients with viral infections of the respiratory tract frequently have superimposed bacterial infections. Several scenarios of the interrelations of viruses and bacteria can be proposed:

> Scenario 1: Simultaneous infections of the respiratory tract by viruses and bacteria are not related except by temporal circumstance.
> Scenario 2: Viral infections alter the host in a manner that promotes superinfection with a bacterium.
> Scenario 3: Bacteria alter the virus in a manner that promotes increased severity of the virus infection.

Although Scenario 3 has been proposed, its clinical significance is not clear; it will not be discussed further (12). In upper respiratory infections, both scenarios 1 and 2 are reasonable possibilities. Bacterial and viral infections are so frequent that simultaneous or closely related occurrences certainly occur. Scenario 2 is probably applicable to otitis media and sinusitis, but it is not clear if this is due to obstruction to the drainage systems of these cavities or to virus-induced changes in the respiratory epithelium facilitating bacterial growth or invasion.

In the lower respiratory tract, the situation is far more complex. With only a few exceptions, bacteria do not appear to cause infections of the larynx,

Table 2 Isolation of Bacteria from Lung Aspirates of Children with Untreated Pneumonia

Location	Age (years)	Positive culture (%)
Recife, Brazil	0–4	60.0
São Paulo, Brazil	0–7	54.1
Zaria, Nigeria	0–8	61.3
Goroka, Papua, New Guinea	0–5	57.8
Newark, NJ	0–15	11.1

Source: Adapted from Ref. 10.

Table 3 Bacteria Isolated from Lung Aspirates of Untreated Children[a]

	% of total positive cultures
Streptococcus pneumoniae	45.0
Haemophilus influenzae	22.8
S. pneumoniae plus H. influenzae	12.9
Staphylococcus aureus	8.7
Other	10.6

[a] 171 of 339 (50.5%) positive.
Source: Adapted from Ref. 10.

trachea, bronchi, or bronchioles. At the level of the alveolus, information is not available which allows clarification of this matter. It has been documented that bacterial superinfections occur in patients with influenza virus infections, but data are lacking to support scenario 2 with the other respiratory viruses (13). Indeed, Hall has reported on the infrequency of bacterial infections in small children with respiratory syncytial virus (RSV) infections (14). Available studies from developing and developed countries (Table 2) suggest that bacterial infections of the lung are far more common in disadvantaged populations (13). Bacteria were isolated on lung aspirations in 54.1–61.3% in children from Brazil, Nigeria, and Papua, New Guinea, as compared to 11.1% in New Jersey. Over 80% of these isolates were *S. pneumoniae* or *H. influenzae* (Table 3). The role of preceding viral infections in those children from developing countries with bacterial pneumonia is unknown.

IV. Role of Respiratory Viruses as Causes of Acute Lower Respiratory Infections in Children

Viruses are clearly the most frequent cause of acute respiratory infections. Results from the Chapel Hill day-care studies (Fig. 2) show that less than 10% of infections involved the lower tract; although the proportion was higher in the youngest children (8). Much is known of the role of individual viruses as causes of childhood ALRI. In most instances, the isolation of these agents from the upper respiratory tract can be correlated with active infections. The most notable exception being the adenoviruses, which can be isolated frequently from the throats of well children. Furthermore, specific clinical syndromes are associated with specific agents. These associations have been confirmed by isolation of the virus and by accurate serological tests that demonstrate specific

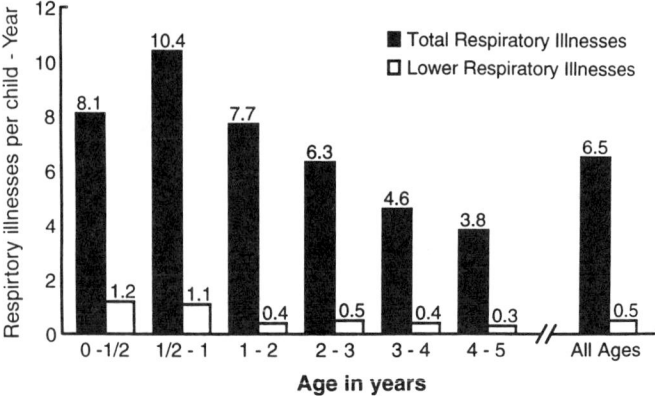

Figure 2 Frequency of respiratory illnesses by age. Frank Porter Graham Child Development Center, Chapel Hill, NC.

antibody responses. The occurrence of ALRI is associated with several important factors: the age of the patient, season of the year, clinical syndrome, infecting agent, and the extent of contact (crowding).

This section addresses these factors, using data from a longitudinal study in a private pediatric practice in Chapel Hill where various factors have been correlated with the occurrence of ALRI. The data and illustrations are considered representative of similar studies reported by others (2,15,16).

A. Age and Gender Incidence

The age- and gender-specific attack rates for total lower respiratory tract infections and four respiratory syndromes are shown in Figure 3. Several important aspects of ALRI are demonstrated. Lower respiratory tract infections are common; in this study, one of every four or five children younger than 1 year of age was taken to the pediatrician each year because of a lower respiratory tract infection (2,16). This rate declined through the late elementary school ages. Lower respiratory tract infections occurred more frequently in young boys than girls. This persisted through the lower elementary school ages both for total lower respiratory tract infections and the specific syndromes. Of the syndromes, croup is the most likely to occur in boys, with a male to female ratio of 1.73 in 6- to 12-month-old infants. As shown in the four lower frames of Figure 3, with the exception of bronchiolitis, the age-specific attack rates for the clinical syndromes were different from those of total lower respiratory

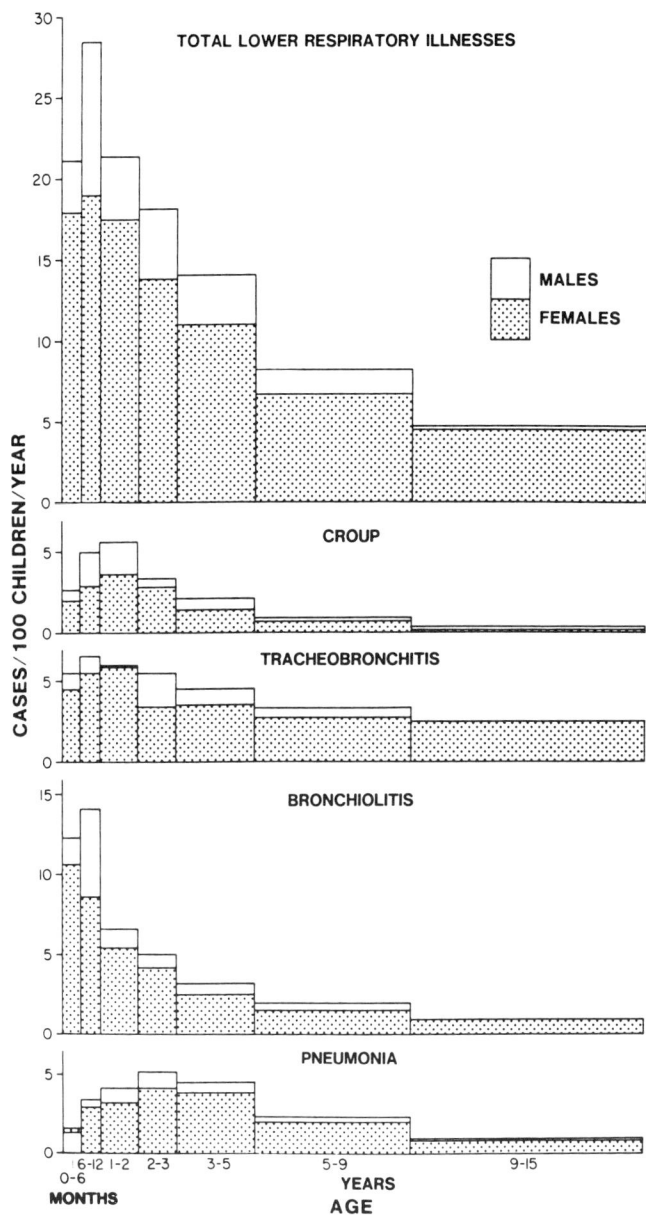

Figure 3 Age- and gender-specific attack rates for total lower respiratory illnesses and four respiratory syndromes, 1964–1975. Rate for boys is represented by entire column and that for girls by stippled portion. Overall rate not shown. Chapel Hill, NC. (From Ref. 37.)

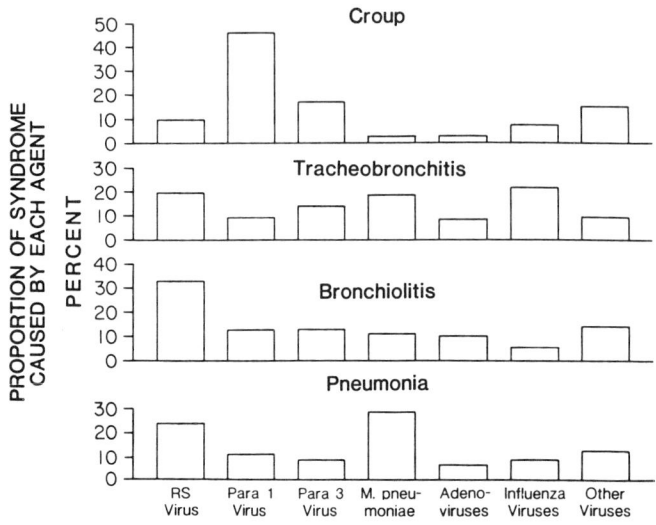

Figure 4 Association between principal agents and four respiratory syndromes. RS virus, respiratory syncytial virus; para 1 virus, parainfluenza virus type 1; para 3 virus, parainfluenza virus type 3. Chapel Hill, NC. (From Ref. 2.)

tract infections and also different from each other. All syndromes occurred less frequently during the first 6 months of life. The incidence of bronchiolitis most nearly resembled the overall incidence of lower respiratory tract infections, peaking in 6- to 12-month-old infants and declining sharply thereafter. Croup peaked in the second year and pneumonia in the third year. Of all the syndromes, tracheobronchitis was most likely to be found in children after the first few years of life.

B. Association of Respiratory Agents and Syndromes

The association between respiratory syndromes and infecting agents is well established and is demonstrated in Figure 4 (2,16). These data show associations across all age groups; with corrections for age, these associations become more dramatic. Croup was caused most frequently by the parainfluenza viruses, especially type 1. Tracheobronchitis was associated with RSV, *M. pneumoniae*, and influenza viruses. The cause of bronchiolitis was most frequently RSV. RSV and *M. pneumoniae* were common causes of pneumonia. In our studies, the influenza viruses were not prominent causes of pneumonia, as reported by Glezen (18,19). Influenza A virus was not isolated as frequently by us; probably because of the relatively insensitive isolation system used.

C. Age Distribution of Lower Respiratory Tract Infections Caused by Specific Infecting Agents

As has been shown, the respiratory infecting agents are associated to some degree with all respiratory syndromes. The age-specific incidence of ALRI caused by specific agents differs, at times to a marked degree, and is shown in Figure 5 (2,16). In all instances, with the exception of the adenoviruses, rates during the first 3 months of life were lower than in later months. The curves for RSV and parainfluenza type 3 are similar except that RSV rates were higher in the first few years. By comparison, parainfluenza virus type 1 occurred in slightly older children, and adenovirus infections occurred almost exclusively in the first 5 years of life. Influenza viruses occurred in all age groups. The rates for *M. pneumoniae* infections show an entirely different age distribution; no isolates were made in children younger than 3 months of age and the peak rates occurred in school-aged children.

D. Seasonal Occurrence of Syndromes and Agents

The respiratory agents, and consequently the associated syndromes, frequently have characteristic seasonal patterns (2,16). An example of this (Fig. 6) shows the monthly occurrence of various agents in relationship to the occurrence of total lower respiratory tract infections in Chapel Hill in 1963–1971 (17). RSV infections occurred in yearly outbreaks in the winter and early spring. There is a close association between the seasonal incidence of bronchiolitis and the isolation of RSV. The occurrence of croup, which is closely associated with the isolation of the parainfluenza viruses, especially type 1, is predominantly in the fall and early winter. Not shown here is that small outbreaks of type 2 parainfluenza viruses occurred in the years when type 1 was absent. Parainfluenza type 3 viruses occurred in a very different pattern. They were the most ubiquitous of the isolates and could be isolated in all seasons. *Mycoplasma pneumoniae* also had a very different pattern of occurrence. Outbreaks associated with pneumonia were unpredictable, usually starting in late summer or fall, and were long lasting. Tracheobronchitis also occurs in seasonal patterns according to the causative agent. It is most closely associated with the influenza viruses, which occur in winter and spring.

V. Role of Various Risk Factors in the Occurrence of Acute Respiratory Infections

Several risk factors that increase the incidence and/or severity of respiratory infections have been identified and are discussed below (16,20).

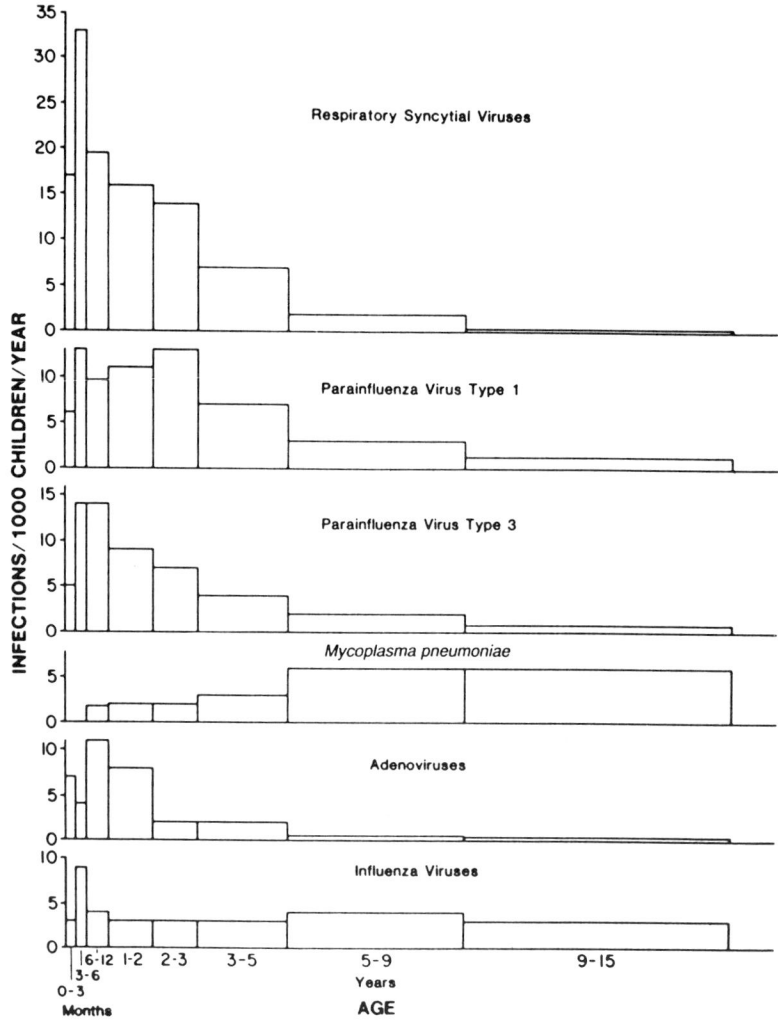

Figure 5 Age-specific attack rates of lower respiratory infections caused by certain agents. Chapel Hill, NC. (From Ref. 37.)

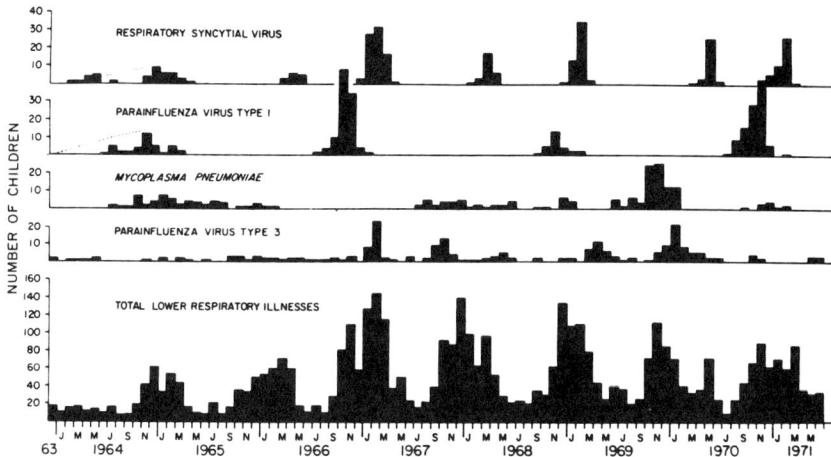

Figure 6 Number of isolations according to month of four major respiratory pathogens from children with lower respiratory illnesses, Chapel Hill, NC. (From Ref. 17.)

A. Age of the Host

As already discussed, all respiratory infections are more frequent in the youngest children and are generally more severe, as indicated by more frequent involvement of the lower respiratory tract.

B. Crowding

Respiratory infections, for the most part, are spread by direct contact or large droplets from the respiratory tract and are thus more likely to occur under conditions that foster close contact. This has been demonstrated for all forms of crowding—number of siblings, room occupancy, population density, and day-care attendance. The role of day care has not been defined as clearly as desirable, but presently available data suggest higher incidence figures for day-care attendees (8,15). Most crowding would be expected to increase the incidence of infection primarily, but it might play a role in increasing severity as well in situations in which crowding is so intense that the infecting dose of microorganisms is large. It is speculated that this might play a role in the increase in severity of acute respiratory infections in developing countries.

C. Gender

The role of gender as a risk factor for respiratory infections has received little attention. Data suggest only slight and probably insignificant differences in incidences between boys and girls for upper respiratory tract infections. There are clear-cut gender differences for ALRI, with a preponderance of disease occurring in boys, suggesting that the risk is to increased severity.

D. Inhaled Pollutants

Inhaled pollutants have received much attention in the past few years (21,22). Although studies vary somewhat in the degree of attributable risk, there is increasingly strong evidence that passive smoking is an important risk factor for increased incidence and for increased severity of ALRI. The impact of passive smoking appears to be greatest in the child younger than 1 year of age and is related most closely with maternal smoking. There is also evidence that wood-burning stoves and possibly the use of gas for cooking are responsible for increasing the risk of acute respiratory infections (23,24).

E. Anatomical Abnormalities, Metabolic and Genetic Diseases, and Immunological Deficiencies

It is clear that abnormalities such as tracheoesophageal fistulas, cystic fibrosis, congenital heart disease, and immunodeficiency syndromes are associated with an increased risk for respiratory infections, both in incidence and severity. However, it is beyond the scope of this chapter to consider these further. The role of atopy and/or reactive airways in increasing the risk for respiratory infection is controversial (25). The relationship between respiratory infections and asthma, in terms of cause and effect, is unclear. The same is true for the relationship between atopy and bronchiolitis. It is commonly believed that the atopic child has more frequent bouts of otitis media and sinusitis, but prospective studies to prove this point have not been reported.

F. Nutrition (Including Breast-Feeding)

It seems probable that malnutrition is important in increasing the risk for acute respiratory infections, especially in developing countries. Because malnutrition is often associated with other risk factors such as crowding and inhaled pollutants, it has not been possible to clearly define its role. The recent report of the role of vitamin A deficiency in the increasing risk for acute respiratory infections is of interest but needs further study to assess its importance (26). Breast-feeding appears to be important in developing countries in reducing the risk for acute respiratory infections, but the data relating to a protective effect of breast-feeding in developed countries are contradictory (27). Results of studies show only small or no reductions in the incidence of all respiratory infections, but they do suggest that the severity of infections may be decreased in young breast-fed infants. It is clear that the effect of nutrition on the risk for acute respiratory infections, including breast-feeding, needs increased attention.

G. Social and Economic Factors

It is difficult, if not impossible, to separate the various social and economic factors that may have an impact on the occurrence of acute respiratory infections, but lower socioeconomic level is linked clearly with increased risk (28). Crowding, malnutrition, and inhaled pollutants, all found in lower socioeconomic classes, especially in developing countries, are contributing factors. The role of stress could also be a contributing factor (29).

VI. Role of Acute Respiratory Infections in Developing Countries

The impact of ALRI in developing countries is much greater than that described above for developed nations (30–34,37). Several aspects of nonindustrialized populations contribute to the magnitude of this problem. One of these aspects is the increased numbers of small children in whom ALRI are a larger problem. For example, in 1991, 89.4% of the 164 million of the world's births were in the developing world, but 98.2% of deaths occurred there (35). The annual causes of these deaths of children under age 5 are shown in Table 4 (36). Respiratory infections and diarrhea accounted for over one half of all deaths. The percentage of distribution of the ALRI-related deaths of children

Table 4 Annual Deaths of Children Under Age 5

Cause of death	Deaths (millions) (no.)	(%)
Respiratory infections		
Pertussis	0.51	4
Measles	1.52	11
Other acute respiratory infections	2.2	15
Neonatal tetanus	0.79	6
Diarrhea	4.0	28
Malaria	1.0	7
Other	4.2	29
Total	14.22	100

Source: Adapted from Ref. 36.

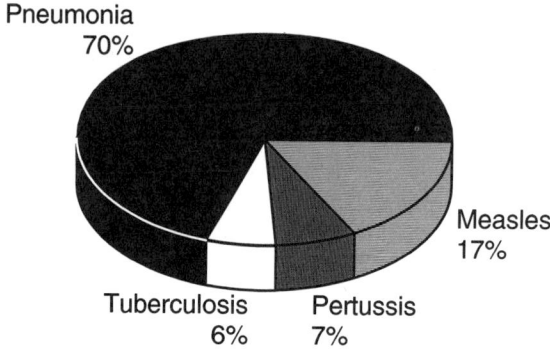

Figure 7 Percentage distribution of ALRI-related deaths of children under five. (Adapted from Ref. 35.)

under age 5 is shown in Figure 7 (35). Pneumonia, responsible for 70% of the ALRI-related deaths, is clearly the big problem in developing world children.

The agents causing acute respiratory illnesses are the same all over the world wherever studies have been done. Thus, RSV, parainfluenza viruses, adenoviruses, and influenza viruses are the principal respiratory viruses found in children with severe ALRI. Rhinoviruses, doubtless a huge problem as a cause of upper respiratory infections, do not appear to be a major cause of ALRI.

One of the most startling aspects of acute respiratory illness in developing nations is that the incidence of total acute respiratory illness is very similar wherever studies have been done (10). Examples of this are shown in Table 5; the incidence rates for India, Costa Rica, Michigan, and Washington are remarkably similar. In sharp contrast are the marked differences in the incidence of severe and fatal acute respiratory illness in both developing and developed countries (10). Table 6 compares the incidence for pneumonia in several advantaged and disadvantaged populations. The rates for pneumonia in Native

Table 5 Incidence of Acute Respiratory Illnesses

Location	Episodes per year		
	Infants	1–2 years	3–5 years
Costa Rica	5.9	7.2	4.2
India	5.6	5.3	4.8
Michigan	6.1	6.1	4.7
Washington	4.5	4.5	4.8

Source: Adapted from Ref. 10.

Table 6 Annual Incidence of Pneumonia in Children

	Cases per 1000 children		
Location	Total	Infants	1–4 years
North Carolina	36	—	40
Washington	30	—	36
Navajos, New Mexico, and Arizona	91.2	291.4	49.9
China	74.6	95.2	53.5
Tari Basin, Papua, New Guinea	—	256	62

Source: Adapted from Ref. 10.

Table 7 Deaths from Pneumonia and Influenza in Children 1–4 Years of Age

Location	Year	No. per 100,000
France	1980	0.7
Netherlands	1981	1.1
Egypt	1979	173.6
Guatemala	1979	251.0

Source: Adapted from Ref. 10.

Table 8 Proportion of Children in Outpatient Services with Acute Respiratory Infections

Location	%
Brazil	41.8
Nigeria	30.1
Thailand	60.7
Iraq	39.3

Source: Adapted from Ref. 10.

Table 9 Proportion of Admissions into Hospital Due to Acute Respiratory Infections in Children Under 15 Years of Age

Location	%
Bangladesh	35.8
Burma	31.5
Pakistan	33.6
Zambia	34.0

Source: Adapted from Ref. 10.

Table 10 Case Fatality of Children Admitted into Hospital Because of Acute Respiratory Infections

Location	%
Bangladesh	12.3
Brazil	10.2
Burma	8.1
Malaysia	2.7
Pakistan	7.3

Source: Adapted from Ref. 10.

American children in the Southwest and in children in the People's Republic of China and Papua, New Guinea, were up to eightfold greater than in children in North Carolina and Washington. The rates for deaths due to pneumonia in developing world children are even more remarkable, being up to several hundred times greater in Egypt and Guatemala than in France and The Netherlands (Table 7) (13). Further examples of the problems presented by acute respiratory illness in developing world children are shown in Tables 8, 9, and 10 (10). The proportion of children presenting with acute respiratory illnesses in outpatient services varied from 30 to 60% (Table 8); the proportion of admissions to hospitals due to acute respiratory illness varied from 31.5 to 35.8% (Table 9); and the case fatality rate of children admitted to hospitals because of acute respiratory illness was as high as 12.3% (Table 10).

VII. Summary and Conclusions

Acute lower respiratory infections occur frequently in children. Most infections are caused by viruses and bacteria; with the greatest proportion being caused by viruses. The viruses most frequently involved are adenoviruses, influenza viruses, parainfluenza viruses, and respiratory syncytial viruses. Acute lower respiratory infections are more common in young children, have rather specific seasonal occurrences, and some agents are associated with specific respiratory syndromes. Risk factors associated with an increased incidence or severity of respiratory infections are occurrence in the very young; crowding; being male; inhaled pollutants; anatomical, metabolic, genetic or immunological disorders; and malnutrition, including vitamin or micronutrient deficiency. Lower respiratory infections are a much greater problem in developing countries than in developed countries; they are the leading causes of death in children under age 5. The same agents cause infections and the incidence of total respiratory infections is the same as in the developed countries. The precise causes of increased morbidity and mortality in the developing world are unclear, but crowding, inhaled pollutants, and malnutrition are likely candidates. The interactive role of viruses and bacteria is not clear, but bacteria appear to play a role in increased severity of respiratory infections in developing countries.

References

1. Loda FA, Clyde WA Jr, Glezen WP, Senior RJ, Sheaffer CI, Denny FW Jr. Studies on the role of viruses, bacteria and *M. pneumoniae* as causes of lower respiratory tract infections in children. J Pediatr 1968; 72:161–176.
2. Denny FW, Clyde WA Jr. Acute lower respiratory tract infections in non-hospitalized children. J Pediatr 1986; 108:635–646.
3. Foy HM, Cooney MK, Maletzky AJ, Grayston JT. Incidence and etiology of pneumonia, croup and bronchiolitis in preschool children belonging to a prepaid medical care group over a four-year period. Am J Epidemiol 1973; 97:80–92.
4. Monto AS, Cavallaro JJ. The Tecumseh study of respiratory illness. II. Patterns of occurrence of infection with respiratory pathogens, 1965–1969. Am J Epidemiol 1971; 94:280–289.
5. Monto AS, Ultman BM. Acute respiratory illness in an American community. JAMA 1974; 227:164–169.
6. Denny FW, Clyde WA Jr, Glezen WP. *Mycoplasma pneumoniae* disease: clinical spectrum, pathophysiology, epidemiology and control. J Infect Dis 1971; 123:74–92.
7. Grayston JT. *Chlamydia pneumoniae* (TWAR) infections in children. Pediatr Infect Dis J 1994; 13:675–685.
8. Loda FA, Glezen WP, Clyde WA Jr. Respiratory disease in group day care. Pediatrics 1972; 49:428–437.
9. Loda FA, Collier AM, Glezen WP, Strangert K, Clyde WA Jr, Denny FW. Occurrence of *Diplococcus pneumoniae* in the upper respiratory tract of children. J Pediatr 1975; 87:1087–1093.
10. Pio A, Leowski J, ten Dam HG. The magnitude of the problem of acute respiratory infections. In: Douglas RM, Kerby-Eaton E, eds. Acute Respiratory Infections in Childhood, Proceedings of an International Workshop, Sydney, August 1984, University of Adelaide, 3–16.
11. Graham NMH. The epidemiology of acute respiratory infections in children and adults: a global perspective (review). Epidemiol Rev 1990; 12:149–178.
12. Scheiblauer H, Reinacher M, Tashiro M, Rott R. Interactions between bacteria and influenza A virus in the development of influenza pneumonia. J Infect Dis 1992; 166:783–791.
13. Leigh MW, Carson JL, Denny FW Jr. Pathogenesis of respiratory infections due to influenza virus: implications for developing countries (review). Rev Infect Dis 1991; 13(suppl 6):S501–S508.

14. Hall CB, Powell KR, Schnabel KC, Gala CL, Pincus PH. Risk of secondary bacterial infection in infants hospitalized with respiratory syncytial viral infection. J Pediatr 1988; 113:266–271.
15. Denny FW, Collier AM, Henderson FW. Acute respiratory infections in day care. Rev Infect Dis 1986; 8:527–532.
16. Denny FW. Acute respiratory infections in children: etiology and epidemiology (review). Pediatr Rev 1987; 9:135–146.
17. Glezen WP, Denny FW. Epidemiology of acute lower respiratory disease in children. N Engl J Med 1973; 288:498–505.
18. Glezen WP. Viral pneumonia as a cause and result of hospitalization. J Infect Dis 1983; 147:765–770.
19. Glezen WP. Serious morbidity and mortality associated with influenza epidemics. Epidemiol Res 1982; 4:25–44.
20. Strope GL, Stempel DA. Risk factors associated with the development of chronic lung disease in children. Pediatr Clin North Am 1984; 31:757–771.
21. Health effects of environmental tobacco smoke exposure in the Health Consequences of Involuntary Smoking: A report of the Surgeon General, US Department of Health and Human Services. Rockville, Maryland, Public Health Service 17–118; 1986.
22. Committee on Passive Smoking, Board of Environmental Studies and Toxicology, National Research Council: Effects of Exposure to Environmental Tobacco Smoke on Lung Function and Respiratory Symptoms in Environmental Tobacco Smoke: Measuring Exposures and Assessing Health Effects. Washington, DC: National Academy Press, 1986:202–209.
23. Honicky RE, Osborne JS III, Akpom CA. Symptoms of respiratory illness in young children and the use of wood-burning stoves for indoor heating. Pediatrics 1985; 75:587–593.
24. Melia RJW, Florey CV, Altman DG, Swan AV. Association between gas cooking and respiratory disease in children. Br Med J 1977; 2:149–152.
25. McIntosh K. Bronchiolitis and asthma: possible common pathogenetic pathways. J Allergy Clin Immunol 1976; 57:595–604.
26. Sommer A, Katz J, Tarwatjo I. Increased risk of respiratory disease and diarrhea in children with pre-existing mild vitamin A deficiency. Am J Clin Nutr 1984; 40:1090–1095.
27. Frank AL, Taber LH, Glezen WP, Kasel GL, Wells CR, Paredes A. Breastfeeding and respiratory virus infection. Pediatrics 1982; 70:239–245.
28. Gardner G, Frank AL, Tabor LH. Effects of social and family factors on viral respiratory infection and illness in the first year of life. J Epidemiol Commun Health 1984; 38:42–48.
29. Graham NMH, Douglas RM, Ryan P. Stress and acute respiratory infection. Am J Epidemiol 1986; 124:389–401.
30. McIntosh K, Halonen P, Ruuskanen O. Report of a workshop on respiratory viral infection; epidemiology, diagnosis, treatment, and prevention. Clin Infect Dis 1993; 16:151–164.
31. Denny FW, Loda FA. Acute respiratory infections are the leading cause of death in children in developing coutnries. Am J Trop Med Hyg 1986; 35:1–2.

32. Berman S. Epidemiology of acute respiratory infections in children in developing countries (review). Rev Infect Dis 1991; 13(suppl 6):S454–S462.
33. Selwyn BJ on behalf of the Coordinated Data Group of BOSTID Researchers: The epidemiology of acute respiratory tract infections in young children: comparison of findings from several developing countries. Rev Infect Dis 1990; 12(suppl 8):S870–S888.
34. McIntosh K. Etiology and epidemiology of acute respiratory tract infections in children in developing countries. Overview of the symposium. J Infect Dis 1990; 12(suppl 8):S867–S869.
35. Grant JP. The State of the World's Children, 1993, published for UNICEF. Oxford, UK: Oxford University Press.
36. Grant JP. The State of the World's Children, 1990, published for UNICEF. Oxford, UK: Oxford University Press.
37. Denny FW, Clyde WE Jr. Acute respiratory tract infections: an overview. Pediatr Res 1983; 17:1026–1029.

3

Viral Pneumonia in Adults

STEPHEN B. GREENBERG

Baylor College of Medicine
and Ben Taub General Hospital
Houston, Texas

I. Introduction

Viral pneumonia is more common in children than in adults. However, both immunocompetent and immunocompromised adults do develop viral pneumonia (1–11). Although most respiratory viruses have been documented in cases of pneumonia, the commonly proven causes are influenza viruses and respiratory syncytial viruses (RSV). Nonrespiratory viruses are also causes of viral pneumonia in adults, especially in immunocompromised hosts (Table 1). Risk factors for pneumonia in adults are similar to those for serious childhood respiratory illnesses and include immune system impairment, underlying respiratory disorders, and increased frequency of exposure (12). In all hospitalized adult patients with community-acquired pneumonia, approximately 8–10% of cases are caused by viruses (13–31). Mixed viral–bacterial infections are commonly identified. Over 50% of community-acquired viral pneumonias in adults are due to influenza virus A. Diagnostic tests are readily available. Antiviral agents are approved for use in herpes virus and influenza virus infections; therefore, rapid diagnostic capabilities are becoming increasingly important to the primary care physician and specialist caring for patients with respiratory illnesses.

Table 1 Etiology of Viral Pneumonia in Adults

Typical respiratory viruses	"Nonrespiratory" viruses
Influenza A and B viruses	Herpes simplex virus (HSV) type 1
Respiratory syncytial virus	Varicella-zoster virus
Parainfluenza virus types 1, 2, and 3	Cytomegalovirus
Adenovirus	Epstein-Barr virus
Coronavirus	HHV-6
Rhinovirus	Measles virus
	Hantavirus

II. Pathogenesis

With few exceptions, viruses spread from the upper to the lower respiratory tract prior to causing pneumonia. The pathological lung changes induced by viral infection are all similar and include necrosis and sloughing of epithelium, with loss of the normal mucosal surface (32–34). Mucus production increases and bronchioles become plugged. Alveoli fill with inflammatory fluid and leukocytes. In peribronchial areas, mononuclear cells increase.

Both specific and nonspecific host defenses are needed for recovery from viral pneumonia. High titers of interferon can be detected in the lungs when viral load is maximal. Antiviral antibody is detected in bronchial secretions by the third day of infection. Cytotoxic T lymphocytes appear around the same time and help clear virus-infected epithelial cells. Full recovery from viral pneumonia, therefore, depends on both humoral and cell-mediated immune responses.

Bacterial superinfection which often occurs following a respiratory viral infection is thought to result from increased adherence and colonization of bacteria on virus-infected epithelial cells (35). It is believed that virus-infected epithelial cells lead to alterations of host cell surfaces, new receptors on exposed surfaces, and/or changes in the extracellular environment allowing for increased bacterial attachment (36–38). In addition, increased bacterial growth and decreased bacterial clearance are indirectly the result of virus-induced suppression of the immune response and phagocytic function, respectively. Studies have demonstrated alterations in bactericidal activity of macrophages and neutrophils where viral replication has occurred. Animal models of viral pneumonia support this concept by demonstrating phagocytic dysfunction in the lower respiratory tract when bacterial superinfection has been reported to develop (35).

III. Comparison of Viral Pneumonia in Children and Adults

Several studies have found 15–30% of proven childhood pneumonias to be viral in etiology (see Chap. 2) (Table 2) (39–48). This is twice as high as the number of cases proven to be of viral etiology in adults. Mixed viral and bacterial pneumonias are frequent in adults, but they are less well defined in children. Epidemiological differences occur in sources of viral transmission between children and adults (49). Schools and day-care centers are thought to be the sources of transmission for young children. In addition, nosocomial transmission is more frequent in hospitalized infants and children than in hospitalized adults (50–51). Adults are more likely to be exposed if there are children where they dwell or if they reside in a closed population such as a prison, military barracks, or nursing home. In infants and children, predisposing medical conditions identified include primary immunodeficiencies, asthma, and sickle cell anemia. Predisposing medical conditions for adults include secondary immunodeficiencies such as transplantation or malignancy, asthma, chronic obstructive pulmonary disease (COPD), and chronic heart disease (52–56). There are no apparent seasonal differences for viral pneumonia between children and adults; both age groups are most likely to develop viral pneumonia during the winter months. There are no reliable diagnostic clinical signs or symptoms in children or adults that differentiate viral from bacterial pneumonias. Radiological patterns are also variable and nonspecific.

IV. Community-Acquired Viral Pneumonia

Over the past 30 years, there have been numerous published studies that have identified the viral causes of pneumonia cases admitted to the hospital (Table 3)

Table 2 Viral Pneumonia in Infants/Children Versus Adults

Factor(s)	Infants/children	Adults
Viruses as cause of pneumonia	Frequent	Uncommon
Mixed viral/bacterial pneumonia	Uncommon	Frequency
Major sources of virus transmission	Schools, day-care centers, hospitals	Children in home, closed populations
Underlying predisposing conditions	1° immunodeficiency, asthma	2° immunodeficiency, asthma, COPD, heart disease
Peak season	November–March	November–March
Clinical manifestations	Not discriminating	Not discriminating
Radiologic patterns	Variable	Variable

Table 3 Community-Acquired Viral Pneumonia in Adults[a]

Study interval	% Viral (no. viral/total)		% Mixed bacterial-viral	Viral culture	Viral serology[b]	Reference
1965–1966	17	(17/100)	71	+	+	13
1967–1968	12	(35/292)	69	+	+	14
1969–1970	9	(13/148)	46	−	+	15
1980	9	(7/81)	?	+	+	16
1980–1981	9	(11/127)	?	−	+	17
1980–1981	7	(12/162)	58	−	+	18
1979–1982	6	(5/80)	?	−	+	19
1982–1983	7	(33/453)	42	−	+	20
1982–1983	10	(15/147)	47	−	+	21
?	15	(22/145)	55	−	+	22
1982–1983	4	(12/274)	?	−	+	23
1984	39	(43/110)	?	−	+	24
1984–1985	13	(31/236)	26	+	+	25
1981–1987	17	(101/588)	?	−	+	26
1987	16	(43/277)	77	+	+	27
1986–1987	8	(10/125)	40	−	+	28
1990–1991	9	(19/206)	32	−	+	29
1991–1992	10.1	(24/237)	?	−	+	30
1991–1993	8	(27/334)	35	−	+	31

[a]Studies in which viral culture or serology was attempted.
[b]Most serology used complement-fixation antibody.

(13–31). The percentage identified as being viral in etiology has ranged from 4 to 39%. The percentage of cases both having bacteria and virus isolated ranged from 26 to 77%. Most of the published studies used various serological assays to detect viral infections. Virus culture techniques were used in less than half of the published series, and no large study employed such newer methods as polymerase chain reaction (PCR) (see Chap. 12). In most of these studies, influenza viruses are the most commonly identified virus. Parainfluenza viruses and RSV are the next most frequently detected viruses.

A. Common Respiratory Viruses

Influenza Viruses

Viral pneumonia in adults is most commonly caused by influenza A and B viruses. Mixed infections with both bacteria and a virus identified contemporaneously are reported often. In pneumonia of viral etiology, influenza A and B viruses have been identified in over 50% of cases (see Chap. 6). Influenzal epidemics are reported every winter throughout the United States. Although influenza is an acute, self-limited disease in most adults, pneumonia is one of several complications (57–68). Four patterns of lower respiratory infection have been described: (1) bronchiolitis, (2) primary influenzal pneumonia, (3) bacterial pneumonia occurring simultaneously with influenzal illness, and (4) bacterial pneumonia following an influenzal illness (69–70). Primary influenzal pneumonia is associated with dyspnea, cyanosis, high fever, and respiratory failure. The most common isolate in those cases with a bacterial course has been *Streptococcus pneumoniae*. *Staphylococcus aureus* has been implicated in approximately 20% of cases of bacterial pneumonia associated with influenza (71). The frequency of pneumonia with acute influenza increases with advanced age, cardiopulmonary disease, and immunosuppression (72–82). Long-term pulmonary sequelae have been reported among survivors of influenzal pneumonia (83–85). In fatal cases of influenzal pneumonia, there is diffuse alveolar damage with variable degrees of fibrosis. In the later stages of nonfatal cases, there may be patchy organization including bronchiolitis obliterans.

Parainfluenza Viruses

Parainfluenza viruses have been documented in approximately 15% of adult viral pneumonias (86–89). Bacterial superinfections are common. Although children are commonly infected, adults can be reinfected and have recurrent clinical respiratory illness that rarely manifests as pneumonia. Recent published series in bone marrow transplant and lung transplant recipients have demonstrated the importance of parainfluenza virus infection as a cause of lower respiratory tract involvement (89,90) (see Chap. 5). Clinical manifestations in transplant recipients included fever, cough, and wheezing. Pulmonary infiltrates were frequent. Respiratory failure leading to death or permanent pulmonary dysfunction was also reported in many infected patients.

Respiratory Syncytial Virus

Pneumonia caused by the respiratory syncytial virus (RSV) is seen in immunosuppressed adults following organ or bone marrow transplantation (91–99) (see Chap. 7). Clinical manifestations have been fever, cough, and rhinorrhea. Wheezing has been reported in 25–50% of these RSV-infected bone marrow transplant patients. Unlike children with RSV, immunocompromised adults uncommonly report otitis media with RSV infections. Mortality rates in RSV-infected transplant patients have ranged from 11 to 78%. Elderly adults in nursing homes and admitted to hospitals have been shown to have severe respiratory illnesses due to RSV and occasionally manifest pneumonia (99–120) (see Chap. 5).

Adenovirus

Adenovirus pneumonia is very uncommon in the immunocompetent adult (121–123) except for that seen among military recruits (124,125). Adenovirus pneumonia has been observed among transplant recipients (126–130). Clinical manifestations have included nonproductive cough, fever, and hypoxia. Radiological findings include bilateral interstitial or alveolar infiltrates. Pleural effusions have been documented (131). In immunocompromised hosts, mortality rates have been as high as 60%. A live vaccine is available and is used in the military but is not widely distributed for civilian use.

Other Respiratory Viruses

Pneumonia due to rhinoviruses or coxsackieviruses have been reported rarely (132–134). These viruses are associated with upper respiratory tract infections and especially the common cold syndrome. With improved diagnostic techniques such as polymerase chain reaction, the true incidence of these viruses as causes of lower respiratory tract disease can be measured more accurately. Because of the difficulty in diagnosing coronavirus infections, the true incidence of lower respiratory tract infections due to this virus is currently incompletely understood (see Chap. 10).

B. Systemic Viral Infections as Causes of Pneumonia

Pneumonia may occur during the course of a systemic viral infection and may be easy to diagnose, because the characteristic clinical presentation is recognized. Measles and varicella viruses can cause pneumonia and are recognized by the characteristic concurrent dermatological findings. However, with those systemic viral infections in which pneumonia occurs during reactivation of a latent or chronic virus, diagnosis may be more difficult. The herpes viruses are a group of DNA viruses which are associated with primary infection, persistent infection, and/or recurrent disease (135). Viral infections with these viruses can cause pneumonia in the settings discussed below.

Herpes Simplex Virus Type 1

The risk factors for herpes simplex virus (HSV) pneumonia include immunosuppression, solid organ transplantation, and damaged respiratory tract epithelium. The incidence of HSV pneumonia in bone marrow transplant patients is approximately 7%. Liver, cardiac, and renal transplant recipients have a 1–10% incidence (136,137). HSV is isolated with increased frequency in mechanically ventilated intensive care unit (ICU) patients (138–141). Recent studies have reported HSV pneumonia post-thoracotomy (142). Damage to the research epithelium by burns, radiation therapy, or endotracheal intubation has been identified in several series of HSV pneumonias. Rarely, immunocompetent elderly adults will develop HSV pneumonia.

There are no specific clinical manifestations that are diagnostic of HSV pneumonia. Fever, cough, dyspnea, and hemoptysis are common signs and symptoms (143–146). Radiological findings include either focal or diffuse interstitial infiltrates. At bronchoscopy, there is evidence of tracheitis and/or mucosal lesions. Pathological material has shown parenchymal necrosis with hemorrhages and mononuclear infiltrates.

Varicella-Zoster Virus

Pneumonia will develop in up to 10–20% of adults with varicella infection and in <1% of patients with disseminated herpes zoster (147–148). Risk factors for pneumonia include pregnancy, smoking, immunosuppression, old age, extent of rash, and COPD (149–167). Patients with varicella pneumonia present with shortness of breath and fever. Diffuse infiltrates are commonly noted on chest radiograph. The pneumonia usually occurs 1–6 days after the onset of rash. Abnormal chest radiographs may be found in asymptomatic patients. Abnormalities in pulmonary function (diffusion capacity or FEF 25–75%) have been detected in subclinical cases. Lung involvement appears to occur by bloodstream infection, not by extension down the respiratory tract.

With recovery, diffuse pulmonary microcalcifications are common. Pathological changes in the lung include endothelial damage of blood vessels with focal hemorrhagic necrosis, mononuclear infiltrates in alveolar walls, and fibrinous exudates with macrophages (168).

In pregnancy, untreated varicella pneumonia has a high mortality rate. Susceptibility of pregnant women to varicella-zoster virus (VZV) is approximately 5%. Varicella occurring within 5 days prior to delivery or 3 days after delivery is associated with a 15–20% neonatal infection and a 11–50% death rate. Up to half of pregnant patients with varicella pneumonia may need short-term mechanical ventilation. Acyclovir is frequently used to treat varicella pneumonia and may be beneficial, although controlled studies of its efficacy in treating varicella pneumonia have not been conducted (169–175).

Cytomegalovirus

Cytomegalovirus (CMV) pneumonia is rarely diagnosed in immunocompetent adults (176–182). However, immunosuppression due to malignancy or transplantation has been associated with an increased number of cases (183–185). Primary infection as well as reactivation of latent virus are each associated with disease activity. Intact cell-mediated immunity appears to be a central mechanism for recovery from CMV infection.

At one cancer center, 20 cases of CMV pneumonia were recently reported over a 25-year period (186). This represents 2.2 cases per 1000 autopsies. All of these patients had fever, dyspnea, and tachypnea during hospitalization. There appeared to be an increased frequency in patients with non-Hodgkin's lymphoma and multiple myeloma. Twelve of the 20 cases had disseminated malignancy at diagnosis and 3 were in complete remission. Disseminated CMV disease was found in 55%, and 70% developed secondary bacterial infections. Mechanical ventilation was needed in seven patients, and 3 patients presented with a shock syndrome. Where radiographs were available for review, 6 of 11 had evidence of consolidation and 4 of 11 had an interstitial pattern.

Among transplant recipients, CMV pneumonia can be a serious complication associated with excess mortality (187–193). Following bone marrow transplantation, CMV pneumonia has been reported in 0.8–7.0% of cases. Although CMV pneumonia is less frequent following autologous transplant compared with allogenic transplant, there is no difference in outcome in these two groups of patients once CMV pneumonia develops. Diagnosis is difficult because of asymptomatic reactivation of latent virus (194–196). Detection of CMV antigen in broncheoalveolar lavage (BAL) samples is predictive of pneumonia developing later; however, approximately one third of patients with CMV detected in BAL will not develop pneumonia. A negative PCR result from BAL fluid has a very high negative predictive value.

The mortality rate from CMV pneumonia in solid organ transplants is still 20–30% even with antiviral therapy. The risk of pneumonia is increased in CMV-seronegative patients who receive organs from seropositive donors.

The combination of CMV with *Pneumocystis carinii* is frequently reported in lung and heart-lung transplant recipients.

A recent report has suggested that CMV may be a significant pathogen in acutely ill patients on mechanical ventilation (197). In 25 cases of CMV pneumonia in mechanically ventilated patients, 17 were diagnosed histologically at autopsy and 7 from open lung biopsy. In 88% of cases, CMV was the sole pathogen. Of those tested on admission to the ICU, 13 of 18 were CMV antibody positive. Blood transfusions were given to 76% of patients. Mechanical ventilation was employed for several days in those diagnosed with CMV pneumonia. Compared with those found not to have CMV pneumonia, patients with the diagnosis had more severe hypoxemia during hospitalization. On review, the investigators could not distinguish CMV from bacterial infection. Usually there were bilateral infiltrates on chest radiograph. Underlying disease was found in most patients and included COPD (25%), malignancy (25%), cardiac surgery (16%), and coma (11%).

Epstein-Barr and Other Herpes Viruses

The Epstein-Barr virus (EBV) has been associated with acute and chronic pneumonitis in adults (198–210). Polymerase chain reaction and immunohistochemistry in desquamative interstitial pneumonitis (DIP) cases have demonstrated evidence of EBV in 30% of cases (211). Rapidly progressive interstitial pneumonitis in cases of polymyositis/dermatomyositis is a rare complication found to be related to EBV (209). What pathogenic role EBV may have in interstitial pneumonitis of polymyositis/dermatomyositis remains to be defined.

Pulmonary manifestations of acute EBV infection are rarely reported. In 5–10% of patients with infectious mononucleosis, chest radiographs will reveal bilateral diffuse infiltrates and occasionally pleural effusion. In patients with symptomatic lung involvement, hypoxemia is common, and respiratory compromise may require mechanical ventilation (212). Recovery is typical, with rare fatalities being reported.

Human herpes virus 6 (HHV-6) has been reported to be associated with pneumonitis in immunocompromised hosts (213–216). This recently discovered herpes virus has similarities to cytomegalovirus in terms of cell susceptibility, latency, and sensitivity to ganciclovir.

Measles

With the widespread use of live attenuated measles vaccine, the number of measles cases has been dramatically reduced during the past 30 years. However, recent community mini-outbreaks of measles have reaffirmed the potential for serious complications. Pneumonia continues to be the most serious complication and leading cause of death with this viral infection (217–226). In measles outbreaks among military recruits, pneumonia was identified in 3–15% of cases. Among those who received the formalin-inactivated measles vaccine in the late 1950s, a severe, atypical measles pneumonitis was observed.

Fatal measles pneumonia in normal adults is rare. However, increased arterial–alveolar (A-a) gradients detected by room air arterial blood gas analyses have been reported in two recently published studies (220,221). In half of the adult patients with measles seen in an emergency center, there were significantly increased A-a gradients. This suggests that hypoxemia is common in measles even when radiographic changes are not detected. In a recent series of six patients with measles pneumonitis treated with intravenous ribavirin, liver function test abnormalities, hypocalcemia, and elevated creatine phosphokinase (CPK) levels were detected (220). Although reported in childhood measles, secondary bacterial pneumonia has been reported infrequently in adults.

Measles in pregnancy has adverse consequences for both mother and fetus. A recently published series found pneumonitis in 7 of 13 pregnant women with measles (227). Adverse fetal outcomes occurred in 4. Ribavirin has teratogenic and mutagenic properties and its use is generally avoided in pregnancy. Whether the potential benefit in measles pneumonitis might outweigh its risk has not been defined.

Immunological abnormalities are known to be common during acute measles infection. Lymphocytopenia and loss of tuberculin skin test reactivity have been recognized. Suppression of delayed-type hypersensitivity and increase in circulating $CD8^+$ cells in peripheral blood have been reported, but only recently have similar changes been detected in lung cells. In five patients with uncomplicated measles who had bronchoalveolar lavage cells tested, an absolute increase in the number of $CD8^+$ and CD11b cells was measured (228). These results point to a role for cell-mediated responses in recovery from measles. It is unknown whether patients with measles pneumonia have an altered local cell-mediated response.

Hantaviruses

In 1993, an outbreak of severe respiratory illness was reported in the southwestern United States (229). The virus documented to be causing this outbreak was a newly described hantavirus. Subsequent to these cases, hantaviruses have been reported in other areas of the United States to cause a similar syndrome. Unlike other hantaviruses which are known to cause hemorrhagic fever with renal syndrome, this zoonosis is characterized by fever and severe noncardiogenic pulmonary edema (230). This hantavirus pulmonary syndrome (HPS) has emerged as a new infectious disease throughout the United States. The hantaviruses which cause this syndrome include Sin Nombre virus, Black

Creek Canal virus, Bayou virus, and Sin Nombre–like viruses (e.g., New York-1) which are not fully characterized. The reservoir appears to be rodents (see also Chap. 11).

Mortality rates from HPS have been >50%. Nonspecific pathological findings are common. The lung demonstrates a mononuclear infiltrate and alveolar edema. The virus is found in endothelial cells by immunohistochemical staining (231).

V. Diagnosis

To diagnose viral pneumonia, both tissue culture cell techniques and serological tests are used (232). Newer diagnostic techniques such as PCR provide rapid identification of specific viruses (233). Specific viral cultures can be employed to recover most of the commonly associated respiratory viruses, but coronaviruses, EBV, and hantaviruses require serological tests (Table 4). Most respiratory viruses can be recovered from nasal wash, throat swab, or sputum specimens if transported rapidly to the laboratory in viral transport medium (234) on ice. Specimens from bronchoscopy secretions or lung biopsy may be used for virus recovery. Nonrespiratory specimens such as stool, urine, or blood may be obtained for virus culture, but the yield is low and positive results should be interpreted carefully. Standard serological tests are available in commercial and governmental laboratories as well as in many hospital laboratories. Acute and convalescent sera are needed to demonstrate a significant antibody rise (see also Chap. 12).

VI. Treatment and Prevention

There are several antiviral agents approved for the treatment of upper respiratory viral infections but most are not yet approved for viral pneumonia (235) (see Chap. 13). Treatment of CMV pneumonia with ganciclovir has been reported to be ineffective (192). Although acyclovir has been administered in HSV and varicella pneumonia, no controlled studies have proven its effectiveness (173). Accordingly, ribavirin has been used in cases of influenza A and B viruses and pneumonia, but the clinical benefit, if any, has not been established. Aerosolized ribavirin is approved for treatment of infants and young children hospitalized with RSV pneumonia. Amantadine/rimantadine also have not been systematically evaluated in influenza A viral pneumonia (236). No approved antivirals are available for measles pneumonia or HPS (237). Interferon-α has not been very effective in reducing clinical symptoms in respiratory viral illness (238).

Table 4 Modes of Detecting Viruses Causing Pneumonia

Virus	Detection by[a]			Comments
	Culture	Direct detection	Serology	
Adenoviruses	+	±	+	Culture and IF are preferred methods of diagnosis. Significance of isolate must be interpreted in relationship to serotype and clinical findings.
Coronaviruses	−	−	+	Diagnosis not routinely available.
Enteroviruses	+	−	−	Significance of isolate must be interpreted in relationship to type isolated and clinical findings.
EBV	−	−	+	Nonspecific heterophilic antibodies (e.g., Monospot) are most readily available but not reliable in children <4 years old. Serology for virus specific antigens is also available.
CMV	+	±	+	Culture is most readily available. Rapid diagnostic methods reported include IF, molecular hybridization, and electron microscopy.
HSV	±	+	+	Culture and IF are both preferred to serology. Significance of isolate must be interpreted in relationship to clinical findings.

Virus				Comments
VZV	±	+	+	Direct detection by nonspecific (e.g., Tzanck preparation, electron microscopy) and specific (e.g., IF) techniques often superior to culture in speed and sensitivity. FAMA is the most sensitive serological method; enzyme immunoassay and anticomplement also are sufficiently sensitive for most uses.
Orthomyxoviruses (influenza A, B, and C) Paramyxoviruses (parainfluenza, RSV)	+	+	+	For RSV, direct detection (IF, ELISA) approaches the sensitivity and specificity of viral culture. For influenza and parainfluenza viruses, direct antigen detection is not as available or as sensitive as viral isolation.
Rhinovirus	+	−	+	Culture is the only routinely available method for rhinovirus detection.
Hantavirus	−	−	+	CDC needed for testing (see Chap. 11)
Measles	+	−	+	Serology is preferred method.

CMV, cytomegalovirus; EB, Epstein-Barr virus; ELISA, enzyme-linked immunosorbent assay; FAMA, fluorescent antibody to membrane antigen; HSV, herpes simplex virus; IF, immunofluorescence; RSV, respiratory syncytial virus; VZV, varicella-zoster virus.
[a] +, Available methods using commercially available reagents; −, not routinely available or not consistently reliable.
Source: From Ref. 8.

Of all the viruses that cause pneumonia, only influenza viruses, VZV, measles virus, and adenoviruses have commercially approved vaccines which can be employed for prevention of infection (239–240). Influenza virus vaccine is updated yearly to reflect the likely current circulating strains of viruses (see Chap. 14). When the circulating virus is antigenetically similar to the vaccine strain, protection against illness is approximately 75%. In addition, hospitalization for pneumonia and influenza syndromes are also reduced by approximately 50%, especially in the elderly. The groups for whom influenza virus vaccines are recommended include those at increased risk for influenza-related complications and those who could transmit the virus to high-risk individuals. Because of the frequent changes in influenza virus strains, yearly vaccination is recommended for these groups. Adenovirus vaccine is used mainly by the military. Other respiratory viruses such as RSV and parainfluenza viruses do not have approved vaccines, although several candidates are under study.

VII. Summary

A wide variety of viruses can cause pneumonia in adults. The relative importance of each varies with the setting in which disease is acquired: the community; closed populations such as the military; health-care facilities where nosocomial spread poses special risks; and immunosuppression as a result of either underlying disease or medication. An understanding of the diagnostic and therapeutic approaches to viral pneumonias is increasingly important in the management of patients with lower respiratory tract illnesses.

References

1. Fransen H. Clinical and laboratory studies on the role of viruses, bacteria, *Mycoplasma pneumoniae* and *Bedsonia* in acute respiratory illness. Scand J Infect Dis 1970: S1:1.
2. Garb JL, Brown RB, Garb JR, Tuthill RW. Differences in etiology of pneumonias in nursing home and community patients. JAMA 1978; 240:2169–2172.
3. Larsen RA, Jacobson JA. Diagnosis of community-acquired pneumonia: experience at a community hospital. Compr Ther 1984; 10:20.
4. Pachon J, Prados MD, Capote PF, Cuello JA, Garnacho J. Severe community-acquired pneumonia. Etiology, prognosis, and treatment. Am Rev Respir Dis 1990; 142:369–373.
5. White RJ, Blainey AD, Harrison KJ, Clarke SD. Causes of pneumonia presenting in a district general hospital. Thorax 1981; 36:566–570.
6. Reichman RC, Dolin R. Viral pneumonias. Med Clin North Am 1980; 64:3: 491–505.

7. Kauffman RS. Viral Pneumonia. Respiratory Infections: Diagnosis and Management. 2nd ed. Pennington JE, ed. New York: Raven Press, 1988:427–442.
8. Greenberg SB. Viral pneumonia. Infect Dis Clin North Am 1991; 5:603–621.
9. Ruben FL. Viral pneumonias. Postgrad Med 1993; 93:57–64.
10. Fang GD, Fine M, Orloff J, Arisumi D, Yu VL, Kapoor W, Grayston JT, Wang SP, Kohler R, Muder RR, et al. New and emerging etiologies for community-acquired pneumonia with implications for therapy. A prospective multicenter study of 359 cases. Medicine 1990; 69:307–316.
11. Glezen WP. Viral pneumonia as a cause and result of hospitalization. J Infect Dis 1983; 147:765.
12. Yang E, Rubin BK. "Childhood" viruses as a cause of pneumonia in adults. Semin Respir Infect 1995; 19:232–243.
13. Fekety FR Jr, Caldwell J, Gump D, Johnson JE, Maxson W, Hulholland. Bacteria, viruses, and mycoplasmas in acute pneumonia in adults. Am Rev Respir Dis 1971; 104:499–507.
14. Sullivan RJ Jr, Dowdle WR, Marine WM, Hierholzer JC. Adult pneumonia in a general hospital. Etiology and host risk factors. Arch Intern Med 1972; 129:935–942.
15. Dorff GJ, Rytel MW, Farmer SG, Scanlon G. Etiologies and characteristic features of pneumonias in a municipal hospital. Am J Med Sci 1973; 266(5):349–358.
16. Prout S, Potgieter PD, Forder AA, Moodie JW, Matthews J. Acute community-acquired pneumonias. S Afr Med J 1983; 64:443–446.
17. Macfarlane JT, Finch RG, Ward MJ, Macrae AD. Hospital study of adult community-acquired pneumonia. Lancet 1982; 2:255–258.
18. Kerttula Y, Leinonen M, Koskela M, Makela PH. The aetiology of pneumonia. Application of bacterial serology and basic laboratory methods. J Infect 1987; 14:21–30.
19. McNabb WR, Shanson DC, Williams TD, Lant AF. Adult community-acquired pneumonia in central London. J Roy Soc Med 1984; 77:550–555.
20. Research Committee of the British Thoracic Society and the Public Health Laboratory Service. Community-acquired pneumonia in adults in British hospitals in 1982–1983: a survey of aetiology, mortality, prognostic factors and outcome. Q. J Med 19887; 62:195.
21. Holmberg H. Aetiology of community-acquired pneumonia in hospital treated patients. Scand J Infect Dis 1987; 19:491.
22. Berntsson E, Blomberg J, Lagergard T, Trollfors. Etiology of community-acquired pneumonia in patients requiring hospitalization. Eur J Clin Microbiol 1985; 4:268–272.
23. Bornstein N, Fleurette J, Bebear C, Chabanon G. Bacteriological and serological diagnosis of community-acquired acute pneumonia, specifically legionnaires' disease: multicenter prospective study of 274 hospitalized patients. Abl Bkt Hyg 1987; 264:93–101.
24. Paun L, Antipa C, Barnaure F, Parvu C, Iacobescu V, Baltiev A, Erscoiu S. Virological investigations in adults with acute pneumonia. Rev Roun Med Virol 1986; 37:23–28.
25. Woodhead MA, Macfarlane JT, McCracken JS, Rose DH. Prospective study of the aetiology and outcome of pneumonia in the community. Lancet 1987; 1:671–674.

26. Morrell RE, Marks MI, Champlin R, Spence L. An outbreak of severe pneumonia due to respiratory syncytial virus in isolated Arctic populations. Am J Epidemiol 1975; 101:231–237.
27. Ortqvist A, Hedlund J, Grillner L, Jalonen E, Kallings I, Leiononen M, Kalin M. Aetiology, outcome and prognostic factors in community-acquired pneumonia requiring hospitalization. Eur Respir J 1990; 3(10):1105–1113.
28. Kauppinen MT, Herva E, Kujala P, Leinonen M, Saikku P, Syrjälä H. The etiology of community-acquired pneumonia among hospitalized patients during a *Chlamydia pneumoniae* epidemic in Finland. JID 1995; 172:1330–1335.
29. Macfarlane JT, Colville A, Guion A, Macfarlane RM, Rose DH. Prospective study of aetiology and outcome of adult lower-respiratory-tract infections in the community. Lancet 1993; 341:511–514.
30. Steinhoff D, Lode H, Ruckdeschel G, Heidrich B, Rolfs A, Fehrenbach FJ, Mauch H, Hoffken G, Wagner J. *Chlamydia pneumoniae* as a cause of community-acquired pneumonia in hospitalized patients in Berlin. Clin Infect Dis 1996; 22: 958–964.
31. Bohte R, van Furth R, van den Broek PJ. Aetiology of community-acquired pneumonia: a prospective study among adults requiring admission to hospital. Thorax 1995; 50:543–547.
32. Aherne W, Bird T, Court SD, Gardner PS, McQuillin J. Pathological changes in virus infections of the lower respiratory tract in children. J Clin Pathol 1970; 23(1): 7–18.
33. Shanley JD. Mechanisms of injury by viral infections of the lower respiratory tract. Med Virol 1995; 5:41–50.
34. Sissons JGP, Borysiewicz LK. Viral immunopathogenesis. Br Bull Med 1985; 41: 31–40.
35. Babiuk LA. Viral-bacterial synergistic interactions in respiratory infections in applied virology. In: Kirstak E, Al-Nakib W, Kirstak C, eds. Applied Virology. New York: Academic Press, 1984:431.
36. Jakab GJ. Mechanisms of bacterial superinfections in viral pneumonias. Schweiz Med Wochenshr 1985; 115:75.
37. Scarpace PJ, Bender BS. Viral pneumonia attenuates adenylate cyclase but not beta adrenergic receptors in murine lung. Am Rev Respir Dis 1989; 140:1602.
38. Tashiro M, Ciborowski P, Klenk HD, Pulverer G, Rott R. Role of Staphylococcus protease in the development of influenza pneumonia. Nature 1987; 325: 536–537.
39. Isaacs D. Problems in determining the etiology of community-acquired childhood pneumonia. Pediatr Infect Dis 1989; 8:143.
40. Murphy TF, Henderson FW, Clyde WA Jr, Collier AM, Denny FW. Pneumonia: an eleven-year study in a pediatric practice. Am J Epidemiol 1981; 113:12–21.
41. Avila M, Salomon H, Carballal G, Ebekian B, Woyskovsky N, Cerqueiro MC, Weissenbacher M. Isolation and identification of viral agents in Argentinian children. Rev Infect Dis 1990; 12:S974–981.
42. Hortal M, Russi JC, Arbiza JR, Canepa E, Chiparelli H, Illarramendi A. Identification of viruses in a study of acute respiratory tract infection in children from Uruguay. Rev Infect Dis 1990; 12:S995.

43. Huq F, Rahman M, Nahar N, Alam A. Acute lower respiratory tract infection due to virus among hospitalized children in Dhaka, Bangladesh. Rev Infect Dis 1990; 12:S982–987.
44. Puthavathana P, Kositanont U, Suwanjutha S, Chantarojanasiri T, Kantakamalakul W, Kantawateera P, Thongcharoen P. A hospital-based study of acute viral infections of the respiratory tract in Thai children, with emphasis on laboratory diagnosis. Rev Infect Dis 1990; 12:S988–994.
45. Rahman M, Huq F, Sach DA, Butler T. Acute lower respiratory tract infections in hospitalized patients with diarrhea in Dhaka, Bangladesh. Rev Infect Dis 1990; 12:S899–986.
46. Suwanjutha S, Chantarojanasiri T, Watthana-Kasetr S, Sirinovin S, Ruangkanchanasetr S, Hotrakitya S, Wasi C, Puthavathana P. A study of nonbacterial agents of acute lower respiratory tract infection in Thai children. Rev Infect Dis 1990; 12: S923–928.
47. Tupasi TE, Lucero MG, Magdangal DM, Mangubat NV, Sunico ME, Torres CU, de Leon LE, Paladin JF, Baes L, Javato MC. Etiology of acute lower respiratory tract infection in children from Alabang, Metro Manila. Rev Infect Dis 1990; 12: S929–939.
48. Weissenbacher M, Carballal G, Avila M, Salomon H, Harisiadi J, Catalano M, Cerqueiro MC, Murtagh P. Etiologic and clinical evaluation of acute lower respiratory tract infections in young Argentinian children: an overview. Rev Infect Dis 1990; 12:S889–898.
49. Mufson MA, Krause HE, Mocega HE, Dawson FW. Viruses, *Mycoplasma pneumoniae* and bacteria associated with lower respiratory tract disease among infants. Am J Epidemiol 1970; 91:192–202.
50. Graman PS, Hall CB. Nosocomial viral respiratory infections. Semin Respir Infect 1989; 4:253.
51. Valenti WM, Hall CB, Menegus MA, Pinus PH, Douglas RG Jr. Nosocomial viral infections. I. Epidemiology and significance. Infect Control 1980; 1:33–37.
52. Anderson DJ, Jordan MC. Viral pneumonia in recipients of solid organ transplants. Semin Respir Infect 1990; 5:38–49.
53. Avery RK. Longworth DL. Viral pumonary infections in thoracic and cardiovascular surgery. Semin Thorac Cardiovasc Surg 1995; 7:88–94.
54. Erice A, Rhame FS, Heussner RC, Dunn DL, Balfour HH Jr. Human immunodeficiency virus infection in patients with solid-organ transplants: report of five cases and review. Rev Infect Dis 1991; 13:537–547.
55. Ruben FL, Nguyen MLT. Viral pneumonitis. Clin Chest Med 1991; 12:223–235.
56. Shanley JD, Jordan MC. Viral pneumonia in the immunocompromised patient. Semin Respir Infect 1986; 1:193–201.
57. Hirschhorn LR, McIntosh K, Anderson KG, Dermody TS. Influenza pneumonia as a complication of autologous bone marrow transplantation. Clin Infect Dis 1992; 14:786–787.
58. Kimball AM, Foy HM, Cooney MK, Allen ID, Matlock M, Plorde JJ. Isolation of respiratory syncytial and influenzaviruses from the sputum of patients hospitalized with pneumonia. J Infect Dis 1983; 147:181–184.

59. Kort BA, Cefalo RC, Baker VV. Fatal influenza A pneumonia in pregnancy. Am J Perinatol 1986; 3:179–182.
60. McKinney WP, Volkert P, Kaufman J. Fatal swine influenza pneumonia during late pregnancy. Arch Intern Med 1990; 150:213–215.
61. Piedra PA. Influenza virus pneumonia; pathogenesis, treatment, and prevention. Semin Respir Infect 1995; 10:216–223.
62. Winterbauer RH, Ludwig WR, Hammar SP. Clinical course, management, and long-term sequelae of respiratory failure due to influenza viral pneumonia. Johns Hopkins Med J 1977; 141:148–155.
63. Stuart-Harris CH. The role of bacterial and viral infection in chronic bronchitis. Arch Environ Health 1968; 16:586–595.
64. Barker WH, Mullooly JP. Pneumonia and influenza deaths during epidemics. Arch Intern Med 1982; 142:85.
65. Karalakulasingam R, Schacht RA, Lansing AM, Raff MJ. Influenza virus pneumonia after renal transplant. Postgrad Med 1977; 62:164–167.
66. Noble RL, Lillington GA, Kempson RL. Fatal diffuse influenza pneumonia premortem diagnosis by lung biopsy. Chest 1973; 63:644.
67. Petersdorf RG, Fusco JJ, Harter DH, et al. Pulmonary infections complicating Asian influenza. AMA Arch Intern Med 1959; 103:264.
68. Ruben FL, Cate TR. Influenza pneumonia. Semin Respir Infect 1987; 2:122.
69. Blumefield HL, Kilbourne ED, Louria DB, et al. Studies on influenza in the pandemic of 1957–58. J Clin Invest 1957; 38:199–212.
70. Schwarzmann SW, Adler JL, Sullivan RJ Jr, Marine WM. Bacterial pneumonia during the Hong King influenza epidemic of 1968–1969. Arch Intern Med 1971; 127:1037–1041.
71. Martin CM, Kunin CM, Gottlieb LS, Finland M. Asian influenza A in Boston, 1957–58. II. Severe staphylococcal pneumonia complicating influenza. Arch Intern Med 1959; 103:532–542.
72. Embrey RP, Geist LJ. Influenza A pneumonitis following treatment of acute cardiac allograft rejection with murine monoclonal anti-CD3 antibody (OKT3). Chest 1995; 108:1456–1459.
73. Hall WN, Goodman RA, Hoble GR, Kendal AP, Steece RS. An outbreak of influenza B in an elderly population. J Infect Dis 1981; 144:297–302.
74. Larsen JW. Influenza and pregnancy. Clin Obstet Gynecol 1982; 25:599–603.
75. Leonardi GP, Leib H, Birkhead GS, Smith C, Costello P, Conron W. Comparison of rapid detection methods for influenza A virus and their value in health-care management of institutionalized geriatric patients. J Clin Microbiol 1994; 32:70–74.
76. Smith CB, Golden CA, Kanner RE, Renzetti AD Jr. Association of viral and *Mycoplasma pneumoniae* infections with acute respiratory illness in patients with chronic obstructive pulmonary diseases. Am Rev Respir Dis 1980; 121:225–232.
77. Knight V, Gilbert BE. Ribavirin aerosol treatment of influenza. Infect Dis Clin North Am 1987; 1:441.
78. Martin CM, Kunin CM, Gottlieb LS, Barnes MW, Liu C, Finland M. Asian influenza A in Boston, 1957–1958. I. Observations in thirty-two influenza-associated fatal cases. AMA Arch Intern Med 1959; 103:515.

79. Osterweil D, Norman D. An outbreak of an influenza-like illness in a nursing home. J Am Geriatr Soc 1990; 38:659–662.
80. Gross PA, Rodstein M, LaMontagne JR, Kaslow RA, Saah AJ, Wallenstein S, Neufeld R, Denning C, Gaerlan P, Quinnan GV. Epidemiology of acute respiratory illness during an influenza outbreak in a nursing home: a prospective study. Arch Intern Med 1988; 148:559–561.
81. Mathur U, Bentley DW, Hall CB. Concurrent respiratory syncytial virus and influenza A infections in the institutionalized elderly and chronically ill. Ann Intern Med 1980; 93:49–52.
82. Falsey AR, Cunningham CK, Barker WH, Kouides RW, Yuen JB, Menegus M, Weiner LB, Bonville CA, Betts RF. Respiratory syncytial virus and influenza A infections in the hospitalized elderly. J Infect Dis 1995; 172:389–394.
83. Yeldandi AV, Colby TV. Pathologic features of lung biopsy specimens from influenza pneumonia cases. Hum Pathol 1994; 25:47–53.
84. Finck ES, Bader I. Pulmonary damage from Hong Kong influenza. Aust NZ J Med 1974; 4:16.
85. Kirshon B, Faro S, Zurawin RK, Samo TC, Carpenter RJ. Favorable outcome after treatment with amantadine and ribavirin in a pregnancy complicated by influenza pneumonia; a case report. J Reprod Med 1988; 33:399–401.
86. Wenzel RP, McCormic DP, Beam WE Jr. Parainfluenza pneumonia in adults. JAMA 1972; 221:294–295.
87. DeFabritus AM, Riggio RR, David DS, Senterfit LB, Cheigh JS, Stenzel KH. Parainfluenza type 3 in a transplant unit. JAMA 1979; 241:384–386.
88. Ross LA, Hitchcock W. Fatal pneumonia caused by parainfluenza type 3 virus. West J Med 1988; 149:223.
89. Akizuki S, Nasu N, Setoguchi M, Yoshida S, Higuchi Y, Yamamoto S. Parainfluenza virus pneumonitis in an adult. Arch Pathol Lab Med 1991; 115:824–826.
90. Wendt CH, Weisdorf DJ, Jordan MC, Balfour HH Jr, Hertz MI. Parainfluenza virus respiratory infection after bone marrow transplantation. N Engl J Med 1992; 326:921–926.
91. Fouillard L, Mouthon L, Laporte JP, Isnard F, Stachowiak J, Aoudjhane M, Lucet JC, Wolf M, Bricourt F, Douay L, et al. Severe respiratory syncytial virus pneumonia after autologous bone marrow transplantation: a report of three cases and review. Bone Marrow Transplant 1992; 9:97–100.
92. Harrington RD, Hooton RM, Hackman RC, Storch GA, Osborne B, Gleaves CA, Benson A, Meyers JD. An outbreak of respiratory syncytial virus in a bone marrow transplant center. J Infect Dis 1992; 165:987–993.
93. Peigue-Lafeuille H, Gazuy N, Mignot P, Deteix P, Beytout D, Baguet JC. Severe respiratory syncytial virus pneumonia in an adult renal transplant recipient: successful treatment with ribavirin. Scand J Infect Dis 1990; 22:87–89.
94. Van Dissel JT, Zijlmans JMJM, Kroes ACM, Fibbe WE. Respiratory syncytial virus, a rare cause of severe pneumonia following bone marrow transplantation. Ann Hematol 1995; 71:253–255.
95. Wendt CH, Hertz MI. Respiratory syncytial virus and parainfluenza virus infections in the immunocompromised host. Semin Respir Infect 1995; 10:4:224–231.

96. Englund JA, Sullivan CJ, Jordan MC, Dehner LP, Vercellotti GM, Balfour HH. Respiratory syncytial virus infection in immunocompromised adults. Ann Intern Med 1988; 109:203–208.
97. Harrington RD, Hooton TM, Hackman RC, Storch GA, Osborne B, Gleaves CA, Benson A, Meyers JD. An outbreak of respiratory syncytial virus in a bone marrow transplant center. J Infect Dis 1992; 165:987–993.
98. Hertz MI, Englund JA, Snover D, Bitterman PB, McGlave PB. Respiratory syncytial virus-induced acute lung injury in adult patients with bone marrow transplants: a clinical approach and review of the literature. Medicine 1989; 68:269–280.
99. Solomon LR, Raftery AT, Mallick NP, Johnson RW, Longson M. Respiratory syncytial virus infection following renal transplantation. J Infect 1981; 3:280–282.
100. Takimoto CH, Cram DL, Root RK. Respiratory syncytial virus infections on an adult medical ward. Arch Intern Med 1991; 151:706–708.
101. Vikerfors T, Grandien M, Olcen P. Respiratory syncytial virus infections in adults. Am Rev Respir Dis 1987; 136:561–564.
102. Zaroukian MH, Kashyap GH, Wentworth BB. Case report: research syncytial virus infection: a cause of respiratory distress syndrome and pneumonia in adults. Am J Med Sci 1988; 295:218–222.
103. Adams JM, Imagawa DT, Zike K. Bronchiolitis and pneumonitis in respiratory syncytial virus. JAMA 1961; 176:1037.
104. Henderson FW. Pulmonary infection with respiratory syncytial virus and the parainfluenza viruses. Semin Respir Infect 1987; 2:112.
105. Dowell SF, Anderson LJ, Gary HE Jr, Erdman DD, Plouffe JF, File TM Jr, Marston BJ, Breiman RF. Respiratory syncytial virus is an important cause of community-acquired lower respiratory infection among hospitalized adults. J Infect Dis 1996; 174:456–462.
106. Sorvillo FJ, Huie SF, Strassburg MA, Butsumyo A, Shandera WX, Fannin SL. An outbreak of respiratory syncytial virus pneumonia in a nursing home for the elderly. J Infect 1984; 9:252–256.
107. Hart RJC. An outbreak of respiratory syncytial virus in an old people's home. J Infect 1984; 8:259–261.
108. Garvie DG, Gray J. Outbreak of respiratory syncytial virus infection in the elderly. Br Med J 1980; 281:1254–1255.
109. Morales F, Calder MA, Inglis JM, Murdoch PS, Williamson J. A study of respiratory infections in the elderly to assess the role of respiratory syncytial virus. J Infect 1983; 7:236–247.
110. Fransen H, Sterner G, Forsgren M, Heigl Z, Wolontis S, Svedmyr A, Tunevall G. Acute lower respiratory illness in elderly patients with respiratory syncytial virus infection. Acta Med Scand 1967; 182:323–330.
111. Levenson RM, Candor OS. Fatal pneumonia in an adult due to respiratory syncytial virus. Arch Intern Med 1987; 147:791–792.
112. Finger R, Anderson LJ, Dicker RC, Harrison B, Doan R, Downing A, Corey L. Epidemic infections caused by respiratory syncytial virus in institutionalized young adults. J Infect Dis 1987; 155:1335–1339.
113. Takimoto CH, Cram DL, Root RK. Respiratory syncytial virus infections on an adult medical ward. Arch Intern Med 1991; 151:706–708.

114. Guidry GG, Black-Payne CA, Payne DK, Jamison RM, George RB, Bocchini JA. Respiratory syncytial virus infection among intubated adults in a university medical intensive care unit. Chest 1991; 100:1377–1384.
115. Agius G, Dindinaud G, Biggar RJ, Peyre R, Vaillant V, Ranger S, Poupet JY, Cisse MF, Castets M. An epidemic of respiratory syncytial virus in elderly people: clinical and serological findings. J Med Virol 1990; 30(2):117–127.
116. Carilli AD, Gold RS, Gordon W. A virologic study of chronic bronchitis. N Engl J Med 1964; 270:123–127.
117. Spelman DW, Stanley PA. Respiratory syncytial virus pneumonitis in adults. Med J Aust 1983; 1:430–431.
118. Sommerville RG. Respiratory syncytial virus in acute exacerbations of chronic bronchitis. Lancet 1963; 2:1247–1248.
119. Hall WJ, Hall CB, Speers DM. Respiratory syncytial virus infection in adults. Ann Intern Med 1978; 88:203–205.
120. Aylward RB, Burdge DR. Ribavirin therapy of adult respiratory syncytial virus pneumonitis. Arch Intern Med 1991; 151:2303–2304.
121. Pearson RD, Hall WJ, Menegus MA, Douglas RG Jr. Diffuse pneumonitis due to adenovirus type 21 in a civilian. Chest 1980; 78:107–109.
122. Komshian SV, Chandrasekar PH, Levine DP. Adenovirus pneumonia in healthy adults. Heart Lung 1987; 16:146–150.
123. Zarraga AL, Kerns FT, Kitchen LW. Adenovirus pneumonia with severe sequelae in an immunocompetent adult. Clin Infect Dis 1992; 15:712–713.
124. Bryant RE, Rhoades ER. Clinical features of adenoviral pneumonia in Air Force recruits. Am Rev Respir Dis 1967; 96:717.
125. Dudding BA, Wagner SC, Zeller JA, Gmelich JT, French GR. Fatal pneumonia associated with adenovirus type 7 in three military trainees. N Engl J Med 1972; 286:1289–1292.
126. Ohori NP, Michaels MG, Jaffe R, Williams P, Yousem SA. Adenovirus pneumonia in lung transplant recipients. Hum Pathol 1995; 26:10:1073–1079.
127. Pingleton SK, Pingleton WW, Hill RH, Dixon A, Sobonya RE, Gertzen J. Type 3 adenoviral pneumonia occurring in a respiratory care unit. Chest 1978; 73:554–555.
128. Shields AF, Hackman RC, Fife KH, Corey L, Meyers JD. Adenovirus infections in patients undergoing bone-marrow transplantation. N Engl J Med 1985; 312:529–533.
129. Zahradnik JM. Adenovirus infection in the immunocompromised patient. Am J Med 1988; 68:725–731.
130. Wright J, Couchonnal G, Hodges GR. Adenovirus type 21 infection. Occurrence with pneumonia, rhabdomyolysis, and myoglobinuria in an adult. JAMA 1979; 241:2420.
131. Speer ME, Schaffer RL, Barrett FF. Adenovirus type 7 pneumonia associated with a large pleural effusion. South Med J 1977; 70:119.
132. Craighead JF, Meier M, Cooley MH. Pulmonary infection due to rhinovirus type 13. N Engl J Med 1969; 281:1403.
133. George RB, Mogabgab WJ. Atypical pneumonia in young men with rhinovirus infections. Ann Intern Med 1969; 71:1073.

134. Jahn CL, Felton AL, Cherry JD. Coxsackie B1 pneumonia in an adult. JAMA 1964; 189:236.
135. Greenberg SB. Respiratory herpesvirus infections. Chest 1994; 106:1S–2S.
136. Schuller D, Spessert C, Frases VJ, Goodenberger DM. Herpes simplex virus from respiratory tract secretions: epidemiology, clinical characteristics, and outcome in immunocompromised and nonimmunocompromised hosts. Am J Med 1993; 94:29–33.
137. Douglas RG Jr, Anderson MS, Weg JG, Williams T, Jenkins DE, Knight V, Beall AC Jr. Herpes simplex virus pneumonia. Occurrence in an allotransplanted lung. JAMA 1969; 210:902–904.
138. Prellner T, Flamholc L, Haidl S, Lindholm K, Widell. Herpes simplex virus—the most frequently isolated pathogen in the lungs of patients with severe respiratory distress. Scand J Infect Dis 1992; 24:283–292.
139. Sherry MK, Klainer AS, Wolff M, Gerhard H. Herpetic tracheobronchitis. Ann Intern Med 1988; 109:229–233.
140. Nash G. Necrotizing tracheobronchitis and bronchopneumonia consistent with herpetic infection. Hum Pathol 1972; 3:284.
141. Tuxen DV, Cade JF, McDonald MI, Buchanan MR, Clark RJ, Pain MC. Herpes simplex virus from the lower respiratory tract in adult respiratory distress syndrome. Am Rev Respir Dis 1982; 126:416.
142. Camazine B, Antkowiak JG, Nava MER, Lipman BJ, Takita H. Herpes simplex viral pneumonia in the postthoracotomy patient. Chest 1995; 108:876–879.
143. Martinez E, de Diego A, Paradis A, Perpiñá, Hernandez M. Herpes simplex pneumonia in a young immunocompetent man. Eur Respir J 1994; 7:1185–1188.
144. Breyer RH, Andrews RI, Mills SA, Cordell AR, Ahl ET. Probable herpes simplex pneumonia after aortic valve replacement. JAMA 1983; 249:1319–1322.
145. Ramsey PG, Fife KH, Hackman RC, Meyers JD, Corey L. Herpes simplex virus pneumonia. Clinical, virologic, and pathologic feature in 20 patients. Ann Intern Med 1982; 97:813–820.
146. Geradts J, Warnock M, Yen TSB. Use of the polymerase chain reaction in the diagnosis of unsuspected herpes simplex viral pneumonia: report of a case. Hum Pathol 1990; 21:118.
147. Weber DM, Pellicchia JA. Varicella pneumonia: study of prevalence in adult men. JAMA 1965; 192:572–573.
148. Clark GPM, Dobson PM, Thickett A, Turner NM. Chickenpox pneumonia, its complication and management. Anaesthesia 1991; 46:376–380.
149. Cox SM, Cunningham FG, Luby J. Management of varicella pneumonia complicating pregnancy. Am J Perinatol 1990; 7:300–301.
150. Duong CM, Munns RE. Varicella pneumonia during pregnancy. J Fam Pract 1979; 8:277–280.
151. Eder SE, Apuzzio JJ, Weiss G. Varicella pneumonia during pregnancy: treatment of two cases with acyclovir. Am J Perinatol 1988; 5:16–18.
152. Ellis ME, Neal KR, Webb AK. Is smoking a risk factor for pneumonia in adults with chickenpox? Br Med J 1987; 294:1002.
153. Esmonde TF, Herdman G, Anderson G. Chickenpox pneumonia; an association with pregnancy. Thorax 1989; 44:812–815.

154. Feldman S. Varicella-Zoster virus pneumonitis. Chest 1994; 106:1:22S–27S.
155. Feldman S, Stokes DC. Varicella zoster and herpes simplex virus pneumonia. Semin Respir Infect 1987; 2:84–94.
156. Gogos CA, Bassaris HP, Vagenakis AG. Varicella pneumonia in adults. A review of pulmonary manifestations, risk factors, and treatment. Respiration 1992; 59: 339–343.
157. Harris RE, Rhoades ER. Varicella pneumonia complicating pregnancy: report of a case and review of literature. Obstet Gynecol 1965; 25:734–740.
158. Hockberger RS. Varicella pneumonia in adults: a spectrum of disease. Ann Emerg Med 1986; 15:931–934.
159. Johnson HN. Visceral lesions associated with varicella. Arch Pathol 1940; 30: 292–307.
160. Preblud SR. Varicella: complications and costs. Pediatrics 1986; 78(suppl):728–735.
161. Rodrigues J, Niederman MS. Pneumonia complicating pregnancy. Clin Chest Med 1992; 13:4:679–691.
162. Schlossberg D, Littman M. Varicella pneumonia. Arch Intern Med 1988; 148: 1630–1632.
163. Triebwasser JH, Harris RE, Bryant RE, Rhoades ER. Varicella pneumonia in adults: report of seven cases and a review of literature. Medicine (Baltimore) 1967; 46:409–423.
164. Waring JJ, Neuberger K, Geever EF. Severe forms of chickenpox in adults with autopsy observations in a case with associated pneumonia and encephalitis. Arch Intern Med 1942; 69:384–408.
165. Weinstein L, Meade R. Respiratory manifestations of chickenpox. Arch Intern Med 1956; 98:91–99.
166. White RG. Chickenpox in pregnancy (letter). Br Med J 1988; 296:864.
167. Zambrano MAR, Martinez A, Minguez JA, Vazquez F, Palencia R. Varicella pneumonia complicating pregnancy. Acta Obstet Gynecol Scand 1995; 74:318–320.
168. Beyer B, Stalder H, Wegmann W. Persistent pulmonary granulomas after recovery from varicella pneumonia. Chest 1986; 89:457–459.
169. Boyd K, Walker E. Use of acyclovir to treat chickenpox in pregnancy. Br Med J 1988; 296:393.
170. Broussard RC, Payne DK, George R. Treatment with acyclovir of varicella pneumonia in pregnancy. Chest 1991; 99:1045–1047.
171. Bryer A, Potgieter P, Moodie J. Acyclovir and varicella pneumonia. S Afr Med J 1984; 66:515.
172. Chitkara R, Gordon R, Khen F. Acyclovir in the treatment of primary varicella pneumonia in non-immunocompromised adults. NY State J Med 1987; 237–238.
173. Smego RA Jr, Asperilla MO. Use of acyclovir for varicella pneumonia during pregnancy. Obstet Gynecol 1991; 78:1112–1116.
174. Van der Meer JWM, Thompson J, Tan WD, Versteeg J. Treatment of chickenpox pneumonia with acyclovir. Lancet 1980(2); 473–474.
175. Lotshaw RR, Keegan JM, Gordon HR. Parenteral and oral acyclovir for management of varicella pneumonia in pregnancy: a case report with review of literature. WV Med J 1991; 87:204–206.

176. Ljungman P. Cytomegalovirus pneumonia; presentation, diagnosis, and treatment. Semin Respir Infect 1995; 10(4):209–215.
177. Raider L. Calcification in chickenpox pneumonia. Chest 1971; 60:504.
178. Klotman ME, Hamilton JD. Cytomegalovirus pneumonia. Semin Respir Dis 1987; 2:95.
179. Lehot JJ, Page Y, Xuan BB, Tardy JC, Chomel JJ, Gibert R, Bosshard S. Severe acute pneumonia associated with cytomegalovirus (CMV). Infection 1983; 11:175–176.
180. Lipton SD, Bryant J, Saed F, Fontillas G. Fatal case of cytomegalovirus pneumonitis in a postpartum woman. Obstet Gynecol 1981; 57:670–673.
181. Cohen JI, Corey GR. Cytomegalovirus infection in the normal host. Medicine (Baltimore) 1985; 64:100–113.
182. Klemola E, Stenström R, von Essen R. Pneumonia as a clinical manifestation of cytomegalovirus infection in previously healthy adults. Scand J Infect Dis 1972; 4:7–10.
183. Buffone GJ, Frost A, Samo T, Demmler GJ, Cagle PT, Lawrence EC. The diagnosis of CMV pneumonitis in lung and heart/lung transplant patients by PCR compared with traditional laboratory criteria. Transplantation 1993; 56:342–347.
184. Duncan AJ, Dummer JS, Paradis IL, Dauber JH, Yousen SA, Zenati MA, Kormos RL, Griffith BP. Cytomegalovirus infection and survival in lung transplant recipients. J Heart Lung Transplant 1991; 10:638–646.
185. Kang EY, Patz EF Jr, Müller NL. Cytomegalovirus pneumonia in transplant patients: CT findings. J Comput Assist Tomogr 1996; 20:295–299.
186. Mera JR, Whimbey E, Elting L, Preti A, Luna MA, Bruner JM, Williams T Jr, Bodey GP, Goodrich JM. Cytomegalovirus pneumonia in adult nontransplantation patients with cancer: review of 30 cases occurring from 1964 through 1990. Clin Infect Dis 1996; 22:1046–1049.
187. Smyth RL, Scott JP, Borysiewicz LK, Sharples LD, Stewart S, Wreghitt TG, Gray JJ, Higenbottam TW, Wallwork J. Cytomegalovirus infection in heart-lung transplant recipients: risk factors, clinical associations, and response to treatment. J Infect Dis 1991; 164:1045–1050.
188. Abdallah PS, Mark JBD, Merigan TC. Diagnosis of cytomegalovirus pneumonia in compromised hosts. Am J Med 1976; 61:326.
189. Elfenbein GJ, Siddiqui T, Rand KH. Successful strategy for prevention of cytomegalovirus interstitial pneumonia after human leukocyte antigen-identical bone marrow transplantation. Rev Infect Dis 1990; 12:S805.
190. Ruutu P, Ruutu T, Volin L, Tukiainen P, Ukkonen P, Hovi T. Cytomegalovirus is frequently isolated in bronchoalveolar lavage fluid of bone marrow transplant recipients without pneumonia. Ann Intern Med 1990; 112:913–916.
191. Emanuel D, Cunningham I, Jules-Elysee K, Brochstein JA, Kernan NA, Laver J, Stover D, White DA, Fels A, Polsky B, et al. Cytomegalovirus pneumonia after bone marrow transplantation successfully treated with the combination of ganciclovir and high-dose intravenous immune globulin. Ann Intern Med 1988; 109:777–782.
192. Reed EC, Bowden RA, Dandliker PS, Lilleby KE, Meyers JD. Treatment of cytomegalovirus pneumonia with ganciclovir and intravenous cytomegalovirus

immunoglobulin in patients with bone marrow transplants. Ann Intern Med 1988; 109:783–788.
193. Peterson PK, Balfour Jr HH, Fryd DS, Ferguson R, Kronenberg R, Simmons RL. Risk factors in the developing of cytomegalovirus-related pneumonia in renal transplant recipients. J Infect Dis 1983; 148:1121.
194. Connolly MG Jr, Baughman RP, Dohn MN, Linnemann CC Jr. Recovery of viruses other than cytomegalovirus from bronchoalveolar lavage fluid. Chest 1994; 105:1775–1781.
195. Crawford SW, Bowden RA, Hackman CR, Gleaves CA, Meyers JD, Clark JG. Rapid detection of cytomegalovirus pulmonary infection by bronchoalveolar lavage and centrifugation culture. Ann Intern Med 1988; 108:180–185.
196. Eriksson BM, Brytting M, Zweygberg-Wirgart B, Hillerdal G, Olding-Stenkvist E, Linde A. Diagnosis of cytomegalovirus in bronchoalveolar lavage by polymerase chain reaction, in comparison with virus isolation and detection of viral antigen. Scand J Infect Dis 1993; 25:421–427.
197. Papazian L, Fraisse A, Garbe L, Zandotti C, Thomas P, Saux P, Gilles P, Gouin F. *Cytomegalovirus*. Anesthesiology 1996; 84:280–287.
198. Myers JL, Peiper SC, Katzenstein AL. Pulmonary involvement in infectious mononucleosis: histopathologic features and detection of Epstein-Barr virus–related DNA sequences. Mod Pathol 1989; 2:444–448.
199. Rodstein M. A case of infectious mononucleosis with atypical pneumonia. Ann Intern Med 1948; 28:1177–1187.
200. Offit PA, Fleisher GR, Koven NL, Plotkin SA. Severe Epstein-Barr virus pulmonary involvement. J Adolesc Health Care 1981; 2:121–125.
201. Mundy GR. Infectious mononucleosis with pulmonary parenchymal involvement. Br Med J 1972; 1:219–220.
202. Andiman WA, McCarthy P, Markowitz RI, Cormier D, Horstmann DM. Clinical, virologic, and serologic evidence of Epstein-Barr virus infection in association with childhood pneumonia. J Pediatr 1981; 99:880–886.
203. Fermaglich DR. Pulmonary involvement in infectious mononucleosis. J Pediatr 1975; 86:93–95.
204. Veal CF Jr, Carr MB, Briggs DD Jr. Diffuse pneumonia and acute respiratory failure due to infectious mononucleosis in a middle-aged adult. Am Rev Respir Dis 1990; 141:502–504.
205. Eaton OM, Little PF, Silver HM. Infectious mononucleosis with pleural effusion. Arch Intern Med 1965; 115:87–89.
206. Vander JB. Pleural effusion in infectious mononucleosis. Ann Intern Med 1954; 41:146–151.
207. O'Donohue WJ, Polly SM, Angelillo VA. Diffuse pneumonia and acute respiratory failure due to infectious mononucleosis. Nebr Med J 1981; 66:245–247.
208. Schooley RT, Carey RW, Miller G, Henle W, Eastman R, Mark EJ, Kenyon K, Wheeler EO, Rubin RH. Chronic Epstein-Barr virus infection associated with fever and interstitial pneumonitis. Ann Intern Med 1986; 104:636–643.
209. Hashimoto Y, Nawata Y, Kurasawa K, Takabayashi K, Oda K, Mikata A, Iwamoto I. Investigation of EB virus and cytomegalovirus in rapidly progressive interstitial pneumonitis in polymyositis/dermatomyositis by *in situ* hybridization

and polymerase chain reaction. Clinical Immunology and Immunopathology 1995; 77(3):298–306.
210. Hogg JC, Hegele RG. Adenovirus and Epstein-Barr virus lung diseases. Semin Respir Infect 1995; 10:244–253.
211. Oda Y, Katsuda S, Okada Y, Kawahara EI, Ooi Akishi, Atsuhiro K, Nakanishi I. Detection of human cytomegalovirus, Epstein-Barr virus, and herpes simplex virus in diffuse interstitial pneumonia by polymerase chain reaction and immunohistochemistry. Am J Clin Pathol 1994; 102:495–502.
212. Haller A, von Segesser L, Baumann PC, Krause M. Severe respiratory insufficiency complicating Epstein-Barr virus infection: case report and review. Clin Infect Dis 1995; 21:206–209.
213. Russler SK, Tapper MA, Knox KK, Liepins A, Carrigan DR. Pneumonitis associated with coinfection by human herpesvirus 6 and Legionella in an immunocompetent adult. Am J Pathol 1991; 138:1405–1411.
214. Pitalion AK, Liu-Yin JA, Freemont AJ, Morris DJ, Fitzmaurice RJ. Immunohistological detection of human herpesvirus 6 in formalin-fixed, paraffin-embedded lung tissues. J Med Virol 1993; 41:103–107.
215. Carrigan DR, Drobyski WR, Russler SK, et al. Interstitial pneumonitis associated with human herpesvirus-6 infection after marrow transplantation. Lancet 1991; 338:147–149.
216. Cone R, Hackman RC, Huang MW, Bowden RA, Meyers JD, Metcalf M, Zeh J, Ashley R, Corey L. Human herpesvirus-6 in lung tissue from patients with pneumonitis after bone marrow transplantation. N Engl J Med 1993; 329: 156–161.
217. Chapnick EK, Gradon JD, Young-doo K, et al. Fatal measles pneumonia in an immunocompetent patient (letter). Clin Infect Dis 1992; 15:377–379.
218. Forni AL, Schluger NW, Roberts RB. Severe measles pneumonitis in adults: evaluation of clinical characteristics and therapy with intravenous ribavirin. Clin Infect Dis 1994; 19:454–462.
219. Germillion DH, Crawford GE. Measles pneumonia in young adults: an analysis of 106 cases. Am J Med 1981; 71:539–541.
220. Henneman PL, Birnbaumer DM, Cairns CB. Measles pneumonitis. Ann Emerg Med 1995; 26:278–282.
221. Ng VL, Boggs JM, York MK, Golden JA, Hollander H, Hadley WK. Fatal measles pneumonia in a immunocompetent patient—case report. Clin Infect Dis 1992; 15:377–379.
222. Rupp ME, Schwartz ML, Bechard DE. Measles pneumonia: treatment of a near-fatal case with corticosteroids and vitamin A. Chest 1993; 103:5:1625–1626.
223. Stein SJ, Greenspoon JS. Rubeola during pregnancy. Obstet Gynecol 1991; 78: 925–929.
224. Hall WJ, Hall CB. Atypical measles in adolescents: evaluation of clinical and pulmonary function. Ann Intern Med 1979; 90:882.
225. Olson RW, Hodges GR. Measles pneumonia. Bacterial suprainfection as a complicating factor. JAMA 1975; 232:363.
226. Sobonya RE, Hiller FC, Pingleton W, Watanabe I. Fatal measles (Rubeola) pneumonia in adults. Arch Pathol Lab Med 1978; 102:366–371.

227. Atmar RL, Englund JA, Hammill H. Complications of measles during pregnancy. Clin Infect Dis 1992; 14:217–226.
228. Myou S, Fujimura M, Yasui M, Ueno T, Matsuda T. Bronchoalveolar lavage cell analysis in measles viral pneumonia. Eur Respir J 1993; 6:1437–1442.
229. Duchin JS, Koster FT, Peters CJ, Simpson GL, Tempest B, Zaki SR, Ksiazek TG, Rollin PE, Nichol S, Umland ET, Moolenaar RL, Reef SE, Nolte KB, Gallaher MM, Butler JC, Breiman RF, and the Hantavirus Study Group. Hantavirus pulmonary syndrome: a clinical description of 17 patients with a newly recognized disease. N Engl J Med 1994; 330:950–1006.
230. Khan AS, Khabbaz RF, Armstrong LR, Holman RC, Bauer SP, Graber J, Strine T, Miller G, Reef S, Tappero J, Rollin PE, Nichol ST, Zaki SR, Bryan RT, Chapman LE, Peters CJ, Ksiazek TG. Hantavirus pulmonary syndrome: the first 100 U.S. cases. J Infect Dis 1996; 173:1297–1303.
231. Warner GS. Hantavirus illness in humans: review and update. South Med J 1996; 89:264–271.
232. Greenberg SB, Krilov LR. Laboratory diagnosis of respiratory viral infections. In: Drew WL, Rubin SJ, eds. Cumitech 21. Washington, DC: American Society of Microbiology, 1986:1.
233. Smith TF, Wold AD, Espy MJ, Marshall WF. New developments in the diagnosis of viral diseases. Infect Dis Clin North Am 1993; 7:183–201.
234. Leland DS, Emanuel D. Laboratory diagnosis of viral infections of the lung. Semin Respir Infect 1995; 10:189–198.
235. Mahmoo W, Sacks SL. Anti-infective therapy for viral pneumonia. Semin Respir Infection 1995; 10:270–281.
236. Dolin R, Reichman RC, Madore HP, Maynard R, Linton PN, Webber-Jones J. A controlled trial of amantadine and rimantadine in the prophylaxis of influenza A infection. N Engl J Med 1982; 307:580–584.
237. Wong RD, Goetz MB, Mathisen G. Clinical and laboratory features of measles in hospitalized adults. Am J Med 1993; 95:377–383.
238. Gwaltney JM Jr. Combined antiviral and antimediator treatment of rhinovirus colds. J Infect Dis 1992; 166:776–782.
239. Centers for Disease Control and Prevention. Prevention and control of influenza. MMWR 44 (RR-3), 1995; April 21:1–10.
240. Mullooly JP, Bennett MD, Hornbrook MC, Barker WH, Williams WW, Patriarca PA, Rhodes PH. Influenza vaccination programs for elderly persons: cost-effectiveness in a health maintenance organization. Ann Intern Med 1994; 121:947–952.

4

Viral Pulmonary Infections in Older Persons

ANN R. FALSEY

University of Rochester School of Medicine and Dentistry and
Rochester General Hospital
Rochester, New York

I. Introduction

Respiratory viruses account for more acute illnesses each year in the United States than any other medical condition and result in nearly 10 billion dollars in medical care costs (1). Although these acute respiratory tract infections are the cause of significant disability and absenteeism in young adults, it is at the extremes of age that the impact of these viruses can be most devastating. Immunosenescence, underlying conditions, and an aging respiratory tract all contribute to the older person's susceptibility to more severe infection (2,3). Pneumonia and influenza together comprise the fifth leading cause of death among persons over the age of 65 (4). Although pneumonia has been referred to as "the old man's friend" by the esteemed physician, Sir William Osler, millions of older persons would strongly disagree. In light of the rapidly aging U.S. population, it is essential to recognize common respiratory viral infections and to know how to diagnose, appropriately treat, and, most importantly, how to prevent them. This chapter will focus on the influenza virus and respiratory syncytial virus (RSV), the two most important pathogens in older persons, and it will include brief descriptions of parainfluenza, coronavirus, and rhinovirus infections.

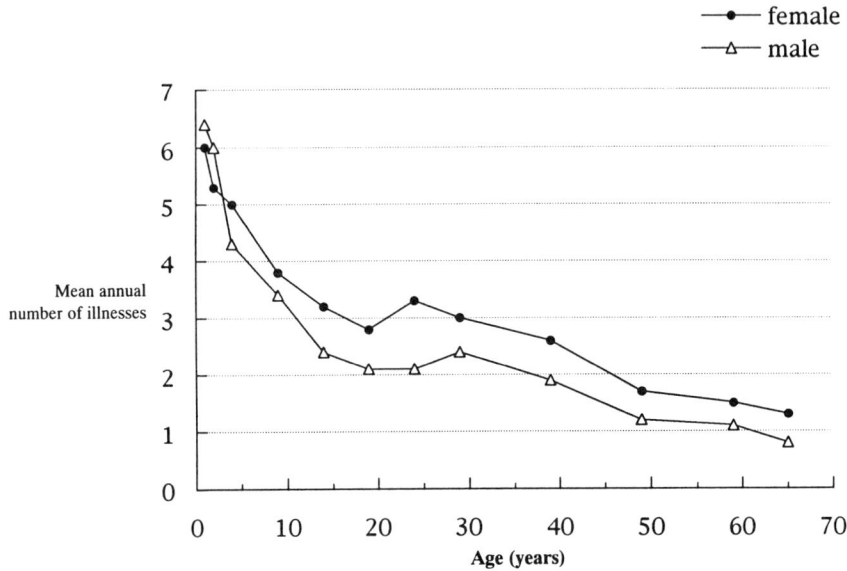

Figure 1 Mean number of respiratory illnesses experienced per year by age group (Tecumseh, MI). (From Ref. 5.)

II. Epidemiology

Rates of acute respiratory tract infections generally decline with advancing age (Fig. 1) (5). Lower rates of infections are presumed to be due to partial immunity and less frequent exposure to respiratory pathogens. In the Tecumseh study, ambulatory individuals over the age of 60 had a mean annual incidence of only 1.3 acute respiratory illnesses, although the number of elderly followed in the study was small (6). More recent studies which focus on older persons suggest that rates of infection depend on place of residence, with those living in congregate settings being at highest risk. In a recent study of community-dwelling older persons by Hodder et al., the overall rate of respiratory infections was 2.5/100 person months. However, rates of infection were significantly higher if they cared for children on a regular basis (3/100 person months) (7). Infection rates in long-term care facilities vary with the season and are unpredictable owing to the epidemic nature of respiratory viruses. The incidence of upper respiratory tract infections (URI) in long-term care facilities is difficult to ascertain because of underreporting, but several studies have estimated rates of approximately 1–3 URI per patient per year (8,9). However, a 1-day prevalence study of skilled nursing homes found the prevalence of respiratory infections to be 1.5%, suggesting that rates are substantially higher (10). A recent study during the winter months at a 590-bed nursing home found the rate of respiratory infections to be 6.3/100 person months, of which 42% were documented to be caused by viruses (11). The highest rates of respiratory infections appear to be in older persons attending senior day-care centers, where rates of 10.8/100 person months have been noted (12). The reasons for high rates of infection in day-care centers are likely multifactorial and include diminished functional status requiring hands-on assistance from staff and increased exposures to pathogens from family, staff, and other day-care participants.

III. Influenza Virus

Since ancient times, outbreaks of influenza virus have caused worldwide pandemics and epidemics of disease. Although morbidity is highest in the young, excess mortality occurs primarily in older persons (13). Influenza viruses are classified as either type A or B, on the basis of stable internal viral proteins. The major surface glycoproteins of influenza, hemagglutinin (H), and neuraminidase (N) are the primary targets of humoral immunity and undergo frequent antigenic changes. Minor changes, known as "drift," are due to spontaneous mutations in the H or N genes and occur in both A and B viruses. Major antigenic changes, known as "shifts," likely occur when the viral genomes of unrelated influenza A viruses reassort and result in a virus with substantially different H or N protein. When these shift viruses circulate widely, pandemics occur in nonimmune populations. Four pandemics have been recorded in this century: 1918 (H1N1), 1957 (H2N2), 1968 (H3N2), and in 1977—reemergence of H1N1. Currently two influenza A viruses, H1N1 and H3N2, in addition to influenza B are circulating in the United States (14). H1N1 viruses do not cause serious problems in older persons, possibly due to immunity acquired in younger life (13,15,16) (see also Chap. 6).

A. Epidemiology

The introduction of influenza into the community typically results in a bell-shaped increase in acute respiratory illnesses lasting 6–8 weeks (13). Infection rates are highest in preschool and school-aged children and decline with advancing age (13,17,18). In studies of nonpandemic influenza by Glezen et al., attack rates were 30% for preschool children, 20% for school-aged children, 15% for adults up to age 45, and 10% for older adults (17).

Despite the high rates of infection in children and young adults, rates of complications and hospitalizations are lowest in persons 5–24 years of age and highest in infants and persons over age 65 (15,19,20). During epidemics of influenza H3N2, hospitalization rates are approximately 6–15/1000 persons over age 65 (19,20). Hospitalization rates are generally lower during influenza B epidemics (15,19). Discharge diagnoses of influenza or pneumonia are traditionally used when calculating hospitalization rates due to influenza. However, influenzal infection can worsen a number of chronic conditions, and more accurate appraisals can be ascertained by using more inclusive cardiopulmonary diagnoses such as congestive heart failure, bronchitis, and chronic obstructive pulmonary disease. Barker and colleagues found that influenza accounted for 11–28% of all hospital admissions for acute cardiopulmonary diseases in persons over age 65 during three winter seasons (15).

B. Risk Factors for Morbidity and Mortality

Mortality from influenza increases dramatically with age (21–23). The age-specific mortality curves typically show a U-shaped pattern with modestly increased case fatality in the very young and increasing case fatality in persons over age 45 (24) (Fig. 2). The susceptibility of older persons to severe disease and complications of influenza may be in part attributable to immunosenescence (25). Evidence suggests that humoral and mucosal immunity is relatively well preserved in older persons (26). However, cell-mediated immunity, which is important for viral clearance, appears to be more significantly affected by aging. The proliferative response of T lymphocytes to influenza antigens is significantly lower in older subjects in comparison with young subjects (25). In addition, diminished lymphocyte interleukin-2 secretion in response to influenza antigen has been observed in elderly volunteers (27). Investigators have also demonstrated that influenza A virus–specific cytotoxic T-lymphocyte activity declines with advancing age (28).

The increased mortality due to influenza in older persons can only partly be explained by direct infection-related complications (23). Barker and Mullooly estimate that only 61% of influenza-related deaths are captured by traditional death certificate coding (29). Deaths due to cardiovascular and cerebrovascular disease also increase significantly during periods of influenza activity. The presence of underlying medical conditions in addition to advanced age contributes significantly to influenza-related mortality (30). In persons over age 65, the presence of one high-risk medical condition (cardiovascular, pulmonary, renal, metabolic, neurological, or malignant disease) increases the risk of influenza-related deaths 39-fold. Barker et al. found that the highest death rates (870/100,000) due to influenza occurred in persons with both chronic cardiac and pulmonary disease. Cardiac disease and pulmonary disease alone were associated with death rates of 104 and 240/100,000, respectively (30). In addition to the suffering caused by influenza, the economic

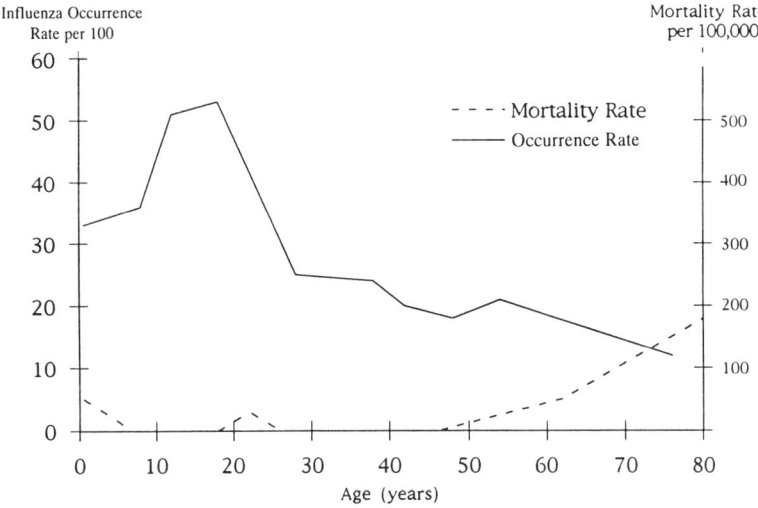

Figure 2 Clinical influenza occurrence rate (Kansas City, 1957) and annual mortality rate for pneumonia and influenza (US, 1957). Clinical influenza may be underestimated in very young children; therefore curve may be falsely low in children less than 10 years old. (From Ref. 24.)

impact of this infection in older persons is enormous (31). Over one billion dollars was reimbursed by Medicare for excess hospitalizations during the 1989–1990 influenza season alone (32). In summary, it is clear that although older persons are less likely to acquire influenza infection than younger persons, they are much more likely to develop complications that result in hospitalization or death.

C. Clinical Manifestations

The clinical manifestations of influenza in older persons may be those of "classic" influenza. Typically, patients present with the abrupt onset of fever, chills, headache, and myalgias. Dry cough, sore throat, and ocular symptoms are also common. Nasal discharge occurs but usually is not as profuse as with other respiratory viruses and is frequently overshadowed by systemic symptoms (14). Fever remains a frequent finding in older persons with influenza, but the height of the fever may be lower than that of children and young adults (14). Although many elderly persons experience classic symptoms, a substantial number will have more subtle presentations. This is particularly true in institutionalized persons where cognitive impairment may prevent patients from offering specific complaints. Infection may be characterized by increased confusion, anorexia, lassitude, unexplained fever, or increased respiratory difficulties (13). In addition, worsening of underlying medical conditions such as congestive heart failure or chronic obstructive pulmonary disease may dominate the clinical picture (33). In a recent study of elderly persons admitted to the hospital with either serologically or culture-confirmed influenza A infection, the principal discharge diagnosis was exacerbation of COPD in 11% of cases and congestive heart failure in 16% of cases (34).

Lower respiratory tract involvement with influenza infection increases with advancing age (14,16). In a study of five influenza epidemics, Fry showed that the rate of pneumonia was 4–8% in persons aged 5–50 but rose steadily to 73% in persons over age 70 (14,35). Influenza pneumonia has classically been divided into three categories: primary viral pneumonia, secondary bacterial pneumonia, and mixed viral–bacterial infection (36). Primary influenzal pneumonia occurs in persons of all ages, most often during pandemics. Influenza-related pneumonia in older persons is most often due to secondary bacterial or mixed viral–bacterial infection. The illness is usually characterized by classic influenza symptoms followed by a 3- to 4-day period of improvement and then sudden recrudescence of fever with the development of worsening respiratory symptoms (36). The most commonly identified bacterial pathogens are *Streptococcus pneumoniae*, *Staphylococcus aureus*, and *Haemophilus influenzae* (14,37).

The devastating impact of influenza on older persons is demonstrated most dramatically during outbreaks of influenza in long-term care facilities. A number of reports document high rates of pneumonia and death during H3N2 and influenza B outbreaks in nursing homes (38–44). H1N1 only rarely causes institutional outbreaks (45). During outbreak situations, attack rates of 20–30% are often observed and rates of pneumonia and hospitalization may be as high as 52% and 29%, respectively (39,41,44). Mortality rates are high among chronically ill, elderly persons, and case fatality rates of up to 30% are not unusual (41). Risk factors for infection in nursing home residents include nonvaccinated status, low preinfection influenza specific antibody titers, and increased functional status (39,42). Paradoxically, higher attack rates are sometimes observed in more functional ambulatory residents; perhaps due to increased opportunity for exposure (42).

D. Diagnosis

Influenzal infection can be diagnosed by a variety of methods. Since the clinical features may be indistinguishable from other respiratory viruses, laboratory confirmation is essential for appropriate therapeutic decisions and infection control policies. Diagnosis of influenza is best made by isolation of the virus from nasopharyngeal secretions or sputum (46). Virus is usually shed for 5–7 days in young adults. On average, older persons shed virus for 3–4 days and have approximately 1000-fold less virus in their secretions (R.F. Betts, personal communication). Influenza virus is reasonably hardy and will survive overnight if specimens are kept on ice; therefore viral culture is a useful diagnostic tool even in nursing home settings (14). Approximately two thirds of positive cultures are detected within 3 days, and with shell vial culture techniques, results may be positive as early as 24 hr (47).

In closed populations where explosive epidemics may occur, the rapid diagnosis of influenza is highly desirable. A number of diagnostic techniques, including polymerase chain reaction (PCR), immunofluorescent assay (IFA), and enzyme immunoassay (EIA), on direct patient specimens have been developed and offer same-day results (48–51). Most studies have examined the utility of these new tools in pediatric or young adult populations. Generally, IFA and EIA are not felt to be sufficiently sensitive to replace viral culture for diagnosis (14). However, EIA rapid antigen testing may have a role in the evaluation of nursing home residents with respiratory infections. A recent study by Leonardi et al. compared the diagnostic utility of IFA, and two commercially available EIA (Directigen FLU-A and Prima EIA) for nasal swab specimens in institutionalized geriatric patients (52). In comparison with culture, the sensitivities of the IFA, Directigen FLU A, and Prima EIA were 92.5, 97.2, 86.8% and the specificities were 99.1, 92.5, 98.1%, respectively. IFA was found to be too labor intensive for practical application in large numbers of nursing homes. Although this study was not controlled, investigators did note that final attack rates of influenza in institutions using combined rapid and culture testing were lower than in institutions using culture alone; suggesting rapid testing was useful for infection control purposes.

Influenzal infection can be confirmed serologically by complement fixation, hemagglutination inhibition assay (HAI), or EIA (46). Since nearly all adults have antibodies against influenza owing to previous infections and/or vaccination, a single elevated titer is not useful for the diagnosis of acute infection. Demonstration of a ≥fourfold rise in influenza-specific IgG in paired acute and convalescent sera can confirm the diagnosis retrospectively.

In summary, viral culture remains the best tool for the diagnosis of influenza in all age groups, including elderly persons. Direct specimen testing may be useful as an adjunct to culture in institutional settings (see also Chap. 12).

E. Treatment

Two antiviral agents, amantadine and rimantadine, are approved in the United States for the treatment and prophylaxis of influenza A infection. Neither drug has activity against influenza B (53). When administered prophylactically, amantadine is 70–90% effective in preventing influenza A illness in studies carried out primarily in young adults (54). These agents can also reduce illness severity, duration of symptoms, and days of viral shedding if they are given within 48 hr of symptom onset (53). Although reasonably well tolerated in young people, central nervous system side effects such as confusion, agitation, and seizures can be problematic in older persons (55–57). Rimantadine produces less central nervous system side effects but is more expensive than amantadine (58). In one study, rimantadine-treated nursing home patients had a more rapid reduction in fever and were prescribed fewer antipyretics, antitussives, and antibiotics (14). Although drug resistance develops rapidly with amantadine or rimantadine treatment, a net therapeutic benefit is preserved (59). Transmission of virus resistant to both agents has been documented; illness due to drug-resistant virus does not appear to be clinically different (60).

Persons over the age of 65 require only half the dose given to young adults to achieve the same plasma levels (53). The appropriate dose of amantadine or rimantadine is 100 mg po daily. Amantadine must be adjusted further for renal insufficiency whereas rimantadine requires dose modification only with far advanced renal disease (53) (see also Chap. 13).

F. Prevention

Infection Control

Outbreaks of influenza in long-term care facilities may be associated with significant morbidity and mortality. Thus prevention of influenza in the nursing home setting is important. Since influenza is spread by small-particle aerosol and residents may be infectious prior to the onset of symptoms, outbreaks tend to be explosive in nature and difficult to control (55). The cornerstone of an effective infection control policy is yearly vaccination for all staff and residents (61,62). Consent for annual influenza vaccination should be obtained from guardians or residents on admission to a long-term care facility (55). When influenza activity has been identified in the community, resident furloughs should be restricted to those that are medically necessary and visitors with respiratory illnesses should be discouraged. Symptomatic residents should be restricted to their rooms with doors closed, and employees should use gloves and masks when entering the rooms of symptomatic patients. If possible, residents and staff from affected wards should be cohorted and vaccination should be offered again to all unvaccinated staff and residents (55,61).

Many authorities, including the Centers for Disease Control (CDC) and Prevention, recommend antiviral prophylaxis once influenza A has been documented within an institution (62,63). Chemoprophylaxis should be given to all residents regardless of their vaccination status and should be continued until 1 week after the onset of the last case of presumed influenza has occurred (63). Although rimantadine is better tolerated than amantadine, the latter is usually selected for prophylaxis because it may be less expensive (14,56,64). For several reasons, these recommendations for prophylaxis have been questioned by some authorities. First, the efficacy of antiviral prophylaxis in nursing homes has not been proven in prospective, controlled studies (55). Second, many influenza-like illnesses in nursing homes are often caused by other respiratory viruses on which amantadine has no effect (11,65,66). Third, the transmission of drug-resistant influenza virus has been documented to occur in nursing homes (67–69). And finally, adverse reactions to amantadine requiring withdrawal of the drug are frequent among elderly persons. Stange and colleagues found that 41% of nursing home residents who received amantadine experienced adverse side effects, of which 22% were classified as severe (57). Falls were reported in 3% of elderly amantadine recipients in one study, and in another study involving 900 institutionalized persons a four- to 8-fold increase in falls was noted during the period of prophylaxis (55). In addition, residents receiving prophylaxis require restraints for agitation and experience an increase in seizure activity more frequently (55). Thus, some authorities prefer a more conservative approach and recommended administration of amantadine only to individuals who have been ill less than 48 hr and to their roommates (55). However, institutionwide prophylaxis should be considered if more than 10% of residents are ill or if there has been a major antigenic shift of the virus.

Vaccination

Influenza vaccine is an effective measure for reducing the impact of influenzal infection in elderly persons and is recommended for all persons over age 65. The current vaccine contains antigens from two type A and one type B viruses, which represent the strains expected to circulate during the upcoming season (62). Mild acute local reactions occur in approximately one third of vaccinees. Systemic reactions such as fever, malaise, and myalgias occur infrequently and are less severe in older persons (70).

The serum antibody response to influenza vaccination is more variable in older persons than in young healthy adults, and a number of vaccine trials have shown a diminished serological response in elderly subjects (71). However, many of these studies suffered from methodological flaws which fail to control for the presence of chronic diseases, prevaccination antibody titers, and previous influenza vaccination status. The serological response of healthy middle-aged and elderly men to influenza vaccine has been shown to be inversely correlated with preimmunization hemagglutination inhibition titers (72). In addition, Gross and colleagues demonstrated that the presence of chronic illness diminished the immune response to influenza vaccine in older persons (73). Although aging per se does not necessarily predict a poor vaccine response, a number of investigators have shown that some healthy older persons have a less vigorous immune response, especially when challenged with a new influenza antigen (74). In elderly vaccine nonresponders, booster doses do not appear to enhance response rates (75,76).

The protective efficacy of influenza vaccine depends on the age and immunocompetence of the subjects as well as the match of vaccine to the circulating epidemic strain. Vaccine efficacy rates for reducing influenza infection in young persons range from 67 to 92% (70). Efficacy rates in elderly persons are generally lower with occasional reports of complete vaccine failures (77). Only one randomized double-blind, placebo-controlled study of influenza vaccine in the elderly has been reported (78). In this study from The Netherlands, investigators found a 50% reduction in serologically proven influenza and a 53% reduction in clinical influenza among vaccinated persons. Most other studies of community-dwelling elderly patients have been case-controlled retrospective analyses in which efficacy was demonstrated by showing reductions of 31–45% in hospitalizations for pneumonia and influenza during periods of influenza virus activity (79–81). In a recent 3-year case-controlled study of 25,000 older persons, Nichol et al. found influenza vaccine to be both efficacious and cost effective (82). Although vaccine recipients had more underlying diseases at baseline than unvaccinated individuals, vaccination was associated with a reduction in hospitalization by 48–57%. Vaccination was also associated with a 37% reduction in hospitalizations for congestive heart failure when influenza A was epidemic. In addition, during the 3 years of study, vaccination was associated with a 39–54% decrease in mortality from all causes (82).

For residents of nursing homes, influenza vaccine is most effective in preventing serious complications of influenza rather than preventing infection itself (62). In this population, vaccination reduces uncomplicated influenzal infection by only 32–45%. However, it has been reported to prevent 50–60% of influenza-related pneumonias and hospitalizations and has reduced death rates by 68–74% (77,83). Furthermore, high rates of vaccination in nursing homes may induce herd immunity and thus benefit unvaccinated residents (62).

In an effort to improve vaccine efficacy in chronically ill, elderly persons, new products, such as live attenuated virus vaccines, hemagglutinin conjugated to diphtheria toxoid, and hemagglutinin incorporated into liposomes, are being developed and evaluated (84–89). Although the older person's response to the current influenza vaccine is variable, there is compelling evidence that the vaccine is both efficacious and cost effective. Annual influenza vaccination is recommended for persons 65 years of age and older as well as for persons with underlying diseases which predispose them to complications of influenza (62) (see also Chaps. 6 and 14).

IV. Respiratory Syncytial Virus

Respiratory syncytial virus (RSV) is well recognized as the leading cause of lower respiratory tract disease in infants and young children. Immunity to RSV is incomplete and reinfections occur throughout adult life, typically causing mild upper respiratory tract infections (90). Although prolonged airway reactivity has been demonstrated following RSV infection, RSV is rarely a cause of serious illness in healthy young adults (91). Since the early 1980s there has been increasing recognition of RSV as a cause of significant illness in elderly persons. It ranks second only to influenza as a major viral pathogen in this age group (34,92) (see also Chap. 7).

A. Epidemiology

RSV was first recognized as a problem in the elderly in institutionalized older persons. Since 1977 there have been nine reports involving 12 institutions of RSV outbreaks in nursing homes and eight prospective studies in which RSV was identified as a common pathogen (8,11,65,66,93–104). Although attack rates as high as 90% have been reported in outbreaks, infection rates are more commonly in the range of 10–40% (93,95,99). In a prospective study of respiratory infections in a long-term facility, RSV accounted for 25% of all acute respiratory tract infections during one winter season (11). RSV has also been shown to be a common cause of infection in seniors attending day-care centers (12). Complication rates of RSV among frail older persons have been variable with rates of pneumonia ranging from 5 to 67% and death from 0 to 20% (11,96,99,101).

RSV infection is also a cause of serious disease in community-dwelling older persons. The incidence of RSV infection in this age group has not been studied and data are limited to case reports of RSV pneumonia and studies of elderly adults requiring hospitalization (105–112). Although the precise incidence is unknown, recent studies indicate that RSV is a cause of excess morbidity and mortality in persons over age 65 at rates similar to those of influenza (34,92). Fleming and Cross compared rates of respiratory illnesses and excess deaths with viral activity in the community during four winter seasons in the United Kingdom. When RSV and influenza activity occurred during different periods, two distinct peaks in the number of respiratory illnesses and deaths were noted (92). Although viral isolates were obtained primarily from children, 81% of all deaths were in persons over age 65. A recent report from the United Kingdom using statistical modeling estimated the mortality associated with RSV over 15 winter seasons was 60–80% more than that associated with influenza (113). Finally, in a recent study of persons over age 65 admitted to the hospital in the winter with acute cardiopulmonary conditions or influenza-like illnesses, RSV was identified in 10% of patients compared with 13% with influenza. RSV cases were identified consistently throughout the winter over a 3-year period in two upstate New York cities, indicating that it is a predictable cause of illness in this age group and not limited to outbreak situations (34).

B. Clinical Manifestations

The clinical manifestations of RSV in older persons can be quite variable, ranging from mild rhinorrhea to severe respiratory distress (11). Early descriptions of RSV in the elderly were limited by selection bias during investigations of outbreaks (95–100). Recent data from prospective studies in day-care and long-term care facilities indicate that the most common symptoms include nasal congestion (92%), cough (90%), sputum production (60%), and constitutional symptoms (53%). Fever was present in about half the patients and wheezing observed in 30–35% (11,12). The impact of RSV illness in those persons requiring hospitalization is significant, as 18% are admitted to an intensive care unit, 10% require ventilatory support, and 10% die (34).

RSV and influenza may circulate at the same time, and it may be difficult to distinguish between the two infections on clinical grounds. Although no feature is diagnostic of RSV infection, certain signs and symptoms may be helpful. Nasal discharge and wheezing are more typical of RSV illness, whereas gastrointestinal complaints, high fevers, and prominent myalgias are more characteristic of influenza (11,34,94,104) (Table 1).

C. Diagnosis

The diagnosis of RSV infection may be accomplished by culture, direct antigen detection, or serological analysis. In older persons, diagnosis during acute infection has been problematic. Although viral culture is the gold standard of diagnosis, RSV is labile and does not survive prolonged transit times, which can be a particular problem in long-term care facilities (114). Direct antigen detection by IFA or commercial colorimetric EIA has been used successfully on nasal wash specimens in children. Nasopharyngeal swabs are the usual specimens collected from older persons, since nasal washes are difficult to obtain from elderly patients, particularly those with diminished capacity for cooperation. In addition, the titer of RSV shed by adults is considerably lower than in children, making diagnosis by culture or antigen detection more difficult (115). When rapid diagnostic tests (IFA and EIA [Directigen]) were compared with culture under optimal conditions and retrospective serology, both methods were very insensitive in elderly persons. IFA detected 1 of 11 infections and EIA missed all cases (116).

Table 1 Clinical Findings in Elderly Patients with Influenza Virus Versus RSV Infection

Finding	Influenza	RSV
Fever >39°C	+++	+
Rhinorrhea	+	+++
Sore throat	++	+
Myalgias	+++	+
Gastrointestinal symptoms	+	0
Wheezing	++	+++

0 = absent; + to +++ indicates mild/common to severe/frequent.
Source: Ref. 162.

Infection with RSV can be demonstrated by a ≥fourfold rise in RSV-specific IgG by either EIA or complement fixation. Since RSV infection in the adult always represents reinfection, a single elevated titer is not reliable evidence of acute RSV infection. Serology by EIA has been found to be both sensitive and specific for RSV infection (103). Eighty-five percent of older persons with culture-proven RSV will mount a ≥fourfold rise in RSV-specific IgG in response to infection as measured by EIA (11). RSV-specific IgM has been detected in 11–81% of older subjects with RSV infection; however its utility for early diagnosis is limited, since antibody response generally requires 5–7 days and rheumatoid factor may interfere with the assay (102,117). Although serological analysis is a valuable method of retrospective diagnosis, new techniques for rapid diagnosis of RSV in the elderly are clearly needed to assist physicians in the management of acute illnesses.

D. Treatment

Treatment of RSV infection in the elderly adult is generally supportive. Ribavirin, a nucleoside analogue with activity against RSV, is approved for young children infected with RSV. Clinical efficacy has been demonstrated in this group with little toxicity (118,119). No controlled trials have been done in adults; however, anecdotal reports in immunocompromised patients and elderly adults suggest that it may be beneficial in selected cases (120,121). The approved method of administration for ribavirin is 20 mg/mL reservoir concentration delivered by continuous aerosol for 12–18 hr a day for 3 days. In the agitated or confused elderly patient, this regimen can be difficult to administer. More recent data from infants indicates that high-dose (60 mg/mL), short-duration ribavirin aerosol given over 2 hr three times a day may be equally effective as standard therapy (122). Clearly, more information in this age group is needed before any general recommendation can be made.

E. Immunity

The risk factors for more severe clinical manifestations of RSV in the elderly adult have not been well defined, but they likely include the presence of underlying heart and lung disease, a declining immune system, and an aging respiratory tract (123,124). The precise roles of humoral, cell-mediated, and secretory immunity have not been thoroughly investigated in the elderly. However, it does appear that most older persons maintain relatively high levels of serum antibody (102,125). No significant difference was found in baseline RSV antibody titers as measured by EIA and neutralization assay among nursing home residents who became infected with RSV versus those who were uninfected (125). There was a trend of less severe disease in subjects with higher serum neutralizing titers; however the difference was not statistically significant. In addition, most elderly persons, even those in nursing homes, maintain a brisk IgG and IgA response to infection (102). Cell-mediated immunity to RSV in the elderly has not been studied.

F. Prevention

At the present time, there is no licensed RSV vaccine; however, as vaccine candidates become available, older persons are a logical target population for immunization. Recent trials with a purified fusion protein (PFP-2) subunit vaccine indicate that healthy persons over age 65 have immune responses similar to the response rates to influenza vaccine with 61% developing a ≥fourfold increase in neutralizing antibody (125a). Frail institutionalized elderly subjects have shown a slightly lower response rate at 47% (125b). Whether such vaccines will offer clinical benefit remains to be demonstrated.

Since an effective vaccine and treatment in this age group remain elusive, the best management is prevention. It is believed that RSV is spread by large droplets and fomites, and thus close contact or contact with contaminated environmental surfaces or skin is necessary for transmission (126,127). In contrast to influenza, which tends to cause explosive outbreaks, nursing home outbreaks of RSV usually occur as a steady trickle of cases over several weeks (11). Although definitive studies are lacking, it is probable that RSV is introduced into the long-term care facility by staff members or visitors. In several outbreaks, investigators noted that cold symptoms were observed among staff members, although none was specifically evaluated (96,98). Handwashing is the single most important infection-control measure for limiting the spread of RSV in the nursing home (128). Because compliance with handwashing is sometimes poor, some authorities have advocated the use of gloves in addition to strict handwashing (127). Since transmission is not by small particle aerosol, respiratory isolation is not necessary.

V. Parainfluenza Viruses

A. Epidemiology and Clinical Manifestations

The parainfluenza viruses (PIV) are members of the paramyxovirus family and four serotypes and two subgroups (1,2,3,4a,4b) are recognized. Infection with parainfluenza viruses is almost universal by age 5, and causes croup, bronchiolitis, and pneumonia in young children. PIV-1 and PIV-2 peak activity occurs most commonly during the fall months, whereas PIV-3 is endemic, occurring throughout the year (129). Similar to RSV, immunity to PIV is incomplete, and reinfection with these viruses occurs throughout life. Epidemiological studies indicate that PIV infections account for approximately 1–15% of acute respiratory tract infections in adults (130–133). Parainfluenzal infections in healthy young adults are generally manifest as mild upper respiratory tract infections. However, occasional outbreaks of PIV-related pneumonias in young adults have been described (134). In addition, PIV infections may be associated with exacerbations of chronic bronchitis (135) (see also Chap. 8).

Comprehensive studies of parainfluenza in community-dwelling older persons are lacking, but current data indicate that, although infection with these viruses is not common, elderly persons may develop serious illness. Fransen et al. found serological evidence of PIV-1 or PIV-3 infection in 11% of persons over age 60 with pneumonia and in 7% with acute respiratory infection (131). In the United Kingdom between 1972 and 1986, a total of 5781 reports of PIV disease were collected (136). Two percent were in persons over age 65 years, of which 56% were diagnosed serologically and 44% were by culture. Most of the infections were PIV-1 (32%) and PIV-3 (65%) with only 3% due to PIV-2. Peak activity of PIV infections among elderly persons followed peak activity in the general population by approximately 1 month, and lower respiratory tract involvement (56%) was more common (136). In a 15-month prospective study of 165 frail seniors attending day care centers, PIV-1 or PIV-3 accounted for only 1% of all acute respiratory illnesses (11).

The impact of PIV appears to be more substantial in institutionalized older persons. Prospective studies of respiratory illnesses in nursing homes have documented PIV infection in 4–14% of cases of respiratory illnesses (8,11,65,137). In addition, several outbreaks of PIV infection in long-term care facilities have been described with high attack rates and substantial morbidity and mortality. Five outbreaks of PIV (four PIV-3 and one PIV-1) in nursing homes were reported in the United Kingdom between 1976 and 1982. Outbreaks were characterized by "chest infections," fever, coryza, and malaise. During one outbreak, four persons died of bronchopneumonia (136). Clusters of PIV types 1 and 3 have also been described in US nursing homes (138). Illnesses were characterized by fever, rhinorrhea, sore throat, and cough. Pneumonia rates were high (17–29%) with several deaths. Attack rates during one outbreak were 22 and 28% in residents and employees, respectively. Employees with direct patient contact had an attack rate of 35% compared with 11% among those without patient contact; suggesting person-to-person spread. Most recently, an outbreak of PIV-3 occurred in a Canadian nursing home affecting 26 of 81 (31%) of residents and 5 of 78 (6%) of staff (139). Lower respiratory tract involvement occurred most commonly in residents requiring extended care (82%) compared with those who were in residential care (27%). Symptoms included rhinorrhea, cough, hoarseness, wheezing, and sore throat. Thirty-one percent were febrile, and one resident was hospitalized with pneumonia. Pneumonia associated with PIV infection in elderly persons does not have distinctive clinical characteristics. Unique histological features are seen in giant cell pneumonia due to PIV invasion of lung tissues and is described in immunocompromised infants and children (see Chap. 5). One case of a 77-year-old woman with lung cancer and giant cell pneumonia with elevated PIV titers has been reported (140).

B. Diagnosis

Diagnosis of PIV infection can be accomplished by viral culture of the nasopharyngeal secretions or sputum. Adults typically shed less virus than do children (129). Serological analysis of acute and convalescent blood by complement-fixation or EIA can establish a diagnosis retrospectively. However, as is true of most other respiratory viral infections, a single elevated titer is not felt to be diagnostic. PIV-1 and PIV-3 infections result in heterologous antibody responses, and therefore it is not possible to distinguish the two infections serologically. Currently, there are no commercially available rapid antigen tests available for the diagnosis of parainfluenza virus.

C. Treatment

Treatment of parainfluenzal infection is supportive. At the present time, there are no available antiviral agents with proven clinical effectiveness against parainfluenza virus (141). Ribavirin has activity in vitro and in vivo, but to date, there have not been randomized, controlled trials of this drug in humans.

D. Infection Control

An effective PIV vaccine has not yet been developed. Therefore, the prevention of PIV infection can only be accomplished by interruption of viral transmission. Although most studies suggest direct person-to-person transmission of parainfluenza, the precise mechanism is unknown. Similar to influenza virus, PIV is stable in small particle aerosols at low humidities found in hospitals;

yet outbreaks tend to proceed more slowly than influenza or other aerosol-spread infections (127). In the long-term care facility, infection control policies are similar to those recommended for RSV and should emphasize handwashing, the use of gloves, and cohorting of cases if possible (see also Chap. 8).

VI. Rhinoviruses

A. Epidemiology

Rhinoviruses are members of the picornavirus family, and at least 100 antigenic types have been identified. These viruses account for approximately 25–50% of upper respiratory tract infections and are the most commonly identified cause of the "common cold" (142). Rhinoviral infections occur sporadically throughout the year, but peaks of activity are seen in the fall and spring (143). Infections with rhinoviruses are common throughout life, and illnesses in healthy young adults are generally mild and are characterized by sneezing, rhinorrhea, and sore throat that last an average of 7–8 days (144). Rhinoviral illnesses may be more severe at the extremes of age, with higher rates of wheezing and prolonged symptoms in persons less than age 5 years or over 40 years of age have been noted (143). Infection with these common viruses may also be more severe in persons with underlying lung disease. Rhinoviruses have been isolated in 3–43% of persons with exacerbations of chronic obstructive pulmonary disease (145–149). Additionally, pulmonary function studies have shown to be abnormal in smokers during rhinoviral infections (147). Pneumonia due to rhinovirus is unusual even in immunocompromised persons and is thought to be related to the virus's inability to replicate at 37°C, which is the temperature of the lower airways (150) (see also Chap. 10).

The precise incidence of rhinoviral infection in healthy independent elderly persons is unknown. However, studies of seniors living in congregate settings such as long-term care facilities or attending senior day-care centers indicate that infection with these viruses is not uncommon (11,12,66). In two prospective studies of acute respiratory illnesses in nursing homes, rhinoviruses were isolated during 6–9% of illnesses (11,66). In addition, rhinoviruses have been isolated from 7% of ill seniors attending day-care centers (150a).

B. Clinical Manifestations

Rhinoviral illnesses in frail elderly persons are characterized most frequently by cough (71–94%), nasal congestion (79–89%), constitutional symptoms (43–91%), and sore throat (21–51%). Three studies have focused on rhinoviral infections in older persons and have produced conflicting data on the severity

Table 2 Clinical Features of Rhinovirus in the Elderly

Features	Comparison of 3 Studies (%)		
	Falsey[a] (N = 14)	Wald[b] (N = 35)	Falsey[c] (N = 33)
Symptoms			
constitutional	43	71	91
nasal congestion	79	60	88
sore throat	21	51	45
cough	71	97	94
dyspnea	14	23	39
Signs			
temperature > 100°F	28	17	18
wheezing	14	34	24
rales	21	28	42
Course			
antibiotics	14	60	40
pneumonia	0	3	0
hospitalization	0	3	3
death	0	3	0

[a]Ref. 11.
[b]Ref. 104.
[c]Ref. 150a.

of these infections in this age group (11,151) (Table 2). Falsey and coworkers described 14 nursing home patients with culture-documented cases and found illnesses to be mild. Patients did not appear to be acutely ill and lower respiratory tract signs, such as wheezing (14%), rales (21%), and rhonchi (14%), were uncommon. No patient had pneumonia or was hospitalized and no deaths occurred (11). In contrast, Wald et al. described an outbreak of 35 documented rhinoviral infections in a nursing home and found illnesses to be more severe. Sixty-six percent of subjects had lower respiratory tract symptoms and 52% had new abnormalities on lung examination. Persons with underlying lung disease had more severe illnesses, with two individuals requiring hospitalization, one radiographically documented pneumonia, and one death secondary to respiratory failure (151). A more recent study of frail older persons in day-care facilities by Falsey et al. found rhinoviral infections to be moderately debilitating; similar to the findings of Wald et al. (152). Illnesses lasted for approximately 2 weeks and 50% had evidence of lower respiratory tract involvement. One subject was hospitalized for worsening congestive heart failure and no deaths occurred (150a).

C. Diagnosis and Treatment

Diagnosis of rhinoviral infection is made by viral culture of nasopharyngeal secretions. Treatment is supportive and aimed toward patient comfort. Particular care should be used when recommending "cold" medications, which frequently contain combinations of drugs, to older persons. Antihistamines and sympathomimetics may cause adverse side effects such as confusion, urinary retention, hypertension, and tachyarrhythmias in elderly persons (151).

D. Infection Control

Clustering of rhinoviral infections in long-term care facilities suggests that nosocomial transmission occurs (11,152). Rhinoviruses are hardy viruses; surviving up to 3 hr on environmental surfaces and skin (153). Virus can be efficiently transferred to hands and infection produced by autoinoculation. Handwashing is the best method to interrupt transmission, and the use of virucidal preparations, such as 2% iodine, may offer additional benefit (154) (see also Chap. 10).

VII. Coronaviruses

A. Epidemiology and Clinical Manifestations

Coronaviruses are common RNA viruses which account for approximately 5–30% of upper respiratory infections (155,156). Two major serogroups, 229E and OC43, have been identified, and peak viral activity tends to occur in the winter and spring (156,157). Primary infection typically occurs in school-aged children, and reinfections are common throughout life (158) (see also Chap. 10).

Similar to rhinoviral infections, infections with coronaviruses generally do not result in serious illness. Symptoms are usually mild and include malaise, headache, sore throat, and nasal congestion (155). Twenty percent of experimentally infected volunteers had low-grade fever. In very young children, coronaviral infection has been associated with wheezy bronchitis and exacerbations of asthma. Additionally, exacerbations of chronic obstructive pulmonary disease have been linked with coronaviral infection in adults (146,147, 159–161).

Few data are available on the impact of coronaviral infections in the elderly, but two recent studies indicate that infection with this virus can also be more severe in frail older persons. In a prospective study by Nicholson et al. of acute respiratory illnesses in 11 nursing homes in the United Kingdom, 13 of 119 episodes were associated with ≥fourfold rises in antibody titers to coronavirus OC43 and one to 229E (66). Illnesses were described as being similar to influenza, and 25% had lower respiratory tract complications defined as dyspnea, wheezing, severe, or productive cough. In a study of frail older persons attending day-care centers, 37 of 451 (8%) respiratory infections were serologically documented to be due to coronavirus 229E (our unpublished data). The most common symptoms were cough (94%), constitutional complaints (88%), and nasal congestion (84%). Lower respiratory tract involvement was also fairly common, with 66% having a productive cough and 34% experiencing dyspnea. Approximately half the patients had rales on lung examination and wheezing was noted in 22%. Illnesses typically lasted 2 weeks, and almost half of the ill persons received antibiotics. Despite being relatively debilitated, all the patients recovered without significant sequelae. In addition, recent work shows infection with coronavirus OC43 to be relatively common in senior day-care centers as well with 49 of 630 (8%) of illnesses due to OC43 (150a).

B. Diagnosis

Unfortunately, the diagnosis of coronaviral infection can only be accomplished in research settings. The organism is extremely fastidious and requires tracheal organ culture for isolation (155). Complement fixation and EIA may be used to diagnose coronaviral infection serologically, but these tests are also not available for commercial use.

C. Management

No antiviral compounds are available for the treatment of coronaviral infections and management is based on providing symptomatic relief. The transmission of coronavirus is unknown and, although no specific comments on infection control policies can be made, good handwashing is recommended (see also Chap. 10).

VIII. Summary

Respiratory viral infections are major causes of mortality and morbidity in the elderly. Influenza viruses and RSV are the two most important viruses in this regard, but other viruses likely contribute to the burden of illness in this age group. The host factors which predispose the elderly to more severe outcomes with viral respiratory infections are not fully elucidated. These factors likely include less vigorous immune responses ("immunosenescence"), decreased mechanical and other clearance functions of the aging respiratory tract, and comorbidities from underlying diseases that might be present. Infection-control measures are important to limit the spread of respiratory viral infections among residents who live in institutions or congregate dwellings, and who are thus at highest risk for these infections. Annual vaccination for influenza A and B, and appropriate use of amantadine or rimantadine for influenza A are important components of programs to control these infections in the elderly.

References

1. Garibaldi RA. Epidemiology of community acquired respiratory tract infections in adults: incidence, etiology and impact. Am J Med 1985; 78:32–37.
2. Dhar S, Shastri SR, Lenora RAK. Aging and the respiratory system. Med Clin North Am 1976; 60:1121–1123.
3. Miller RA. The aging immune system: primer and prospectus. Science 1996; 273: 70–74.
4. Centers for Disease Control. Hospitalizations for the leading causes of death among the elderly—United States 1987. MMWR 1990; 39:777–779.
5. Monto AS, Ullman BM. Acute respiratory illness in am American community: the Tecumseh study. JAMA 1974; 227:164–169.
6. Monto AS, Cavallaro JJ. The Tecumseh study of respiratory illness. II. Patterns of occurrence of infection with respiratory pathogens. 1965–1969. Am J Epidemiol 1971; 94:280–289.
7. Hodder SL, Ford AB, FitzGibbon PA, Jones PK, Kumar ML, Mortimer EAJ. Acute respiratory illness in older community residents. J Am Geriatr Soc 1995; 43:24–29.
8. Arroyo JC, Jordan W, Milligan L. Upper respiratory tract infection and serum antibody responses in nursing home patients. Am J Infect Control 1988; 16: 152–158.
9. Scheckler WE, Peterson PJ. Infections and control among residents of eight rural Wisconsin nursing homes. Arch Intern Med 1985; 146:1981–1984.
10. Garibaldi RA, Brodine S, Matsumiya S. Infections among patients in nursing homes: policies, prevalence and problems. N Engl J Med 1981; 305:731–735.
11. Falsey AR, Treanor JJ, Betts RF, Walsh EE. Viral respiratory infections in the institutionalized elderly: clinical and epidemiologic findings. J Am Geriatr Soc 1992; 40:115–119.
12. Falsey AR, McCann RM, Hall WJ, Tanner MA, Criddle MM, Formica MA, et al. Acute respiratory tract infection in daycare centers for older persons. J Am Geriatr Soc 1995; 43:30–36.
13. Cate TR. Clinical manifestations and consequences of influenza. Am J Med 19887; 82:15–19.
14. Betts R. Influenza Virus. In: Mandell GL, Gennett JF, Dolin R, eds. Principles and Practices of Infectious Diseases. 4th ed. New York: Churchill Livingstone, 1199:1546–1567.
15. Barker WH, Menegus MA, Hall CB, Betts RF, Freundlich CB, Long CE, et al. Communitywide laboratory-based influenza surveillance focused on older persons, 1989–1992. Am J Prev Med 1995; 11:149–155.

16. Foy HH, Cooney MK, Allan I, Kenny GE. Rates of pneumonia during influenza epidemics in Seattle 1964–1975. JAMA 1979; 241:253–258.
17. Glezen WP, Couch RB. Interpandemic influenza in the Houston area, 1974–76. N Engl J Med 1978; 298:587–592.
18. Fox JP, Cooney MK, Hall CE, Foy HM. Influenza virus infections in Seattle families, 1975–1979. II. Pattern of infection in invaded households and relation of age and prior antibody to occurrence of infection and related illness. Am J Epidemiol 1982; 116:228–242.
19. Perrotta DM, Decker M, Glezen WP. Acute respiratory disease hospitalizations as a measure of impact of epidemic influenza. Am J Epidemiol 1985; 122:468–476.
20. Glezen WP, Payne AA, Snyder DN, Downs TD. Mortality and influenza. J Infect Dis 1982; 146:313–321.
21. Glezen WP, Payne AA, Snyder DN, Downs, TD. Mortality and influenza. J Infect Dis 1982; 146:313–321.
22. Barker WH, Mullooly JP. Impact of epidemic A influenza in a defined adult population. Am J Epidemiol 1980; 112:798–811.
23. Sprenger MJ, Mulder PGH, Beyer WEP, Van Strik R, Masurel N. Impact of influenza on mortality in relation to age and underlying disease, 1967–1989. Int J Epidemiol 1993; 22:334–340.
24. Monto AS. Influenza: quantifying morbidity and mortality. Am J Med 1987; 82:20–25.
25. Powers DC. Immunity to influenza in the elderly. In: Powers DC, Morley JE, Coe RM, eds. Aging, Immunity and Infection. New York: Springer, 1994:41–55.
26. Powers DC, Murphy BR, Fries LF, Adler WH, Clements ML. Reduced infectivity of cold adapted influenza A H1N1 viruses in the elderly: correlation with serum and local antibodies. J Am Geriatric Soc 1992; 40:163–167.
27. McElhaney JE, Beattie BL, Devine R, Grynoch R, Toth EL, Bleakley RC. Age-related decline in interleukin 2 production in response to influenza vaccine. J Am Geriatr Soc 1990; 38:652–658.
28. Powers DC. Influenza A virus–specific cytotoxic T lymphocyte activity declines with advancing age. J Am Geriatr Soc 1993; 41:1–5.
29. Barker WH, Mullooly JP. Underestimation of the role of pneumonia and influenza in causing excess mortality. Am J Public Health 1981; 71:643–645.
30. Barker WH, Mullooly JP. Pneumonia and influenza deaths during epidemics—implications for prevention. Arch Intern Med 1982; 142:85–89.
31. Schoenbaum SC. Economic impact of influenza—the individual's perspective. Am J Med 1987; 82:26–30.
32. McBean AM, Babish JD, Warren JL. The impact and cost of influenza in the elderly. Arch Intern Med 1993; 153:2105–2111.
33. Buscho RO, Shultz PS, Finch E, Mufson MA, Saxtan D. Infections with viruses and mycoplasma pneumoniae during exacerbations of chronic bronchitis. J Infect Dis 1978; 137:377–383.
34. Falsey AR, Cunningham CK, Barker WH, Kouides RW, Yuen JB, Menegus M, et al. Respiratory syncytial virus and influenza A infections in the hospitalized elderly. J Infect Dis 1995; 172:389–394.
35. Fry J. Influenza 1959, the story of an epidemic. Br Med J 1959; 2:135.

36. Louria DE, Blumenfeld HL, Ellis JT, Kilbourne ED, Rogers DE. Studies on influenza in the pandemic of 1957–1958. II. Pulmonary complications of influenza. J Clin Invest 1959; 38:213–265.
37. Scheiblauer H, Reinacher M, Tashiro M, Rott R. Interactions between bacteria and influenza A virus in the development of influenza pneumonia. J Infect Dis 1992; 166:783–791.
38. Center for Disease Control. Outbreaks of influenza among nursing home residents—Connecticut, United States. MMWR 1985; 34:478–482.
39. Center for Disease Control. Outbreak of influenza A in a nursing home—New York, December 1991–January 1982. MMWR 1992; 41:129–131.
40. Ruben FL, Johnston F, Streiff EJ. Influenza in a partially immunized aged population. Effectiveness of killed Hong Kong vaccine against infection with the England strain. JAMA 1974; 230:863–866.
41. Goodman RA, Orenstein WA, Munro TF, Smith SC, Sikes K. Impact of influenza A in a nursing home. JAMA 1982; 247:1451–1453.
42. Hall WN, Goodman RA, Noble GR, Kendal AP, Steece RS. An outbreak of influenza B in an elderly population. J Infect Dis 1981; 144:297–302.
43. Ikeda RM, Drabkin PD. Influenza A outbreaks in nursing homes (letter). J Am Geriatr Soc 1992; 40:1288–1289.
44. Coles FB, Balzano GJ, Morse DL. An outbreak of influenza A (H3N2) in a well-immunized nursing home population. J Am Geriatr 1992; 40:589–592.
45. Mather U, Bentley DW, Hall CB, Roth FK, Douglas RG Jr. Influenza A/Brazil/78 (H1N1) infection in the elderly. Am Rev Respir Dis 1981; 123:633–635.
46. Wiselka M. Influenza: diagnosis, management, and prophylaxis. Br Med J 1994; 308:1341–1345.
47. Schirm J, Luijt DS, Pastoor DW, Mandema JM, Schroder FP. Rapid detection of respiratory viruses using mixtures of monoclonal antibodies on shell viral cultures. J Med Virol 1992; 38:147–151.
48. Waner JL, Todd SJ, Shalaby H, Murphy P, Wall LV. Comparison of Directigen FLU-A with viral isolation and direct immunofluorescence for the rapid detection and identification of influenza A virus. J Clin Microbiol 1991; 29:479–482.
49. Doller G, Schuy W, Tjhen KY, Stekeler B, Gerth HJ. Direct detection of influenza virus antigen in nasopharyngeal specimens by direct enzyme immunoassay in comparison with quantitating virus shedding. J Clin Microbiol 1992; 30:866–869.
50. Cherian T, Bobo L, Steinhoff MC, Karron RA, Yolken RH. Use of PCR-enzyme immunoassay for identification of influenza A virus matrix RNA in clinical samples negative for cultivable virus. J Clin Microbiol 1994; 32:623–628.
51. Chomel CC, Pardon D, Thouvetd, Allard JP. Comparison of three rapid methods for direct diagnosis of influenza and conventional isolation procedure. Biological 1991; 19:287–292.
52. Leonardi GP, Leib H, Birkhead GS, Smith C, Costello P, Conron W. Comparison of rapid detection methods for influenza A virus and their value in health care management of institutionalized geriatric patients. J Clin Microbiol 1994; 32:70–74.
53. Douglas RG. Prophylaxis and treatment of influenza. N Engl J Med 1990; 322:443–450.

54. Dolin R, Reichman RC, Madore HP, Maynard R, Linton PN, Webber-Jones J. A controlled trial of amantadine and rimantadine in the prophylaxis of influenza A infection. N Engl J Med 1982; 307:580–584.
55. Gravenstein S, Miller BA, Drinka P. Prevention and control of influenza A outbreaks in long term care facilities. Infect Control Hosp Epidemiol 1992; 13:49–54.
56. Guay DRP. Amantadine and rimantadine prophylaxis of influenza A in nursing homes. Drugs Aging 1994; 5:8–19.
57. Stange K, Little DW, Blatnik B. Adverse reactions to amantadine prophylaxis of influenza in a retirement home. J Am Geriatr Soc 1991; 39:700–705.
58. Anonymous. Rimantadine for prevention and treatment of influenza. Med Lett 1993; 35:109–110.
59. Hayden FG, Sperber SJ, Belshe RB, Clover RS, Hay AJ, Pyke S. Recovery of drug-resistant influenza A virus during therapeutic use of rimantadine. Antimicrol Agents Chemother 1991; 35:1741–1747.
60. Hayden FG, Belshe RB, Clover RD, Hay AJ, Oakes MG, Soo W. Emergence and apparent transmission of rimantadine-resistant influenza A virus in families. N Engl J Med 1989; 321:1696–1702.
61. Gomolin IH, Leib HB, Arden NH, Sherman FT. Control of influenza outbreaks in the nursing home: guidelines for diagnosis and management. J Am Geriatr Soc 1995; 43:71–74.
62. Anonymous. Prevention and control of influenza—recommendations of the Advisory Committee on Immunization Practices. MMWR 1996; 45 RR-5:1–24.
63. Monto AS. Using antiviral agents to control outbreaks of influenza A infection. Geriatrics 1994; 49:30–34.
64. Patriarca P, Kater N, Kendal. Safety of prolonged administration of rimantadine hydrochloride in the prophylaxis of influenza A virus infections in nursing homes. Antimicrob Agents Chemother 1984; 26:101–103.
65. Gross PA, Rodstein M, LaMontagne JR, Kaslow RA, Saah AJ, Wallenstein S, et al. Epidemiology of acute respiratory illness during an influenza outbreak in a nursing home. Arch Intern Med 1968; 148:559–561.
66. Nicholson KG, Baker DJ, Farquhar A, Hurd D, Kent J, Smith SH. Acute upper respiratory tract viral illness and influenza immunization in homes for the elderly. Epidemiol Infect 1990; 105:609–618.
67. Degelau J, Somani SK, Cooper SL, Guay DRP, Crossley KB. Amantadine-resistant influenza A in a nursing facility. Arch Intern Med 1992; 152:390–392.
68. Houck P, Hemphill M, Lacroix S, Hirsh D, Cox N. Amantadine-resistant influenza A in nursing homes. Arch Intern Med 1995; 155:533–537.
69. Mast EE, Harmon MW, Gravenstein S, Wu SP, Arden NH, Circo R, et al. Emergence and possible transmission of amantadine resistant viruses during nursing home outbreaks of influenza A (H3N2). Am J Epidemiol 1991; 134:988–997.
70. Bentley DW. Vaccinations. Clin Geriatr Med 1992; 8:745–760.
71. Beyer WEP, Palache AM, Baljet M, Masurel N. Antibody induction by influenza vaccines in the elderly: a review of the literature. Vaccine 1989; 7:385–394.
72. Wenzel RP, Hendley JO, Sande MA, Gwaltney JM. Bivalent influenza vaccine: serum and nasal antibody responses to parenteral vaccination. JAMA 1973; 226:435–438.

73. Gross PA, Quinnan GVJ, Weksler ME, Setia U, Douglas RG Jr. Relation of chronic disease and immune response to influenza vaccine in the elderly. Vaccine 1989; 7:303–309.
74. McElhaney JE, Meneilly GS, Lechelt KE, Beattie BL, Bleackley CR. Antibody response to whole-virus and split-virus vaccines in successful aging. Vaccine 1993; 11:1055–1060.
75. Brandriss M, Betts RF, Mathur U, Douglas RG. Responses of elderly subjects to monovalent A/USSR/77 (H1N1) and trivalent A/USSR/77 (H1N1)-A/Texas/77 (H3N2)-B/Hong Kong/72 vaccines. Am Rev Respir Dis 1981; 124:681–684.
76. Gross PA, Weksler ME, Quinnan GW, Douglas RG, Gaerlan PF, Denning C. Immunization of elderly people with two doses of influenza vaccine. J Clin Microbiol 1987; 25:1763–1765.
77. Gross PA, Hermogenes AW, Sacks HS, Lau J, Levandowski RA. The efficacy of influenza vaccine in elderly persons—a Meta-analysis and review of the literature. Ann Intern Med 1995; 123:518–527.
78. Govaert TME, Thijs CTMCN, Masurel N, Sprenger MJW, Dinant GJ, Knottnerus JA. The efficacy of influenza vaccination in elderly individuals—a randomized double-blind placebo-controlled trial. JAMA 1994; 272:1661–1665.
79. Anonymous. Perspectives in disease prevention and health promotion: final results: Medicare influenza vaccine demonstration—selected states, 1988–1992. MMWR 1993; 42:602–604.
80. Mullooly JP, Bennett MD, Hornbrook MC, Barker WH, Williams WW, Patriarca PA, et al. Influenza vaccination programs for elderly persons: cost-effectiveness in a health maintenance organization. Ann Intern Med 1994; 121:947–952.
81. Foster DA, Talsma A, Furumoto-Dawson A, Ohmit SE, Margulies JR, Arden NH, et al. Influenza vaccine effectiveness in preventing hospitalization for pneumonia in the elderly. Am J Epidemiol 1992; 136:296–307.
82. Nichol KL, Margolis KL, Wuorenma J, Von Sternberg T. The efficacy and cost effectiveness of vaccination against influenza among elderly persons living in the community. N Engl J Med 1994; 331:778–784.
83. Strassburg MA, Greenland S, Sorvillo FJ, Lieb LE, Habel LA. Influenza in the elderly: report of an outbreak and a review of vaccine effectiveness reports. Vaccine 1986; 4:38–44.
84. Powers DC, Hanscome PJ, Freda Pietrobon PJ. Cytotoxic T lymphocyte responses to a liposome-adjuvant influenza A virus vaccine in the elderly. J Infect Dis 1995; 162:1103–1107.
85. Gluck R, Mischler R, Finkel B, Que JU, Scarpa B, Cryz SJ Jr. Immunogenicity of new virosome influenza vaccine in elderly people. Lancet 1994; 344: 160–163.
86. Gorse GJ, Otto EE, Powers DC, Chambers GW, Eickhoff CS, Newman FK. Induction of mucosal antibodies by live attenuated and inactivated influenza virus vaccines in the chronically ill elderly. J Infect Dis 1996; 173:285–290.
87. Treanor JJ, Mattison HR, Dumyati G, Yinnon A, Erb S, O'Brien D, et al. Protective efficacy of combined live intranasal and inactivated influenza A virus vaccines in the elderly. Ann Intern Med 1992; 117:625–633.

88. Treanor JJ, Dumyati G, O'Brien D, Riley MA, Riley G, Erb S, et al. Evaluation of cold-adapted, reassortant influenza B virus vaccines in elderly and chronically ill adults. J Infect Dis 1994; 169:402–407.
89. Gravenstein S, Drinka P, Duthie EH, Miller BA, Brown CS, Hensley M, et al. Efficacy of an influenza hemagglutinin-diphtheria toxoid conjugate vaccine in elderly nursing home subjects during an influenza outbreak. J Am Geriatr Soc 1994; 42:245–251.
90. Johnson KM, Bloom HH, Mufson MA, Chanock RM. Natural infection of adults by respiratory syncytial virus: possible relation to mild upper respiratory disease. J Infect Dis 1962; 267:68–72.
91. Hall WJ, Hall CB, Speers DM. Respiratory syncytial virus infection in adults: clinical, virologic, and serial pulmonary function studies. Ann Intern Med 1978; 88: 203–205.
92. Fleming DM, Cross KW. Respiratory syncytial virus or influenza? Lancet 1993; 342:1507–1510.
93. Center for Disease Control. Epidemiologic notes and reports: respiratory syncytial virus—Missouri. MMWR 1977; 26:351.
94. Mathur U, Bentley DW, Hall CB. Concurrent respiratory syncytial virus and influenza A infections in the institutionalized elderly and chronically ill. Ann Intern Med 1980; 93:49–52.
95. Garvie DG, Gray J. Outbreak of respiratory syncytial virus infection in the elderly. Br Med J 1980; 281:1253–1254.
96. Public Health Laboratory Service Communicable Diseases Surveillance Centre. Respiratory syncytial virus infection in the elderly 1976–1982. Br Med J 1983; 287:1618–1619.
97. Morales F, Calder MA, Inglis JM, Murdoch PS, Williamson J. A study of respiratory infection in the elderly to assess the role of respiratory syncytial virus. J Infect 1983; 7:236–247.
98. Hart RJC. An outbreak of respiratory syncytial virus infection in an old people's home. J Infect 1984; 8:259–261.
99. Sorvillo FJ, Huie SF, Strassburg MA, Butsumyo A, Shandera WX, Fannin SL. An outbreak of respiratory syncytial virus pneumonia in a nursing home for the elderly. J Infect Dis 1984; 9:252–256.
100. Mandal SK, Joglekar VM, Khan AS. An outbreak of respiratory syncytial virus infection in a continuing-care geriatric ward. Age Ageing 1985; 14:184–186.
101. Osterweil D, Norman D. An outbreak of an influenza-like illness in a nursing home. J Am Geriatr Soc 1990; 38:659–662.
102. Agius G, Dindinaud G, Biggar RJ, Peyre R, Valiant V, Ranger S, et al. An epidemic of respiratory syncytial virus in elderly people: clinical and serological findings. J Med Virol 1990; 30:117–127.
103. Falsey AR, Walsh EE, Betts RF. Serologic evidence of respiratory syncytial virus infection in nursing home patients. J Infect Dis 1990; 162:568–569.
104. Wald TG, Miller BA, Shult P, Drinka P, Langer L, Gravenstein S. Can respiratory syncytial virus and influenza A be distinguished clinically in institutionalized older persons? J Am Geriatr Soc 1995; 43:170–174.

105. Zaroukian MH, Kashyap GH, Wentworth BB. Case report: respiratory syncytial virus infection a cause of respiratory distress syndrome and pneumonia in adults. Am J Med Sci 1988; 295:218–222.
106. Levenson RM, Kantor OS. Fatal pneumonia in an adult due to respiratory syncytial virus. Arch Intern Med 1987; 147:791–792.
107. Multz AS, Keil K, Karpel JP. Respiratory syncytial virus infection in an adult with Wegener's granulomatosis. Chest 1992; 101:1717–1718.
108. Vikerfors T, Grandien M, Olcen P. Respiratory syncytial virus infections in adults. Amer Rev Respir Dis 1987; 136:561–564.
109. Fransen H, Sterner G, Gorsgren M, Heigl Z, Wolontis S, Svedmyr A, et al. Acute lower respiratory illness in elderly patients with respiratory syncytial virus infection. Acta Med Scand 1967; 182:323–329.
110. Kimball AM, Foy HM, Conney MK, Allan ID, Matlock M, Plorde JJ. Isolation of respiratory syncytial and influenza viruses from the sputum of patients hospitalized with pneumonia. J Infect Dis 1983; 147:181–184.
111. Zaroukian MH, Leader I. Community-acquired pneumonia and infectiion with respiratory syncytial virus. Ann Intern Med 1988; 109:515–516.
112. Spelman DW, Stanley PA. Respiratory syncytial virus pneumonitis in adults. Med J Aust 1983; 1:430–431.
113. Nicholson KG. Impact of influenza and respiratory syncytial virus on mortality in England and Wales from Jaunuary 1975 to December 1990. Epidemiol Infect 1996; 116:51–63.
114. Walsh EE, Hall CB. Respiratory syncytial virus in diagnostic procedures for viral rickettsial and chlamydial infections. In: Schmidt NJ, Emmons RW, eds. APHA. Washington, DC: APHA, 1989:693–712.
115. Englund JA, Piedra PA, Jewell A, Baxter BB, Whimbey E. Rapid diagnosis of RSV in immunocompromised adults (abstr). 34th ICAAC 1995; 1436.
116. Falsey AR, McCann RM, Hall WJ, Criddle MM. Evaluation of four methods for the diagnosis of respiratory syncytial virus infection in older adults. J Am Geriatr Soc 1996; 44:71–73.
117. Vikerfors T, Grandien M, Johansson M, Pettersson C. Detection of an immunoglobulin M response in the elderly for early diagnosis of respiratory syncytial virus infection. J Clin Microbiol 1988; 26:808–811.
118. Smith DW, Frankel LR, Mathurs LH, Tang ATS, Ariagno RL, Prober CG. A controlled trial of aerosolized ribavirin in infants receiving mechanical ventilation for severe respiratory syncytial virus infection. N Engl J Med 1991; 325:24–29.
119. Hall CB, McBride JT, Walsh EE, Bell DM, Gala CL, Hildreth S, et al. Aerosolized Ribavirin treatment of infants with Respiratory Syncytial virus infection. N Engl J Med 1983; 308:1443–1447.
120. Aylward RB, Burdge DR. Ribavirin therapy of adult respiratory syncytial virus pneumonitis. Arch Intern Med 1991; 151:2303–2304.
121. Harrington RD, Hooton TM, Hackman RC, Storch GA, Osborne B, Gleaves CA, et al. An outbreak of respiratory syncytial virus in a bone marrow transplant center. J Infect Dis 1992; 165:987–993.
122. Englund JA, Piedra PA, Ahn Y, Gilbert BE, Hiatt P. High-dose, short-duration ribavirin aerosol therapy compared with standard ribavirin therapy in

children with suspected respiratory syncytial virus infection. J Pediatr 1994; 125: 635–641.
123. Saltzman RL, Peterson PK. Immunodeficiency of the elderly. Rev Infect Dis 1987; 9:1127–1139.
124. Pfitzenmeyer P, Brondel L, d'Athis P, Lacroix S, Didier JP, Gaudet M. Gerontol 1993; 39:267–275.
125. Falsey AR, Walsh EE. Humoral immunity to respiratory syncytial virus infection in the elderly. J Med Virol 1992; 36:39–43.
125a. Falsey AR, Walsh EE. Safety and immunogenicity of a respiratory syncytial vaccine (PFP-2) in ambulatory adults over age 60. Vaccine 1996; 14(13):1212.
125b. Falsey AR. Safety and immunogenicity of a respiratory syncytial virus subunit vaccine (PFP-2) in the institutionalized elderly. Vaccine 1997; 15(10):1130–1132.
126. Hall CB, Douglas RG Jr, Gelman JM. Possible transmission of fomites of respiratory syncytial virus. J Infect Dis 1980; 141:98–102.
127. Graman PS, Hall CB. Epidemiology and control of nosocomial viral infections. Infect Dis Clin North Am 1989; 3:815–841.
128. Falsey AR. Noninfluenza respiratory virus infection in long-term care facilities. Infect Control Hosp Epidemiol 1991; 12:602–608.
129. Hall CB. Parainfluenza viruses. In: Feigin RD, Cherry JD, eds. Textbook of Pediatric Infectious Diseases. 3rd ed. Philadelphia: Saunders, 1992:1613–1625.
130. Mufson MA, Chang V, Gill V, Wood SC, Romansky MJ, Chanock RM. The role of viruses, mycoplasmas and bacteria in acute pneumonia in cilivian adults. Am J Epidemiol 1967; 86:526–543.
131. Fransen H, Heigl Z, Wolontis S, Forsgren M, Svedmyr A. Infections with viruses in patients hospitalized with acute respiratory illness, Stockholm 1963–1967. Scand J Infect Dis 1969; 1:127–136.
132. Stanek J, Heinz F. On the epidemiology and etiology of pneumonia in adults. J Hyg Epidemiol Microbiol 1988; 1:31–38.
133. Monto AS, Sullivan KM. Acute respiratory illnesses in the community. Frequency of illness and the agents involved. Epidemiol Infect 1993; 110:145–160.
134. Wenzel RP, McCormick DP, Beam WEJ. Parainfluenza pneumonia in adults. JAMA 1972; 221:294–295.
135. Fagon J, Chastre J. Severe exacerbations of COPD patients: the role of pulmonary infections. Semin Respir Infect 1996; 11:109–118.
136. Public Health Laboratory Service Communicable Disease Surveillance Centre. Parainfluenza infections in the elderly 1976–82. Br Med J 1983; 287:1619.
137. Hornsleth A, Siggaard-Andersen J, Hjort L. Epidemiology of herpesvirus and respiratory virus infections. Part 1. Serologic findings. Geriatrics 1975; 61–68.
138. Anonymous Epidemiologic Notes and Reports. Parainfluenza outbreaks in extended care facilities—United States. MMWR 1978; 27:475–476.
139. Glasgow KW, Tamblyn SE, Blair G. A respiratory outbreak due to parainfluenza virus type 3 in a home for the aged—Ontario. Can Commun Dis Rep 1995; 21: 57–61.
140. Akizuki S, Nasu N, Setoguchi M, Yoshida S, Higuchi Y, Yamamoto S. Parainfluenza virus pneumonitis in an adult. Arch Pathol Lab Med 1991; 115: 824–826.

141. Treanor JJ. Viral infections of the respiratory tract: prevention and treatment. Int J Antimicrobial Agents 1994; 4:1–22.
142. Gwaltney JM, Hendley JO, Simon G, Jordan WS. Rhinovirus infections in an industrial population - I. the occurrence of illness. N Engl J Med 1966; 275: 1261–1268.
143. Monto A, Bryan ER, Ohmit S. Rhinovirus infections in Tecumseh, Michigan: frequency of illness and number of serotypes. J Infect Dis 1987; 156:43–49.
144. Gwaltney JM, Hendley JO, Simon G, Jordan WS. Rhinovirus infections in an industrial population: II Characteristics of illnesses and antibody response. JAMA 1967; 202:158–164.
145. Smith CB, Golden CA, Kanner RE, Renzetti AD. Association of viral and mycoplasma pneumoniae infections with acute respiratory illness in patients with chronic obstructive pulmonary diseases. Am Rev Respir Dis 1980; 121: 225– 232.
146. Wiselka MJ, Kent J, Cookson JB, Nicholson KG. Impact of respiratory virus infection in patients with chronic chest disease. Epidemiol Infect 1993; 111: 337–346.
147. Eadie MB, Scott EJ, Grist NR. Virological studies in chronic bronchitis. Br Med J 1966; 2:671–673.
148. McNamara MJ, Phillips IA, Williams OB. Viral and mycoplasma pneumoniae infections in exacerbations of chronic lung disease. Am Rev Respir Dis 1969; 100:19–24.
149. Gump DW, Phillips CA, Forsyth BR, McIntosh K. Lamborn KR, Stouch WH. Role of infection in chronic bronchitis. Am Rev Respir Dis 1976; 113:465–474.
150. Gwaltney JM. Rhinoviruses. Principles and Practices of Infectious Diseases. 4th ed. 1995:1656–1662.
150a. Falsey AR, McCann RM, Hall WJ, Criddle MM, Formica MA, Wycoff D, Kolassa JE. The "common cold" in frail older persons: impact of rhinovirus and coronavirus in a senior daycare center. JAGS 1997; 45:706–711.
151. Ziment I. Management of respiratory problems in the aged. J Am Geriatr Soc 1982; 30:S36–S44.
152. Wald TG, Shult P, Krause P, Miller BA, Drinka P, Gravenstein S. A rhinovirus outbreak among residents of a long-term care facility. Ann Intern Med 1995; 123:588–593.
153. Hendley J, Wenzel RP, Gwaltney JM. Transmission of rhinovirus colds by self-inoculation. N Engl J Med 1973; 288:1361–1364.
154. Gwaltney JM, Hoskalski PB, Hendley JO. Interruption of experimental rhinovirus transmission. J Infect Dis 1980; 142:811–815.
155. Larson HE, Reed SE, Tyrrell DAJ. Isolation of rhinoviruses and coronaviruses from 38 colds in adults. J Med Virol 1980; 5:221–229.
156. Isaacs D, Flowers D, Clarke JR, Valman HB, MacNaughton MR. Epidemiology of coronavirus respiratory infections. Arch Dis Child 1983; 58:500–503.
157. McIntosh K, Kapikian AZ, Turner HC, Hartley JW, Parrott RH, Chanock RM. Seroepidemiologic studies of coronavirus infection in adults and children. Am J Epidemiol 1970; 91:585–592.

158. Cavallaro JJ, Monto AS. Community-wide outbreak of infection with a 229E-like coronavirus in Tecumseh, Michigan. J Infect Dis 1970; 122:272–279.
159. McIntosh K. Ellis EF, Hoffman LS, Lybass TG, Eller JJ, Fulginiti VA. The association of viral and bacterial respiratory infections with exacerbations of wheezing in young asthmatic children. J Pediatr 1973; 82:579–590.
160. McIntosh K. Chao RK, Krause HE, Wasil R, Mosega HE, Mufson MA. Coronavirus infection in acute lower respiratory tract disease in infants. J Infect Dis 1974; 130:502–507.
161. Fridy WW, Ingram RH, Hierholzer JC, Coleman MT. Airways function during mild viral respiratory illnesses. Ann Intern Med 1974; 80:150–155.
162. Betts RF, Falsey AR, Hall CB, Treanor JJ. Viral Pneumonias. In: Mandell GL, Simberkoff MS, eds. Atlas of Infectious Diseases. Philadelphia: Churchill Livingstone, 1996.

5

Respiratory Viral Infections in Immunocompromised Patients

RAPHAEL DOLIN

Harvard Medical School
Boston, Massachusetts

I. Introduction

Viral infections of the lung have been recognized as important clinical problems in immunocompromised patients, particularly those undergoing bone marrow or solid organ transplantation or intensive antitumor therapy. Until relatively recently, the viruses which have been recognized as causative agents of these infections have been primarily herpes viruses, particularly cytomegalovirus, and occasionally adenoviruses (1). However, substantial new information has emerged to indicate that "community" respiratory viruses, such as influenza virus, respiratory syncytial virus, and parainfluenza virus, may be important pathogens in immunocompromised patients. The recently generated data regarding community respiratory viral infections, along with approaches to the prevention and therapy of these infections, will be the primary topic of this chapter. Pulmonary infections with herpesviruses in immunocompromised patients, now well recognized, will be dealt with briefly, and the reader is referred to excellent reviews of this latter subject (2–4).

The discussion of respiratory viral infections in immunocompromised patients will be presented according to the major causes of the underlying immunosuppression.

II. Cancer and Leukemia

The impact of infections with community respiratory viruses in patients with underlying malignancies, admittedly a large and heterogeneous group, is incompletely understood. Risk factors, such as the nature and stage of the underlying disease, and the type and duration of therapeutic regimens, have not been analyzed in detail. Nonetheless, several studies have suggested that these infections are associated with significant morbidity and, on occasion, mortality in this group of patients. A large-scale epidemiological study carried out by the Centers for Disease Control (CDC) from 1957–1966 in patients with neoplasms reported "excess mortality" associated with the three most severe influenza outbreaks that occurred during that time (5). This excess mortality was substantially less than that observed in patients with chronic cardiopulmonary diseases. Nonetheless, patients with underlying malignancies have been generally assumed to be at increased risk for complications of influenza, presumably because of immunosuppression, and on that basis, annual influenza vaccination of such patients has been recommended by the Public Health Service (6). Feldman et al., at St. Jude's Children's Research Hospital (Memphis, Tennessee), reported that illness with influenza viral infection was prolonged in 20 children and young adults (ages 2–23 years) who were receiving immunosuppressive therapy (7). Other than prolonged duration, illness was not reported to be "unusual" compared with that in normal children, although three patients developed secondary bacterial infections, one of whom had pneumonia. Kempe et al. prospectively studied a group of unvaccinated children with cancer, and they noted that the incidence of influenzal infection was higher in such children (23 of 73, or 32%) than in nonimmunosuppressed matched controls (10 of 70, or 14%) (8). No differences were noted in illness patterns between the two groups, although two cancer patients with influenza were hospitalized with fever and neutropenia compared with none of the controls. Craft et al. studied 64 children with acute lymphocytic leukemia, aged 1.5 to 14.0 years over a 2- to 30-month period (9). Influenza A–associated illness developed in 11 of these children, of whom two also had pneumonitis. Two children had influenza B–associated illness, which was apparently mild. Prolonged shedding of influenza viruses was also reported in the study. Occasional individual cases have also been reported in which severe influenza A infection occurred in children and adults with underlying tumors, including a fatal case in an adult with malignant lymphoma (10) and in an adult with progressive Hodgkin's disease from whom virus was isolated from the lung at autopsy (11).

More recently, Whimbey and colleagues reported that community respiratory viral infections occurred in 60 of 335 (18%) adults hospitalized with leukemia at MD Anderson Cancer Center (MDCC), Houston, Texas, over an 18-month period (12). Most of these patients had acute myelogenous leukemia. The majority of infections were caused by influenza viruses (32%) and respiratory syncytial virus (RSV) (30%), followed by picornaviruses (17%), parainfluenza viruses (10%), and adenoviruses (3%). The epidemiological pattern of viral infections in these patients was similar to that seen in the community. In this patient population, 38 (63%) of these respiratory viral infections were complicated by pneumonia with an associated mortality of 47%. Twenty-two patients (36%) manifested a typical upper respiratory tract illness without associated mortality.

The majority of pneumonias associated with community respiratory viral infections were preceded by signs and symptoms of an upper respiratory tract illness (rhinorrhea, nasal and sinus congestion, or sore throat). Investigators believe this to be an important presenting feature which distinguishes these pneumonias from those caused by other infections in immunosuppressed patients (12).

In Whimbey's study, patients with influenza had a high rate of pneumonia (78%) and mortality (43%). Autopsies performed on eight of these patients with influenza A showed histopathology in the lung which was interpreted as "consistent" with viral pneumonia (12). An additional patient had influenza A isolated from pulmonary tissue. RSV infections were also associated with high rates of pneumonia (71%) and mortality (53%). Neutrophil counts of $\leq 500/mL$ were an important risk factor for severe disease. Pulmonary histopathology of fatal cases was consistent with RSV pneumonia, although other pulmonary pathogens were also found in 3 of 10 cases. Infections with parainfluenza viruses were reported less frequently, but high rates of associated pneumonia (6 of 9, or 67%) and mortality (66%) were also noted.

Picornaviruses (mostly rhinoviruses) were frequently detected (17%) in cultures from patients with underlying malignancies who have respiratory illnesses (12). This is not surprising because of the frequency of such infections in the community in general. Many of the illnesses associated with these infections appear to be limited to the upper respiratory tract, but some patients had virus isolated in the setting of pneumonias caused by bacterial or fungal organisms, and a few had otherwise unexplained severe and even fatal pneumonias. Additional studies are needed to define the significance of rhinoviral infections in patients with underlying malignancies, as well as infections caused by other "common cold" viruses, such as coronaviruses.

III. Bone Marrow Transplantation

The group of immunocompromised patients in whom the significance of community respiratory viral infections has been most clearly defined are patients

Table 1 Relative Frequency of Community Respiratory Viral Infections in Bone Marrow Transplant Patients

Site	Virus (%)[a]				
	Influenza	RSV	PIV	Rhinovirus[b]	Ref.
Fred Hutchinson Cancer Center	11	35	30	25	25
MD Anderson Cancer Center	18	49	9	18	12
European Group for Blood and Bone Marrow Transplantation	27	29	20	—	26

RSV, respiratory syncytial virus; PIV, parainfluenza virus.
[a]Individual virus/total respiratory virus isolates.
[b]Isolates described as picornaviruses are included.

who have undergone bone marrow transplantation (13–20). Investigators at MDCC have conducted studies in bone marrow transplant patients similar to those described above in patients with leukemia (12). Over two consecutive winter seasons (November 1992–May 1994), 67 of 271 (31%) adult bone marrow transplant patients who were hospitalized for an acute respiratory illness had community respiratory viral infections as determined by viral culture or antigen detection. RSV was the most common virus detected (49%) followed by influenza (18%), picornaviruses (18%), parainfluenza viruses (9%), and adenoviruses (6%) (Table 1). The temporal distribution of these infections was similar to that seen in the community. Infections occurred in patients with either autologous or allogeneic transplants, and they were seen both during pre-engraftment and postengraftment periods. The clinical patterns of respiratory illness were similar to those seen in patients with leukemias. Twenty-eight (42%) patients had an upper respiratory tract illness as manifested by rhinorrhea, nasal and sinus congestion, sore throat, and/or cough. Thirty-nine (58%) patients had pneumonia associated with their viral infection. The pneumonias were either "primary viral" or associated with bacterial or fungal pathogens. The overall mortality associated with these pneumonias ranged from 42% in allogeneic transplant patients to 60% in autologous transplant recipients. Autopsies performed on 12 patients showed histopathological and immunochemical evidence of RSV pneumonia in seven patients, one of whom also had *Candida* in the lung. Two of three patients who died with influenza had histopathology consistent with viral pneumonia and did not have other pathogens identified. Two patients who died with picornaviral infections also had histopathological evidence of viral pneumonia and had no other pathogens isolated from the lung (12).

The importance of RSV infections in bone marrow transplants had been initially reported by Englund et al. at the University of Minnesota (21) and subsequently confirmed by studies at the Fred Hutchinson Cancer Research Center (FHCRC), Seattle, Washington, and elsewhere (13–15,22,23). In these studies, the frequency of associated pneumonia appeared to be highest in preengraftment transplant recipients, but the mortality was similar in both pre- and postengraftment transplant settings. Subsequent studies from the MDCC suggested that RSV disease may be somewhat more severe in the immediate postengraftment period (12). At MDCC, outbreaks of RSV infection have been somewhat less frequent in recent years, which has been attributed to more aggressive and effective infection-control measures (see below).

In the MDCC experience, influenza was also associated with significant morbidity and mortality in bone marrow transplant (BMT) patients (12). Fourteen of 20 (70%) BMT recipients had pneumonia associated with influenza viral infection, and five died (36%). The clinical patterns of illnesses were again similar to those noted in patients with leukemia. Of 10 patients who died with influenzal infections and underwent autopsy examinations, 8 had histopathology consistent with viral pneumonia, and 3 of these also had other respiratory tract pathogens. The other two patients had bacterial and/or fungal pneumonias at autopsy (12).

Parainfluenza viruses have also been recognized as causes of severe infection in bone marrow transplant recipients (12,19,24). The overall clinical course of parainfluenza viral infections in these patients appears to be similar to that described above in patients with parainfluenza viral infection and leukemia. High rates of pneumonia and mortality were observed, and most pneumonias were preceded by signs of upper respiratory tract illness. Autopsies of seven patients who died of parainfluenza viral infection revealed histopathology consistent with viral pneumonia in six patients, four of whom also were infected with other opportunistic pathogens (12). Parainfluenza infections were seen throughout the year in a pattern similar to the occurrence of these infections in the community.

Bowden, at the FHCRC, recently reported her experience with community respiratory viral infections in bone marrow transplant patients from 1990 to 1996 (25). The most frequent infections were caused by RSV (35% of all respiratory viral infections), followed by parainfluenza viruses (30%), rhinoviruses (25%), and influenza viruses (11%) (see Table 1). In patients with RSV infections, virus was isolated only from the upper respiratory tract by nasopharyngeal/throat washings in 51% and from the lower respiratory tract in the other 49%. Parainfluenza virus was isolated from the lower respiratory tract by bronchoalveolar lavage (BAL) in approximately 22% of patients. On the other hand, influenza viruses were infrequently isolated from the lower respiratory tract, and only one rhinoviral isolate was obtained through BAL.

Mortality associated with RSV outbreaks in 1990 and 1994 reported by this group was high (approximately 80%), although an outbreak in 1996 had a somewhat lower mortality (25). Mortality associated with parainfluenza pneumonia was similar to that reported for RSV pneumonia. There were too few patients with influenza pneumonia in the FHCRC series to assess mortality rates. An earlier study of 19 bone marrow transplant patients who had parainfluenza pneumonia from the University of Minnesota, also reported a high mortality rate (32%) (19).

The European Group for Blood and Bone Marrow Transplantation recently reported their experience with community respiratory viral infections in bone marrow transplant patients (26). Information was obtained via a questionnaire distributed to centers in Europe, three of which, in Sweden, France, and The Netherlands, were routinely examining clinical specimens from bone marrow transplant patients for the presence of respiratory viruses. Over the period 1989–1996, a total of 66 cases were reported, 39 of which came from Huddinge University Hospital, Huddinge, Sweden. The overall frequency of infections ranged from 4.0 to 7.1%. The most frequent infection was caused by RSV (29%), followed by adenoviruses (24%), influenza A viruses (20%), parainfluenza viruses (20%), and influenza B viruses (8%) (see Table 1). RSV infections were associated with a high rate of pneumonia (15 of 19 patients), and 6 of the 15 patients with pneumonia died. RSV infections were diagnosed both prior to and after engraftment. Two of 13 patients with influenzal infection had pneumonia and died. Both of these patients were diagnosed prior to engraftment. Ten patients with influenzal infection diagnosed after engraftment apparently did well, although eight of these had chronic graft-versus-host disease. Of the five patients with influenza B viral infection, one developed pneumonia and died. At autopsy, viral pneumonia and pericardial aspergillosis were reported. All 16 patients with adenoviral infection apparently also had pneumonia, and there was associated mortality of 75%. Many of these patients had disseminated adenoviral infection outside of the respiratory tract (26).

IV. Solid Organ Transplantation

Community respiratory viral infections have also been recognized as causes of severe disease in solid organ transplant recipients (27), although these infections have not been studied as extensively in this patient population as they have been in bone marrow transplant recipients. Since the late 1980s, case reports have appeared of RSV and other community respiratory viral infections in liver (28–30), cardiac (31,32), lung (33–35), and renal transplant patients (36,37). Pohl et al. reported 17 cases of RSV infection in pediatric liver transplant patients occurring over a 6-year period (30). Many of these cases appeared to be nosocomial in origin, and 71% had lower respiratory tract involvement. Twelve percent of patients with RSV-associated pneumonia had respiratory failure, and the overall mortality rate was 12%.

Wendt et al. reported that lung transplant recipients may be at particular risk for morbidity and mortality associated with RSV and parainfluenza viral infections (27). She described 10 cases of parainfluenza viral infection and 9 cases of RSV infection, which represented 21% of all lung transplants that were performed at the University of Minnesota between 1986 and 1993. Lower respiratory tract involvement was common in these patients, and pulmonary infiltrates were seen in 10 of 18 patients who received chest radiographs. Infections were frequently associated with abnormal pulmonary function tests, particularly abnormal spirometric findings. Overall mortality attributed to these community respiratory viral infections was 5%, which was somewhat lower than that reported in liver transplant patients. Wendt suggested that the high rates of community respiratory viral infections in lung transplants may reflect impaired host defenses in the transplanted lung itself, as well as a general immunocompromised state of the patient (27).

Variable rates and severity of illnesses associated with influenza viral infections have also been reported in organ transplant recipients. Ljungman reported on 12 cases of influenza A (30) and Aschan reported 5 cases of influenza B (38) in renal transplant recipients in which disease was relatively self-limited and mild. Mauch reported 12 cases of influenza B in children with organ transplants in whom disease was more severe and prolonged, with lower respiratory tract involvement occurring in 5 of the 12 children (39). Of interest, 5 of these 12 patients had neurological disease, including one who died of cerebral herniation.

Adenoviral pulmonary infections in solid organ transplant recipients have also been reported. Breinig et al. reported four cases of adenoviral infection in liver transplant recipients, who may be at particular risk for severe infection of the liver with adenoviruses (28). Renal transplant recipients appear to be at risk for the development of acute hemorrhagic cystitis caused by adenovirus type 11 (40,41).

In addition to the morbidity of the above infections themselves, it has been suggested that viral infections may increase the risk of organ rejection (27). Support for this suggestion has come primarily from observations in renal transplant patients, and systematic studies of the relationship between viral respiratory infections and acute rejection in other solid organ recipients have not been carried out.

V. Human Immunodeficiency Virus Infection

Patients infected with human immunodeficiency virus (HIV) have host-defense defects which predispose them to serious respiratory tract infections, including both humoral and cell-mediated immune defects (42). Many patients with HIV infection also have chronic pulmonary and cardiac diseases which increase the risk of severe respiratory tract infections. Consistent with this, bacterial pneumonias have been reported to be more frequent and severe in HIV-infected patients than in the general population (43). However, epidemiologically based systematic studies of the frequency and severity of community respiratory viral infections in HIV-infected patients have not been carried out. In 1988, the Centers for Disease Control (CDC) and Prevention reported an increase in pneumonia-associated mortality among young adults (ages 25–44) during months when influenza was prevalent in cities with a high rate of HIV infection (44). This was interpreted as a possible indication of increased severity of influenza in HIV-infected patients, although no direct causal link was presented. The remaining reports in the literature consist of small series of cases or individual case reports which have noted variable severities of illness, and in some cases, prolonged shedding of virus. Safrin et al. reported six cases of influenza in HIV-infected adults (two with influenza A/H1N1 and two with influenza B), with overall unremarkable clinical courses except for the presence of somewhat prolonged fever (45). Thurn reported a case of influenza A H3N2 in an HIV-infected adult with evidence of lower respiratory tract illness (pneumonitis) (46). Two fatal cases have been reported in HIV-infected children with A/H3N2 infection. One child had underlying cardiomyopathy and shed virus for "at least 3½ weeks" (47). The other child also had *Pneumocystis carinii* and cytomegalovirus (CMV) present in the lung (48). Another HIV-infected child was reported to have a prolonged illness associated with influenza A, and shed virus for at least 2 months (49). A seizure which was associated with influenza B infection in an HIV-infected child has been reported, but the child had an otherwise unremarkable illness (47).

King et al. conducted a prospective study in which he described 10 respiratory syncytial viral (RSV) infections in HIV-infected children (50). The severity of RSV-associated illness was similar to that seen in a cohort of non–HIV-infected children. HIV-infected children were more likely to have pneumonia, but non–HIV-infected children were more likely to have wheezing. No deaths associated with RSV were reported among the HIV-infected children. However, prolonged shedding of virus was seen (median 30 days; range 1–199 days), and was associated with advanced HIV disease. Another series by Chandwani et al. reported 10 HIV-infected children who were hospitalized with RSV infection, two of whom died, both with concurrent bacterial infections (51). This series also noted that wheezing was relatively uncommon in HIV-infected children. Three children had prolonged shedding of RSV from 30 to 90 days.

Sixteen cases of RSV infection in HIV-infected children were reported by McIntosh (47). The illness in 14 of the 16 children was described as being unremarkable, but 2 children died; one of the fatal cases was also infected with CMV and *P. carinii*, whereas no other pathogen was identified in the other case. Prolonged shedding was also reported in this series. Other case reports include an HIV-infected adult who had a prolonged lower respiratory tract infection associated with RSV, and who also shed virus for 17 days (52), and an HIV-infected child who had severe lower respiratory tract illness, and was simultaneously infected with RSV, parainfluenza type 3, and *P. carinii* (53). The child recovered and shed RSV for at least 3 weeks.

McIntosh also reported five cases of HIV-infected children who had parainfluenzal infection (47). One of these children was asymptomatic, one had wheezing, and two had pneumonia, of which one was a fatal case in which *P. carinii* also was present. Two of these children shed parainfluenza type 3 for 2 and 9 months. Another child had status asthmaticus associated with parainfluenza type 2, which was shed for approximately 1 year. An additional case was reported in that series of an HIV-infected child with severe lower respiratory tract infection associated with infection with parainfluenza 3, adenovirus, and *P. carinii* (47). Parainfluenza virus was shed for 1–3 months in these last two cases. Another HIV-infected child was reported with pneumonia associated with parainfluenza type 3 infection, who also had concomitant *P. carinii* infection. This child recovered from the respiratory illness (54). A fatal case of an HIV-infected child was reported in which a measles giant cell pneumonia was present along with CMV and parainfluenza type 3 (55). Measles pneumonitis has been reported following live measles-mumps-rubella vaccine administration to a patient with advanced HIV infection (55a).

Adenoviruses have also been reported to cause severe infections in HIV-infected patients. A fatal case in an HIV-infected adult with pneumonia associated with adenovirus type 29 has been described (56). Two HIV-infected children and one adult were reported to have fatal disseminated adenoviral infection, including hepatic necrosis, associated with adenovirus types 1, 2, and 3 (57). A fatal adenovirus type 5 disseminated infection has also been reported in an HIV-infected child (58). An untyped adenoviral infection was found in a 6-month-old infant with likely HIV infection and a fatal hemorrhagic illness (47).

Rhinoviral or coronaviral infections associated with severe illness or prolonged virus shedding in HIV-infected patients have not been reported.

VI. Prevention

Nosocomial spread of community viral respiratory infections is well documented. Up to two of three of hospitalized bone marrow transplant recipients (59) and more than half of leukemia patients (60) have been reported to have acquired their RSV infection nosocomially. Thus, control of nosocomial transmission of respiratory viruses is important in the prevention of these infections in immunosuppressed patients. RSV is transmitted primarily by direct person-to-person contact, most commonly from hands contaminated with infected secretions, followed by inoculation through the conjunctival or nasal mucosa of the host (see Chap. 7). Contact with fomites and other environmental sources contaminated with RSV-containing secretions is also an important link in the chain of spread of RSV infection. Aerosol transmission of infection by RSV appears to be much less important, although infection via large particle droplets (>5 μm) has been implicated. Since large particle droplets usually travel relatively short distances (<1 m), transmission by this route also requires close contact.

Infection-control measures to prevent transmission of RSV by the above routes include contact isolation of RSV-infected patients and requirements for washing of hands and wearing of gowns on entering a patient's room (61, 62). In some centers, masks are also recommended to reduce the possibility of transmission via droplets (63). Early identification, isolation, and cohorting of patients with RSV are also essential measures to control nosocomial spread. Rapid diagnostic methods are available to detect RSV infection, of which the most widely used is antigen detection in nasopharyngeal washings (see Chap. 12). Another important measure is the prohibition of contact between immunocompromised patients and staff or visitors who have symptoms of upper respiratory tract infections. Restriction of visits by children less than 12 years of age has also been advocated because of the high rate of viral respiratory infections in that age group (61–63).

Other measures to prevent RSV infection include prophylaxis with RSVIG, a human immunoglobulin enriched for RSV neutralizing antibody. RSVIG, administered at a high dose (750 mg/kg), protected high-risk infants and children against lower respiratory tract disease caused by RSV and reduced rates of hospitalization, and it is approved for that use (64). RSVIG prophylaxis requires monthly administration, and it is associated with transient fever, reversible fluid overload, and a decrease in oxygen saturation. The efficacy of RSVIG in the prophylaxis of RSV infection in immunocompromised patients has not been studied systematically, although it is being employed for that purpose currently in a number of transplant centers.

Nosocomial outbreaks of parainfluenza viral infection can also occur, and since the modes of transmission of parainfluenza viral infections are believed to be similar to that of RSV, the same control measures described above for RSV are recommended (61–63).

In transmission of influenza virus, small-particle aerosols are believed to be important, although spread via large-particle aerosols, by direct contact, and by fomites can also occur. Therefore, in addition to the infection-control measures noted above, respiratory isolation of cases has been advocated to control nosocomial spread (63). A particularly important part of the overall control strategy for influenza is the use of influenza vaccine. Annual immunization should be offered to all immunocompromised patients along with health care workers, family members, and other individuals likely to come in close contact with immunocompromised patients. Immunization with inactivated influenza vaccine appears to be safe in immunocompromised patients, including transplant recipients. However, immune responses may be suboptimal in such patients, particularly those with advanced underlying diseases, such as malignancies and HIV-associated illnesses (65,66) and in those receiving cancer chemotherapy (67). Responses in bone marrow transplant patients appear to be poor within 6 months of transplantation but return to normal over the next 18 months (68). Variable responses in renal transplant recipients have been reported, and poor responses have been associated with intensive immunosuppression regimens, poor allograft function, and high levels of azotemia (69–72). Immune responses to influenza vaccines also appear to be lower in patients with heart, lung, or liver transplants (67,73). Immunization of patients prior to transplantation, if possible, is one approach to improve immune responses to influenza vaccination. Administration of a second ("booster") dose of vaccine may occasionally augment responses, but this has not been generally effective in patients with advanced HIV-associated disease or in cardiac transplant recipients (65,68,74).

Another approach to the prevention of influenza A infection is chemoprophylaxis with amantadine or rimantadine. These drugs have been demonstrated to be highly effective in the prevention of influenza A infection and associated illness in immunocompetent adults and children (see Chap. 13), but their efficacy in immunocompromised patients has not been established. However, the drugs are generally well tolerated, and they may provide particular benefit in immunocompromised patients who have not been immunized or whose immune responses to vaccination are expected to be suboptimal. Prophylaxis may also be useful if vaccination is performed late; that is, when influenza A virus is already circulating in the community. Prophylaxis with amantadine or rimantadine may also provide additive protection to that conferred by vaccination, and it thus can be considered even when responses to the vaccine are anticipated to be "normal." Prophylaxis may be particularly important when circulating influenza A strains are significantly different antigenically from those in the vaccines. Since amantadine and rimantadine are active only against influenza A virus, prophylaxis should be instituted only when evidence of influenza A activity exists in the community. Prophylaxis should be continued for the duration of influenza A activity (usually 6–8 weeks) or at least during the period of peak activity, which is ordinarily several weeks. Chemoprophylaxis may also be considered for individuals, vaccinated or not, who are likely to come in close contact with immunocompromised patients.

Table 2 Antiviral Therapy of Influenza A or B Infections in Transplant Recipients[a]

Antiviral therapy	Patients	Survivors (%)
Amantadine/rimantadine	15	15 (100)
Ribavirin[b]	9	6 (67)
Not specified	17	14 (82)
No antiviral therapy	55	47 (85)

[a]Includes both bone marrow and solid organ transplant recipients.
[b]Includes two patients who received IV ribavirin.
Source: Adapted from Ref. 75.

VII. Treatment

Amantadine and rimantadine have been demonstrated to be effective in the treatment of uncomplicated influenza A–associated illness in healthy young adults and children, although rimantadine is not currently approved for treatment in children (see Chap. 13). However, the efficacy of these drugs in the treatment of influenza A in immunocompromised patients has not been established, and only anecdotal reports of their use for that purpose have appeared in the literature (Table 2) (75). Therapy with amantadine or rimantadine has been associated with the emergence of resistant viruses in both immunocompetent (76) and immunosuppressed patients (77), and transmission of resistant viruses may occur. Despite the above limitations, many investigators believe that the potential benefit/risk ratio is sufficiently favorable to use amantadine or rimantadine to treat influenza A infections in immunosuppressed patients, particularly in the absence of effective alternative therapy.

Ribavirin is a broad-spectrum antiviral which is approved for aerosolized administration to children hospitalized with RSV (see Chap. 13). It is active in vitro against influenza A and B viruses, and it has been reported to provide modest benefit when administered via aerosol to immunocompetent children with influenzal infection (78). Its use via aerosol administration has also been reported in small numbers of immunosuppressed patients with influenza A or B infection, but its overall benefit is uncertain (Table 2) (75). Intravenous ribavirin is available as an investigational agent, and it has been used anecdotally to treat influenza-associated pneumonia (79) and myocarditis (80). Aerosolized ribavirin has also been used to treat RSV and parainfluenza viral infections in immunosuppressed patients, including bone marrow transplant recipients, solid organ transplant recipients, leukemia patients, and patients with a variety of other immunosuppressive disorders (81). Therapeutic responses have been generally disappointing when infections have progressed to pneumonia or to respiratory distress. However, some investigators have suggested that benefits may occur if therapy were administered early when symptoms were limited to the upper respiratory tract (25). The use of RSVIG combined with aerosolized ribavirin has also been reported in small numbers of immunocompromised patients with RSV infection, and a possible benefit of treatment initiated early has also been suggested (81,82). Studies are underway to examine the effect of various dosage regimens for ribavirin, with and without RSVIG, in these infections. Appropriately controlled large-scale trials will be needed to assess the efficacy of ribavirin and RSVIG in immunocompromised patients.

Ribavirin, with and without concomitant IgG, has been used anecdotally to treat adenoviral infections in immunocompromised patients, but the clinical benefit, if any, has also not been established (83).

VIII. Cytomegaloviral and Other Herpes Viral Infections

As noted earlier, cytomegaloviruses are well established as causes of pulmonary infections in immunocompromised patients (2–4) and will only be reviewed briefly here. In contrast to infections with the community respiratory viruses described above, clinical manifestations of cytomegaloviral infections lie most frequently outside of the respiratory tract. However, pulmonary infections with CMV can occur and carry extensive morbidity and mortality. CMV infections, including those involving the lung, present the greatest problem in bone marrow transplant patients (4). With the widespread use of CMV seronegative blood products, the major source of CMV infections in these patients is reactivation of latent CMV either in the recipient or from donor marrow (4). The pathogenesis of CMV pneumonia is incompletely understood, but it appears to have a component of alloreactivity, since pneumonia is more frequent in allogeneic than in autologous transplant recipients (85). CMV-associated pneumonia most frequently presents 50–60 days after bone marrow transplantation with fever, tachypnea, and a nonproductive cough. Hypoxia is usually present and interstitial pneumonia with either diffuse or localized patterns are seen on chest radiography. However, a variety of other radiographic findings have also been reported, including localized infiltrates in a segmental or lobar distribution and nodular patterns (86). Diagnosis is established by demonstration of CMV in pulmonary tissue along with characteristic histopathology consisting of thickened alveolar membranes and a mononuclear cellular infiltrate. Detection of CMV by bronchoalveolar lavage in the presence of a compatible clinical setting is also frequently used to make the diagnosis of CMV pneumonia. Commonly, other pulmonary pathogens may be present as well, and in that case, it is difficult to be certain of the role of CMV in the pneumonic process. CMV pneumonia is associated with high rates of mortality in bone marrow transplant patients, and treatment with ganciclovir alone has been disappointing (4,87,88). Many transplant centers use combined ganciclovir and intravenous immune globulin, with an intensive initial (induction) phase of therapy followed by a maintenance phase (4). Emphasis is placed on initiating therapy early; that is, before the establishment of extensive pneumonia. This has led to various strategies of "preemptive" therapy in which treatment is initiated when CMV is first detected in blood or in respiratory secretions (89). Some centers are also employing "prophylactic" therapy with ganciclovir at the peak period of risk of CMV disease around the time of engraftment, sometimes preceded by the use of acyclovir during the period before engraftment (4,90).

In solid organ transplant recipients, CMV pneumonia appears to be a particularly important problem in lung and heart–lung transplant recipients, although it also occurs in recipients of other organ transplants (3,91). The use of antithymocyte or antilymphocyte serum or globulin is an important risk factor in the development of severe CMV disease. The approaches to treatment and prevention of CMV disease are similar to those described above (3).

Infection with herpes simplex virus (HSV) in immunosuppressed patients is primarily manifested by mucocutaneous signs and symptoms, usually involving the oropharynx or the genital tract. Lower respiratory tract involvement, including tracheitis, tracheobronchitis, and pneumonitis, has also been described but is much less common (see Chap. 3) (92,93). The likely pathogenesis of HSV pneumonitis appears to be retrograde spread of virus from the oropharynx. Because HSV pharyngeal lesions and/or shedding of virus is so common in immunosuppressed patients, unequivocal establishment of the diagnosis of HSV pneumonitis requires demonstration of HSV in pulmonary tissue. HSV pneumonitis is usually treated with intravenous acyclovir at a dose of 5 mg/kg q8hr for adults.

Varicella-zoster virus (VZV) can involve the lung as part of primary infection (varicella or chickenpox). This occurs more frequently in adults compared with children, and it can be particularly fulminant and life threatening in immunosuppressed patients (see Chap. 3) (94,95). Pulmonary involvement with reactivated infection (herpes zoster) even with dissemination is rare. Treatment is also with intravenous acyclovir given at higher doses than for HSV infections (10 mg/kg q8hr in adults).

IX. Summary

Respiratory viral infections are important causes of morbidity and mortality in immunosuppressed patients. Their significance has been most clearly established in leukemia and bone marrow transplant patients, but solid organ transplant recipients are affected as well. Respiratory syncytial virus appears to have the greatest impact, but parainfluenza and influenza viruses are also important. The significance of respiratory viruses in HIV-infected patients is less clear, although some cases of severe disease and prolonged shedding have been reported. Infection-control measures to prevent nosocomial transmission of respiratory viruses are important to reduce the spread of these infections among hospitalized patients. Amantadine, rimantadine, and ribavirin are available for treatment of respiratory viral infections, but their efficacy in immunosuppressed patients has not been established.

References

1. Dolin R. Pneumonia caused by viruses other than herpesviruses. In: Shellhamer J, Pizzo PA, Parillo JE, Masur H, eds. Respiratory Disease in the Immunosuppressed Host. Philadelphia: Lippincott, 1991:398–408.
2. Dummer JS, Ho M, Simmons RL. Infections in solid organ transplant recipients. In: Mandell GL, Bennett JE, Dolin R, eds. Principles and Practice of Infectious Diseases. 4th ed. New York: Churchill Livingstone, 1995:2722–2732.
3. Hibbard PL, Snydman DR. Cytomegalovirus infection in organ transplant recipients. Infect Dis Clin North Am 1995; 9:863–877.
4. Zaia JA, Forman SJ. Cytomegalovirus infection in the bone marrow transplant recipient. Infect Dis Clin North Am 1995; 9:879–900.
5. Housworth J, Langmuir AD. Excess mortality from epidemic influenza, 1957–1966. Am J Epidemiol 1974; 100:40–48.
6. Prevention and Control of Influenza. MMWR 1997; 46(No. RR-9):1–25.
7. Feldman S, Webster RG, Sugg M. Influenza in children and young adults with cancer. Cancer 1977; 39:350–353.
8. Kempe A, Hall CB, MacDonald NE, Foye HR, Woodin KA, Cohen HJ, Lewis ED, Gullace M, Gala CL, Dulberg CS. Influence in children with cancer. J Pediatr 1989; 115:33–39.
9. Craft AW, Reid MM, Gardner PS, Jackson E, Kernahan J, McQuillin J, Noble TC, Walker W. Virus infections in children with acute lymphoblastic leukemia. Arch Dis Child 1979; 54:755–759.
10. Skeggs DBL. Complications associated with radiotherapy of thymic tumors. Proc R Soc Med 1966; 66:155–157.
11. Smith TF, Burgert EO Jr, Dowdle WR, Noble GR, Campbell RJ, Van Scoy RE. Isolation of swine influenza virus from autopsy lung tissue of man. N Engl J Med 1976; 294:708–710.
12. Whimbey E, Englund JA, Couch RB. Community respiratory virus infections in immunocompromised patients with cancer. Am J Med 1997; 102:10–18.
13. Hertz MI, Englung JA, Snover D, Bitterman PB, McGlave PB. Respiratory syncytial virus-induced acute lung injury in adult patients with bone marrow transplants: a clinical approach and review of the literature. Medicine 1989; 68:269–281.

14. Fouillard L, Mouthon L, Laporte JP, Ishard F, Stachowiak J, Aoudjhane M, Lucet JC, Wolf M, Bricourt F, Douay L. Severe respiratory syncytial virus pneumonia after autologous bone marrow transplantation: a report of three cases and review. Bone Marrow Transplant 1992; 9:97–100.
15. Harrington RD, Hooton RD, Hackman RC, Storch GA, Osborne B, Gleaves CA, Benson A, Meyers JD. An outbreak of respiratory syncytial virus in a bone marrow transplant center. J Infect Dis 1992; 165:987–993.
16. Bowden RA. Other viruses after marrow transplantation. In: Forman SJ, Blume KG, Thomas ED, eds. Bone Marrow Transplantation. Cambridge, MA: Blackwell, 1994:443–453.
17. Hirschhorn LR, McIntosh K, Anderson KG, Dermody TS. Influenza pneumonia as a complication of autologous bone marrow transplantation. Clin Infect Dis 1992; 14:786–787.
18. Sable CA, Hayden FG. Orthomyxoviral and paramyxoviral infections in transplant patients. Infect Dis Clin North Am 1995; 9:987–1003.
19. Wendt CH, Weisdorf DJ, Jordan MC, Balfour HH Jr, Hertz MI. Parainfluenza virus respiratory infection after bone marrow transplantation. N Engl J Med 1992; 326:921–926.
20. Lewis V, Champlin R, Englund J, Couch R, Goodrich JM, Rolston K, Przepiorka D, Mirza MQ, Yousuf HM, Luna M, Bodey GP, Whimbey E. Respiratory disease due to parainfluenza virus in adult bone marrow transplant recipients. Clin Infect Dis 1996; 23:1033–1037.
21. Englund JA, Sullivan CJ, Jordan C, Dehner LP, Vercellotti GM, Balfour HH Jr. Respiratory syncytial virus infections in immunocompromised adults. Ann Intern Med 1988; 109:203–208.
22. Martin MA, Bock MJ, Pfaller MA, Wenzel RP. Respiratory syncytial virus infections in adult bone marrow transplant recipients. Lancet 1988; 1:1396–1397.
23. Winn N, Mitchell D, Pugh S, Russell NH. Successful therapy with ribavirin of late onset respiratory syncytial virus pneumonitis complicating allogeneic bone marrow transplantation. Clin Lab Haematol 1992; 14:29–32.
24. Whimbey E, Vartivarian SE, Champlin R, Elting LS, Luna M, Bodey GP. Parainfluenza virus infection in adult bone marrow transplant patients. Eur J Clin Microbiol Infect Dis 1993; 12:699–701.
25. Bowden RA. Respiratory virus infections after marrow transplant: the Fred Hutchinson Cancer Research Center experience. Am J Med 1997; 102:27–30.
26. Ljungman P. Respiratory virus infections in bone marrow transplant recipients: the European perspective. Am J Med 1997; 102:44–47.
27. Wendt CH. Community respiratory viruses: organ transplant recipients. Am J Med 1997; 102:31–36.
28. Breinig MK, Zitelli B, Starzl TE, Ho M. Epstein-Barr virus, cytomegalovirus, and other infections in children after liver transplantation. J Infect Dis 1987; 156: 273–279.
29. Salt A, Sutehall G, Sargaison M, Woodward C, Barnes ND, Calne RY, Wreghitt TC. Viral and toxoplasma gondii infections in children after liver transplantation. J Clin Pathol 1990; 43:63–67.

30. Pohl C, Green M, Wald ER, Ledesma-Medina J. Respiratory syncytial virus infections in pediatric liver transplant recipients. J Infect Dis 1992; 165:166–169.
31. Berbari N, Johnson DH, Cunha BA. Respiratory syncytial virus pneumonia in a heart transplant recipient presenting as fever of unknown origin diagnosed by gallium scan. Heart Lung 1995; 24:257–259.
32. Sinnott JT, Cullison JP, Sweeney MS, Hammond M, Holt DA. Respiratory syncytial virus pneumonia in a cardiac transplant recipient. J Infect Dis 1988; 158:650–751.
33. Doud JR, Hinkamp T, Garrity ER Jr. Respiratory syncytial virus pneumonia in a lung transplant recipient: case report. J Heart Lung Transplant 1995; 11:479–485.
34. Murrin-Espin M, Didier A, Carre P, Icart J, Henry S, Leophante P. Continuous aerosolized ribavirin for respiratory syncytial virus infection in lung transplant recipients. Lancet 1993; 341:897.
35. Wendt CH, Fox JMK, Hertz MI. Parzmyxovirus infection in lung transplant recipients. J Heart Lung Transplant 1995; 14:479–485.
36. Briggs KD, Timbury MC, Paton AM, Bell PR. Viral infection and renal transplant rejection. Br Med J 1972; 4:520–522.
37. Peigue-Lafeuille H, Gazuy N, Mignot P, Detreix P, Beytout D, Baguet JC. Severe respiratory syncytial virus pneumonia in an adult renal transplant recipient: successful treatment with ribavirin. Scand J Infect Dis 1990; 22:87–89.
38. Aschan J, Ringden O, Ljungman P, Andersson J, Lewensohn-Fuchs S, Forsgren M. Influenza B in transplant patients. Scand J Infect Dis 1989; 21:349–350.
39. Mauch TJ, Bratton S, Myers T, Krane E, Gentry SR, Kashtan CE. Influenza B virus infection in pediatric solid organ transplant recipients. Pediatrics 1994; 994:225–229.
40. Harnett GB, Bucens MR, Clay SJ, Saker BM. Acute haemorrhagic cystitis caused by adenovirus type 11 in a recipient of a transplanted kidney. Med J Aust 1982; 1:565–567.
41. Shindo K, Kitayama T, Ura T, Matsuya F, Kusaba Y, Kanetake H, Saito Y. Acute hemorrhagic cystitis caused by adenovirus type 11 after renal transplantation. Urol Int 1986; 41:152–155.
42. Stanley SK, Fauci AS. Immunology of AIDS and HIV infection. In: Mandell GL, Bennett JE, Dolin R, eds. Principles and Practice of Infectious Diseases. 4th ed. New York: Churchill Livingstone, 1995:1203–1217.
43. Hirschtick RE, Glassroth J, Jordan MC, Wilcosky TC, Wallace JM, Kvale PA, Karkowitz N, Rosen MJ, Mangura BT, Hopewell PC. Bacterial pneumonia in persons infected with the human immunodeficiency virus. N Engl J Med 1995; 333:845.
44. Increase in pneumonia mortality among young adults and the HIV epidemic—New York City, United States. MMWR 1988; 37:593–596.
45. Safrin S, Rush JD, Mills J. Influenza in patients with human immunodeficiency virus infection. Chest 1990; 98:33–37.
46. Thurn JR, Henry K. Influenza A pneumonitis in a patient infected with the human immunodeficiency virus (HIV). Chest 1989; 95:807–810.
47. McIntosh K. Respiratory viral infections. In: Pizzo PA, Wilfert CM, eds. Pediatric AIDS. The Challenge of HIV Infection in Infants, Children and Adolescents. Baltimore: Williams & Wilkins, 1994:365–376.

48. Cohen-Abbo A, Wright PF. Complex etiology of pneumonia in infants perinatally infected with human immunodeficiency virus 1. Pediatr Infect Dis J 1991; 10:545–547.
49. Evans KD, Kline MW. Prolonged influenza A infection responsive to rimantadine therapy in a human immunodeficiency virus–infected child. Pediatr Infect Dis J 1995; 14:332–334.
50. King JC. Community respiratory viruses in individuals with human immunodeficiency virus infection. Am J Med 1997; 102:19–24.
51. Chandwani S, Borkowsky W, Krasinski K, Lawrence R, Welliver R. Respiratory syncytial virus infection in human immunodeficiency virus-infected children. J Pediatrics 1990; 117:251–254.
52. Murphy D, Rose RC. Respiratory syncytial virus pneumonia in a human immunodeficiency virus-infected man. JAMA 1989; 261:1147.
53. Josephs S, Kim H, Brandt CD, Parrott RH. Parainfluenza 3 virus and other common respiratory pathogens in children with human immunodeficiency virus infection. Pediatr Infect Dis J 1988; 7:207–209.
54. de Blic J, Blanche S, Danel C, LeBourgeois M, Caniglia M, Scheinmann P. Bronchoalveolar lavage in HIV-infected patients with interstitial pneumonitis. Arch Dis Child 1989; 64:1246–1250.
55. Nadel S, McGann K, Kodinka RL, Rutstein R, Chatten J. Measles giant cell pneumonia in a child with human immunodeficiency virus infection. Pediatr Infect Dis J 1991; 10:542–544.
55a. CDC. Measles pneumonitis following measles-mumps-rubella vaccination of a patient with HIV infection. MMWR 1996; 45:603–606.
56. Valainis GT, Carlisle JT, Daroca DJ, Gohd RS, Enelow TJ. Respiratory failure complicated by adenovirus serotype 29 in a patient with AIDS. J Infect Dis 1989; 160:349–351.
57. Krilov LR, Rubin LG, Frogel M, Gloster E, Ni K, Kaplan M, Lipson SM. Disseminated adenovirus infection with hepatic necrosis in patients with human immunodeficiency virus infection and other immunodeficiency states. Rev Infect Dis 1990; 12:303–307.
58. Janner D, Petru AM, Belchis D, Azimi PH. Fatal adenovirus infection in a child with acquired immunodeficiency syndrome. Pediatr Infect Dis J 1990; 9:434–436.
59. Whimbey E, Champlin RE, Englund JA, Mirza NQ, Pedra PA, Goodirch JM, Przepiorka D, Luna MA, Morice RC, Neumann JL. Combination therapy with aerosolized and intravenous immunoglobulin for respiratory syncytial virus disease in adult bone marrow transplant recipients. Bone Marrow Transplant 1995; 16:393–399.
60. Whimbey E, Couch RB, Englund JA, Andreef M, Goodrich JM, Raad II, Lewis V, Mirza N, Luna MA, Baxter B. Respiratory syncytial virus pneumonia in hospitalized adult patients with leukemia. Clin Infect Dis 1995; 21:376–379.
61. Tablan OC, Anderson LJ, Arden NH, Breiman RF, Butler JC, McNeil MM. Guideline for prevention of nosocomial pneumonia. Part 1. Issues on prevention of nosocomial pneumonia—1994. Am J Infect Control 1994; 22:247–292.
62. Garner JS, and the Hospital Infection Control Practices Advisory Committee. Guidelines for isolation precautions in hospitals. Infect Control Hosp Epidemiol 1996; 17:53–80.

63. Raad I, Abbas J, Whimbey E. Infection control of nosocomial respiratory viral disease in the immunocompromised host. Am J Med 1997; 102:48–52.
64. Groothius JR, Simose EAF, Levin MJ, Hall CB, Long CE, Rodriguez WJ, Arrobio J, Meissner HC, Fulton DR, Welliver RC. Prophylactic administration of respiratory syncytial virus immune globulin to high-risk infants and young children. N Engl J Med 1993; 329:1524–1530.
65. Miotti PG, Nelson KE, Dallabetta GA, Farzadagan H, Margolick J, Clements ML. The influence of HIV infection on antibody responses to a two-dose regimen of influenza vaccine. JAMA 1989; 262:779–783.
66. Nelson KE, Clements ML, Miotti P, Cohn S, Polk BF. The influence of human immunodeficiency virus (HIV) infection on antibody responses to influenza vaccines. Ann Intern Med 1988; 109:383–388.
67. Gross PA, Lee H, Wolff JA, Hall CB, Minnefore AB, Lazicki ME. Influenza immunization in immunosuppressed children. J Pediatr 1978; 92:30–35.
68. Engelhard D, Nagler A, hardan I, Morag A, Aker M, Maciu H, Strauss N, Parag G, Naparstek E, Ravid Z. Antibody response to a two-dose regimen of influenza vaccine in allogeneic T cell-depleted and autologous BMT recipients. Bone Marrow Transplant 1993; 11:1–5.
69. Pabico RC, Douglas RG, Betts RF, McKenna BA, Freeman RB. Antibody response to influenza vaccination in renal transplant recipient. Ann Intern Med 1976; 85:431–436.
70. Rytel MW, Nubojewski RA, Rosenkranz MA, Sedmak G. Humoral and cell mediated immune response to bivalent influenza A/NJ/76 and A/Vict/75 vaccine in renal allograft recipients. Dev Biol Stand 1977; 39:225–230.
71. Versluis DJ, Beyer WEP, Masurel N, Wenting GJ, Weimar W. Impairment of the immune response to influenza vaccination in renal transplant recipients by cyclosporine, but not azathioprine. Transplantation 1986; 42:376–379.
72. Kumar SS, Ventura AK, Vanduwex B. Influenza vaccination in renal transplant recipients. JAMA 1978; 239:840–842.
73. Kobashigawa JA, Warner-Stevenson L, Johnson BL, Mariguchi JD, Kawata N, Drinkwater DC, Laks H. Influenza vaccine does not cause rejection after cardiac transplantation. Transplant Proc 1993; 25:2738–2739.
74. Blumberg EA, Albano C, Pruett T, Isaacs R, Fitzpatrick J, Bergin J, Crump C, Hayden F. The immunogenicity of influenza virus vaccine in solid organ transplant recipients. Clin Infect Dis 1996; 22:295–302.
75. Hayden FG. Prevention and treatment of influenza in immunocompromised patients. Am J Med 1997; 102:55–60.
76. Hayden FG. Amantadine and rimantadine—clinical aspects. In: Richman DR, ed. Antiviral Drug Resistance. Chichester, UK: Wiley, 1996:59–77.
77. Englund JA, Champlin RE, Yousuf H, Wyde PR, Atmar RL, Regnery H, Klimov A, Cox N, Whimbery E. Disease due to rimantadine/amantadine–resistant influenza (R-Flu) virus in bone marrow transplant recipients (BMT): a prospective study. Abstracts of the 36th ICAAC, 1996. Abstract H8:164.
78. Rodriguez WH, Hall CB, Elliver R, Simoes EA, Ryan ME, Stutman H, Johnson G, Van Dyke R, Groothius JR, Arrobio J. Efficacy and safety of aerosolized

ribavirin in young children hospitalized with influenza: a double-blind, multicenter, placebo-controlled trial. J Pediatr 1994; 125:129–135.
79. Hayden FG, Sable CA, Connor JD, Lane J. Intravenous ribavirin by constant infusion for serious influenza and parainfluenzavirus infection. Antiviral Ther 1996; 1:51–56.
80. Ray CG, Icenogle TB, Minnich LL, Copeland JG, Grogan TM. The use of intravenous ribavirin to treat influenza virus-associated acute myocarditis. J Infect Dis 1989; 159:829–836.
81. Englund JA, Piedra PA, Whimbey E. Prevention and treatment of respiratory syncytial virus and parainfluenza viruses in immunocompromised patients. Am J Med 1997; 102:61–70.
82. Gruber WC, Wilson SZ, Throop BJ, Wyde PR. Immunoglobulin administration and ribavirin therapy; efficacy in respiratory syncytial virus infection of the cotton rat. Pediatr Res 1987; 21:270–274.
83. Carrigan DR. Adenovirus infections in immunocompromised patients. Am J Med 1997; 102:71–74.
84. Meyers JD. Prevention of cytomegalovirus infection after marrow transplantation. Rev Infect Dis 1989; 11:s1691–s1705.
85. Wingard JR, Chen DY-H, Burns WH, Fuller DJ, Braine HG, Yeager AM, Kaiser H, Burke PJ, Graham ML, Santos GW. Cytomegalovirus infection after autologous bone marrow transplantation with comparison to infection after allogeneic bone marrow transplantation. Blood 1988; 71:1432–1437.
86. Beschorner WE, Hutchins GM, Burns WH, Saral R, Tutschka PJ, Santos GW. Cytomegalovirus pneumonia in bone marrow transplant recipients: miliary and diffuse patterns. Am Rev Respir Dis 1980; 122:107–114.
87. Erice A, Jordan MC, Chace BA, Fletcher C, Chinnock BJ, Balfour HH. Ganciclovir treatment of cytomegalovirus disease in transplant recipients and other immunocompromised hosts. JAMA 1987; 257:3082–3087.
88. Shepp DH, Dandliker PS, de Miranda P, Burnette TC, Cederberg DM, Kirk LE, Meyers JD. Activity of 9-(2-hydroxyl-1-[hydroxymethyl], ethoxymethyl) guanine in the treatment of cytomegalovirus pneumonia. Ann Intern Med 1985; 103:368–373.
89. Goodrich HM, Mori M, Gleaves CA, DuMond C, Cays M, Ebeling DF, Buhles WC, DeArmond B, Meyers JD. Early treatment with ganciclovir to prevent cytomegalovirus disease after allogeneic bone marrow transplantation. N Engl J Med 1991; 325:1601–1607.
90. Winston DJ, Ho WG, Bartoni K, DuMond C, Ebeling DF, Buhles WC, Champlin RE. Ganciclovir prophylaxis of cytomegalovirus infection and disease in allogeneic bone marrow transplant recipients. Ann Intern Med 1993; 118:179–184.
91. Calhoun NH, Nichols L, Davis R, Bryant CL, Levine SM, Zamora CA, Anzueta A, Lum CT, Grover FL, Trinkle JK. Single lung transplantation: factors in postoperative cytomegalovirus infection. J Thoracic Cardiovasc Surg 1992; 103:21.
92. Douglas RG Jr, Anderson MS, Weg JG, Williams T, Jenkins DE, Knight V, Beall AC Jr. Herpes simplex virus pneumonia. Occurrence in an allotransplant lung. JAMA 1969; 210:902–904.

93. Schuller D, Spessert C, Frases VJ, Goodenberger DM. Herpes simplex virus from respiratory tract secretions: epidemiology, clinical characteristics, and outcome in immunocompromised and nonimmunocompromised hosts. Am J Med 1993; 94: 29–33.
94. Weber DM, Pellicchia JA. Varicella pneumonia: study of prevalence in adult men. JAMA 1965; 192:572–573.
95. Clark GPM, Dobson PM, Thickett A, Turner NM. Chickenpox pneumonia, its complication and management. Anaesthesia 1991; 46:376–380.

Part Two

VIRUSES CAUSING RESPIRATORY INFECTIONS

6

Influenza A and B Viruses

JOHN J. TREANOR
University of Rochester School of Medicine and Dentistry
Rochester, New York

I. Introduction

The influenza viruses are classified into three distinct types, influenza A virus, influenza B virus, and influenza C virus, based on major antigenic differences in the nucleoprotein and matrix proteins. In addition, there are significant differences in genetic organization, structure, host range, epidemiology, and clinical characteristics between the three influenza virus types, which are summarized in Table 1. However, all three viruses share certain characteristics which are fundamental to their biological behavior, including the presence of a host cell–derived envelope, envelope glycoproteins of critical importance in viral entry and egress from cells, and a segmented genome of negative sense (i.e., opposite of message sense) single-stranded RNA. The standard nomenclature for influenza viruses includes the influenza type, place of initial isolation, strain designation, and year of isolation. For example, the current influenza A virus vaccine strain initially isolated in Nanchang, China, in 1996 and given strain designation 933 is designated as the influenza A/Nanchang/993/96 virus.

Table 1 Differences Between Influenza A, B, and C Viruses

	Influenza A	Influenza B	Influenza C
Genetics	8 gene segments	8 gene segments	7 gene segments
Structure	10 viral proteins M2 unique	11 viral proteins NB unique	9 viral proteins HEF unique
Host range	Humans, swine, equine, avian, marine mammals	Humans only	Humans and swine
Epidemiology	Antigenic shift and drift Drift is generally linear	Antigenic drift only More than one variant may cocirculate	Antigenic drift only Multiple variants
Clinical features	May cause large pandemics with significant mortality in young disease	Severe disease generally confined to elderly or those at high risk; pandemics not seen	Mild disease without seasonality

Each of the RNA gene segments of the influenza viruses encodes one or two viral proteins which are distributed between the envelope and the non-envelope structural proteins or are nonstructural. A diagrammatic representation of the influenza A virus is shown in Figure 1; differences in structure between influenza A, B, and C viruses that exist are noted.

II. Viral Replication

Influenza A and B virions attach to susceptible cells through the interaction of the hemagglutinin (HA) with cell surface sialic acid–containing receptors and are internalized into endosomal vesicles. Influenza C viruses attach to receptors containing 9-O-acetyl-N-acetylneuraminic acid using an analogous envelope glycoprotein, the HEF protein. In the low pH of the endosome, the HA undergoes a conformational change which liberates the fusion peptide present on the amino terminus of HA_2 (1,2), resulting in fusion of the viral envelope and the endosomal membrane. Previous proteolytic cleavage of the HA is critical, because this conformational change and membrane fusion can only take place if the HA has been cleaved into HA_1 and HA_2 subunits.

Following fusion of the viral and cell membranes, the contents of the virion enter the cell. Influenza viruses are unusual among RNA viruses in that transcription and replication of the viral genome takes place in the nucleus (3).

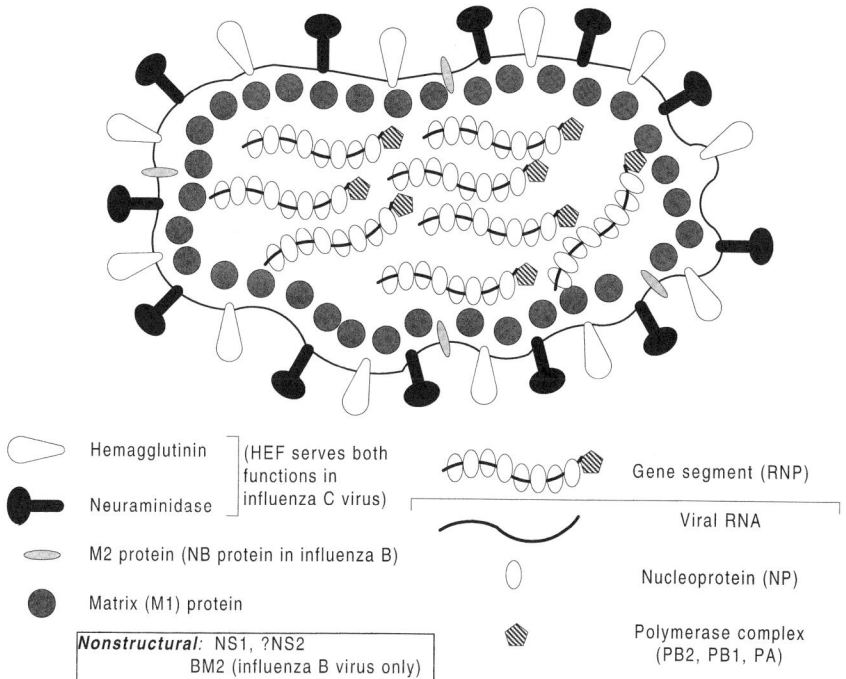

Figure 1 Influenza viruses are enveloped viruses with a segmented, negative-sense RNA genome. The three virus types, A, B, and C, share a common general structure; specific differences are shown here and in Table 1.

Therefore, after entry into the cell, the viral ribonucleoproteins (RNP), containing viral RNA, nucleoprotein, and polymerase proteins, are transported to the nucleus (4). Cytoplasmic to nuclear transport of the RNP requires that the association between the M1 protein and the RNP in the virion be disrupted. The mechanism of uncoating has been studied most intensively for influenza A viruses. The low pH of the endosome triggers the pH-dependent ion channel activity of the influenza A virus M2 protein (5) resulting in transport of H+ ions into the virion and lowering of the intravirionic pH. The lower intravirionic pH in turn disrupts the RNP–M1 interaction and allows transport of the RNP to the nucleus (6). The influenza B virus M2 protein (BM2) is a cytosolic protein of uncertain function (7). Instead, influenza B virus encodes the NB protein, a unique protein which is transcribed from the neuraminidase gene segment using an alternative start codon (8). Similar to the influenza A M2, the influenza B NB protein is a cationic channel present in small quantities on the surface of the virion (9,10), and it likely serves the same role in virus replication, although this has not been studied as intensively. Mechanisms of uncoating of influenza C viruses have not been described in detail.

In the nucleus, three species of virus-specific RNA are made: positive-sense viral messenger RNA (mRNA), positive-sense templates (complementary RNA, cRNA) for replication of the viral genome, and negative-sense daughter virion RNAs (vRNA). Synthesis of viral mRNA is initiated with primers derived from newly synthesized capped cellular mRNAs and terminates at a polyadenylation site situated 15–22 nucleotides from the 5' end of the virion RNA (11,12). Synthesis of cRNA is initiated without a primer and continues through the polyadenylation site to result in a full-length copy of the genomic RNA which can be used as a template for synthesis of daughter vRNA. Readthrough of the polyadenylation site (antitermination) requires the presence of free nucleoprotein (NP) (13). Finally, synthesis of daughter vRNA segments from cRNA is also initiated without a primer.

The functions of transcription and replication are performed by the viral polymerase, a complex of three proteins (PB1, PB2, and PA) (14,15) in which each protein has specific function(s). The PB2 protein is responsible for recognition and endonucleolytic cleavage of capped host cell mRNAs (14,16), whereas the PB1 protein has the RNA-dependent RNA polymerase function (14). The role of the PA protein is less clearcut, but may act as an allosteric modulator to change the polymerase complex from a mRNA to a vRNA-synthesizing form (17). The rate of synthesis of each of these RNA species is tightly regulated during productive viral infection.

Influenza virus mRNA represent the only example of mRNA which are not synthesized by eukaryotic RNA polymerase II which are able to use the cellular splicing machinery. In fact, two of the viral mRNA are spliced: the M1 mRNA is spliced to form the M2 mRNA and the NS1 mRNA is spliced to form the NS2 mRNA. In most productively infected cells, the levels of both M1 and NS1 mRNA splicing are regulated so that the ratio of unspliced to spliced viral mRNAs in the cytoplasm is approximately 10:1. The rate of splicing of influenza virus mRNA is largely controlled by sequences within the mRNA (18), whereas the ratio of spliced to unspliced mRNA in the cytoplasm appears to depend largely on the rate of transport of the unspliced mRNA out of the nucleus (19). The influenza virus NS1 and M1 mRNA are also unique, along with certain retroviral mRNA, in that pre-mRNA which are capable of interacting with the splicing apparatus are also used in unspliced form as messages (19). The mechanism by which some of these mRNA avoid interaction with the splicing machinery and are efficiently transported out of the nucleus is unclear, however. Recent evidence suggests that the NS1 protein plays an important role in the regulation of transport of mRNA from the nucleus to the cytoplasm and in the splicing of pre-mRNA (20,21). After replication of the viral RNA, newly formed daughter RNA strands are assembled into daughter

RNP. In contrast to the situation when infection is initiated, the daughter RNP now must be reassociated with M1 protein in order to be transported from the nucleus back to the cytoplasm (22).

While the viral RNA is being replicated, the envelope proteins (HA, NA, M2, and NB) are synthesized on membrane-bound ribosomes and transported to the cell surface by the trans Golgi apparatus. During synthesis and transport, N-linked carbohydrate is added, and these proteins undergo further maturation, including cleavage of the HA in cells with appropriate proteases. During this process, regulation of the pH of the Golgi apparatus by the M2 protein is critical in preventing a premature (and irreversible) conformational change of the HA to the low pH form (23,24). The influenza B NB may play a similar role.

Viral envelope proteins begin to accumulate on the cell membrane and associate with other components of the virus in an as yet undetermined fashion. Membrane-associated M1 protein may play a role in this process (25). The formation of infectious progeny viruses requires the incorporation of at least one of each gene segment into the virions. Evidence favoring both random and directed strategies exists (26,27). Viruses then form by budding, and they must be released from the cell membrane (Fig. 2). Since the viral envelope is derived from the host cell membrane, which contains sialic acid glycoproteins, newly formed viral particles would remain attached to the host cell and to each other unless some means were available to cleave receptor sites from these membranes. Mutant viruses which lack NA activity form large, multimeric aggregates, which suggests that release of virus from cells and each other is an important function of the viral NA (28,29). The receptor-destroying activity of the HEF protein is a neuramiate-O-acetyl esterase, and it appears to play the same role as the NA of influenza A and B viruses (30).

III. Pathogenesis and Host Response

A. Pathogenesis

Nature of Cellular Injury

Infection of permissive cells by influenza viruses is associated with the typical viral cytopathic effect (CPE), including rounding of cells, clumping of nuclear chromatin, development of intracytoplasmic inclusions composed of the virus NS1 protein and cellular ribosomal RNA, and cell lysis. There is also a dramatic shutoff of host–cell protein synthesis which occurs at several levels. Newly synthesized cellular mRNA are degraded, probably because cleavage by the viral cap endonuclease renders these transcripts susceptible to hydrolysis by cellular nuclease (31), whereas translation of already synthesized cytoplasmic

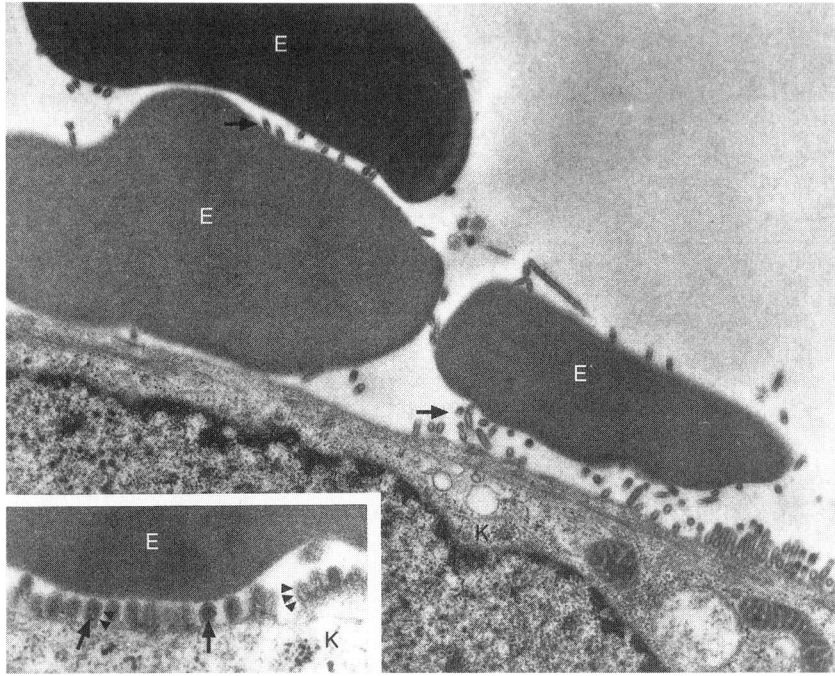

Figure 2 Virions of influenza A virus (arrows) are seen budding from the surface of Rhesus monkey kidney cells (K). In the inset, the dense nucleoprotein core of the virus (arrows) can be distinguished from the lighter fringe of individual hemagglutinin and neuraminidase spikes (arrowheads). Guinea pig erythrocytes (E) are being aggregated to the cell surface and to each other by the HA. The hemagglutination reaction, and its inhibition by specific antibody (hemagglutination-inhibition) are described in the text. (From Winn WC Jr, Westenfeld FW. Images in Medicine. N Engl J Med 305:912.)

mRNA is blocked at both initiation and elongation (32). Finally, expression of the influenza virus PA protein has been shown to induce generalized degradation of coexpressed proteins through an unknown mechanism (33). Ultimately, the loss of critical cellular proteins likely contributes to cell death.

In addition to effects leading to cell necrosis, there is increasing evidence that infection of cells with influenza A and B viruses may cause cell death by apoptosis (34,35), a form of cell death characterized by fragmentation of nuclear DNA. Bronchiolar epithelial and alveolar cells harvested from experimentally infected mice also exhibit apoptotic changes suggesting that this mechanism of cell death may be important in the pathogenesis of influenza in vivo (36). The specific mechanism by which influenza virus induces apoptosis is unclear, but it may be related to induction of the Fas antigen by double-stranded RNA during viral replication (37).

Influenza viral infection of peripheral blood mononuclear cells, including polymorphonuclear leukocytes (PML), lymphocytes, and monocytes, is non-productive but associated with measurable defects in cellular function which may be relevant to the pathogenesis of influenza-related infectious complications. These include defects in PML chemotaxis and phagocytosis (38) as well as decreased proliferation and costimulation by mononuclear cells (39,40). The effects are mediated both by viral replication as well as possibly by a direct toxic effect of certain viral proteins, including the hemagglutinin, neuraminidase (41,42), and the nucleoprotein (43). It has been noted that the short portion of the sequence of the influenza A virus NP is homologous to a naturally occurring peptide found in normal bronchoalveolar lavage (BAL) fluid which inhibits polymorphonuclear neutrophil (PMN) chemotaxis and oxidative burst (44).

Pathophysiology

Initial infection of the respiratory tract with influenza viruses may take place by direct inoculation or by inhalation of small-particle aerosols containing virus. Challenge studies in human volunteers have demonstrated that virus is approximately 100-fold more infectious by the aerosol route than when administered by nasal drops (45). It is not clear which mode of infection plays the greatest role in nature.

Following initial infection, there is widespread involvement of the trachea, bronchi, and lower airways. Bronchoscopy of individuals with typical, uncomplicated acute influenza has revealed diffuse inflammation of the larynx, trachea, and bronchi with mucosal injection and edema (46,47). Biopsy in these cases has revealed a range of histological findings from vacuolization of columnar cells with cell loss to extensive desquamation down to the basal layer of cells (47,48). Viral antigen can be demonstrated in epithelial cells but is not seen in the basal cell layer (49). Generally, the tissue response becomes more prominent as one moves distally in the airway (47). Epithelial damage is accompanied by cellular infiltrates primarily composed of lymphocytes and histiocytes (47). Histological findings on autopsy of more severe cases show extensive necrotizing tracheobronchitis with ulceration and sloughing of the bronchial mucosa (48,50). Recovery is associated with rapid regeneration of the epithelial cell layer and pseudometaplasia. These findings can be reproduced to a large extent in a murine model in which infection with a low dose of virus leads to desquamation of ciliated cells over 2–3 days followed by regeneration from an undifferentiated basal layer of cells (51) (Fig. 3).

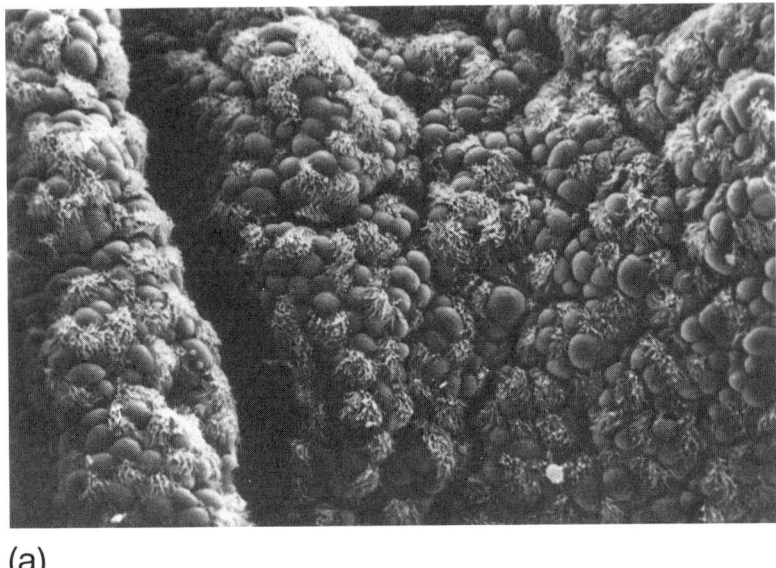

(a)

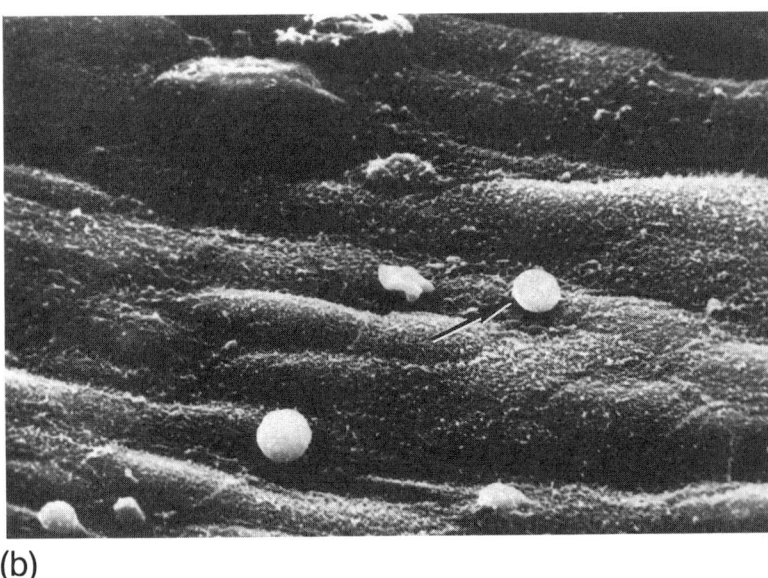

(b)

Figure 3 Scanning electron micrograph of mouse tracheal epithelium showing pathological changes induced by influenza. (a) Normal mouse trachea with tracheal epithelial cells and cilia. (b) Mouse trachea 5 days after influenza virus infection. The epithelial cells have been sloughed, revealing the intact basement membrane. (From Ref. 66.)

Abnormalities of pulmonary function are frequently demonstrated in otherwise healthy, nonasthmatic young adults with uncomplicated (nonpneumonic) acute influenza. Demonstrated defects include diminished forced-flow rates, increased total pulmonary resistance, and decreased density-dependent forced-flow rates consistent with generalized increased resistance in airways less than 2 mm in diameter (52,53) as well as increased responses to bronchoprovocation (52). In addition, abnormalities of carbon monoxide diffusing capacity (54) and increases in the alveolar–arterial oxygen gradient (55) have been seen. Of note, pulmonary function defects can persist for weeks after clinical recovery. Influenza in asthmatics (56) or patients with chronic obstructive disease (57) with influenza may result in acute declines in forced vital capacity (FVC) or forced expiratory volume in 1 sec (FEV_1). Individuals with acute influenza may be more susceptible to bronchoconstriction from air pollutants such as nitrates (58).

Primary viral pneumonia is an uncommon but often severe complication of acute influenza. In this situation, viral infection reaches the lung either by contiguous spread from the upper respiratory tract or by inhalation. The trachea and bronchi contain bloody fluid, and the mucosa is hyperemic (59). Tracheitis, bronchitis, and bronchiolitis are seen with loss of normal ciliated epithelial cells. Submucosal hyperemia, focal hemorrhage, edema, and cellular infiltrate are present. The alveolar spaces contain varying numbers of neutrophils and mononuclear cells admixed with fibrin and edema fluid. The alveolar capillaries may be markedly hyperemic with intra-alveolar hemorrhage. Acellular, hyaline membranes line many of the alveolar ducts and alveoli (59). Pathological findings seen by biopsy of lung in nonfatal cases are similar to those described in fatal cases (60).

Bacterial superinfection is a well-recognized complication of viral pneumonia and accounts for a large proportion of the morbidity and mortality of viral lower respiratory tract disease, especially in adults. Consequently, the spectrum of disease and pathophysiology of bacterial superinfection has been studied intensively, and a number of factors have been identified in viral respiratory disease which could play a role in increasing the risk of bacterial infection (61). Uncomplicated influenza is associated with significant abnormalities in ciliary clearance mechanisms (62,63). In addition, increased adherence of bacteria to virus-infected epithelial cells has been demonstrated (64,65). The disruption of the normal epithelial cell barrier to infection and loss of mucociliary clearance undoubtedly contribute the enhancement of bacterial pathogenesis (47,66). Alterations in polymorphonuclear leukocytes and mononuclear cells described above may also contribute to enhanced bacterial infection (39,67,68). Finally, bacteria themselves may enhance the replication of some viruses such as influenza viruses by the release of proteases which cleave the viral hemagglutinin (69).

Viral Factors Which Influence Pathogenicity

Clinical characteristics of illness during the 1918 influenza pandemic differed from those of subsequent pandemics and with higher mortality rates in young adults. Since the virus responsible for this pandemic is not available for further study, it is impossible to know what viral factors, if any, might have been responsible for this behavior. Since that time there has been little direct evidence for major inherent differences in viral strains in regard to the pathogenic potential in humans. Recent H1N1 viruses do appear to cause relatively milder illness compared with recent H3N2 viruses (70,71). However, for the most part, the severity of most epidemics is likely to be determined largely by the status of immunity in the population.

In contrast, multiple influenza viruses with altered levels of pathogenicity in animal models have been described. A variety of classic genetic and molecular biological techniques have been used to evaluate the role of specific viral genes or gene products in determining the virulence of influenza viruses in these models. An exhaustive review of these studies is beyond the scope of this chapter, but the studies have generally shown that virulence is a multigenic trait whose specific basis varies between virus strains and the models used (72–74).

An exception to this has been the elegant demonstration of the role of hemagglutinin cleavability in the virulence of avian influenza A viruses in domesticated birds. Infection of fowl with avian influenza viruses can result in a relatively avirulent asymptomatic infection limited to the respiratory and gastrointestinal mucosa or a virulent, rapidly progressive, fatal systemic infection with involvement of the brain and other visceral organs. Comparison of the HAs of virulent and avirulent strains of H5 and H7 subtype influenza A viruses has shown that the structure of the HA cleavage site is critical in determining the virulence phenotype in this model. Proteases capable of cleaving the HA of avirulent viruses, such as tryptase Clara (75), are restricted in distribution to cells of the respiratory and gastrointestinal mucosa, thereby limiting replication to these areas. However, the addition of several basic amino acids to the cleavage site (76) coupled with the absence of a nearby glycosylation site (77) renders the hemagglutinin capable of being cleaved by ubiquitous cellular furin-like proteases (78) and allows these viruses to escape the confines of the mucosa and replicate systemically (79). Variability in HA cleavage has not as yet been demonstrated to be a factor in the pathogenicity of influenza viruses in humans.

B. Mechanisms of Protection from Reinfection and Amelioration of Severity

Epidemiological and experimental observations in humans have shown that infection with influenza virus results in long-lived resistance to reinfection with the homologous virus (80). In addition, variable degrees of cross protection within a subtype have been observed, but infection induces essentially no protection across subtypes (81). Infection induces both systemic and local antibody as well as cytotoxic T-cell responses, each of which plays a role in recovery from infection and resistance to reinfection.

Antibody Responses

Systemic Responses

Infection with influenza virus results in the development of antibody to the influenza virus envelope glycoproteins HA and NA as well as to the structural M and NP proteins. Some individuals may develop antibody to the M2 protein as well (82). As measured by enzyme-linked immunosorbent assay (ELISA), serum IgM, IgA, and IgG antibody to the HA appear simultaneously within 2 weeks of inoculation of virus (83). Although responses to the HA develop after primary infection, responses to the NA appear to require previous infection (81). Peak antibody responses are seen at 4–7 weeks after infection and decline slowly thereafter; titers can still be detected years after infection even without reexposure.

Antibody to the HA can be measured by standard hemagglutination inhibition (HAI) tests or a variety of ELISA, and neutralizes viral infectivity (84). Antihemagglutinin antibody protects against both disease and infection with the homologous virus (85). However, antibody-deficient mice show complete protection on rechallenge, showing that antibody also is not absolutely necessary for protection in the lethal challenge mouse model (86).

Antibody to the NA can be measured by NA inhibition or ELISA. In contrast to anti-HA antibody, anti–NA antibody does not neutralize viral infectivity but instead reduces efficient release of virus from infected cells resulting in decreased plaque size in in vitro assays (87). Observations on the relative protection of those with anti–N2 antibody during the A/Hong Kong/68 (H3N2) pandemic (88,89) as well as experimental challenge studies in humans (90) have shown that anti–NA antibody can be protective against disease and results in decreased viral shedding but is infection permissive (91). Passive transfer studies in mice have also suggested that antibody to the M2 protein of influenza A viruses may have a similar effect to that of anti–NA antibody (92). Antibody to internal viral proteins such as M or NP is nonneutralizing and does not appear to be protective.

Mucosal Responses

The majority of studies of mucosal responses to influenza in humans have concentrated on the measurement of HA responses by ELISA. These studies have demonstrated significant mucosal responses to infection with wild-type virus or live attenuated influenza vaccines. Both IgA and IgG are found in nasal secretions. Nasal HA-specific IgG is predominantly IgG_1 and correlates well with serum levels of HA-specific IgG_1, suggesting that nasal IgG originates by passive diffusion from the systemic compartment (93). Nasal HA-specific IgA is predominantly polymeric and IgA_1, suggesting local synthesis. Serum HA specific IgA is also mostly polymeric IgA_1. The origin of serum IgA after mucosal infection is unclear but may be due to seeding of peripheral lymphoid tissue by memory cells derived from the mucosa (85).

Studies in mice and ferrets have emphasized the importance of local IgA antibody in the resistance to infection, particularly in the protection of the upper respiratory tract. Polymeric IgA was shown to be specifically transported into the nasal secretions of mice and to protect against nasal challenge. Protection could be abrogated by intranasal administration of antiserum against IgA but not IgM or IgG (94). Local antibody has also been shown to play a role in protection against antigenic variants in mice (95). Studies in humans have also suggested that the resistance to reinfection induced by viral infection is mediated predominantly by local HA-specific IgA, whereas that induced by parenteral immunization with inactivated virus also depends on systemic IgG (90,96). Importantly, either modality can be protective if present in high enough concentrations.

Cellular Responses

Antibody responses to the HA are T-cell–dependent (97–99), and class II restricted, $CD4^+$ cells provide help (Th) to B cells for the production of antibody to the HA and NA. Both CD4 cells which recognize epitopes on the HA molecule as well as CD4 cells recognizing epitopes on M, NP, or PB2 may provide help for HA antibody production (100). The epitopes on HA recognized by Th cells are distinct from those recognized by neutralizing antibody (102) and may be cross-reactive within a subtype. Influenza-specific Th cells also promote the generation of virus-specific $CD8^+$ cytotoxic T lymphocytes (103, 104).

Recently, it has been recognized that Th responses can be further classified as type 1 (Th1) or type 2 (Th2) responses based on the profile of cytokines produced on in vitro challenge. Influenza viral infection of mice generates a strong Th1-type response (105). Th2-type cytokines (interleukins IL-4, IL-5, IL-6, IL-10) have been also described in the lungs of mice infected with influenza virus (106,107). Circumstantial evidence suggests that protective immune responses to influenza are associated with Th1-like responses. Adoptive transfer of anti-influenza T-cell clones secreting cytokines of the Th2 type fails to promote viral clearance (108), and administration of interferon-γ (INF-γ) delays viral clearance and the development of cytotoxic T lymphocytes (CTl) in influenza virus–infected mice (109). Of note, blockade of INF-γ by INF antibody does not effect development of CTL responses but results in reduced migration of PMN to the lung in the murine model (110). In addition, administration of IL-4 to infected mice promotes Th2-type responses and results in markedly delayed viral clearance (111).

Influenza virus–infected cells can be lysed by antibody in the presence of complement, by antibody-dependent cellular cytotoxicity (112), or by the action of CTL. Generally, CTL express CD8 and are restricted by class I. Such cells may recognize either HA or internal proteins such as M, NP, or PB2 (113). Therefore, CTL may be subtype specific, or in the case of those which recognize internal proteins, they may be broadly cross-reactive, lysing cells infected with influenza A but not influenza B virus (114,115). In addition, class II–restricted cells may exhibit cytotoxic activity similar to that shown by class I–restricted cells (115).

Extensive adoptive transfer experiments have shown that virus-specific CTL can mediate recovery from influenza viral infection (116–121), including both HA-specific and cross-reactive CTL. However, studies in mice lacking major histocompatibility complex (MHC) class I have shown that CTL are not absolutely required for recovery (122–124).

CTL responses to influenza also develop in humans following influenza virus infections, generally peaking on about day 14 after infection (125). Although not studied extensively, the presence of virus-specific prechallenge class I–restricted Tc lymphocytes has been shown to correlate with reductions in the duration and level of viral replication in adults with low levels of serum HA and NA antibody who were challenged with influenza A virus (126). The role of CTL directed against internal viral proteins in protection against severe disease in humans is unclear, as the internal viral proteins were shared between viruses causing the pandemics of 1957 and 1968 and the viruses in circulation immediately prior to these pandemics (127,128). Memory CTL responses may play a role in ameliorating the severity of disease and speeding recovery following infection, as suggested by the finding of more severe influenza in individuals with severe defects in cell-mediated immunity (129).

IV. Epidemiology

A. Disease Impact

Influenza epidemics are regularly associated with excess morbidity and mortality (130), usually expressed in the form of excess rates of pneumonia- and influenza-associated hospitalizations during influenza epidemics (130,131). Both influenza A and B can be associated with severe illness (132). During interpandemic years, influenza is usually associated with a U-shaped epidemic

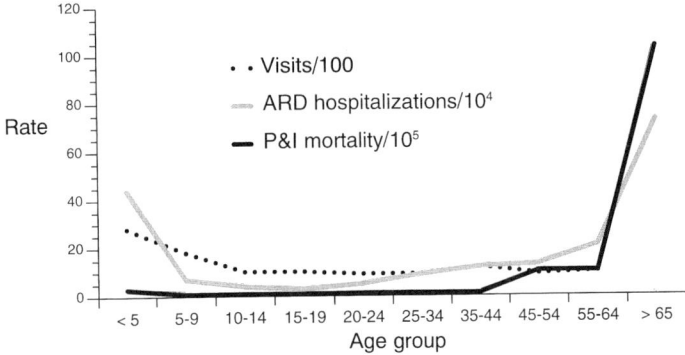

Figure 4 Typical epidemic curve in the interpandemic era showing the rates of medically attended illness, hospitalizations for acute respiratory disease, and pneumonia- and influenza-related mortality by age for several seasons of influenza in Houston, Texas. Attack rates and hospitalizations occur at both extremes of age, but mortality occurs largely in those over age 65. P&I, pneumonia and influenza. (Data from Ref. 133.)

curve. Attack rates are generally highest in the young, whereas mortality is generally highest in the elderly (130,133) (Fig. 4). Excess morbidity and mortality are particularly high in those with certain "high-risk" medical conditions, such as adults and children with cardiovascular and pulmonary conditions, including asthma, or those requiring regular medical care because of chronic metabolic disease, renal dysfunction, hemoglobinopathies, or immunodeficiency (134,135,136) (Table 2). Of note, the majority of individuals hospitalized during influenza epidemics are ambulatory and leading productive lives prior to the acute illness (134).

Table 2 Pneumonia and Influenza (P&I) Deaths During Influenza Epidemics

Age	No. high-risk conditions	No. of P&I deaths	P&I deaths per $10^6 \pm$ SE
15–44	Without HR	0	0
	1 HR	0	0
	≥ 2 HR	0	0
45–64	Without HR	1	2 ± 2
	1 HR	7	10 ± 13
	≥ 2 HR	4	377 ± 195
≥65	Without HR	1	9 ± 9
	1 HR	14	217 ± 59
	≥ 2 HR	11	306 ± 257

Source: Adapted from Ref. 134.

Much of the impact of influenza is related to the malaise and consequent disability that it produces even in young, healthy individuals. It has been estimated that a typical case of influenza, on average, is associated with 5–6 days of restricted activity, 3–4 days of bed disability, and about 3 days lost from work or school (137,138). The average number of medical visits for cases in which medical attention was sought was from 1.1 to 3.6 visits depending on year of the outbreak and age of the patient. It is worth noting that direct medical costs of illness account for only about 20% of the total expenses of a case of influenza, with a major proportion (30–50%) of the economic impact due to loss of productivity.

B. Seasonality

A familiar characteristic of influenza is the concentration of cases in the winter months in both the Northern and Southern hemispheres. The reasons for these seasonal changes are not entirely clear. Computer modeling studies suggest that the effect can mostly be explained by postulating seasonal effects on viral transmissibility (139). Such effects could be the result of more favorable environmental conditions for viral survival (140) or behavioral changes that increase transmission, such as indoor crowding. It is interesting to note that pandemics are often accompanied by disruption of the normal restriction of cases to the winter months.

C. Evolution of Influenza Viruses

As described earlier, infection with the influenza virus effectively induces immune resistance to reinfection which is long-lived. Thus, in order to sustain replication in human hosts, the influenza viruses undergo rapid evolution of the main envelope antigens, HA and NA, which allows the virus to escape from these protective responses. The study of these evolutionary pathways of HA, and to a lesser extent NA, has provided important insights into the immunology, biology, and genetics of these viruses (141).

Two patterns of epidemiological behavior of influenza have been observed in humans (142) (Fig. 5). Geographically limited outbreaks, or epidemics, of influenza occur each year with varying severity. These epidemics are associated with viruses containing antigenically variant HA, which are able partially to escape immunity generated by previously circulating strains, a phenomenon referred to as antigenic drift. The mechanism of antigenic drift is the accumulation of point mutations in one or more of the five antigenic sites on the HA molecule (143,144). Comparison of the HA gene sequences of influenza viruses isolated in successive years reveals differences in the patterns of evolution of the HA between influenza A, B, and C viruses. Generally, a

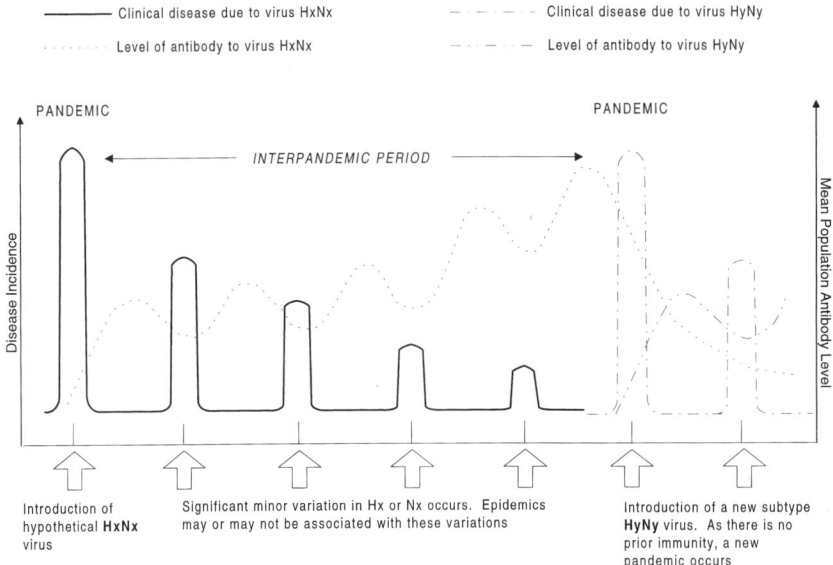

Figure 5 Model of the epidemic behavior of influenza in humans. H1N1 viruses are introduced into a population with little or no prior immunity in 1918, and a severe, worldwide epidemic, or pandemic, occurs. As the population recovers from the pandemic, the level of immunity to H1 and N1 increases, so that subsequent outbreaks, or epidemics, are of variable severity but less than that of the pandemic. These epidemics are associated with antigenic variants that generally differ from the variant of the preceding year by a few amino acids in H or N. In 1957, the H1N1 viruses are replaced by the H2N2 virus, and the process repeats itself. (Modified from Ref. 142.)

single, or relatively few lineages of HA circulate in humans, and the accumulation of point mutations is linear with each strain replacing the previously circulating one. In contrast, multiple lineages of influenza C virus cocirculate based on sequence comparisons of the HEF gene. The evolution of influenza B viruses is somewhere between these two examples, with relatively few, but more than one, lineage of HA gene cocirculating (145). Relatively less information is available regarding the evolution of NA gene sequences, but these appear to follow a similar pattern (146).

At infrequent intervals, much more severe, worldwide outbreaks, or pandemics, of influenza occur. Pandemics are usually associated with influenza viruses with HA or NA so radically different from those of previous strains as to constitute an entirely new subtype. Under these circumstances, the virus enters a population which is for all purposes completely susceptible, and severe disease with rapid spread results. This phenomenon is referred to as antigenic shift, and is only seen with influenza A viruses. Recent pandemics have included those of 1918 when the H1N1 viruses replaced previously circulating H3N8 viruses; in 1957, when H2N2 replaced H1N1 viruses; and 1968, when H3N2 viruses replaced H2N2 virus. In 1977, H1N1 viruses reappeared after a 20-year absence. However, instead of replacing H3N2 viruses, H1N1 and H3N2 viruses have since cocirculated.

The degree of genetic difference between subtypes, 30% or greater, precludes emergence by simple point mutation, and the origin of new pandemic strains has been the subject of intense interest and study for obvious reasons. The most plausible explanation for their origin takes into account three features of this phenomenon: (1) the virus has a segmented genome, (2) pandemics only occur with influenza A viruses, and (3) influenza A viruses, but not other influenza viruses, maintain a large reservoir of genetic diversity in animals.

Influenza A viruses infect a variety of animals, including humans, swine, horses, marine mammals, and, in particular, avian species. In fact, no less than 15 unique HA subtypes (H1–H15) (147) and 9 NA subtypes (N1–N9) (148) have been identified in avian influenza viruses. Fortunately, avian influenza A viruses themselves appear to be relatively restricted to their ability to replicate in humans, possibly because of the divergent evolution of the "internal" viral genes during adaptation to their avian hosts (128). However, the ability of the segmented influenza virus to reassort gene segments during mixed infection provides a mechanism to introduce these novel HA and NA subtypes into human viruses. Simultaneous infection of a susceptible cell with both a human and avian virus could result in production of a reassortant virus containing gene segments derived from the human virus which allow efficient replication in human cells and genes encoding the novel HA or NA from the avian virus allowing efficient spread in the face of previous immunity (Fig. 6).

Extensive sequence analysis of the genes of avian and human influenza viruses has provided indirect evidence supporting this hypothesis. These studies have shown significant sequence similarity between the HA, NA, and PB1 gene segments of the pandemic H2N2 virus and avian viruses (127,149) and between the H3 and PB1 gene segments of the pandemic H3N2 virus and avian viruses (149,150). Reassortment would be facilitated by the presence of a third species which is susceptible to infection with both avian and human viruses, and pigs meet this requirement. This is an especially attractive concept, because it would explain the observation that new pandemics often arise in the Far East, where humans, pigs, and aquatic fowl live in close proximity. There have been several recent intriguing observations suggesting interspecies transmission in the Far East (151,152) as well as demonstration of naturally occurring avian-human reassortment viruses in pigs (153). It is likely, however, that such events occur rarely.

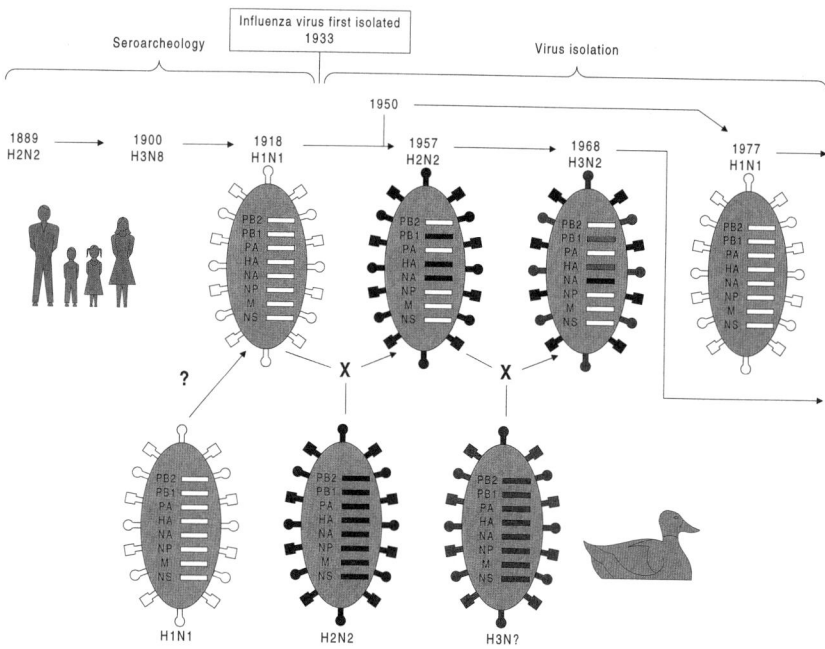

Figure 6 Pandemic influenza is associated with replacement of previously circulating influenza A viruses with viruses containing divergent HA, NA, and other genes (shown as shaded squares). Nucleotide sequence analysis has suggested that the new genes are derived by genetic reassortment between human and animal influenza A viruses, which contribute the novel HA and NA genes to the antigenically shifted viruses. (Note: data for 1918 strains of H1N1 virus are inferred from 1933 H1N1 viruses, the year in which influenza virus was first isolated.) Phylogenetic analysis has suggested that the 1918 virus possessed eight gene segments from an avian virus and was transmitted to humans and pigs before 1918. (Modified from Ref. 14.)

There is obviously great interest in predicting the possibilities for a new pandemic influenza, a disease which can be considered the prototype of an emerging (or reemerging) infection (154). The serological observation that infection of humans appears to be limited to viruses of the H1, H2, and H3 subtype HA and N1, N2, and possibly N8 subtype NA suggests that there may be limitations on the possible makeup of such a virus (128). If so, then one might predict that the next pandemic would arise when the pool of individuals susceptible to H2 viruses, which last circulated in 1968, reaches sufficient size. Of interest, H2 subtype viruses are very common in birds, and they have been isolated from birds sold in live bird markets in New York City (155). The final answer to the question is unclear; in the meantime, considerable planning is underway for the almost inevitable occurrence of the next pandemic (156).

V. Clinical Features

A. Disease Manifestations

The onset of influenza is typically, but not invariably, abrupt, and many individuals can recall the exact hour of onset of illness. A characteristic of acute influenza is the predominance of systemic symptoms, including fever, prostration, and malaise, which can be quite disabling even in previously healthy subjects. Generalized myalgias are typical, and myalgias of the extraocular muscles with pain on lateral gaze are frequently encountered. Headache is common. Respiratory symptoms may be relatively minimal, particularly early in the course, and include nasal complaints, sore throat, hoarseness, and nonproductive cough. Because of the involvement of the tracheal epithelium in infection, complains of burning throat and substernal pain may be seen. Other than fever, there are usually few findings on physical examination. Affected individuals may exhibit rhinitis, pharyngitis, conjunctival injection, and tracheal tenderness. The chest is usually clear in uncomplicated cases. Most acute symptoms resolve in 3–5 days, but complete recovery may take weeks. The clinical features of influenza A and B viral infection are similar.

B. Influenza in Children

Influenza is an important cause of acute febrile illness in children during epidemics. Generally, symptoms of influenza are similar to those in adults, although children may have higher fever with febrile seizures. Influenza is associated with otitis media (157), and influenza virus can be isolated from middle ear fluid in affected children (158). Influenza A viruses are also an important cause of croup (acute laryngotracheobronchitis) during influenza epidemics (159,160), with relatively more severe disease than with other viral causes (159).

C. Influenza in Immunocompromised Hosts

Influenza and other RNA viruses are being increasingly recognized as causes of lower respiratory tract disease in immunocompromised individuals. Influenza may result in more severe disease with prolonged viral shedding in those infected with human immunodeficiency virus (HIV), although the overall impact of HIV infection on disease caused by influenza viruses is unclear (see Chap. 5) (136). Pneumonitis in recipients of bone marrow transplantation has been reported with parainfluenza, respiratory syncytial, and influenza virus infections (161). Influenzal infection of transplant recipients is frequently nosocomially acquired (129).

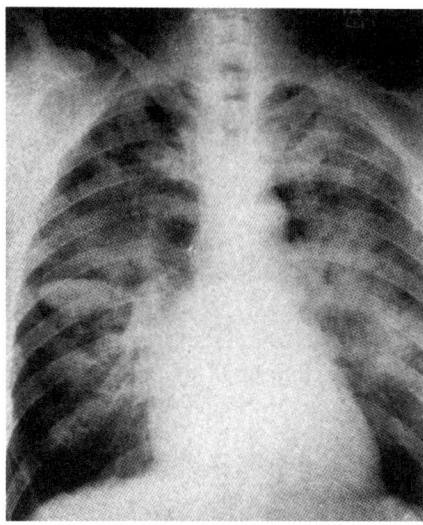

Figure 7 Chest radiograph of a 49-year-old man with primary influenza virus pneumonia superimposed on rheumatic heart disease with mitral stenosis and insufficiency. The density in the right mid-lung field represents a loculated interlobar effusion that was present prior to the acute illness. Diffuse interstitial infiltrates are seen bilaterally. (From Ref. 59 by copyright permission of The American Society for Clinical Investigation.)

VI. Complications

A. Pulmonary Complications

Classically, four types of lower respiratory complications of acute influenza have been described (59). Primary viral pneumonia is seen predominantly in those with prior cardiac disease. The patient presents with typical features of acute influenza but experiences a rapid progression of dyspnea, cough and cyanosis, and the development of adult respiratory distress syndrome. Chest radiographs reveal bilateral interstitial infiltrates (Fig. 7), sputum production is scanty, and Gram stain reveals few organisms. Secondary bacterial pneumonia often presents 1–2 weeks after apparent recovery from an acute influenza episode with recurrence of fever and signs and symptoms of typical lobar pneumonia. Common respiratory bacterial pathogens, including *Streptococcus pneumoniae*, β-hemolytic streptococci, and *Haemophilus influenzae* are often isolated. In addition, the incidence of *Staphylococcus aureus*, which is otherwise an uncommon pulmonary pathogen, is much increased (162). Mixed viral-bacterial pneumonia may also occur with features common to both syndromes. Finally, dyspnea and lower respiratory signs, such as rales, rhonchi, and wheezes, may be seen without visible radiographic infiltrates.

B. Extrapulmonary Complications

Extrapulmonary complications appear to be uncommon. Myositis with myoglobinuria and elevated serum creatine phosphokinase has been seen predominantly with influenza B in children (163). Both myocarditis and pericarditis have also been associated with influenza (164). The toxic shock syndrome has been reported following influenza; presumably reflecting colonization of the damaged respiratory tract with toxin-producing *S. aureus* (165). Encephalitis has also been reported in acute influenza. Of note, Reye's syndrome, an illness of unknown cause characterized by mental status changes and hepatic failure, has been associated with influenza, particularly influenza B, as well as with other respiratory viral infections (166). The use of aspirin increases the risk of Reye's syndrome (167), and aspirin should not be administered to children with acute respiratory disease. (This proscription has been associated with a marked decrease in the incidence of Reye's syndrome.) Acetaminophen and non-steroidal antiinflammatory drugs have not been associated with an increased risk of Reye's syndrome.

VII. Diagnosis

The constellation of typical clinical symptoms during periods of significant influenza epidemic activity is highly suggestive of influenza. Isolation of virus in cell cultures from samples of respiratory secretions such as nasopharyngeal swabs, washes, or throat gargles remains the gold standard of specific viral diagnosis. Renal epithelial cells, such as Madin-Darby canine kidney (MDCK) or Rhesus monkey kidney (RhMK) cells are generally used; alternatively, virus can be isolated in embryonated hen's eggs. Viral isolation and identification requires 3–5 days.

A variety of techniques have been employed in order to speed this process. Centrifugation of samples directly onto cells in shell vials with detection of the production of viral antigens by immunofluorescence (IF) or enzyme immunoassay (ELISA) can reduce the time needed to detect virus to 1 or 2 days (168). Rapid detection of viral antigen directly in respiratory secretions can be accomplished by a variety of techniques including IF (169), time-resolved immunofluorescence (TRFIA) (170), radioenzyme immunoassay (171), and ELISA (172). The most rapid of the ELISA can produce results in less than 1 hr with sensitivity and specificity approaching that of cell culture under optimal conditions. Available formats include filter immunoassays (Directigen FLU-A, Becton Dickenson Microbiology Systems, Cockeysville, MD) (173) and microtiter plate assays (Enzygnost Influenza A and B, Behringwerke AG, Marburg, Germany) (174). The sensitivity of such tests may be higher with NP washes and swabs than with other samples (175). Recently, polymerase chain reaction (PCR) techniques have been described for rapid detection of influenza virus RNA in clinical samples (176, 177); such techniques may also be useful for direct characterization of viral genes without alterations introduced by virus isolation techniques (178).

VIII. Prevention and Therapy

A. Vaccines

Both inactivated vaccines and live attenuated viral vaccines have been developed to stimulate humoral and, to a lesser extent, cellular immunity to influenza (see Chap. 14). The major focus of influenza immunization has generally been the stimulation of local and systemic antibody to the HA and NA (179).

Inactivated Influenza Vaccine

Currently, inactivated influenza vaccines, consisting of either whole virus, detergent-treated "split-product," or subunit HA/NA vaccines are licensed for the prevention of influenza. Because influenza viruses A (H1N1) and A (H3N2) and influenza B viruses cocirculate, a trivalent vaccine is generally used.

Randomized, placebo-controlled trials of modern influenza vaccines have demonstrated these vaccines to be well tolerated in all age groups. Mild local reactions occur in a minority of subjects, and systemic symptoms, such as malaise, headache, or myalgias, occur at a low rate similar to placebo (180–182). Reactions to whole virus and split-product vaccines at current doses are similar in adults (183), but whole virus vaccines are unacceptably reactogenic in children (184) and should not be used in those under 12 years of age. In children, two doses of vaccine are required with primary immunization.

Inactivated influenza vaccines are immunogenic when administered at the currently recommended dose of approximately 15 μg of each HA antigen in healthy adults, and result in increases in hemagglutination-inhibition (HI) antibody in about 90% of recipients (180,181,183). Antibody to the NA is seen less frequently, partially because the relative lability of the NA during the inactivation process. In addition, animal studies have suggested that anti–NA responses are impaired when this antigen is presented in association with an HA to which the animal is primed (so-called intravirionic competition) (185,186). Both systemic and local antibody responses have been observed (187,188). The dose–response curve appears to be fairly flat (182,183), with an increase in local reactions being seen with higher doses (189). Purified preparations of HA may allow the use of increased doses without increasing reactogenicity and may result in somewhat increased antibody responses (190–192). Only a single dose of vaccine is required in individuals who have been previously vaccinated or who have experienced prior infection with a related subtype, but a two-dose schedule is required in unprimed individuals (182,184). In addition, previous exposure significantly affects the breadth of the serum antibody response (193). Generally, the responses of children with high-risk conditions are similar to those of age-matched controls (194–197).

Inactivated influenza vaccine has been shown to be effective in the prevention of influenza A in several randomized or semirandomized controlled studies conducted in young adults, with levels of protection of 70–90% when there is a good antigenic match between vaccine and epidemic viruses (198–200). However, when the antigenic relatedness of the vaccine strain and epidemic strain is low, the effectiveness of inactivated vaccine effectiveness is considerably lower (199,201,202). Vaccination of young adults is associated with decreased absenteeism from work or school and is significantly cost saving (203).

Relatively few prospective trials of protective efficacy have been conducted in high-risk populations. In one recent randomized, placebo-controlled trial in an elderly population, inactivated vaccine was approximately 58% effective in preventing laboratory-documented influenza (204). In addition, numerous retrospective case-controlled studies are available which have documented the effectiveness of inactivated influenza vaccines in these individuals (134,202,205–210). Vaccine is protective against influenza- and pneumonia-related hospitalizations in the elderly, and it is even accompanied by a decrease in all-cause mortality (211). It has been estimated that among elderly persons living in the community, influenza vaccination is associated with a direct savings of $117 per year per person vaccinated (212).

Several groups of adults with potentially decreased responses to inactivated influenza vaccine have been identified. Individuals with chronic renal disease may respond less well to influenza vaccine (213), although not all studies have seen such an effect (214,215). Diminished immune responses to vaccination may occur in renal transplant recipients (216–218). Such impaired responses are associated with both the degree of azotemia and the degree of immunosuppression (216,219). Cyclosporin A, a potent suppressor of T cells, is associated with significantly more impaired immune responses to vaccination (219,220).

Influenza vaccination is safe in individuals with rheumatoid arthritis (221) and systemic lupus erythematosus (222,223), and it is not associated with exacerbations of disease. The response to vaccination in HIV-infected individuals is related to the degree of immunosuppression (224). It has been suggested that the immune activation associated with influenza immunization may transiently stimulate HIV replication (225). The clinical significance of these observations is unclear.

Most patients with chronic lung disease respond reasonably well to vaccination, and steroids at doses commonly used to treat reactive airways disease do not appear to preclude vaccine responses (226,227). Importantly, vaccination is safe, and it is not associated with worsening pulmonary function (227, 228). Although vaccine is usually not administered to patients with true egg allergy, such individuals can be desensitized and safely vaccinated if necessary (229).

Despite studies which support the use of inactivated vaccines in the elderly, the protective efficacy of vaccination appears to be lower in individuals over age 65 than in younger adults (202,204,207,230–232); possibly because of decreased antibody responsiveness to influenza vaccine in this age group (181, 191,233–236). The specific factors in aging which result in decreased immune responses to vaccination are not completely clear. Aged animals clearly have diminished responses to vaccination compared with young animals. However, in human studies, multiple factors may be involved. Not all studies have shown diminished responses to vaccination in the elderly, with the effect of the specific antigen outweighing any effect of age (237). The effect of age may be primarily in effecting the subclass of HA-specific IgG produced (238), which is consistent with an effect of aging on numbers of naive T cells. In some studies, the presence of chronic disability rather than age per se appears better able to predict the lack of responsiveness (239). Malnutrition, also a common problem in the disabled elderly, does not appear to play an important role (240). Although whole virus vaccines may be more reactogenic (241), there is concern that split-product vaccines may be less immunogenic in the elderly (242,243), with subunit vaccines being the least immunogenic (244). Current recommendations for the use of inactivated influenza vaccines are shown in Table 3.

Several problematic areas remain regarding current licensed vaccines. Current inactivated vaccines do not protect the upper respiratory tract and may have limited efficacy in altering the epidemiology of influenza (245). These vaccines also do not appear to provide significant protection against antigenically drifted viruses. The duration of protective immunity also appears to be limited, particularly in the elderly (246). Thus, current inactivated vaccines must be administered yearly. In some situations, yearly administration has been reported to result in decreased effectiveness (247). Recent studies suggest that prior immunization does not adversely affect immune responses to vaccination or the protection afforded by inactivated vaccine, at least in healthy adults (248). However, vaccines with a longer duration of protective effect would be highly desirable.

Finally, there is concern that use of eggs for the production of vaccine may be suboptimal. Influenza viruses, whether growing in cell culture or replicating within an animal, should be considered to be populations of individual viral lineages. Passage of such "quasispecies" under selective conditions can result

Table 3 Target Groups for Influenza Vaccination

Groups at increased risk for influenza-related complications:
  persons ≥65 years of age
  residents of chronic-care facilities
  adults and children with chronic pulmonary or cardiovascular disorders
  adults and children with chronic metabolic disease (including diabetes), renal dysfunction, hemoglobinopathies, or immunosuppression
  children and adolescents receiving long-term aspirin therapy
Groups that can transmit influenza to high-risk persons defined above:
  physicians, nurses, and other health-care workers
  employees of hospitals and chronic-care facilities
  providers of home care to high-risk persons
  household contacts of high-risk persons
In addition, vaccination should be considered in:
  pregnant women
  individuals with human immunodeficiency virus (HIV) infection
  individuals who provide essential community services
  individuals who wish to reduce their chance of acquiring influenza infection

Source: Adapted from Ref. 135.

in a change in the distribution of the population from one predominant type to another. An example of such a phenomenon is the observation of selection of antigenically variant influenza A viruses on passage in embryonated hen's eggs.

Significant antigenic differences between the HA of viruses isolated in mammalian cells (e.g., MDCK cells) and those of viruses isolated in avian cells (embryonated eggs) have been demonstrated for viral clones isolated from the same individual. Direct PCR amplification of viruses in nasal secretions has documented that the HA of the major population of virus shed from the nasopharynx of infected humans is identical to that isolated in MDCK cells and significantly different from that isolated in eggs. Although these differences may amount to only a few amino acids, the MDCK cell–grown virus is clearly more effective than egg-grown virus as an inactivated vaccine for protection of experimental animals (249,250). Antigenic differences of this type have been documented for H3N2, H1N1, and influenza B viruses (178,251–257). Thus, continued attention should be paid to the possibility that current inactivated influenza vaccines, which are selected for high-yield growth in eggs, may not be optimally antigenically representative of the viruses which are infecting humans. In addition, the production of vaccine requires the ready availability of specific pathogen–free eggs. For these reasons, alternative substrates for growth of influenza viruses for vaccine production are currently being developed (258). The use of recombinant DNA techniques to generate vaccine antigen also allows control over the sequence of the HA used. Recently, HA antigens generated in insect cells by recombinant baculoviruses were shown to be safe and immunogenic in young adults and the elderly and to provide protection against laboratory documented influenza A in young adults (259–261).

Live Virus Vaccines

Live virus vaccines for influenza have also been intensively evaluated in humans. The use of live attenuated viruses as influenza vaccines offers several potential advantages over parenteral inactivated vaccines, including induction of a mucosal immune response which closely mimics that induced by natural influenza viral infection (245). In addition, the superiority of such vaccines in protection of the upper respiratory tract (262) could potentially also be useful in strategies to limit the spread of virus within the population (263). In practical terms, the use of a nasal rather than a parenteral route of administration might be more acceptable to patients, particularly in certain age groups. A key requirement for the development of attenuated influenza vaccines is the ability rapidly to attenuate new antigenic variants. The most widely used approach takes advantage of the segmented nature of the influenza virus genome to generate reassortant viruses in which the gene segments encoding attenuation are derived from a well-characterized master donor vaccine virus, and the gene segments encoding the HA and NA are derived from the new antigenic variant (264,265). In the past, extensive studies were performed to evaluate the use of temperature-sensitive (266) or avian (267) influenza viruses as donors of attenuating genes. However, these approaches were not successful either because of genetic instability (268) or unreliable attenuation (269,270). Importantly, such deficiencies in the safety profile of these approaches to live attenuated influenza vaccine were only detected when studies were performed in young children, who are generally most susceptible to infection by the vaccine viruses.

The most promising approach to the development of a master donor virus has been the use of cold-adapted (CA) viruses. The process of cold adaptation refers to the repetitive passage of a virus at gradually decreasing temperature until a virus is isolated which replicates efficiently at a low temperature at which the replication of the original wild-type virus is significantly restricted (271). During this process, additional mutant phenotypes are frequently acquired.

The CA influenza A/Ann Arbor/6/60 virus (271) has been extensively evaluated as a donor of attenuating genes for the generation of CA vaccine viruses. A large number of CA A/AA/60 reassortant influenza A viruses have been evaluated in young adults and children and in high-risk groups, and they have been found to be attenuated and immunogenic (reviewed in Ref. 272). Importantly, genetic reversion to virulence has not been demonstrated even in seronegative young children. This is likely because the genetic basis of attenuation resides on at least three gene segments—PB1, PB2, and PA gene segments (273,274). In addition, since none of these gene segments would be expected to interact with the HA or NA of the wild-type donor virus, the attenuation of CA reassortant viruses would not be expected to vary significantly from reassortant to reassortant. A similarly derived CA influenza B/Ann Arbor/1/66 virus has been used as a donor of attenuating genes for the generation of CA influenza B vaccine viruses (271). A variety of CA B/AA/66 reassortant viruses have been evaluated in young adults and in children (275–279), and they also appear to be nonreactogenic, immunogenic, and genetically stable (280).

Reassortant CA influenza A (96,262) and B (276,277) viruses provide protection against homologous wild-type challenge in young adults at least equal to that provided by inactivated vaccines. Recently, reassortant CA viruses have been shown to protect against natural wild-type influenzal infection in randomized, controlled field trial evaluations conducted in children (281, 282) and adults (283) with levels of protection similar to those provided by inactivated vaccine.

Several issues remain to be determined with these viruses. Both CA influenza A and B viruses manifest relatively limited replication and immunogenicity in the elderly, which may limit their effectiveness in this important target population (284–286). However, combinations of local live attenuated influenza vaccine and parenteral inactivated vaccine administered together may be helpful (287). In addition, significant interference between individual reassortant viruses may occur when administered together (288,289), which may complicate formulation of effective multivalent preparations.

A variety of additional live attenuated influenza viruses have been evaluated. Perhaps the most intriguing, novel approach has utilized techniques for the reverse genetic engineering of specific mutations in the genome of influenza A and B viruses (290–292). An influenza A virus in which the 3' and 5' ends of the neuraminidase gene segment were replaced by the corresponding regions of an influenza B virus was recently shown to replicate but to manifest attenuated virulence in a murine model (293). Attenuation has also been achieved by manipulation of the stalk of the NA (294,295) and by direct introduction of attenuating mutations into the PB2 gene (296). Further development of such viruses may lead to a second generation of potential live viral vaccine candidates as well as providing a vector for the administration of additional immunogenic epitopes (297,298).

DNA Vaccines

An advantage of live viral vaccines is that they result in endogenous, intracellular synthesis of viral antigen and presentation in the context of MHC class I. An alternative means to induce intracellular synthesis of viral antigens is the delivery of the genes encoding the antigen of interest by a heterologous foreign vector. Recently, it has been recognized that, under certain circumstances, foreign DNA could be delivered directly to the cells of an intact animal and be taken up and expressed, and that the animal would manifest an immune response to the foreign gene product (299). Immunization of mice with DNA encoding the HA as well as the internal M and NP proteins of influenza A induces long-lived humoral and cellular immune responses (300, 301) which are protective against viral infection and disease. Recently, immunization of African green monkeys with DNA encoding a combination of three HA and other influenza virus genes was shown to induce serum antibody against all three HA (302), and studies of similar candidate DNA vaccines have been initiated in humans.

B. Antiviral Chemotherapy

Given the well-recognized public health impact of influenza and the large body of knowledge regarding the basic virology of this virus, it is not surprising that the development of antiviral agents active against the influenza viruses has been a subject of intense interest and effort. However, only amantadine (1-adamantanamine hydrochloride) and the related drug rimantadine (α-methyl-1-adamantane methyl-amine hydrochloride) are currently licensed for the prevention and treatment of influenza (303) (see Chap. 13).

Amantadine and Rimantadine

Amantadine and rimantadine are active against all strains of influenza A virus in a variety of cell culture systems and animal models (303). In cell culture, inhibitory levels for influenza A virus range from 0.2 to 0.4 μg/mL for amantadine and 0.1 to 0.4 μg/mL for rimantadine (304). Both drugs are active only against influenza A virus at clinically achievable levels. The antiviral activity of these drugs is due to interaction with the M2 protein of susceptible viruses based on analysis of drug-resistant mutants (305–307). Binding of these drugs to the M2 protein interferes with the function of the M2 as an ion channel which can be measured by in vitro assays of channel activity (5). In turn, this inhibits the pH-dependent release of RNP, which is manifested by inhibition of uncoating in cell culture assays (308–311). The drugs may also effect HA maturation of certain strains of virus.

Amantadine and rimantadine are effective in the prophylaxis of both experimentally induced and naturally acquired influenza A with an efficacy of approximately 70–90%; values that are approximately equal to that of inactivated vaccine. However, rimantadine is associated with fewer side effects. For

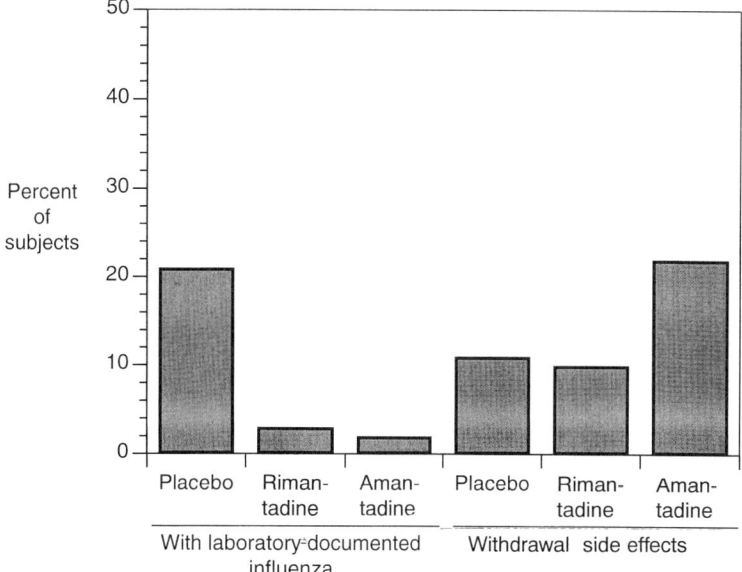

Figure 8 Prophylaxis of influenza with amantadine and rimantadine. Both rimantadine and amantadine prevented laboratory documented influenza, but rimantadine was associated with significantly fewer side effects. (Data from Ref. 312.)

example, when both drugs were compared in healthy adults at doses of 200 mg per day versus placebo during an epidemic of predominantly H1N1 influenza A virus, amantadine and rimantadine were equally effective in the prevention of laboratory-documented influenza A, but withdrawal rates, primarily due to minor central nervous system (CNS) side effects, were significantly higher among amantadine recipients (Fig. 8) (312). Amantadine has been shown to be effective in the prophylaxis of experimental influenza A (H1N1) in young adults when administered at 100 mg per day (313) with decreased CNS side effects. Relatively less is known about the effectiveness of these drugs in the prevention of influenza in high-risk subjects. However, preliminary data suggest that rimantadine is effective in the prevention of influenza A in the elderly and that the protective effect is additive to that provided by inactivated influenza vaccine (314).

In order to avoid the need to administer drug to large numbers of subjects for prolonged periods, the use of amantadine in prophylaxis of family contacts of index cases during influenza outbreaks has also been evaluated. In one trial, in which both the index case and family members were treated with amantadine, there was no evidence of protection against influenza A (H3N2)

(315). In contrast, in a second study performed by the same investigators, but in which the index case was not treated, the rate of laboratory-documented influenza A (H3N2) in household contacts was reduced by 63% (316). More recently, a similar study was performed in which rimantadine was administered to both index cases and family members during outbreaks of H1N1 and H3N2 influenza A. However, there was no difference in the rates of laboratory-documented influenza A infection in family contacts receiving rimantadine compared with contacts receiving placebo (317). Importantly, the failure of rimantadine under these circumstances appeared to be the result of the selection and transmission of influenza A viruses which had become resistant to the antiviral action of rimantadine (317). Illness caused by resistant virus was clinically similar to that caused by sensitive virus.

Amantadine is currently recommended for use during institutional outbreaks of influenza A; a situation that has been compared with an outbreak in a large family (318). Although no placebo-controlled, randomized trials have been done to evaluate the use of amantadine under these circumstances, retrospective analyses of such outbreaks support this recommendation (319,320). These studies have suggested efficacy of amantadine during nosocomial outbreaks among high-risk patients in hospitals as well as in multiple outbreaks in nursing homes. Amantadine-resistant virus has also been isolated under these circumstances, however, with transmission to others, a finding which could diminish the effectiveness of the drug in institutional prophylaxis (321, 322). Amantadine must be administered at a low dose (i.e., 100 mg per day) to avoid CNS toxicity in elderly individuals.

Both amantadine and rimantadine are active in the treatment of experimentally induced and naturally acquired influenza A, with most studies showing a reduction in clinical symptom scores, a more rapid reduction of fever, and a reduction in the levels and duration of viral shedding when compared with placebo (323,324). Amantadine was also shown to be slightly more effective than aspirin in the reduction of clinical symptoms of naturally acquired influenza A in young adults (325). In addition, treatment with amantadine results in significantly more rapid improvement in small airways dysfunction in healthy adults with uncomplicated influenza (Fig. 9) (52,326). Rimantadine has also been evaluated in the treatment of influenza A in children, and it has been shown to reduce the level of viral shedding early in infection when compared with acetaminophen (327,328). More variable effects on clinical symptom scores have been seen, with one study showing a decrease in scores and fever compared with acetaminophen (327), and the other, in which illness was relatively mild, showing no significant difference (328). In both studies, viral shedding was relatively prolonged in those receiving rimantadine, and resistant virus was shed late in the course of illness. Illness associated with shedding of resistant virus was similar to that associated with drug-sensitive virus.

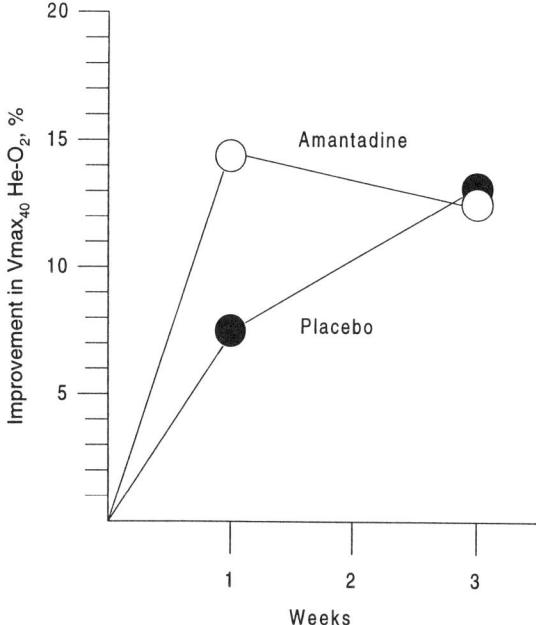

Figure 9 Improvement in pulmonary function with amantadine treatment of uncomplicated influenza A in young adults. There was a statistically significant difference between amantadine and placebo recipients in the degree of improvement of pulmonary function after 1 week. (Modified from Ref. 326.)

Comparative studies of the efficacy of amantadine or rimantadine in the treatment of more complicated influenza infection; for example, in hospitalized patients or those with pneumonia have not been reported. However, most authorities would support the use of amantadine or rimantadine in the treatment of complicated influenza A viral infection even late in the course of illness (329).

Antiviral drug resistance has been one factor which has limited the more widespread use of these drugs (318). Amantadine- and rimantadine-resistant viruses emerge fairly frequently in treated individuals (317,330), although resistant virus is seen infrequently in individuals unexposed to these drugs (331). Resistant virus can be transmitted to and cause disease in susceptible contacts (317,322,330), and drug-resistant virus retains full pathogenic potential in experimental animals (332,333). Although the use of combined vaccination and amantadine can decrease the generation and transmission of resistant viruses (334,335), the problem of drug resistance remains an important consideration which may limit the more widespread use of these agents. However, the M2 protein remains an attractive target for the development of antiviral agents, because it is so specific for influenza virus and because highly accurate in vitro screening assays are available (336).

Ribavirin

The antiviral drug ribavirin (1B-D-ribofuranosyl-1,2,3-triazole-3-carboxamide) is active against influenza A and B virus in human challenge models when administered by small-particle aerosol (337,338). However, the relatively limited efficacy of the drug (339) and the cumbersome method of administration have limited its utility in this situation. Intravenous ribavirin has been reported to be useful for the treatment of influenza virus–associated acute myocarditis (340).

Sialidase Inhibitors

The determination of the crystal structure of the neuraminidase complexed with its substrate, sialic acid (341), has allowed the development of a series of sialic acid analogues with neuraminidase-inhibiting activity (342). The most active of these compounds, 4-guanidino-2,4-dideoxy-2,3-dehydro-N-acetylneuraminic acid (4-guanidino-Neu5Ac2en, GG167) is a highly potent and selective inhibitor of the neuraminidase of influenza A and B viruses. GG167 has significant antiviral activity against a wide variety of laboratory and clinical influenza A and B isolates in cell culture and in the mouse and ferret models (342,343). The drug is not orally bioavailable and is not effective when administered parenterally in animals; apparently because therapeutic levels are not achieved in respiratory secretions (344). Therefore, effective use of this agent requires topical administration to the respiratory tract.

Limited studies in humans have also indicated the efficacy of GG167 (345). Intranasal GG167 was effective in the prophylaxis and therapy of influenza in a model in which relatively susceptible young adults were experimentally infected by intranasal drops containing the A/Texas/36/91 (H1N1) virus. GG167 was 82% effective in preventing infection and 95% effective in preventing febrile illness when administered beginning 4 hr before viral challenge. In addition, both early treatment (beginning 26–32 hr after challenge) and late treatment (beginning 50 hr after challenge) were effective in reducing viral shedding compared with placebo, and early treatment also reduced symptom scores (345). Preliminary results of treatment of healthy subjects with early, uncomplicated, naturally acquired influenza have also been encouraging (346).

Because GG167 interacts with highly conserved residues within the influenza virus neuraminidase, it was hoped that antiviral resistance would be a limited problem. In fact, truly resistant viruses have not been isolated from humans treated with GG167 in clinical trials to date. Viruses resistant to the in vitro antiviral activity of GG167 have been isolated after passage in cell culture. The majority of these viruses remain sensitive to the neuraminidase-inhibiting activity of GG167, and infections with such viruses remain susceptible to treatment in animal models. Genetic analysis suggests that such pseudoresistant viruses may contain altered HA with relatively decreased affinity for sialic acid–containing receptors (347). Such mutant viruses may be less dependent on neuraminidase for release from cells. After further passage in the presence of GG167, it is possible to isolate viruses which are resistant to the NI activity of the drug associated with a point mutation (Glu-119-Ala) in the NA gene (347). Thus it appears that the development of antiviral resistance to GG167 may require prolonged exposure to the inhibitor. Because of the very exciting results with this compound, considerable efforts to develop other NA-inhibiting agents, potentially with oral activity, are currently underway (348).

Other Antiviral Drugs

A number of other antiviral drugs have been developed and shown to be active against influenza in cell culture and animal models. Intranasal INF-α2, administered as a large-particle aerosol, resulted in decreased viral replication and clinical symptoms scores in young adults challenged with influenza A virus (349). However, drug administration was associated with significant local toxicity, which has limited further development of this approach. Other approaches currently in use include the development of in vitro assays of influenza virus polymerase function which allow rapid screening of compounds for polymerase-inhibiting activity, the use of bispecific monoclonal antibodies (350), or potential interruption of recently described interactions between the NP (351) and NS1 (352) proteins and cellular proteins which are probably critical in replication of these viruses.

IX. Summary

Influenza viruses cause outbreaks of acute respiratory disease with systemic symptoms. The outbreaks vary in severity depending on the viral strain and on levels of preexisting immunity in the community. Mortality occurs primarily in the elderly and in certain other high-risk groups. The structure and replicative cycle of influenza viruses have been intensively studied and provide targets for the development of antiviral drugs. Reassortment of the segmented genome is being used to produce stable, live, attenuated vaccines, and high-yielding strains for the production of inactivated vaccines. Despite advances in our knowledge, the factors leading to the emergence of pandemic strains of virus remain incompletely understood.

References

1. Wharton J, Weis W, Skehel J, Wiley D. Structure, function, and antigenicity of the hemagglutinin of influenza virus. In: Krug RN, ed. The Influenza Viruses. New York: Plenum Press, 1989:153–169.
2. Skehel J, Bayley P, Brown E. Changes in the conformation of the influenza virus hemagglutinin at the pH optimum of virus mediated fusion. Proc Natl Acad Sci (USA) 1982; 79:968–972.
3. Herz C, Stavnezer E, Krug RM, Gurney TJ. Influenza virus, an RNA virus, synthesizes its messenger RNA in the nucleus of infected cells. Cell 1981; 26:391–400.
4. Martin K, Helenius A. Transport of incoming influenza virus nucleocapsids into the nucleus. J Virol 1991; 65:232–244.
5. Pinto LH, Holsinger LJ, Lamb RA. Influenza virus M2 protein has ion channel activity. Cell 1992; 69:517–528.
6. Bui M, Whittaker G, Helenius A. Effect of M1 protein and low pH on nuclear transport of influenza virus ribonucleoproteins. J Virol 1996; 70:8391–8401.
7. Horvath CM, Williams MA, Lamb RA. Eukaryotic coupled translation of tandem cistrons: identification of the influenza B virus BM2 polypeptide. EMBO J 1990; 9:2639–2647.
8. Shaw MW, Choppin PW, Lamb RA. A previously unrecognized influenza B virus glycoprotein from a bicistronic mRNA that also encodes the viral neuraminidase. Proc Natl Acad Sci (USA) 1983; 80:4879–4883.
9. Brassard DL, Leser GP, Lamb RA. Influenza B virus NB glycoprotein is a component of the virion. Virology 1996; 220:350–360.
10. Sunstrom NA, Premkumar LS, Premkumar A, Ewart G, Cox GB, Gage PW. Ion channels formed by NB, an influenza B protein. J Membr Biol 1996; 150:127–132.
11. Robertson J, Schubert M, Lazzarini R. Polyadehylation sites for influenza virus mRNA. J Virol 1981; 38:157–163.
12. Ye Z, Baylor N, Wagner R. Transcription-inhibition and RNA-binding domains of influenza A virus matrix protein mapped with anti-idiotypic antibodies and synthetic peptides. J Virol 1989; 63:3586–3594.
13. Beaton AR, Krug RM. Transcription antitermination during influenza viral template RNA synthesis requires the nucleocapsid protein and the absence of a 5′ capped end. Proc Natl Acad Sci (USA) 1986; 83:6282–6286.
14. Braam J, Ulmanen I, Krug RM. Molecular model of a eukaryotic transcription complex: functions and movement for influenza P proteins during capped RNA-primed transcription. Cell 1983; 34:609–618.
15. Detjen BM, St. Angelo C, Katze MG, Krug RM. The three influenza virus polymerase (P) proteins not associated with viral nucleocapsids in the infected cell are in the form of a complex. J Virol 1987; 61:13–22.
16. Blass D, Patzelt E, Kuecler E. Cap-recognizing protein of influenza virus. Virology 1982; 116:339–348.

17. Nakagawa Y, Oda K, Nakada S. The PB1 subunit alone can catalyze cRNA synthesis, and the PA subunit in addition to the PB1 subunit is required for viral RNA synthesis in replication of the influenza virus genome. J Virol 1996; 70:6390–6394.
18. Plotch SJ, Krug RM. In vitro splicing of influenza viral NS1 mRNA and NS1-beta globin chimeras: possible mechanisms for the control of viral mRNA splicing. Proc Natl Acad Sci (USA) 1986; 83:5444–5448.
19. Alonso-Caplan FV, Krug RM. Regulation of the extent of splicing of influenza virus NS1 mRNA: role of the rates of splicing and of the nucleocytoplasmic transport of NS1 mRNA. Mol Cell Biol 1991; 11:1092–1098.
20. Lu Y, Quian XY, Krug RM. The influenza virus NS1 protein: a novel inhibitor of pre-mRNA splicing. Genes Dev 1994; 8:1817–1828.
21. Qui Y, Krug RM. The influenza virus NS1 protein is a poly A-binding protein that inhibits the nuclear export of mRNAs containing poly A. J Virol 1994; 68:2425–2432.
22. Martin K, Helenius A. Nuclear transport of influenza virus ribonucleoproteins: the viral matrix protein (M1) promotes export and inhibits import. Cell 1991; 67: 117–130.
23. Takeuchi K, Lamb RA. Influenza virus M2 protein ion channel activity stabilizes the native form of Fowl plague virus hemagglutinin during intracellular transport. J Virol 1994; 68:911–919.
24. Shimbo K. Brassard DL, Lamb RA, Pinto LH. Ion selectivity and activation of the M2 ion channel of influenza virus. Biophys J 1996; 70:1335–1346.
25. Kretzschmar E, Bui M, Rose JK. Membrane association of influenza virus matrix protein does not require specific hydrophobic domains or the viral glycoproteins. Virology 1996; 220:37–45.
26. Duhaut SD, McCauley JW. Defective RNAs inhibit the assembly of influenza virus genome segments in a segment-specific manner. Virology 1996; 216:326–337.
27. Enami M, Sharma G, Benham C, Palese P. An influenza virus containing nine different RNA segments. Virology 1991; 185:291–298.
28. Garcia-Sastre A, Palese P. The cytoplasmic tail of the neuraminidase protein of influenza A virus does not play an important role in the packaging of this protein into viral envelopes. Virus Res 1995; 37:37–47.
29. Mitnaul LJ, Castrucci MR, Murti KG, Kawaoka Y. The cytoplasmic tail of influenza A virus neuraminidase (NA) affects NA incorporation into virions, virion morphology, and virulence in mice but is not essential for virus replication. J Virol 1996;70:873–879.
30. Hofling K, Brossmer R, Klenk H, Herrier G. Transfer of an esterase-resistant receptor analog to the surface of influenza C virions results in reduced infectivity due to aggregate formation. Virology 1996; 218:127–133.
31. Katze M, Krug R. Metabolism and expression of RNA polymerase II transcripts in influenza virus infected cells. Mol Cell Biol 1984; 4:2198–2206.
32. Katze M, DeCorato D, Krug R. Cellular mRNA translation is blocked at both initiation and elongation after infection by influenza virus or adenovirus. J Virol 1986; 60:1027–1039.
33. Sanz-Esquerro JJ, De La Luna S, Ortin J, Nieto A. Individual expression of the influenza virus PA protein induces degradation of expressed proteins. J Virol 1995; 69:2420–2426.

34. Hinshaw VS, Olsen CW, Dybdahl-Sissoko N, Evans D. Apoptosis: a mechanism of cell killing by influenza A and B viruses. J Virol 1994; 68:3667–3673.
35. Takizawa T, Shigeru M, Higuchi Y, Nakamura S, Nakanishi Y, Fukuda R. Induction of programmed cell death (apoptosis) by influenza virus infection in tissue culture cells. J Gen Virol 1993; 74:2347–2355.
36. Mori I, Komatsu T, Takeuchi K, Nakakuki K, Sudo M, Kimura Y. In vivo induction of apoptosis by influenza virus. J Gen Virol 1995; 76:2869–2873.
37. Takizawa T, Fukuda R, Miyawaki T, Ohashi K, Nakanishi Y. Activation of the apoptotic Fas antigen-encoding gene upon influenza virus infection involving spontaneously produced beta-interferon. Virology 1995; 209:288–296.
38. Larson HE, Parry RP, Tyrrell DAJ. Impaired polymorphonuclear leucocyte chemotaxis after influenza virus infection. Br J Dis Chest 1980; 74:56–62.
39. Roberts NJ, Steigbigel RT. Effect of in vitro virus infection on response of human monocytes and lymphocytes to mitogen stimulation. J Immunol 1978; 121:1052–1058.
40. Roberts NJ, Prill AH, Mann TN. Interleukin 1 and interleukin 1 inhibitor production by human macrophages exposed to influenza virus or respiratory syncytial virus: respiratory syncytial virus is a potent inducer of inhibitory activity. J Exp Med 1986; 163:511–519.
41. Suzuki H, Kurita T, Kakinuma K. Effects of neuraminidase on O_2 consumption and release of O_2 and H_2O_2 from phagocytosing human polymorphonuclear leukocytes. Blood 1982; 60:446–453.
42. Cassidy LF, Lyles DS, Abramson JS. Depression of polymorphonuclear leukocyte functions by purified influenza virus hemagglutinin and sialic acid-binding lectins. J Immunol 1989; 142:4401–4406.
43. Cooper JA Jr, Carcelen R, Culbreth R. Effects of influenza A nucleoprotein on polymorphonuclear neutrophil function. J Infect Dis 1996; 173:279–284.
44. Cooper JA Jr, Culbreth RR. Characterization of a neutrophil inhibitor peptide harvested from human bronchiolar lavage: homology to influenza A nucleoprotein. Am J Respir Cell Mol Biol 1996; 15:207–215.
45. Alford RH, Kasel JA, Gerone PJ, Knight V. Human influenza resulting from aerosol inhalation. Proc Soc Exp Biol Med 1966; 122:800–804.
46. Martin CM, Kunin CM, Gottlieb LS, Barnes MW, Liu C, Finland M. Asian influenza A in Boston, 1957–1958. Arch Intern Med 1959; 103:516–531.
47. Walsh JJ, Dietlein LF, Low FN, Burch GE, Mogabgab WJ. Bronchotracheal response in human influenza. Arch Intern Med 1961; 108:376–388.
48. Hers JFP, Mulder J, Masurel N, Kuip LVD, Tyrrell DAJ. Studies on the pathogenesis of influenza virus pneumonia in mice. J Pathol Bacteriol 1962; 83:207–217.
49. Mulder J, Hers JF. Influenza. Groningen, The Netherlands: Wolters-Noordhoff, 1979.
50. Oseasohn R, Adelson L, Kaji M. Clinocopathologic study of 33 fatal cases of Asian influenza. N Engl J Med 1959; 260:509.
51. Ramphal R, Cogliano RC, Shands JWJ, Small PAJ. Serum antibody prevents lethal murine influenza pneumonitis but not tracheitis. Infect Immun 1979; 25:992–997.

52. Little JW, Hall WJ, Douglas RG Jr, Mudholkar GS, Speers DM, Patel K. Airway hyperreactivity and peripheral airway dysfunction in influenza A infection. Am Rev Respir Dis 1978; 118:295–303.
53. Hall WJ, Douglas RG Jr, Hyde RW, Roth FK, Cross AS, Speers DM. Pulmonary mechanics after uncomplicated influenza A infection. Am Rev Respir Dis 1976; 113:
54. Horner GJ, Gray FD Jr. Effect of uncomplicated, presumptive influenza on the diffusing capacity of the lung. Am Rev Respir Dis 1973; 108:866–869.
55. Johanson WGJ, Pierce AK, Sanford JP. Pulmonary function in uncomplicated influenza. Am Rev Respir Dis 1969; 100:141–146.
56. Kondo S, Abe K. The effects of influenza virus infection on FEV1 in asthmatic children. Chest 1991; 100:1235–1238.
57. Smith CB, Kanner RE, Goldern CA, Klauber MR, Renzetti AD Jr. Effect of viral infections on pulmonary function in patients with chronic obstructive pulmonary diseases. J Infect Dis 1980; 141:271–279.
58. Utell MJ, Aquilina AT, Hall WJ, Speers DM, Douglas RGJ, Gibb FR, Morrow PE, Hyde RW. Development of airway reactivity to nitrates in subjects with influenza. Am Rev Respir Dis 1980; 121:233–241.
59. Louria DB, Blumenfeld HL, Ellis JT, Kilbourne ED, Rogers DE. Studies on influenza in the pandemic of 1957–1958. II. Pulmonary complications of influenza. J Clin Invest 1959; 38:213–265.
60. Yelandi AV, Colby TV. Pathologic features of lung biopsy specimens from influenza pneumonia cases. Hum Pathol 1994; 25:47–53.
61. Greenberg SB. Viral pneumonia. Infect Dis Clin North Am 1991; 5:603–621.
62. Levandowski RA, Gerrity TR, Garrard CS. Modifications of lung clearance mechanisms by acute influenza A infection. J Lab Clin Med 1985; 106:428–432.
63. Camner P, Jarstrand C, Philipson K. Tracheobronchial clearance in patients with influenza. Am Rev Respir Dis 1973; 108:131–135.
64. George RC, Broadbent DA, Drasar BS. The effect of influenza virus on the adherence of *Haemophilus influenzae* to human cells in tissue culture. Br J Exp Pathol 1983; 64:655–659.
65. Babiuk LA. Viral-bacterial synergistic interactions in respiratory infections in applied virology. In: Kurstak E, Al-Nakib W, Kurstak C, eds. Applied Virology. New York: Academic Press, 1984:431.
66. Ramphal R, Fischschweiger W, Shands JWJ, Small PA. Murine influenzal tracheitis: a model for the study of influenza and tracheal epithelial repair. Am Rev Respir Dis 1979; 120:1313–1324.
67. Cassidy LF, Lyles DS, Abramson JS. Synthesis of viral proteins in polymorphonuclear leukocytes infected with influenza A virus. J Clin Microbiol 1988; 26:1267–1270.
68. Abramson JS, Wheeler JG, Parce JW, Rowe MJ, Lyles DS, Seeds M, Bass DA. Suppression of endocytosis in neutrophils by influenza A virus in vitro. J Infect Dis 1986; 154:456–463.
69. Akaike T, Molla A, Ando M, Araki S, Maeda H. Molecular mechanism of complex infection by bacteria and virus analyzed by a model using Serratia protease and influenza virus in mice. J Virol 1989; 63:2252–2259.

70. Frank AL, Taber LH, Wells JM. Comparison of infection rates and severity of illness for influenza A subtypes H1N2 and H3N2. J Infect Dis 1985; 151:73–80.
71. Wright PF, Thop[son J, Karzon DT. Differing virulence of H1N1 and H3N2 influenza strains. Am J Epidemiol 1980; 112:814–819.
72. Brown EG. Increased virulence of a mouse-adapted variant of influenza A/FM/1/47 virus is controlled by mutations in genome segments 4, 5, 7, and 8. J Virol 1990; 64:4523–4533.
73. Li S, Schulman J, Itamura S, Palese P. Glycosylation of neuraminidase determines the neurovirulence of influenza A/WSN/33 virus. J Virol 1993; 67:6667–6673.
74. Schlesinger RW, Bradshaw GL, Barbone F, Reinacher M, Rott R, Husak P. Role of hemagglutinin cleavage and expression of M1 protein in replication of A/WS/33, A/PR/8/34, and WSN influenza viruses in mouse brain. J Virol 1989; 63:1695–1703.
75. Kido H, Yokogoshi Y, Sakai K, Tashiro M, Kishion Y, Fudutomi A, Katunoma N. Isolation and characterization of a novel trypsin-like protease found in rat bronchiolar Clara cells: a possible activator of the viral fusion glycoprotein. J Biol Chem 1992; 267:13573–13579.
76. Kawaoko Y, Webster RG. Sequence requirements for cleavage activation of influenza virus hemagglutinin expressed in mammalian cells. Proc Natl Acad Sci (USA) 1988; 85:324–328.
77. Kawaoko Y, Webster RG. Interplay between carbohydrate in the stalk and the length of the connecting peptide determined the cleavability of influenza virus hemagglutinin. J Virol 1989; 63:3296–3300.
78. Stieneke-Grober A, Vey M, Angliker H, Shaw E, Thomas G, Roberts C, Klenk H-D, Garten W. Influenza virus hemagglutinin with multibasic cleavage site is activated by furin, a subtilisin-like endoprotease. EMBO J 1992; 11:2407–2414.
79. Horimoto T, Kawaoka Y. Reverse genetics provides direct evidence for a correlation of hemagglutinin cleavability and virulence of an avian influenza A virus. J Virol 1994; 68:3120–3128.
80. Noble GR. Epidemiologic and clinical aspects of influenza. In: Beare AS, ed. Basic and Applied Influenza Research. Boca Raton, FL: CRC Press, 1982:1179.
81. Couch RB, Kasal JA. Immunity to influenza in man. Ann Rev Microbiol 1983; 37:529–549.
82. Black RA, Rota PA, Gorodkova N, Klenk H-D, Kendal AP. Antibody response to the M2 protein of influenza A virus expressed in insect cells. J Gen Virol 1993; 74:143–146.
83. Murphy BR, Nelson DL, Wright PF, Tierney EL, Phelan MA, Chanock RM. Secretory and systemic immunologic response in children infected with live attenuated influenza A virus. Infect Immun 1982; 36:1102–1108.
84. Virelizier J-L. Host defenses against influenza virus: the role of anti-hemagglutinin antibody. J Immunol 1975; 115:434–439.
85. Murphy BR, Clements ML. The systemic and mucosal immune response of humans to influenza A virus. Curr Top Microbiol Immunol 1989; 146:107–116.
86. Bot A, Reichlin A, Isobe H, Bot S, Schulman J, Yokoyama WM, Bona CA. Cellular mechanisms involved in protection and recovery from influenza virus infection in immunodeficient mice. J Virol 1996; 70:5668–5672.

87. Webster RG, Reay PA, Laver WG. Protection against lethal influenza with neuraminidase. Virology 1988; 164:230–237.
88. Murphy BR, Kasel JA, Chanock RM. Association of serum antineuraminidase antibody with resistance to influenza in man. N Engl J Med 1972; 286:1329–1332.
89. Monto AS, Kendal AP. Effect of neuraminidase antibody on Hong Kong influenza. Lancet 1973; I:623–625.
90. Clements ML, Betts RF, Tierney EL, Murphy BR. Serum and nasal wash antibodies associated with resistance to experimental challenge with influenza A wild-type virus. J Clin Microbiol 1986; 24:157–160.
91. Johansson BE, Grajower B, Kilbourne ED. Infection-permissive immunization with influenza virus neuraminidase prevents weight loss in infected mice. Vaccine 1993; 11:1037–1039.
92. Treanor JJ, Tierney EL, Zebedee SL, Lamb RA, Murphy BR. Passively transferred monoclonal antibody to the M2 protein inhibits influenza A virus replication in mice. J Virol 1990; 64:1375–1377.
93. Wagner DK, Clements ML, Reimer CB, Snyder M, Nelson DL, Murphy BR. Analysis of immunoglobulin G antibody responses after administration of live and inactivated influenza A vaccine indicates that nasal wash immunoglobulin G is a transudate from serum. J Clin Microbiol 1987; 25:559–562.
94. Renegar KB, Small PAJ. Passive transfer of local immunity to influenza virus by IgA antibody. J Immunol 1991; 146:1972–1978.
95. Liew FY, Russel SM, Appleyard G, Brand CM, Beale J. Cross-protection in mice infected with influenza A virus by the respiratory route is correlated with local IgA antibody rather than serum antibody or cytotoxic T cell activity. Eur J Immunol 1984; 14:409–413.
96. Clements ML, Betts RF, Tierney EL, Murphy BR. Resistance of adults to challenge with influenza A wild-type virus after receiving live or inactivated virus vaccine. J Clin Microbiol 1986; 23:73–76.
97. Virelizier J-L, Allison AC, Shild GC. Antibody responses to antigenic determinants of influenza virus hemagglutinin. II. Original antigenic sin: A bone marrow–derived lymphocyte memory phenomenon modulated by thymus-derived lymphocytes. J Exp Med 1974; 140:1571–1578.
98. Burns WH, Billups LC, Notkins AL. Thymus dependence of viral antigens. Nature 1975; 256:654–656.
99. Lucas SJ, Barry DW, Kind P. Antibody production and protection against influenza in immunodeficient mice. Infect Immun 1978; 20:115–119.
100. Lamb JR, Woody JN, Hartzman RD, Eckels DD. In vitro influenza virus–specific antibody production in man: antigen-specific and HLA-restricted induction of helper activity mediated by cloned human T lymphocytes. J Immunol 1982; 129:1465–1470.
101. Lamb JR, Woody JN, Hartzman RJ, Eckels DD. In vitro influenza virus specific antibody production in man: antigen-specific and HLA-restricted induction of helper activity mediated by cloned human T lymphocytes. J Immunol 1982; 129:1465–1470.
102. Hackett CJ, Deitzschold B, Gerhard W, Knorr R, Gillessen D, Melchers F. Influenza virus site recognized by a murine helper T cell specific for H1 strains:

localization to a nine amino acid sequence in the hemagglutinin molecule. J Exp Med 1983; 158:294–302.
103. Biddison WE, Sharrow SO, Shearer GM. T cell subpopulations required for the human cytotoxic T lymphocyte response to influenza virus: evidence for T cell help. J Immunol 1981; 127:487–491.
104. Reiss CS, Burakoff SJ. Specificity of the helper T cell for the cytotoxic T lymphocyte response to influenza viruses. J Exp Med 1981; 154:541.
105. Topham DJ, Tripp RA, Sarawar SR, Sangster MY, Doherty PC. Immune $CD4^+$ T cells promote the clearance of influenza virus from major histocompatibility complex class II -/- respiratory epithelium. J Virol 1996; 70:1288–1291.
106. Baumgarth N, Brown L, Jackson D, Kelso A. Novel features of the respiratory tract T-cell response to influenza virus infection: lung T cells increase expression of gamma interferon mRNA in vivo and maintain high levels of mRNA expression for interleukin-5 (IL-5) and IL-10). J Virol 1994; 68:7575–7581.
107. Sarawar SR, Carding SR, Allan W, McMickle A, Gujihashi D, Kiyono H, McGhee JR, Doherty PC. Cytokine profiles in bronchoalveolar lavage cells from mice with influenza pneumonia: consequences of CD4+ and CD8+ T cell depletion. Reg Immunol 1993; 5:142–150.
108. Graham MB, Braciale VL, Braciale TJ. Influenza virus-specific CD4+ T helper type 2 T lymphocytes do not promote recovery from experimental virus infection. J Exp Med 1994; 180:1273–1282.
109. Sarawar SR, Sangster M, Coffman RL, Doherty PC. Administration of anti–IFN-γ antibody to B2-microglobulin–deficient mice delays influenza virus clearance but does not switch the response to a Tc helper cell 2 phenotype. J Immunol 1994; 153:1246–1253.
110. Baumgarth N, Kelso A. In vivo blockade of gamma interferon affects the influenza virus–induced humoral and the local cellular immune response in lung tissue. J Virol 1996; 70:4411–4418.
111. Moran TM, Isobe H, Fernandez-Sesma A, Shulman JL. Interleukin-4 causes delayed virus clearance in influenza virus–infected mice. J Virol 1996; 70:5230–5235.
112. Hashimoto G, Wright PF, Karzon DT. Antibody-dependent cell-mediated cytotoxicity against influenza virus–infected cells. J Infect Dis 1983; 148:785–794.
113. Fleischer B, Becht H, Rott R. Recognition of viral antigens by human influenza A virus–specific T lymphocyte clones. J Immunol 1985; 165:2800–2804.
114. Braciale TJ. Immunologic recognition of influenza virus–infected cells. II. Expression of influenza A matrix protein on the infected cell surface and its role in recognition by cross-reactive cytotoxic T cells. J Exp Med 1977; 146:673–689.
115. Yewdell JW, Hackett CJ. The specificity and function of T lymphocytes induced by influenza A viruses. In: Krug R, ed. The Influenza Viruses. New York: Plenum Press, 1989:361–429.
116. Lin Y-L, Askonas BA. Biologic properties of an influenza A virus–specific killer T cell clone. Inhibition of virus replication in vivo and induction of delayed-type hypersensitivity reactions. J Exp Med 1981; 154:225–234.
117. Lukacher AE, Braciale VL, Braciale TJ. In vivo effector function of influenza virus–specific cytotoxic T lymphocyte clones is highly specific. J Exp Med 1984; 160:814–826.

118. Taylor PM, Askonas BA. Influenza nucleoprotein–specific cytotoxic T-cell clones are protective in vivo. Immunology 1986; 58:417–420.
119. Yap KL, Ada GL, McKenzie IFC. Transfer of specific cytotoxic T lymphocytes protects mice inoculated with influenza virus. Nature 1978; 273:238–239.
120. MacKenzie CD, Taylor PM, Askonas BA. Rapid recovery of lung histology correlates with clearance of influenza virus by specific $CD8^+$ cytotoxic cells. Immunology 1989; 67:375–381.
121. Reiss CS, Schulman JL. Cellular immune responses of mice to influenza virus infection. Cell Immunol 1980; 56:502–506.
122. Eichelberger M, Allan W, Zijlstra M, Jaenisch R, Doherty PC. Clearance of influenza virus respiratory infection in mice lacking class I major histocompatibility complex–restricted T cells. J Exp Med 1991; 174:875–880.
123. Scherle PA, Palladino G, Gerhard W. Mice can recover from pulmonary influenza virus infection in the absence of class-I–restricted cytotoxic T cells. J Immunol 1992; 148:212–217.
124. Epstein SL, Misplon JA, Lawson CM, Subbarao EK, Connors M, Murphy BR. Beta 2-microglobulin–deficient mice can be protected against influenza A infection by vaccination with vaccinia-influenza recombinants expressing hemagglutinin and neuraminidase. J Immunol 1993; 150:5484–5493.
125. Ennis FA. Some newly recognized aspects of resistance against and recovery from influenza. Arch Virol 1982; 73:207–217.
126. McMichael AJ, Gotch FM, Noble GR, Beare PAS. Cytotoxic T-cell immunity to influenza. N Engl J Med 1983; 309:13–17.
127. Treanor J, Kawaoka Y, Miller R, Webster RG, Murphy BR. Nucleotide sequence of the avian influenza A/Mallard/NY/6750 virus polymerase genes. Virus Res 1980; 14:257–270.
128. Treanor JJ, Murphy B. Genes involved in the restriction of replication of avian influenza A viruses in primates. In: Kirstak E, ed. Virus Variability, Epidemiology, and Control. New York: Plenum Press, 1990:159–176.
129. Whimbey E, Eling LS, couch RB, Lo W, Williams L, Champlin RE, Bodey GP. Influenza A virus infection among hospitalized adult bone marrow transplant recipients. Bone Marrow Transplant 1994; 13:437–440.
130. Glezen WP. Serious morbidity and mortality associated with influenza epidemics. Epidemiol Rev 1982; 4:24–44.
131. Perrotta DM, Decker M, Glezen WP. Acute respiratory disease hospitalizations as a measure of impact of epidemic influenza. Am J Epidemiol 1985; 122:468–476.
132. Blaine WB, Luby JP, Martin SM. Severe illness with influenza B. Am J Med 1980; 68:181–189.
133. Glezen WP, Keitel WA, Taber LH, Piedra PA, Clover RC, Couch RB. Age distribution of patients with medically-attended illnesses caused by sequential variants of influenza A/H1N1: comparison to age-specific infection rates, 1978–1989. Am J Epidemiol 1991; 133:296–304.
134. Barker WH, Mullooly JP. Impact of epidemic type A influenza in a defined adult population. Am J Epidemiol 1980; 112:798–813.
135. CDC. Prevention and control of influenza: recommendations of the Immunization Practices Advisory Committee (ACIP). MMWR 1992; 41:1–17.

136. Safrin S, Rush JD, Mills J. Influenza in patients with human immunodeficiency virus infection. Chest 1990; 98:33–37.
137. Schoenbaum SC. Impact of influenza in persons and populations. In: Brown LE, Hampson AW, Webster RG, eds. Options for the Control of Influenza III. New York: Elsevier, 1996:17–25.
138. Kavet J. A perspective on the significance of pandemic influenza. Am J Public Health 1977; 67:1063–1070.
139. Yorke MA, Nathanson N, Pianigiani G, Martin J. Seasonality and the requirements for perpetuation and eradication of viruses in populations. Am J Epidemiol 1979; 109:103–123.
140. Schaffer FL, Soergel ME, Straube DC. Survival of airborne influenza virus: effects of propagating host, relative humidity, and composition of spray fluids. Arch Virol 1976; 54:263–273.
141. Webster RG, Bean WJ, Gorman OT, Chambers TM, Kawaoka Y. Evolution and ecology of influenza A viruses. Microbiol Rev 1992; 56:152–179.
142. Kilbourne ED. Influenza. New York: Plenum Press, 1987.
143. Stevens DJ, Douglas AR, Skehel JJ, Wiley DC. Antigenic and amino acid sequence analysis of the variants of H1N1 influenza virus in 1986. Bull WHO 1987; 65:177–180.
144. Webster RG, Kendal AP, Gerhard W. Analysis of antigenic drift in recently isolated influenza A (H1N1) viruses using monoclonal antibody preparations. Virology 1979; 96:258–264.
145. Yamashita M, Krystal M, Fitch WM, Palese P. Influenza B virus evolution: co-circulating lineages and comparison of evolutionary patterns with those of influenza A and C viruses. Virology 1988; 163:112–122.
146. Xu X, Cox NJ, Bender CA, Regnery HL, Shaw MW. Genetic variation in the neuraminidase genes of influenza A (H3N2) viruses. Virology 1996; 224:175–183.
147. Rohm C, Zhou N, Suss J, Mackenzi J, Webster RG. Characterization of a novel influenza hemagglutinin, H15: criteria for determination of influenza A subtypes. Virology 1996; 217:508–515.
148. Colman PM, Ward CW. Structure and diversity of influenza virus neuraminidase. Curr Top Microbiol Immunol 1985; 11:177–255.
149. Kawaoka Y, Krauss S, Webster RG. Avian-to-human transmission of the PB1 gene of influenza A viruses in the 1957 and 1968 pandemics. J Virol 1989; 63:4603–4608.
150. Bean WJ, Schell M, Katz J, Kawaoka Y, Naeve C, Gorman O, Webster RG. Evolution of the H3 hemagglutinin from human and nonhuman hosts. J Virol 1992; 66:1129–1138.
151. Shu LL, Zhou NN, Sharp GB, He SQ, Zhang TJ, Webster RG. An epidemiological study of influenza viruses among Chinese farm families with household ducks and pigs. Epidemiol Infect 1996; 117:179–188.
152. Zhou N, He S, Zhang T, Zhou W, Shu L, Sharp GB, Webster RG. Influenza infection in humans and pigs in southeastern China. Arch Virol 1996; 141:649–661.
153. Castrucci MR, Donatelli I, Sidoli I, Barigazzi G, Kawaoka Y, Webster RG. Genetic reassortment between avian and human influenza A viruses in Italian pigs. Virology 1993; 193:503–506.

154. Webster RG, Wright SM, Castrucci MR, Bean WJ, Kawaoka Y. Influenza—a model of an emerging virus disease. Intervirology 1993; 35:16–25.
155. Schafer JR, Kawaoka Y, Bean WJ, Suss J, Senne D, Webster RG. Origin of the pandemic 1957 H2 influenza A virus and the persistence of its possible progenitors in the avian reservoir. Virology 1993; 194:781–788.
156. Shortridge KF. The next pandemic influenza virus? Lancet 1995; 346:1210–1212.
157. Henderson FW, Collier AM, Sanyal MA, Watkins JM, Fairclough DL, Clyde WA Jr, Denny FW. A longitudinal study of respiratory viruses and bacteria in the etiology of acute otitis media with effusion. N Engl J Med 1982; 306:1377–1383.
158. Chonmaitree T, Howie V, Truant A. Presence of respiratory viruses in middle ear fluids and nasal wash specimens from children with acute otitis media. Pediatrics 1986; 77:698–702.
159. Howard JB. Influenza A2 virus as a cause of croup requiring tracheostomy. J Pediatr 1972; 81:1148–1150.
160. Kim HW, Brandt CD, Arrobio JO, Murphy B, Chanock RM, Parrott RH. Influenza A and B virus infection in infants and young children during the years 1957–1976. Am J Epidemiol 1979; 109:464–479.
161. Sable CA, Hayden FG. Orthomyxoviral and paramyxoviral infections in transplant recipients. Infect Transplant 1995; 9:987–1003.
162. Schwarzmann SW, Adler JL, Sullivan RFJ, Marine WM. Bacterial pneumonia during the Hong King influenza epidemic of 1968–1969. Arch Intern Med 1971; 127:1037–1041.
163. Dietzman DE, Schaller JG, Ray CG, Reed ME. Acute myositis associated with influenza B infection. Pediatrics 1976; 57:255–258.
164. Hildebrandt HM, Massab HF, Willis PWI. Influenza virus pericarditis. Am J Dis Child 1962; 104:579–582.
165. MacDonald KL, Osterholm MT, Hedberg CW, Schrock CG, Peterson GF, Jentzen JM, Lenoard SA, Schlievert PM. Toxic shock syndrome: a newly recognized complication of influenza and influenza like illness. JAMA 1987; 257:1053–1058.
166. Hurwitz ES, Nelson DB, Davis C, Morens D, Schonberger LN. National surveillance for Reye's syndrome: a five-year review. Pediatrics 1982; 70:895–900.
167. Barrett MJ, Hurwitz ES, Schonberger LB, Rogers MF. Changing epidemiology of Reye's syndrome in the United States. Pediatrics 1986; 77:598–602.
168. Espy MJ, Smith TF, Harmon MW, Kendal AP. Rapid detection of influenza virus by shell vial assay with monoclonal antibodies. J Clin Microbiol 1986; 24:677–679.
169. Daisy JA, Lief FS, Friedman HW. Rapid diagnosis of influenza A infection by direct immunofluorescence of nasaopharyngeal aspirates in adults. J Clin Microbiol 1979; 9:688–692.
170. Walls HH, Johansson KH, Harmon MW, Halonen PE, Kendal AP. Time-resolved fluoroimmunoassay with monoclonal antibodies for rapid diagnosis of influenza infections. J Clin Microbiol 1986; 24:907–912.
171. Coonrod JD, Betts RF, Linnema– CC Jr, Hsu LC. Etiologic diagnosis of influenza A virus by enzymatic radioimmunoassay. J Clin Microbiol 1984; 19:361–365.
172. Harmon MW, Pawlik KM. Enzyme immunoassay for direct detection of influenza type A and adenovirus antigens in clinical specimens. J Clin Microbiol 1982; 15:5–11.

173. Waner JL, Todd SJ, Shalaby H, Murphy M, Wall LV. Comparison of directigen FLU-A with viral isolation and direct immunofluorescence for the rapid detection and identification of influenza A virus. J Clin Microbiol 1991; 29:479–482.
174. Doller G, Schuy W, Tjhen KY, Stekeler B, Gerth H-J. Direct detection of influenza virus antigen in nasopharyngeal specimens by direct enzyme immunoassay in comparison with quantitating virus shedding. J Clin Microbiol 1992; 30:866–869.
175. Ryan-Pourier KA, Katz JM, Webster RG, Kawaoka Y. Application of directigen FLU-A for the detection of influenza A virus in human and non-human specimens. J Clin Microbiol 1992; 30:1072–1075.
176. Class ECJ, Sprenger MJW, Kleter GEM, van Beek R, Quint WGV, Masurel N. Type-specific identification of influenza viruses A, B, and C by the polymerase chain reaction. J Virol Methods 1992; 39:1–13.
177. Pisareva M, Bechtereva T, Plyusnin A, Dobretsova A, Kisselev O. PCR-amplification of influenza A virus specific sequences. Arch Virol 1992; 125:313–318.
178. Katz JM, Wang M, Webster RG. Direct sequencing of the HA gene of influenza (H3N2) reveals sequence identity with mammalian cell-grown virus. J Virol 1990; 64:1808–1811.
179. Kilbourne ED. Comparative efficacy of neuraminidase-specific and conventional influenza virus vaccines in induction of antibody to neuraminidase in humans. J Infect Dis 1976; 134:384–394.
180. Cate TR, Couch RB, Parker D, Baxter B. Reactogenicity, immunogenicity, and antibody persistence in adults given inactivated influenza virus vaccines—1978. Rev Infect Dis 1983; 5:737–747.
181. Quinnan GV, Schooley R, Dolin R, Ennis FA, Gross P, Dwaltney JM Jr. Serologic responses and systemic reactions in adults after vaccination with monovalent A/USSR/77 and trivalent A/USSR/77, A/Texas/77, B/Hong Kong/72 influenza vaccines. Rev Infect Dis 1983; 5:748–757.
182. Wright PF, Cherry JD, Foy HM, Glezen WP, Hall CB, McIntosh K, Monto AS, Parrott RH, Protnoy B, Taber LH. Antigenicity and reactogenicity of influenza A/USSR/77 virus vaccine in children—a multicenter evaluation of dosage and toxicity. Rev Infect Dis 1983; 5:758–764.
183. LaMontagne JR, Noble GR, Quinnan GV, Curlin GT, Blackwelder WC, Smith JI, Ennis FA, Bozeman FM. Summary of clinical trials of inactivated influenza vaccine—1978. Rev Infect Dis 1983; 5:723–736.
184. Wright PF, Thompson J, Vaughn WT, Folland DS, Sell SHW, Karzon DT. Trials of influenza A/New Jersey/76 virus vaccine in normal children: an overview of age-related antigenicity and reactogenicity. J Infect Dis 1977; 136:S731–S741.
185. Johansson BE, Moran TM, Bona CA, Kilbourne DE. Immunologic responses to influenza virus neuraminidase is influenced by prior experience with the associated viral hemagglutinin. III. Reduced generation of neuraminidase-specific helper T cells in hemagglutinin-primed mice. J Immunol 1987; 139:2015–2019.
186. Johansson BE, Kilbourne ED. Dissociation of influenza virus hemagglutinin and neuraminidase eliminates their intravirionic antigenic competition. J Virol 1993; 67:5721–5723.

187. Wenzel RP, Hendley JO, Sande MA, Gwaltney JM Jr. Revised (1972–1973) bivalent influenza vaccine: serum and nasal antibody responses to parenteral vaccination. JAMA 1973; 226:435–438.
188. Clements ML, Murphy BR. Development and persistence of local and systemic antibody responses in adults given live attenuated or inactivated influenza A virus vaccine. J Clin Microbiol 1986; 23:66–72.
189. Mostow RA, Schoenbaum SC, Dowdle WR, Coleman MT, Kaye HS, Hierholzer JC. Studies on inactivated influenza vaccine II effect of increasing dosage on antibody response and adverse reactions in man. Am J Epidemiol 1970; 92:248–256.
190. Sullivan KM, Monto AS, Foster DA. Antibody response to inactivated influenza vaccines of various antigenic concentrations. J Infect Dis 1990; 161:333–335.
191. Remarque EJ, van Beek WC, Ligthart GJ, Borst RJA, Nagelkerken L, Palache AM, Sprenger MJW, Masurel N. Improvement of the immunoglobulin subclass response to influenza vaccine in elderly nursing-home residents by the use of high-dose vaccines. Vaccine 1993; 11:649–654.
192. Keitel WA, Couch RB, Cate TR, Hess KR, Baxter B, Quarles JM, Atmar RL, Six HR. High doses of purified influenza A virus hemagglutinin significantly augment serum and nasal secretion antibody responses in healthy young adults. J Clin Microbiol 1994; 32:2468–2473.
193. Levandowski RA, Regnery HL, Staton E, Burgess BG, Williams MS, Groothuis JR. Antibody responses to influenza B viruses in immunologically unprimed children. Pediatrics 1991; 88:1031–1036.
194. Allison JE, Glezen WP, Taber LH, Paredes A, Webster RG. Reactogenicity and immunogenicity of bivalent influenza A and monovalent influenza B virus vaccines in high-risk children. J Infect Dis 1977; 136 Suppl:S672–S676.
195. Hillman BC, Jamison RM, Kirkpatrick CJ. Reactivity and antibody response to vaccination with bivalent influenza A/Victoria/75-A/New Jersey/76 vaccines in children with chronic pulmonary diseases. J Infect Dis 1977; 136(suppl):S638–S644.
196. Hall CB, Modlin JF, Hilman BC, Boyer KM, Cherry JD, Lauer BA, Lerman SJ, McIntosh K, Gross PA, Bacum RJ. Response of children with cardiac disease to the bivalent influenza A vaccines. J Infect Dis 1977; 136 Suppl:S632–S637.
197. Groothuis JR, Levin MJ, Rabalais GP, Meiklejohn G, Lauer BA. Immunization of high-risk infants younger than 18 months of age with split-product influenza vaccine. Pediatrics 1991; 87:823–828.
198. Meiklejohn G, Eickhoff TC, Graves P, Josephine I. Antigenic drift and efficacy of influenza virus vaccines, 1976–1977. J Infect Dis 1978; 138:618–624.
199. Meiklejohn G. Viral respiratory disease at Lowry Air Force Base in Denver, 1952–1982. J Infect Dis 1983; 148:775–783.
200. Ruben FL. Prevention and control of influenza: role of vaccine. Am J Med 1987; 82:31–33.
201. Barker WH, Mullooly JP. Influenza vaccination of elderly persons: reduction in pneumonia and influenza hospitalizations and deaths. JAMA 1980; 244:2547–2549.
202. Ruben FL, Johnston F, Streiff EJ. Influenza in a partially immunized population: effectiveness of killed Hong King vaccine against infection with the England strain. JAMA 1974; 230:863–866.

203. Nichol KL, Lind A, Margolis KL, Murdoch M, McFadden R, Hauge M, Magnan S, Drake M. The effectiveness of vaccination against influenza in healthy, working adults. N Engl J Med 1995; 333:889–893.
204. Govaert TM, Thijs CT, Masurel N, Sprenger MJ, Dinant GJ, Knottnerus JA. The efficacy of influenza vaccination in elderly individuals. A randomized double-blind placebo-controlled trial. JAMA 1994; 270:1956–1961.
205. Paul WS, Cowan J, Jackson GG. Acute respiratory illness among immunized and nonimmunized patients with high-risk factors during a split season of influenza A and B. J Infect Dis 1988; 157:633–639.
206. Patriarca PA, Weber JA, Parker RA, Hall WN, Kendal AP, Bregman DJ, Schonberger LB. Efficacy of influenza vaccine in nursing homes: reduction in illness and complications during an influenza A (H3N2) epidemic. JAMA 1985; 253:1136–1139.
207. Saah AJ, Neufeld R, Rodstein M, La Montagne JR, Blackwelder W, Bross P, Quinnan G, Kaslow R. Influenza vaccine and pneumonia mortality in a nursing home population. Arch Intern Med 1986; 146:2353–2357.
208. Patriarca PA, Weber JA, Parker RA, Orenstein WA, Hall WN, Kendal AP, Schonberger LB. Risk factors for outbreaks of influenza in nursing homes: a case-control study. Am J Epidemiol 1986; 124:114–119.
209. Gross PA, Quinnan GV, Rodstein M, LaMontagne JR, Kaslow RA, Saah AJ, Wallenstein S, Neufeld R, Denning C, Gaerlan P. Association of influenza immunization with reduction in mortality in an elderly population: a prospective study. Arch Intern Med 1988; 148:562–565.
210. Betts RF, Dolin R, Treanor JJ, Roth FK, O'Brien D, Erb S. Inactivated influenza vaccine reduces frequency and severity of illness in the elderly (abstr 289). In: 24th Interscience Conference on Antimicrobial Agents and Chemotherapy. Washington, DC: American Society for Microbiology, 1984.
211. Fedson DS, Wajda A, Nicol JP, Hammond GW, Kalser DL, Roos LL. Clinical effectiveness of influenza vaccination in Manitoba. JAMA 1993; 270:1956–1961.
212. Nichol KL, Margolis KL, Wuorenma J, Von Sternberg T. The efficacy and cost effectiveness of vaccination against influenza among elderly persons living in the community. N Engl J Med 1994; 331:778–784.
213. Pabico RC, Douglas RG Jr, Betts RF, McKenna BA, Freeman RB. Influenza vaccination of patients with glomerular diseases: effects on creatinine clearance, urinary protein excretion, and antibody response. Ann Intern Med 1974; 81:171–177.
214. Osanloo EO, Berlin BS, Popli S, Ing TS, Cummings JE, Gandhi VC, Geis WP, Hano JE. Antibody responses to influenza vaccination in patients with chronic renal failure. Kidney Int 1978; 14:614–618.
215. Jordan MC, Rousseau WE, Tegtmeier GE, Noble GR, Muth RG, Chin TD. Immunogenicity of inactivated influenza virus vaccine in chronic renal failure. Ann Intern Med 1973; 79:790–794.
216. Pabico RC, Douglas RG Jr, Betts RF, McKenna BA, Freeman RB. Antibody response to influenza vaccination in renal transplant patients: correlation with allograft function. Ann Intern Med 1976; 85:431–436.

217. Stiver HG, Graves P, Meiklejohn G, Schroter G, Eickhoff TC. Impaired serum antibody response to inactivated influenza A and B vaccine in renal transplant recipients. Infect Immun 1977; 16:738–741.
218. Kumar SS, Ventura AK, VanderWerf B. Influenza vaccination in renal transplant recipients. JAMA 1978; 239:840–842.
219. Versluis DJ, Beyer WE, Masurel N, Wenting GJ, Weimar W. Impairment of the immune response to influenza vaccination in renal transplant recipients by cyclosporine, but not azathioprine. Transplantation 1986; 42:376–379.
220. Huang KL, Armstron JA, Ho M. Antibody response after influenza immunization in renal transplant patients receiving cyclosporin A or azathioprine. Infect Immun 1983; 40:421–424.
221. Chalmers A, Scheifele D, Patterson C, Williams D, Weber J, Shuckett R, Teufel A. Immunization of patients with rheumatoid arthritis against influenza: a study of vaccine safety and immunogenicity. J Rheumatol 1994; 21:1203–1206.
222. Brodman R, Gilfillan R, Glass D, Schur PH. Influenzal vaccine response in systemic lupus erythematosis. Ann Intern Med 1978; 88:735–740.
223. Williams GW, Steinberg AD, Reinertsen JL, Klassen LW, Decker JL, Dolin R. Influenza immunization in systemic lupus erythematosus: a double-blind trial. Ann Intern Med 1978; 88:729–734.
224. Nelson KE, Clements ML, Miotti P, Cohn S, Polk BF. The influence of human immunodeficiency virus (HIV) infection on antibody resonses to influenza vaccines. Ann Intern Med 1988; 109:383–388.
225. O'Brien WA, Ferbas-Grovit K, Namazi A, Ovcak-Derzic S, Wnag H-J, Park J, Yermian C, Mao S-H, Zack JA. Human immunodeficiency virus-type 1 replication can be increased in peripheral blood of seropositive patients after influenza vaccination. Blood 1995; 86:1082–1089.
226. Kubiet MA, Gonzelez-Rothi RJ, Cottey R, Bender BS. Serum antibody response to influenza vaccine in pulmonary patients receiving corticosteroids. Chest 1996; 110:367–370.
227. Park CL, Frank AL, Sullivan M, Jindal P, Baxter BD. Influenza vaccination of children during acute asthma exacerbation and concurrent prednisone therapy. Pediatrics 1996; 98:196–200.
228. Stenius-Aarniala B, Huttunen JK, Pyhala R, Haahtela T, Jokela P, Jukkara A, Karakorpi T, Kataja M, Kava T, Kussisto P, Lahdensuo A, Mansury L, Niemisto M, Taivianen A, Vaara S, Vesterinen E. Lack of clinical exacerbations in adults with chronic asthma after immunication with killed influenza virus. Chest 1986; 89:786–789.
229. Davies R, Pepys J. Egg allergy, influenza vaccine, and immunoglobulin E antibody. J Allergy Clin Immunol 1976; 57:373–383.
230. Carter ML, Renzulio PO, Helgerson SD, Martin SM, Jekel JF. Influenza outbreaks in nursing homes: how effective is influenza vaccine in the institutionalized elderly? Infect Control Hosp Epidemiol 1986; 11:473–478.
231. Arden NH, Patriarca PA, Kendal AP. Experiences in the use and efficacy of inactivated influenza vaccine in nursing homes. In: Options for the Control of Influenza. Keystone, CO: Liss, 1986:155–168.

232. Arroyo JC, Postic B, Brown A, Harrison K, Birgenheier R, Dowda H. Influenza A/Philippines/2/82 outbreak in a nursing home: limitations of influenza vaccination in the aged. Am J Infect Control 1984; 12:329–334.
233. Powers DC, Belshe RB. Effect of age on cytotoxic T lymphocyte memory as well as serum and local antibody responses elicited by inactivated influenza vaccine. J Infect Dis 1993; 197:584–592.
234. Nicholson KG, Baker DJ, Chakraverty P, Parquhar A, Hurd D, Kent J, Litton PA, Smith SH. Immunogenicity of inactivated influenza vaccine in residential homes for elderly people. Age Ageing 1992; 21:182–188.
235. Coles FB, Balzano GJ, Morse DL. An outbreak of influenza A (H3N2) in a well immunized nursing home population. J Am Geriatr Soc 1992; 40:589–592.
236. Treanor J, Dumyati G, O'Brien D, Riley MA, Riley G, Erb S, Betts R. Evaluation of cold-adapted, reassortment influenza B virus vaccines in elderly and chronically ill adults. J Infect Dis 1994; 169:402–407.
237. Glathe H, Bigl S, Grosche A. Comparison of humoral immune responses to trivalent influenza split vaccine in young, middle-aged and elderly people. Vaccine 1993; 11:702–705.
238. Powers DC. Effect of age on serum immunoglobulin G subclass antibody responses to inactivated influenza virus vaccine. J Med Virol 1994; 43:57–61.
239. Gross PA, Quinnan GV, Weksler ME, Setia U, Douglas RG Jr. Relation of chronic disease and immune response to influenza vaccine in the elderly. Vaccine 1989; 7:303.
240. Pozzetto B, Odelin MF, Bienvenu J, Defayolle M, Aymard M. Is there a relationship between malnutrition, inflammation, and post-vaccinal antibody response to influenza viruses in the elderly? J Med Virol 1993; 41:39–43.
241. al-Mazron A, Scheiflele DW, Soong T, Bjornson G. Comparison of adverse reactions to whole-virion and split virion influenza vaccines in hospital personnel. Can Med Assoc J 1991; 145:213–218.
242. McElhaney JE, Meneilly GS, Lechelt KE, Beattie BL, Bleackley RC. Antibody response to whole-virus and split-virus influenza vaccines in successful ageing. Vaccine 1993; 11:1055–1060.
243. McElhaney JE, Meneilly GS, Lechelt KE, Bleackley RC. Split-virus influenza vaccines: do they provide adequate immunity in the elderly? J Gerontol 1994; 49:M37–M43.
244. Zei T, Neri M, Iorio AM. Immunogenicity of trivalent subunit and split influenza vaccines (1989–90 winter season) in volunteers of different groups of age. Vaccine 1991; 9:613–617.
245. Johnson PR, Feldman S, Thompson JM, Mahoney JD, Wright PF. Immunity to influenza A virus infection in young children: a comparison of natural infection, live cold-adapted vaccine, and inactivated vaccine. J Infect Dis 1986; 154:121–127.
246. MacKenzie JS. Influenza subunit vaccine: antibody response to one and two doses of vaccine and length of response, with particular reference to the elderly. Br Med J 1977; 1(6055):200–202.
247. Hoskins TW, Davies JR, Smith AJ, Miller CL, Allchin A. Assessment of inactivated influenza A vaccine after three outbreaks of influenza A at Christ's Hospital. Lancet 1979; 1:33–35.

248. Keitel WA, Cate TR, Couch RB. Efficacy of sequential annual vaccination with inactivated influenza virus vaccine. Am J Epidemiol 1988; 127:353–364.
249. Katz JM, Webster RG. Efficacy of inactivated influenza A virus (H3N2) vaccines grown in mammalian cells or embryonated eggs. J Infect Dis 1989; 160: 191–198.
250. Wood JM, Oxford JS, Dunleavy U, Newman RW, Major D, Robertson JS. Influenza A (H1N1) vaccine efficacy in animal models is influenced by two amino acid substitutions in the hemagglutinin molecule. Virology 1989; 171:214–221.
251. Robertson JS, Bootman JS, Newman R, Oxford JS, Daniels RD, Webster RG, Shcild GC. Structural changes in the haemagglutinin which accompany egg adaptation of an influenza A (H1N1) virus. Virology 1987; 160:31–37.
252. Robertson JS, Bootman JS, Nicolson C, Major D, Robertson EW, Wood JM. The hemagglutinin of influenza B virus present in clinical material is a single species identical to that of mammalian cell-grown virus. Virology 1990; 179:35–40.
253. Robertson JS, Nicolson C, Bootman JS, Major D, Robertson EW, Wood JM. Sequence analysis of the haemagglutinin (HA) of influenza A (H1N1) viruses present in clinical material and comparison with the HA of laboratory-derived virus. J Gen Virol 1991; 72:2671–2677.
254. Rocha EP, Xu X, Hall EH, Allen JR, Regnery HL, Cox NJ. Comparison of 10 influenza A (H1N1 and H3N2) haemagglutinin sequences obtained directly from clinical specimens to those of MDCK cell- and egg-grown viruses. J Gen Virol 1993; 74:2513–2518.
255. Wang M, Katz JM, Webster RG. Extensive heterogeneity in the hemagglutinin of egg-grown influenza viruses from different patients. Virology 1989; 171: 275–279.
256. Katz JM, Webster RG. Antigenic and structural characterization of multiple subpopulations of H3N2 influenza virus from an individual. Virology 1988; 165: 446–456.
257. Katz JM, Webster RG. Amino acid sequence identity between the HA1 of influenza A (H3N2) viruses grown in mammalian and primary chick kidney cells. J Gen Virol 1992; 73:1159–1165.
258. Govorkova EA, Kaverin NV, Gubareva LV, Meignier B, Webster RG. Replication of influenza A viruses in a green monkey continuous cell line (Vero). J Infect Dis 1995; 172:250–253.
259. Powers DC, Smith GE, Anderson EL, Kennedy DJ, Hackett CS, Wilkinson BE, Volvovitz F, Belshe RB, Treanor JJ. Influenza A virus vaccines containing purified recombinant H3 hemagglutinin are well-tolerated and induce protective immune responses in healthy adults. J Infect Dis 1995; 171:1595–1598.
260. Treanor JJ, Betts RF, Smith GE, Anderson EL, Hackett CS, Wilkinson BE, Beshe RB, Powers DC. Evaluation of a recombinant hemagglutinin expressed in insect cells as an influenza vaccine in young and elderly adults. J Infect Dis 1996; 173: 1467–1470.
261. Lakey DL, Treanor JJ, Betts RF, Smith GE, Thompson J, Sannella E, Reed G, Wilkinson BE, Wright PF. Recombinant baculovirus influenza A hemagglutinin vaccines are well tolerated and immunogenic in healthy adults. J Infect Dis 1996; 174:838–841.

262. Clements ML, Betts RF, Murphy BR. Advantage of live attenuated cold-adapted influenza A virus over inactivated vaccine for A/Washington/80 (H3N2) wild-type virus infection. Lancet 1984; 1:704–708.
263. Rudenko LG, Slepushkin AN, Monto AS, Kendal AP, Grigorieva EP, Burtseva EP, Rekstin AR, Beljaev AL, Bragina VE, Cox N, Ghendon YZ, Alexandrova GI. Efficacy of live attenuated and inactivated influenza vaccines in schoolchildren and their unvaccinated contacts in Novgorod, Russia. J Infect Dis 1993; 168:881–887.
264. Chanock RM, Murphy BR. Use of temperature-sensitive and cold-adapted mutant viruses in the immunoprophylaxis of acute respiratory tract disease. Rev Infect Dis 1980; 2:421–432.
265. Wright PF, Karzon DT. Live attenuated influenza vaccines. Prog Med Virol 1987; 34:70–88.
266. Murphy BR, Wood FT, Massicot JG, Spring SB, Chanock RM. Temperature-sensitive mutants of influenza virus. XV. The genetic and biologic characterization of a recombinant influenza virus containing two *ts* lesions produced by mating two complementing, single lesion *ts* mutants. Virology 1978; 88:231–243.
267. Murphy BR, Buckler-White AJ, London WT, Harper J, Tierney EL, Miller NT, Reck LJ, Chanock RM, Hinshaw VS. Avian-human reassortant influenza V viruses derived by mating avian and human influenza A viruses. J Infect Dis 1984; 150:841–850.
268. Tolpin MD, Massicot JG, Mullinix MG, Kim HW, Parrott RH, Chanock RM, Murphy BR. Genetic factors associated with loss of the temperature-sensitive phenotype of the influenza A/Alaska/77-*ts*-1A2 recombinant g\during growth *in vivo*. Virology 1981; 112:505–517.
269. Steinhoff MC, Halsey NA, Wilson MH, Burns BA, Samorodin RK, Fries LF, Murphy BR, Clements ML. Comparison of live, attenuated cold-adapted and avian-human influenza A/Bethesda/85 (H3N2) reassortant virus vaccines in infants and children. J Infect Dis 1990; 162:394–401.
270. Steinhoff MC, Halsey NA, Wilson MH, King J, Burns BA, Samorodin RK, Perkis V, Murphy Br, Clements ML. The A/Mallard/6750/78 avian-human, but not the A/Ann Arbor/6/60 cold-adapted, influenza A/Kawasaki/ (H1N1) reassortant virus vaccine retains partial virulence for infants and children. J Infect Dis 1991; 165:1023–1028.
271. Maassab HF, DeBorde DC. Development and characterization of cold-adapted viruses for use as live virus vaccines. Vaccine 1985; 3:335–369.
272. Murphy BR. Use of live, attenuated cold-adapted influenza A reassortant virus vaccines in infants, children, young adults, and elderly adults. Infect Dis Clin Pract 1993; 2:176–181.
273. Snyder MH, Betts RF, DeBorde D, Tierney EL, Clements ML, Herrington D, Sears SD, Dolin R, Maassab HF, Murphy BR. Four viral genes independently contribute to attenuation of live influenza A/Ann Arbor/6/60 (H2N2) cold-adapted reassortant virus vaccines. J Virol 1988; 62:488–495.
274. Subbarao EK, Perkins M, Treanor JJ, Murphy BR. The attenuation phenotype conferred by the M gene of the influenza A/Ann Arbor/6/60 cold-adapted virus

(H2N2) on the A/Korea/82 (H3N2) reassortant virus results from a gene constellation effect. Virus Res 1992; 25:37–50.
275. Anderson EL, Newman FK, Maassab HF, Belshe RB. Evaluation of a cold-adapted influenza B/Texas/84 reassortant virus (CRB-87) vaccine in young children. J Clin Microbiol 1992; 30:2230–2234.
276. Keitel WA, Couch RB, Cate TR, Six HR, Baxter BD. Cold-recombinant influenza B/Texas/1/84 virus vaccine: attenuation, immunogenicity, and efficacy against homotypic challenge. J Infect Dis 1990; 161:22–26.
277. Clements ML, Snyder MH, Sears SD, Maassab HF, Murphy BR. Evaluation of the infectivity, immunogenicity, and efficacy of live cold-adapted influenza B/Ann Arbor/1/86 reassortant virus in adult volunteers. J Infect Dis 1990; 161:869–877.
278. Edwards KM, King JC, Steinhoff MD, Thompson J, Clements ML, Wright PF, Murphy BR. Safety and immunogenicity of live attenuated cold adapted influenza B/Ann Arbor/1/86 virus vaccine in infants and children. J Infect Dis 1991; 163:740–745.
279. Treanor JJ, Betts RF. Evaluation of live attenuated cold-adapted influenza B/Yamagata/16/88 reassortant virus vaccine in healthy adults. J Infect Dis 1993; 168:455–459.
280. Snyder MH, London WT, Maassab HF, Murphy BR. Attenuation and phenotypic stability of influenza B/Texas/1/84 cold-adapted reassortant virus: studies in hamsters and chimpanzees. J Infect Dis 1989; 160:604–610.
281. Piedra PA, Glezen WP. Influenza in children: epidemiology, immunity, and vaccines. Semin Pediatr Infect Dis 1992; 2:140–146.
282. Gruber WC, Belshe RB, King JC, Treanor JJ, Piedra PA, Wright PF, Reed GW, Anderson E, Newman F. Evaluation of live attenuated influenza vaccines in children 6–18 months of age: safety, immunogenicity, and efficacy. J Infect Dis 1996; 173:1313–1319.
283. Edwards KM, Dupont WD, Westrich MK, Plummer WDJ, Palmer PS, Wright PF. A randomized controlled trial of cold-adapted and inactivated vaccines for the prevention of influenza A disease. J Infect Dis 1994; 169:68–76.
284. Powers DC, Fries LF, Murphy BR, Thumar JB, Clements ML. In elderly persons live attenuated influenza A virus vaccines do not offer an advantage over inactivated virus vaccine in inducing serum or secretory antibodies or local immunologic memory. J Clin Microbiol 1991; 29:498–505.
285. Gorse GJ, Belshe RB, Munn NJ. Local and systemic antibody responses in high-risk adults given live attenuated and inactivated influenza A virus vaccines. J Clin Microbiol 1988; 26:911–918.
286. Powers DC, Sears SD, Murphy BR, Thuman B, Clements ML. Systemic and local antibody responses in elderly subjects given live or inactivated influenza A virus vaccines. J Clin Microbiol 1989; 27:2666–2671.
287. Treanor JJ, Mattison HR, Dumyati G, Yinnon A, Erb S, O'Brien D, Dolin R, Betts RF. Protective efficacy of combined live intranasal and inactivated influenza A virus vaccines in the elderly. Ann Intern Med 1992; 117:625–633.
288. Keitel WA, Couch RB, Quarles JM, Cate TR, Baxter B, Maassab HF. Trivalent attenuated cold-adapted influenza virus vaccine: reduced viral shedding and serum antibody responses in susceptible adults. J Infect Dis 1993; 167:305–311.

289. Piedra PA, Glezen WP, Mbawuike I, Gruber WC, Baxter BD, Boland FJ, Byrd RW, Fan LL, Lewis JK, Rhodes LJ, Whitney SE, Taber LH. Studies on reactogenicity and immunogenicity of attenuated bivalent cold-recombinant influenza type A (CRA) and inactivated trivalent influenza vaccines (TI) in infants and young children. Vaccine 1993; 11:718–724.
290. Enami M, Luytjes W, Krystal M, Palese P. Introduction of site-specific mutations into the genome of influenza virus. Proc Natl Acad Sci (USA) 1990; 87:3802–3805.
291. Luytjes W, Krystal M, Enami M, Parvin JD, Palese P. Amplification, expression, and packaging of a foreign gene by influenza virus. Cell 1989; 59:1107–1113.
292. Barclay WS, Palese P. Influenza B viruses with site-specific mutation introduced into the HA gene. J Virol 1995; 69:1275–1279.
293. Muster T, Sabbarao EK, Enami M, Murphy BR, Palese P. An influenza A virus containing influenza B virus 5' and 3' noncoding regions on the neuraminidase gene is attenuated in mice. Proc Natl Acad Sci 1991; 88:5177–5181.
294. Cstrucci MR, Bilsel P, Kawaoka Y. Attenuation of influenza A virus by insertion of a foreign epitope into the neuraminidase. J Virol 1992; 66:4647–4653.
295. Castrucci MR, Kawaoka Y. Biologic importance of neuraminidase stalk length in influenza A viruses. J Virol 1993; 67:759–764.
296. Subbarao EK, Park EJ, Lawson CM, Chen AY, Murphy BR. Sequential addition of temperature-sensitive missense mutations into the PB2 gene of influenza A transfectant viruses can effect an increase in temperature sensitivity and attenuation and permits the rational design of a genetically engineered live influenza A virus vaccine. J Virol 1995; 69:5969–5977.
297. Li S, Polonis V, Isobe H, Zaghouani H, Guinea R, Moran T, Bona C, Palese P. Chimeric influenza virus induces neutralizing antibodies and cytotoxic T cells against human immunodeficiency virus type 1. J Virol 1993; 67:6659–6666.
298. Muster T, Ferko B, Klima A, Purtscher M, Trkola A, Schulz P, Grassauer A, Englehardt OG, Garcia-Sastre A, Palese P, Katinger H. Mucosal model of immunization against human immunodeficiency virus type 1 with a chimeric influenza virus. J Virol 1995; 69:6678–6686.
299. Wolff JA, Malone RW, Williams P, Chong W, Acsadi G, Jani A, Felgner PL. Direct gene transfer into mouse muscle in vivo. Science 1990; 247:1465–1468.
300. Ulmer JB, Donnelly JJ, Parker SE, Rhodes GH, Felgner PL, Dwarki VJ, Gromkowski SH, Deck RR, DeWitt CM, Friedman A, Hawe LA, Leander KR, Martinez D, Perry HC, Shiver JW, Montgomery DL, Liu MA. Heterologous protection against influenza by injfection of DNA encoding a viral protein. Science 1993; 259:1745–1749.
301. Robinson HL, Hunt LA, Webster RG. Protection against a lethal influenza virus challenge by immunization with a haemagglutinin-expressing plasmid DNA. Vaccine 1993; 11:957–960.
302. Donnelly JJ, Friedman A, Martinez D, Montgomery DL, Shiver JW, Motzel SL, Ulmer JB, Liu MA. Preclinical efficacy of a prototype DNA vaccine: enhanced protection against antigenic drift in influenza virus. Nature Med 1995; 1:583–587.
303. Dolin R. Antiviral chemotherapy and chemoprophylaxis. Science 1985; 227:1296–1303.

304. Douglas RG Jr. Prophylaxis and treatment of influenza. N Engl J Med 1990; 322:443–450.
305. Lubeck MD, Shulman JL, Palese P. Susceptibility of influenza A viruses to amantadine is influenced by the gene coding for the M protein. J Virol 1978; 28: 710–716.
306. Hay AJ, Wolstenholme AJ, Skehel JJ, Smith MH. The molecular basis of the specific anti-influenza action of amantadine. EMBO J 1985; 4:3021–3024.
307. Belshe RB, Smith MH, Hall CB, Betts R, Hay AJ. Genetic basis of resistance to rimantadine emerging during treatment of influenza virus infection. J Virol 1988; 62:1508–1512.
308. Richman DD, Yazaki P, Hoestetler KY. The intracellular distribution and antiviral activity of amantadine. Virology 1981; 112:81–90.
309. Richman DD, Hostetler KY, Yazaki PJ, Clark S. Fate of influenza A virion proteins after entry into subcellular fractions of LLC cells and the effect of amantadine. Virology 1986; 151:200–210.
310. Bukrinskaya AG, Vorkunova NK, Kornilayeva GV, Narmanbetova RA, Vorkunova GK. Influenza virus uncoating in infected cells and effect of rimantadine. J Gen Virol 1982; 60:49–59.
311. Ruigrok RWH, Hirst EMA, Hay AJ. The specific inhibition of influenza A virus maturation by amantadine: an electron microscopic examination. J Gen Virol 1991; 72:191–194.
312. Dolin R, Reichman RC, Madore HP, Maynard R, Linton PN, Webber-Jones J. A controlled trial of amantadine and rimantadine in the prophylaxis of influenza A in humans. N Engl J Med 1982; 307:580–584.
313. Sears SD, Clements ML. Protective efficacy of low-dose amantadine in adults challenged with wild-type influenza A virus. Antimicrob Agents Chemother 1987; 31:1470–1473.
314. Betts RF, Treanor JJ, Braman P, Bentley D, Dolin R. Antiviral agents to prevent or treat influenza in the elderly. J Respir Dis 1987; 8:S56–S59.
315. Galbraith AW, Oxford JS, Schild GC, Watson GI. Study of 1-adamantanamine hydrochloride used prophylactically during the Hong Kong influenza epidemic in the family environment. Bull WHO 1969; 41:677–682.
316. Galbraith AW, Oxford JS, Schild GC. Protective effect of 1-adamantanamine hydrochloride on influenza A2 in the family environment. Lancet 1969; 2:1026–1028.
317. Hayden FG, Belshe RB, Clover RD, Hay AJ, Oakes MG, Soo W. Emergence and apparent transmission of rimantadine-resistant influenza A virus in families. N Engl J Med 1989; 321:1696–1702.
318. Monto AS, Arden NH. Implications of viral resistance to amantadine in control of influenza A. Clin Infect Dis 1992; 15:362–367.
319. Atkinson WL, Arden NH, Patriarca PA, Leslie N, Liu K-J, Gohd R. Amantadine prophylaxis during an institutional outbreak of type A (H1N1) influenza. Arch Intern Med 1986; 146:1751–1756.
320. Arden NH, Patriarca PA, Fasano MB, Liu K-J, Harmon MW, Kendal AP, Rimland D. The roles of vaccination and amantadine prophylaxis in controlling an outbreak of influenza A (H3N2) in a nursing home. Arch Intern Med 1988; 148:865–868.

321. Mast EE, Harman MW, Gravenstein S, Wu S-P, Arden NH, Circo R, Tyska G, Kendal AP, Davis JP. Emergence and possible transmission of amantadine-resistant viruses during nursing home outbreaks of influenza A (H3N2). Am J Epidemiol 1991; 134:988–997.
322. Degelau J, Somani SK, Cooper SL, Guay DRP, Crossley KB. Amantadine-resistant influenza A in a nursing facility. Arch Intern Med 1992; 152:390–392.
323. Hayden FG, Monto AS. Oral rimantadine hydrochloride therapy of influenza A virus H3N2 subtype infection in adults. Antimicrob Agents Chemother 1986; 29: 339–341.
324. Van Voris JP, Betts RF, Hayden FG, Christmas WA, Douglas RG Jr. Successful treatment of naturally occurring influenza A/USSR/77 H1N1. JAMA 1981; 245: 1128–1131.
325. Younkin SW, Betts RF, Roth FK, Douglas RG Jr. Reduction in fever and symptoms in young adults with influenza A/Brazil/78 H1N1 infection after treatment with aspirin or amantadine. Antimicrob Agents Chemother 1983; 23:577–582.
326. Little J, Hall W, Douglas RGJ, Hyde RW, Speers DM. Amantadine effect on peripheral airways abnormalities in influenza. Ann Intern Med 1976; 85:177–182.
327. Hall CB, Dolin R, Gala CL, Markovitz DM, Zhang YQ, Madore PH, Disney FA, Talpey WB, Green JL, Francis AB, Pichichero ME. Children with influenza A infection: treatment with rimantadine. Pediatrics 1987; 80:275–282.
328. Thompson J, Fleet W, Lawrence E, Pierce E, Morris L, Wright P. A comparison of acetaminophen and rimantadine in the treatment of influenza A infection in children. J Med Virol 1987; 21:249–255.
329. Douglas RG Jr. Treatment of influenza (letter). N Engl J Med 1992; 322:1753.
330. Hayden FG, Sperber SJ, Belshe RB, Clover RD, Hay AJ, Pyke S. Recovery of drug-resistant influenza A virus during therapeutic use of rimantadine. Antimicrob Agents Chemother 1991; 35:1741–1747.
331. Belshe RB, Burk B, Newman F, Curruti RL, Sim I. Resistance of influenza A virus to amantadine and rimantadine: results of one decade of surveillance. J Infect Dis 1989; 159:430–435.
332. Bean WJ, Threlkeld SC, Webster RG. Biologic potential of amantadine-resistant influenza A virus in an avian model. J Infect Dis 1989; 159:1050–1056.
333. Sweet C, Hayden FG, Jakeman KJ, Grambas S, Hay AJ. Virulence of rimantadine-resistant human influenza A (H3N2) viruses in ferrets. J Infect Dis 1991; 164:969–972.
334. Webster RG, Kawaoka Y, Bean WJ, Beard CW, Brugh M. Chemotherapy and vaccination: a possible strategy for the control of highly virulent influenza virus. J Virol 1985; 55:173–176.
335. Webster RG, Kawaoka Y, Bean WJ. Vaccination as a strategy to reduce the emergence of amantadine- and rimantadine-resistant strains of A/Chick/Pennsylvania/83 (H5N2) influenza virus. J Antimicrob Chemother 1986; 18:157–164.
336. Tu Q, Pinto LH, Luo G, Shaughnessy MA, Jullaney D, Kurtz S, Krystal M, Lamb RA. Characterization of inhibition of M2 ion channel activity by BL-1743, an inhibitor of influenza A virus. J Virol 1996; 70:4246–4252.
337. Gilbert BE, Wilson SZ, Knight V, Couch RB, Quarles JM, Dure L, Hayes N, Willis G. Ribavirin small-particle aerosol treatment of infections caused by

influenza virus strains A/Victoria/7/83 (H1N1) and B/Texas/1/84. Antimicrob Agents Chemother 1985; 27:309–313.
338. Wilson SZ, Gilbert BE, Quarles JM, Knight V, McClung HW, Moore RV, Couch RB. Treatment of influenza A (H1N1) virus infection with ribavirin aerosol. Antimicrob Agents Chemother 1984; 26:200–203.
339. Bernstein DI, Reuman PD, Sherwood JR, Young EC, Schiff GM. Ribavirin small-particle aerosol treatment of influenza B virus infection. Antimicrob Agents Chemother 1988; 32:761–764.
340. Ray CG, Icenogle TB, Minnich LL, Copeland JG, Grogan TM. The use of intravenous ribavirin to treat influenza virus-associated acute myocarditis. J Infect Dis 1989; 159:829–836.
341. Varghese JN, Laver WG, Colman PM. Structure of the influenza glycoprotein antigen neuraminidase at 2.9A resolution. Nature 1983; 303:35–40.
342. von Itzstein M, Wu W-Y, Kok GB, Pegg MS, Dyason JC, Jin B, Phan TV, Smythe ML, White HF, Oliver SW, Colman PM, Varghese JN, Ryan DM, Woods JM, Bethell RC, Hotham VJ, Cameron JM, Penn CR. Rational design of potent sialidase-based inhibitors of influenza virus replication. Nature 1993; 363:418–423.
343. Woods JM, Bethell RC, Coates JAV, Healy N, Hiscox SA, Pearson BA, Ryan DM, Ticehurst J, Tilling J, Walcott SM, Penn CR. 4-guanidino-2,4-dideoxy-2,3-dehydro-N-acetylneuraminic acid is a highly effective inhibitor both of the sialidase (neuraminidase) and of growth of a wide range of influenza A and B viruses in vitro. Antimicrob Agents Chemother 1993; 37:1473–1479.
344. Ryan DM, Tucehurst J, Dempsey MH, Penn CR. Inhibition of influenza virus replication in mice by GG167 (4-guanidino-2,4-dideoxy-2,3,dehydro-N-Acetylneuraminic acid) is consistent with extracellular activity of viral neuraminidase (sialidase). Antimicrob Agents Chemother 1994; 38:2270–2275.
345. Hayden FG, Treanor JJ, Betts RF, Lobo M, Esinhart JD, Hussey EK. Safety and efficacy of the neuraminidase inhibitor GG167 in experimental human influenza. JAMA 1996; 275:295–299.
346. Matsumoto K, Nerome K, Numasaki Y, Oguri K, Fukuda T. Inhaled and intranasal GG167 in the treatment of influenza A and B: preliminary results. In: Bron LE, Hampson AW, Webster RG, eds. Options for the Control of Influenza III. Amsterdam: Elsevier, 1996:713–717.
347. Gubareva LV, Bethell R, Hart GJ, Murti KG, Penn CR, Webster RG. Characterization of mutants of influenza A selected with the neuraminidase inhibitor 4-guanidino-Neu5Ac2en. J Virol 1996; 70:1818–1827.
348. Murakami M, Ikeda K, Achiwa K. Chemoenzymatic synthesis of neuraminic acid analogs structurally varied at C-5 and C-9 as potential inhibitors of the sialidase from influenza virus. Carbohydrate Res 1996; 280:101–110.
349. Treanor J, Dolin R, Betts RF, Erb S, Roth F, Reichman RC. Intranasal interferon as prophylaxis against experimentally induced influenza in humans. J Infect Dis 1987; 156:379–383.
350. Fernandez-Sesma A, Schulman JL, Moran TM. A bispecific antibody recognizing influenza A virus M2 protein redirects effector cells to inhibit virus replication in vitro. J Virol 1996; 70:4800–4804.

351. O'Neill RE, Palese P. NPI-1, the human homolog of SRP-1, interacts with influenza virus nucleoprotein. Virology 1995; 206:116–125.
352. Wolff T, O'Neill RE, Palese P. Interaction cloning of NS1-I, a human protein that binds to the nonstructural NS1 proteins of influenza A and B viruses. J Virol 1996; 70:5363–5372.

7

Respiratory Syncytial Virus

EDWARD E. WALSH

University of Rochester School of
Medicine and Dentistry and
Rochester General Hospital
Rochester, New York

BARNEY S. GRAHAM

Vanderbilt University School of Medicine
Nashville, Tennessee

I. Introduction and History

In 1955, a unique virus was isolated from a laboratory chimpanzee with a respiratory illness and named "chimpanzee coryza agent" (1). In the following winter, an identical virus was recovered from two infants hospitalized with lower respiratory tract symptoms, and the virus was renamed respiratory syncytial virus (RSV) by Chanock to reflect the giant syncytia which developed during growth in tissue culture (2). During the subsequent 15 years, RSV was proven to be the most important cause of serious lower respiratory tract infection in infants and young children, causing an estimated 90,000 hospitalizations and 4500 deaths annually in the United States (3–7). The virus is also considered a significant cause of infant morbidity and mortality in developing countries (8,9). Recently, RSV has been implicated as a serious pathogen in certain adult populations, such as bone marrow transplant recipients, the frail elderly, and those with underlying cardiopulmonary diseases (10–12). Finally, primary RSV infection is suspected as a possible cause of long-term pulmonary dysfunction, especially childhood asthma (13–17).

Despite 40 years of investigation, many facets of RSV infection are not fully understood, including the pathophysiology of disease and protective immune mechanisms. Development of a vaccine is considered the most practical prospect for disease control, since antiviral therapy for RSV is costly, cumbersome to administer, and marginally efficacious (18). Unfortunately, the search for an RSV vaccine has been foiled by repeated failures and unanticipated setbacks; most notably the disastrous results of immunization with a formalin-inactivated whole virus vaccine in the 1960s (19–22). Nevertheless, recent advances in the understanding of viral genome structure and replication, the nature and function of the viral proteins, and the pathogenesis and immunology of infection support current optimism that control of RSV is possible.

II. Viral Structure and Replication

Human RSV is an enveloped RNA virus of the genus *Pneumovirus* within the family *Paramyxoviridae* and consists of two antigenically distinct groups, designated A and B (23). Other members of this genus include bovine and caprine RSV strains, pneumonia virus of mice, and turkey rhinotracheitis virus. The *Paramyxoviridae* also includes the genus *Morbillivirus* (measles virus) and *Paramyxovirus* (parainfluenza viruses 1–4 and mumps virus).

By electron microscopy, RSV has a pleomorphic spherical or filamentous form 80–350 nm in diameter and up to 10 μm in length (24). Glycoprotein spikes protrude from the lipid envelope which surrounds a tightly coiled nucleocapsid complex containing single-stranded negative-sense RNA (23). Each of the 10 viral proteins is encoded by a single gene, although two genes (M2 and G) overlap. In addition, the G protein gene contains a second open reading frame which is used during viral replication (25,26). Eight of the viral proteins are found in virions, whereas the remaining two are nonstructural proteins found only in infected cells (27).

There are two major and one minor transmembrane envelope glycoproteins. A heavily glycosylated G protein serves as the viral attachment protein, and it may exist as a homotrimer (28,29a,b). Its counterpart, the cellular receptor for RSV, has yet to be identified. The 298–amino acid backbone predicts a size of 33 kDa, although the mature protein is 85–90 kDa (30). This discrepancy is the result of posttranslational O-glycosylation which occurs at the >70 potential glycosylation sites provided by its uniquely high (30.6%) serine and threonine content (30–33). This unusual glycosylation pattern is characteristic of mucinous proteins secreted by respiratory epithelium, and it appears to be important for viral infectivity and antigenicity (34–36). Significantly, the nucleotide and amino acid sequences of the G protein from group A and B viruses contain substantial differences in the extracytoplasmic region, which allows ready strain classification by monoclonal antibody reactivity or gene sequence analysis (37–40). Antibody to G neutralizes virus in vitro, and immunization with G partially protects animals from challenge, although protection is highly group specific (41,42a). In addition to full-size G, infected cells secrete a slightly smaller soluble form of G (Gs), which is identical to virion G minus the transmembrane and intracytoplasmic regions (25,26). The role of Gs in virus infection is unknown, but recent studies suggest that it potentiates the induction of IL-5 and eosinophilia (42b). It has also been shown that G is not required for cell entry, although virus with G deleted is attenuated in its virulence (42c).

The second major transmembrane protein, the fusion protein (F) promotes fusion of the viral and cell membranes after viral attachment, allowing the viral replicative complex to enter the cell cytoplasm where transcription and translation of viral RNA occurs (43,44). During replication, expression of F protein on the cell surface induces cell-to-cell fusion, permitting viral spread without exposure to the extracellular environment (43). The F protein has a molecular weight of 70 kDa and exists as a noncovalently linked dimer (45,46). During synthesis, F is cleaved into disulfide-linked fragments (F_1 and F_2) at a cleavage-activation site (amino acids 131–136). This exposes a hydrophobic domain on F_1 which may be important in membrane fusion, cell tropism, and pathogenicity (45). The F protein carries several neutralizing epitopes, two of which are related to fusion activity, and which are highly conserved among isolates of both RSV groups (47,48). The F protein is also a target for cytotoxic T lymphocytes (CTL) (49–52). Immunization with F protein induces protective immunity to both RSV groups in experimental animals (53,54).

The third transmembrane protein is a small (7.5 kDa) hydrophobic (SH) protein which exists as multimers in infected cells and purified virions (55,56). The SH protein, in concert with the F and G proteins, contributes to the fusogenic property of the virus (57). SH does not carry neutralizing epitopes.

Unique among the paramyxoviruses, RSV has two membrane-associated matrix proteins, M and M2, which, by analogy to other paramyxoviruses, are thought to be important in virion assembly and membrane stabilization (23,58). Collins has shown that the mRNA of the 5' proximal open reading frame of M2 is a transcription-elongation factor required for viral replication, a finding important for development of live vaccines based on infectious DNA clones (59–61). Finally, the M2 protein is a target for CTL in the mouse model of RSV infection and in humans. Immunization of animals with vaccinia virus expressing M2 protein provides transient (<30 days) protection from challenge with either group A or B viruses (62–65).

The viral replicative machinery includes the N protein, a phosphorylated (P) protein, and the large (L) polymerase protein, which are bound tightly to viral RNA in a nucleocapsid complex (23,66,67). The N protein, but not P or

L, has been identified as a target of CTL (64). The two nonstructural proteins, NS1 and NS2, have no recognized functional role and do not apparently participate in the host immune response (23).

RSV grows well in many standard cell lines including HEp-2, HeLa, Vero, and fibroblasts and replicates to a lesser degree in macrophages (68). The virus also replicates well in primary human nasal and bronchial epithelial cells (69). RSV absorbs to cells relatively slowly, requiring 2 hr at room temperature for maximal attachment which parallels the cell binding kinetics of the G protein (28). Replication occurs entirely in the cell cytoplasm and virus buds from the cell membrane. Viral release begins at about 24 hr, and peak titers are approximately 10^{7-8} pfu/mL in the culture supernatant when cytopathic effect is maximal. RSV is thermolabile and 99% of infectivity is lost at 37°C in 2 days. For maximal recovery, virus should be fast frozen in dry ice–alcohol and stored at −70°C with stabilizers, such as 25% sucrose (68,70).

III. Epidemiology

A. Transmission

Humans are the only recognized natural hosts of human RSV, although bovine and ovine RSV strains are economically important causes of respiratory illness in cattle and sheep (71). There is no evidence of natural cross-species infection, although many experimental animals, such as the mouse, cotton rat, ferret, sheep and several primate species, are readily infected experimentally with human RSV (68). Infection results from direct contact with secretions from infected persons or their secretions. RSV is generally introduced into the home by school-aged children with upper respiratory symptoms, and it rapidly spreads to other members of the family, including 63% of newborns and 43% of the adults (72). Transmission is most efficient by large-particle fomites rather than by fine aerosol droplets, which is in contrast to the influenza virus (73). Thus, RSV outbreaks in closed populations tend to spread slowly rather than explosively as with influenza. Despite its relative thermolability, RSV is stable on various surfaces sufficiently long to allow dissemination from the environment (74). Inoculation of the eye or nasal mucosa by contaminated hands is considered the most common mechanism of transmission, and the use of gloves, gowns, and goggles and handwashing can interrupt nosocomial spread (75,76). Once inoculated, RSV replicates locally with an incubation period of 5 days before symptoms begin. Hospitalized infants generally shed virus for 7 days, but it can be for up to 21 days (77). Immunocompromised infants may shed virus for 30 days or more, sometimes in the absence of recognizable symptoms (78). During reinfection, viral shedding is brief; generally 1–4 days (72,79,80). In primary infection, virus titers frequently exceed 10^4

50% tissue culture infective doses ($TCID_{50}$) per milliliter of nasal wash fluid (77). Young adults shed lower quantities (10^3 $TCID_{50}$) of virus than children (72). Even lower titers of virus in nasal wash (15 pfu/mL) and bronchoalveolar lavage fluid (714 pfu/mL) from RSV-infected adult bone marrow transplant recipients have been reported by Englund (81).

B. Seasonality and Incidence

RSV causes annual winter epidemics which began in late fall and continue through early spring in temperate climates (3–6,82). In the subtropics, outbreaks occur during the rainy season. Summertime infection is considered rare, although one study from Louisiana found that 21% of infants with summer respiratory infections had RSV (83). During peak outbreak periods, other viruses with epidemic potential, such as influenza virus and parainfluenza virus 1, are usually absent from the community. This viral interference phenomena is not always apparent and mixed outbreaks, including dual infections, may occur. Fifty to 70% of infants are infected during the first year of life, with the remainder being infected by their second birthday (5). The majority of primary infections are relatively mild, although approximately 0.5–1.0% of infected infants require hospitalization with severe lower respiratory tract illness (3,85). In virtually every epidemiological investigation, RSV is the single most important cause of pneumonia and bronchiolitis in infants under the age of 1 year, accounting for 5–40% of all pneumonias, 40–90% of bronchiolitis, and 3–10% of croup cases which require hospitalization (86,87). During the peak of RSV epidemics, the virus is responsible for 70% of bronchiolitis and 55% of pneumonia cases requiring hospitalization (6).

Factors predisposing to more severe disease, but not increased infection rates, are underlying cardiopulmonary disorders (especially bronchopulmonary dysplasia and cyanotic congenital heart disease), age <3 months, prematurity, and male sex (3,6,78,88). In a study from Canada involving 1584 hospitalized infants, 16% had cardiac conditions, 13% had lung disease, 24% were premature, and 24% were less than 6 weeks of age (89). In addition, lower socioeconomic status, household crowding, exposure to cigarette smoke, and lack of breast feeding have also been associated with more serious disease.

C. Reinfections

Reinfection with RSV occurs in all age groups and reflects incomplete immunity to this virus (72,79,90). In a prospective analysis in a day-care center, Henderson found that 65–75% of previously infected infants were reinfected on reexposure (90). Although generally less severe than primary infection, 17–25% still developed signs of lower respiratory tract involvement. Underlying cardiopulmonary disease or treatment for malignancy increases the severity of reinfection (91). Infection in adults always represents reinfection, and it is generally symptomatic. In a study of nosocomial transmission of RSV on pediatric wards, half of the exposed medical staff became infected and 82% developed clinical illness (92).

In contrast to healthy young adults, immunocompromised adults and the frail elderly are at significant risk of serious complications of RSV infection (10–12,84,93–96). Between 11 and 18% of adult bone marrow transplant recipients are infected each winter (95,96). In one study, RSV accounted for half of the pathogens recovered from bone marrow transplant recipients with respiratory symptoms (96). In approximately half of these patients, the infection progressed to pneumonia with an attendant mortality of 62% overall (84,93–96). Illness severity is greatest prior to engraftment of the transplanted marrow. Among elderly adults, RSV is a significant cause of excess morbidity and mortality in both community-dwelling and institutionalized persons (10, 11,97,98). RSV outbreaks are well documented in nursing homes, and attack rates can reach 40% (99,100). In one prospective study, RSV accounted for 27% of viral respiratory illnesses in a long-term care facility during the winter (10). Illness can be severe, with rates of pneumonia ranging from 5 to 67% and mortality from 0 to 53% (10,99,100). Although the impact of RSV in the elderly is less readily apparent than in the newborn, evidence is accumulating which suggests that among community-dwelling elderly, RSV may be as serious as nonpandemic influenza (11,97,98). In England during 1991–1994, excess respiratory morbidity was temporally associated with peak RSV activity, whereas another study from the same country encompassing a 15-year period estimated that mortality associated with RSV was 60–80% more than that associated with influenza (97,98). During a 3-year period in western New York State, recent RSV infection was associated with hospitalization of elderly persons for cardiopulmonary symptoms during the winter nearly as often as influenza virus (10 vs 13%, respectively) (11). A recent study of community-acquired pneumonia in adults from Ohio identified RSV as the third most frequent cause—behind pneumococcal and influenza pneumonia (101).

D. Nosocomial Infection

Nosocomial spread of RSV is a serious concern on pediatric units during the winter months. Health-care personnel have been implicated in the transmission of virus from infected to uninfected infants, which can reach 45% of infants hospitalized longer than 1 week (92,102). Bone marrow transplant units are also prime locations for the spread of RSV with serious consequences (12,93,94). Infection-control measures can significantly reduce nosocomial infection rates.

E. Strains

During epidemics, viral strains representing both groups A and B can be isolated (37,103–112). In one study, the proportions of group A to group B viruses recovered from infected infants in 14 US cities varied markedly, suggesting that epidemics are local rather than national or global in their spread (110). Overall group A isolates are more frequent than group B viruses. In Rochester, New York, over a 15-year period (1974–1990), 71% of the isolates were group A and in only four winters were group B viruses dominant (108). Since a temporal pattern of group A and group B dominance could not be clearly discerned, immune pressure is probably not solely responsible for RSV group dynamics within a community. The effect of strain variation on clinical illness is controversial, although several studies strongly suggest that group A RSV infections are more severe than group B infections (108,111,113). In two studies from Rochester, the relative risk of severe disease was 3.3- to 6.6-fold greater for hospitalized group A–infected infants than for group B–infected infants (111,113). The mechanism of increased pathogenicity of group A strains is unknown. The role of strain variation in immunity is unclear, although one small study of 13 reinfections suggested that reinfection with the homologous virus group was less common than with a heterologous strain virus (114).

IV. Nonadaptive Immune Response to Infection

A. Epithelium

Upper airway epithelial cells are where RSV first encounters the host and leads to the release of proinflammatory cytokines and initiation of nonadaptive immune responses. A number of in vitro studies show that pulmonary epithelial cell lines produce interleukin-6 (IL-6), IL-8, IL-11, granulocyte-macrophage colony-stimulating factor (GM-CSF), and soluble tumor necrosis factor (TNF) receptor after RSV infection (115–122). Support for the in vitro data are found in studies of natural RSV infection, in which high levels of IL-6, IL-8, TNF-α, and IL-1β were detected in nasal washes from children with acute RSV lower respiratory tract disease (Neuzil, submitted) (123). In addition, children with RSV-associated otitis had increased levels of IL-1β, IL-6, and TNF-α mRNA in middle ear fluid (124). These proinflammatory cytokines have local effects on airway epithelium, and they may have direct antiviral effects (125). TNF-α reduces RSV replication in HEp-2 cells, human cord and adult blood monocytes, and alveolar macrophages in vitro (125–127). Furthermore, inhibition of TNF-α in RSV-infected mice exacerbates disease, resulting in greater weight loss and delayed recovery (125). However, the major influence of epithelium-derived proinflammatory cytokines may be on downstream immunological events, since they affect expression of cell surface adhesion molecules and major histocompatibility complex (MHC) antigens I and II and influence differentiation and activation of effectors in the adaptive immune response.

B. Interferon and Natural Killer Cells

Interferon, the prototypic innate antiviral, is poorly induced by RSV in contrast to influenza (128–130). Although interferon-α (IFN-α) is detectable in >50% of nasal wash samples of children with RSV, levels are less than half those found in influenza-infected children (126). Similarly, measurable serum IFN-α levels are less frequent and lower than with influenza (126,130,131). IFN-α levels often correlate with natural killer (NK) cell activity, but direct measurement of NK activity in RSV-infected humans has not been done. In mice, NK-cell activity occurs early after RSV challenge, peaking on day 3 following infection (132). The role of NK cells in the pathogenesis and defense of RSV has not been defined (132).

C. Macrophages

Macrophages can influence RSV-induced disease in their role as antigen-presenting cells, as a source of cytokines, and their susceptibility to infection. Human alveolar macrophages infected with RSV in vitro produce IL-6, TNF-α, and IL-8 (134). Macrophages in bronchoalveolar lavage fluid from children with RSV express IL-1β and TNF-α, and those from RSV-infected adult transplant recipients express viral proteins, class II MHC molecules, and IL-1β (135). RSV-infected human alveolar macrophages also produce IL-10 in vitro, which is an important immunoregulatory cytokine known to inhibit a variety of factors, including cytokine production, MHC class II expression, and Th1 CD4 lymphocyte differentiation (136–138). RSV-infected peripheral blood mononuclear cells also produce an uncharacterized substance that inhibits IL-1 activity; an effect not seen in influenza infected peripheral blood mononuclear cells (PBMC) (139).

D. Eosinophils

Severe RSV-induced disease is associated with eosinophilia. Products of eosinophil degranulation are found in nasal wash and serum in children with severe primary infection (139b,c,d), and children with vaccine-enhanced disease had blood eosinophilia (20). Eosinophils have been induced in murine models by priming with F1-RSV or with formulations containing the RSV G glycoprotein. Immunization with G induces more eosinophils than F, regardless of adjuvant. Recombinant vaccinia viruses expressing G induce eosinophils particularly when G is secreted (42a). The region of G associated with induction of eosinophilia is near the immunogenic domain (139e,f,g). Increasing the activation of IFN-8 producing $CD8^+$ CTL can effectively reduce the magnitude of eosinophilia induced by RSV G (139h,i).

V. Adaptive Immune Response to Infection

During the 5- to 7-day incubation period during which virus reaches the lower respiratory tract by progressive cell-to-cell spread or aspiration of infectious secretions, the adaptive components of the immune system respond through both humoral and cell-mediated mechanisms. Although disease manifestations can result from direct viral cytopathology, there is growing evidence that the immunopathology resulting from the process of viral clearance is more important. Understanding the pathogenesis of RSV-induced disease has been the subject of intense investigation over the last 2 decades.

A. Antibody

At birth, infants possess neutralizing IgG antibody passively acquired in utero. Antibody levels depend on the maternal level and gestational age, since transfer of specific IgG subclasses begin at about 30 weeks' gestation and become maximal at 38–40 weeks. After birth, RSV-specific antibody declines with a half-life of 21–28 days. Glezen has shown that higher levels of maternal antibody correlate with reduced severity of RSV infection during the first year of life (140). In addition, protection has been correlated with levels of serum IgG to F protein as well as with serum neutralizing antibody titer (141).

In primary infection, infants respond with secretory and serum neutralizing antibody, directed at the F and G envelope glycoproteins, and internal proteins (142–145). In young infants (< 8 months), the serum IgG response is less than that of IgA (142,146). IgG1 and IgG3 are the dominant subclasses produced to F and G proteins in children, whereas IgG1 and IgG2 are the predominant subclass response to G in adults during reinfection (146,147). This difference is probably due to young infants' diminished recognition of carbohydrate antigens. In general, the antibody response to primary RSV infection is weak and of short duration. This poor response is attributed to two major factors: the presence of maternal antibody and immaturity of the infant immune system. Response to the F glycoprotein is influenced more by the presence of maternally acquired antibody than age, whereas the reverse is true for the G response (142,148a). After repeated infections, antibody titers are sustained at a relatively constant level which approximate adult levels. Nevertheless, reinfection is common. In adult volunteer challenge studies, wild-type

RSV can be isolated from nasal secretions in two thirds of subjects and half experience a "cold" syndrome (149). Moreover, three quarters of subjects can be reinfected at least twice within a 2-year period. Although serum neutralizing activity correlated with protection, even those with the highest titers have a 25% reinfection rate (79). Natural reinfection of the upper airway with RSV is reported to be independent of preinfection serum neutralizing antibody in both adults and children (90,133,150,151). However, in a longitudinal, prospective study of children followed from birth to age 5, the rate of reinfection was inversely correlated with the serum neutralizing titer and the number of previous infections (140). Nevertheless, reinfection of the upper airway occurs in the presence of measurable serum neutralizing antibody (140). The importance of mucosal antibody in the prevention of reinfection has also been investigated. Although adults with low levels of neutralizing activity in nasal secretions are more likely to be reinfected with RSV, reinfection can occur in the presence of nasal wash neutralizing activity (79,152,153).

The importance of antibody for viral clearance after primary infection has been addressed in mouse models. RSV-specific antibody is first detected on day 10 after challenge, whereas T-cell responses peak earlier and are temporally associated with viral clearance (132). Although antibody is not necessary for termination of RSV replication after primary infection, mice without antibody demonstrated enhanced pulmonary histopathology and experienced more severe illness than mice with an intact antibody response (154). In contrast, antibody is necessary for complete protection of the lung from reinfection in the mouse model (154,155). Human studies and animal experiments indicate that passively acquired antibody is sufficient for protection from severe lower respiratory tract infection (156,160–165).

B. CD8$^+$ Cytotoxic T Lymphocytes

CTL control acute viral infection directly by destroying virus-producing cells and possibly by releasing cytokines with antiviral activity, such as IFN-γ and TNF-α. RSV-specific HLA class I–restricted CTL have been derived from adult peripheral blood mononuclear cells and from children following acute RSV infection (166–169). Following experimental infection of mice or calves, the natural occurrence of the CTL response correlates with viral clearance and recovery (132,155,170,171).

In addition to antiviral activity, CD8$^+$ CTL are also capable of causing immunopathology in murine models of RSV (172). Cannon found that in persistently infected immunodeficient (nu/nu) BALB/c mice, RSV replication is terminated by infusion of low numbers ($<10^6$) of RSV-specific CTL without inducing illness, yet transfer of a larger number of CTL results in hemorrhagic pneumonitis (173–175). Other investigators, however, have not noted this effect (176). The major antigenic target for memory CTL for humans is the N protein (52,166). Other targets for CTL response in humans and mice include SH, F, and M2 proteins (49–52,62,63,166,177,178). Although CTL appear to be important for clearing virus after primary infection, They are not sufficient by themselves to prevent reinfection in mice immunized with recombinant vaccinia virus expressing either the M2 or N protein (64,180).

C. CD4$^+$ T Helper Lymphocytes

CD4$^+$ T helper (Th) lymphocytes are critical for the initiation of new immune responses. They respond to the environment and to signals derived from antigen-presenting cells, undergo selective activation and differentiation, and translate information to other cellular effectors in the immune response through their expression of surface adhesion molecules and cytokines. In general, T-helper responses to antigenic stimulation are characterized as Th1- or Th2-like based on the cytokines produced. Th1 cytokines (IL-2, IFN-γ, TNF-β) are associated with induction of CD8$^+$ CTL and class-switching to IgG1 in humans. In contrast, Th2 cytokines (IL-4, IL-5, IL-6, IL-10, IL-13) are associated with reduced CTL activity and isotype switching to IgG$_4$ (in humans) and IgE. The pathways for CD4$^+$ T-cell differentiation are autostimulatory and cross-inhibitory. The pattern of differentiation is influenced by a variety of factors including host phenotype, mechanisms of antigen presentation, nature of the specific antigen or epitope, and the cytokine milieu induced by the antigenic stimuli.

CD4$^+$ lymphocyte responses in humans, determined in vitro by lymphoproliferation or in vivo by skin testing, have been detected in normal children following RSV infection, although there was no correlation of magnitude or protein specificity with age or severity of disease (181,182). Conclusions about the potential role of CD4$^+$ lymphocytes in the pathogenesis of RSV infection are inferred from studies in animals. Passive transfer of CD4$^+$ T-cell clones in mice can clear RSV infection but not as efficiently as CD8$^+$ clones (183). Nevertheless, CD4$^+$ T lymphocytes are critical for the induction of RSV-specific antibody and are necessary for the lung pathology associated with reinfection or infection following vaccination of mice and calves (155,171,184).

VI. Disease Pathogenesis
A. Bronchiolitis and Pneumonia

The characteristic pathology associated with fatal RSV infection in normal infants is localized in the 75- to 300-μm diameter bronchioles (185,186). There is necrosis of bronchiolar epithelium, syncytium formation, loss of ciliated cells, and increased production of mucus. In addition, there is infiltration of the underlying submucosa with mononuclear cells, predominantly lymphocytes. The epithelial damage, mucus, and inflammatory cells produce a plug that effectively obstructs the small airways leading to air trapping. In some infants, the process extends into the lining cells of the alveolar space leading to interstitial lymphoid infiltrates and alveolar edema. Airway obstruction leading to ventilation-perfusion mismatching and thickening of alveolar septa are thought to cause hypoxia. In typical bronchiolitis there are relatively few virus-infected cells detected by immunofluorescence, which suggests that disease is primarily the result of immunopathology (153,185). This general paradigm of bronchiolitis being an immune-mediated disease is consistent with findings in children with acquired immunodeficiency syndrome (AIDS), who can shed RSV for over 6 months, yet have few clinical manifestations of bronchiolitis (187). Nevertheless, in patients with severe T- and B-cell deficiency, such as severe combined immunodeficiency syndrome, the disease process is dominated by direct virus-mediated cytopathology with high quantities of virus and large syncytial cells containing typical eosinophilic cytoplasmic inclusions (95,188,189). Patients whose immunodeficiency is restricted to either B or T cells do not appear to be as susceptible to this frequently fatal disease syndrome.

Additional insight into the role the immune response plays in disease pathogenesis can be gleaned from results of prior RSV vaccine trials. In the 1960s, a formalin-inactivated alum-precipitated whole virus vaccine (FI-RSV) was administered parenterally to infants and children. Not only did the vaccine fail to protect against RSV infection, but illness in vaccinees following subsequent RSV infection was unusually severe with a high rate of hospitalization and some deaths (19–22). In contrast, vaccine trials using parenteral live virus were not associated with enhanced illness (190). Several theories have been advanced to explain the pathogenesis of the FI-RSV–enhanced illness. One suggests that formalin inactivation diminished the immunogenicity of the F protein and that virus was free to spread by cell-to-cell fusion during subsequent infection. When sufficient viral antigen reacted with antibody, it was postulated that an Arthus-like, immune complex–mediated reaction occurred (191). Children who experienced vaccine-enhanced illness had antibody responses to F and G measured by enzyme immunoassay (EIA) but lacked neutralizing and antifusion activity (192,193). Another theory has implicated a heightened delayed-type hypersensitivity (DTH) response similar to that seen in recipients of the inactivated measles vaccine which led to the atypical measles syndrome (194,195). Children immunized with FI-RSV were found to have a heightened lymphocyte proliferative response (179). A third proposal was that an exaggerated $CD8^+$ CTL response occurred; based on the murine model where passive transfer of large numbers of $CD8^+$ CTL is associated with enhanced pathology (174,175). However, it is unlikely that immunization with a formalin-inactivated vaccine could induce $CD8^+$ MHC class I–restricted

RSV-specific CTL, since inactivated antigens are usually unable to enter the MHC class I antigen processing pathway.

The clinical features of the vaccine-enhanced illness included symptoms associated with bronchiolitis (wheezing, cough, coryza), but there was more lower respiratory tract disease and evidence of pneumonia on chest radiographs. Hospitalization rates and illness severity were highest in the youngest group of children, who were 2–7 months of age at the time of immunization (19). Vaccine-induced immune responses were therefore more likely to produce enhanced illness when the first exposure to RSV antigen was through vaccination, since there was no enhanced illness when the vaccination was given after 24 months of age (21). Pulmonary pathology included neutrophils, not usually a component of the histological infiltrate associated with natural RSV infection, and a high frequency of eosinophilia (19,20).

Experimental animals immunized with the formalin-inactivated vaccine, but not with live RSV, also develop excess pathology on live virus challenge (196–198). Immunization with FI-RSV or purified RSV protein subunits primes mice for dominant expression of IL-4 mRNA relative to IFN-γ mRNA (a Th2-like response) (197). In contrast, priming with live RSV leads to dominant expression of IFN-γ mRNA relative to IL-4 mRNA (a Th1-like response) (197). The FI-RSV–primed Th2 response includes the production of IL-5 (197). This complements the finding of eosinophilia in RSV-infected mice primed intradermally with FI-RSV or live recombinant vaccinia expressing the RSV G glycoprotein (198). Additionally, priming with recombinant vaccinia virus expressing the G protein tended to induce lymphocytes with Th2 cytokine profiles, whereas vaccinia vectors expressing other RSV proteins induced lymphocytes with Th1 cytokine secretion profiles (201,202). In experiments using $CD4^+$ T-cell lines derived from mice primed with recombinant vaccinia vectors, it was shown that Th2 $CD4^+$ T-cell lines specific for G caused increased weight loss and delayed viral clearance in comparison with Th1 $CD4^+$ T cell lines from vaccinia-F–primed mice (203).

These experimental results provide a basis for a working model for the pathogenesis of RSV vaccine–enhanced illness, which holds that immunization with inactivated whole RSV induces a subset of $CD4^+$ lymphocytes that results in nonprotective immunopathological responses after subsequent infection with wild-type RSV. This may be the result of a dominant Th2 response with production of IL-4, IL-5, and related cytokines. This response inhibits Th1 differentiation, perpetuates Th2 responses to subsequent infection with poor viral clearance, and production of mediators linked with airway hyperresponsiveness (204). Subsequent studies suggest that although an exaggerated Th2 response may be "bad," an exaggerated Th1 response may not necessarily be "good" (205,206a,b). The precise cause of RSV vaccine–enhanced illness is still an area of considerable controversy and ongoing research.

Immune mechanisms may also play a role in RSV-associated clinical phenomena, such as apnea and hyporetinolemia (207–209). The former may occur early in infection and may be related to specific cytokine patterns seen in some infants with RSV infection (210–213). Low plasma vitamin A levels are often present in infants on hospitalization with lower respiratory tract infection (209). Theoretical causes are increased utilization for respiratory epithelial cell repair and cytokine-mediated impaired release of retinol binding protein from liver (214). Unlike the case in measles, treatment of RSV-infected infants with vitamin A does not appear to significantly affect disease severity (214,215).

B. Asthma and Atopy

Severe RSV infection is strongly associated with childhood asthma and repeated episodes of bronchospastic bronchitis which can persist into adulthood (216). There is also evidence that RSV is an important determinant of aeroallergen sensitization (type I hypersensitivity) during the first years of life (216,217). Although the mechanisms underlying the propensity of RSV to promote allergic responses have not been completely defined, there is evidence that virus-specific IgE and IgG4 levels are increased and histamine and other mast cell products are released in children with RSV-associated wheezing (218,219). The IgE response and wheezing could potentially be IL-4 mediated, a Th2 cytokine, and provide a partial explanation for severe illness in children undergoing primary RSV infection. Openshaw found that immunization of mice with RSV G protein, but not F protein, results in an influx of eosinophils into the alveoli following viral challenge (198).

A bovine model of allergic inflammation supports the concept that the cytokine milieu resulting from aeroallergen sensitization alters the immunological outcome and illness manifestations of RSV infection (220). Calves exposed to aerosolized *Micropolyspora faeni* (Mf) and subsequently infected with RSV had increased induction of RSV-specific IgE, worsened lung pathology, and heightened clinical disease expression on reexposure to Mf antigen compared with calves that received either Mf aerosolization alone or RSV infection alone. There is also evidence in mice that RSV infection modulates the immune response to other aerosolized antigens with increased IgE production (221). RSV-infected BALB/c mice exposed to aerosolized ragweed develop earlier and higher ragweed-specific IgE and IgG when reexposed to ragweed than do noninfected controls. Similarly, mice given ovalbumin (ova) intranasally after RSV infection developed ova-specific IgE (222).

Class switching by B lymphocytes to produce IgE is promoted by IL-4, a Th2 cytokine. IL-4 also increases vascular cell adhesion molecule-1 (VCAM-1) expression on endothelial cells, which in turn regulates eosinophil and lymphocyte migration. The level of eosinophil cationic protein found in nasal washes of children correlates with bronchiolitis and wheezing (223–225a). This supports the concept that the inflammation associated with RSV in children with severe disease is an allergy-like process that is similar to that found in persons with chronic asthma. New models for measuring airway hyperresponsiveness in the setting of RSV infection and allergic airway inflammation may eventually provide insight into basic mechanisms of RSV-induced wheezing and lead to new intervention strategies (225b,c,d,e).

VII. Clinical Manifestations

A. Primary Infection

Asymptomatic RSV infection is considered to be rare. Except in very young neonates, illness almost always begins with upper respiratory symptoms. Nasal congestion with mucoid or clear discharge is present in over 90% of cases. Pharyngitis and fever (38–40°C) are nearly as common, as are systemic symptoms of irritability and poor feeding. Conjunctivitis is noted in one quarter of infants and concurrent otitis media is not uncommon (226–228). After several days of upper respiratory symptoms, signs of lower respiratory involvement often become predominant. The incidence of lower respiratory signs and symptoms is high, ranging from 30 to 70% (86). Cough is the most common finding (80%), and it may be severe and paroxysmal but without the characteristics of whooping cough. Dyspnea, tachypnea, and signs of respiratory distress may develop manifested by intercostal muscle retractions and in some cases by cyanosis. In bronchiolitis, audible wheezing is usually evident. The severity of symptoms and physical findings can vary over time, and it may be difficult to assess accurately clinical change by infrequent examinations over short periods. Virtually all patients with primary RSV infection have some degree of hypoxemia. In one study of hospitalized infants, the average arterial oxygen saturation was 87% (equivalent to a PaO_2 of 53 mmHg) (229). However, the degree of oxygen desaturation correlates poorly with other clinical measurements of severity such as respiratory rate, lethargy, and wheezing and only weakly with observed cyanosis (229,230). Nevertheless, determination of arterial oxygen saturation may be the single best, and simplest, tool to assess degree of illness (231).

Apnea is noted in 18% of RSV-infected infants, and it is associated with young postnatal age, prematurity, and a history of apnea of prematurity (232). Among these infants, 28% ultimately required ventilatory support. Apnea is not simply a response to more severe disease, since a study of neonatal RSV infection found that apnea was most common among the very young (<3 weeks) in contrast to older infants, who had more wheezing and signs of lower respiratory tract involvement (234).

In hospitalized infants, the most prevalent chest radiographic findings are hyperinflation (87%), parahilar peribronchial infiltrates (92%), and local areas of atelectasis (41%) (233). Middle or upper lobe consolidation has been reported to occur in one quarter of cases, but atelectasis may account for this appearance (229,233). Diffuse interstitial infiltrates, nodular infiltrates, pleural effusion, and adenopathy may occur but are all unusual (233). The radiographic appearance does not discriminate RSV from other viral infections or from bacterial superinfection, although several studies suggest that the presence of atelectasis is indicative of more severe disease (231,233).

Except for approximately 10% of infants who require ventilatory support, the clinical course of hospitalized infants is of slow improvement after 1 or 2 days, and the average duration of hospitalization for otherwise healthy infants without complications is 3–5 days (229). Once improvement is clearly evident, subsequent deterioration is uncommon despite persistence of significant hypoxemia at discharge (229). Rare cases of severe repeat infection within the same RSV season, generally with a different viral strain, can occur (personal observation).

Age at infection clearly influences the severity and incidence of specific symptoms. Hospitalization is uncommon under 3–4 weeks of age; implying that illness is mild in this age group, perhaps a result of high levels of maternally transmitted neutralizing antibody (5). In a study of 23 neonatal infections, Hall found that neonates <3 weeks of age were less likely to have pneumonia (7 vs 56%) and more likely to have nonspecific signs (29 vs 0%) than older neonates (234). The incidence of bronchiolitis and pneumonia peaks between 2 and 6 months of age. In a prospective study of primary RSV infection in a day-care center, 71% of 2- to 6-month-old infants, 54% of 6- to 12-month-old infants, and 42% of 1- to 2-year-old children had evidence of lower respiratory disease (90). Severity is also increased by the presence of underlying diseases. Infants with congenital heart disease, bronchopulmonary dysplasia, or those who are receiving cytotoxic drugs for malignancy required intensive care unit (ICU) treatment in 63, 36, and 60%, respectively, in contrast to 10–20% of normal infants (78,88,235). Infants infected with the human immunodeficiency virus (HIV) may have a higher incidence of interstitial pneumonia rather than bronchiolitis (236).

Except for otitis media, coinfection with another virus or bacteria is uncommon, although it appears to be associated with a worse outcome (237). The most frequent coinfecting viral agent is adenovirus. Bacterial superinfection occurs in 1% of infants, although the routine use of antibiotics for RSV infection can increase this incidence slightly (238).

B. Reinfection in Children

Reinfection is generally milder than primary infection RSV infection, although infants with underlying diseases may still require hospitalization (91,239). In normal children >3 years of age, reinfection primarily causes upper respiratory symptoms and fever. Otitis media with middle ear effusion is a common complication. In one study, RSV infection was complicated by otitis media in one third, greater than that associated with adenovirus (28%), influenza (28%), or rhinoviral (10%) infections (227). In a Finnish study of 137 infants with otitis media, RSV antigen was detected in 15% of middle ear effusions; in half as the sole pathogen (226). In a recent study from Galveston, Texas, RSV infection was implicated by culture or antigen detection in 51 of 271 children aged 2 months to 7 years with otitis media (228). In three quarters of the cases, pathogenic bacteria were also recovered. Longer duration of symptoms and failure to respond to antibiotic treatment was associated with the presence of both RSV and bacteria.

C. Reinfection in Adults

Reinfection in adults is generally mild, although fever, pharyngitis, and cough are common (102). Lower respiratory tract signs are uncommon; however, illness is severe enough to result in work absenteeism in half of an infected medical staff. In addition, pulmonary function tests demonstrated increased airway reactivity with carbachol challenge for at least 8 weeks (80). Three populations of adults are at significant risk for severe RSV infection; the frail elderly, adults with chronic obstructive pulmonary disease (COPD) or congestive heart failure (CHF), and those receiving immunosuppressive therapy after solid organ or bone marrow transplantation (10–12,84,93–96,98,100,240). Residents of long-term care facilities appear to be at greatest risk for severe disease (see Chap. 4). Sorvillo noted that 22 of 40 (55%) cases of RSV infection developed radiographically confirmed pneumonia, evenly divided between patchy lower lobe pneumonitis and consolidation, with 20% mortality (100). Agius noted an 11.5% mortality rate in another institutional outbreak which was characterized by fever and cough in 96% of the infections and signs of bronchopneumonia in 42% (240). In a prospective study from Rochester, New York, RSV infection was confirmed in 40 residents of a nursing home during a single winter (10). Fever was present in half of the subjects, nasal congestion in 92%, and wheezing and rales were heard in 35–40%. Pneumonia was diagnosed in 10% of these patients and 5% died.

Community-dwelling elderly are also at risk for severe RSV infection. In a 3-year analysis of 1580 persons over 65 years of age hospitalized for acute cardiopulmonary disease or influenza-like illness, Falsey identified recent RSV infection in 10% and influenza in 13% (11). Clinical signs and symptoms were indistinguishable from influenza on admission, and both groups required ICU care and ventilatory support equally. Notably, RSV-infected patients were more likely to be treated for bronchospasm and had a higher overall mortality

(10 vs 6%). RSV infection has also been linked to exacerbations of COPD (241,242). In a recent literature review of viral infection and acute bronchitis, RSV was identified as the first or second most common viral agent associated with acute flares of bronchitis (243).

Adult organ transplant recipients, especially those receiving bone marrow grafts, are subject to devastating RSV infection, and nosocomial acquisition is a serious problem (see Chap. 5) (93). Early symptoms of nasal congestion, rhinorrhea, fever, and cough are the rule and should be viewed with concern during the winter season (12,94,96). Approximately half of RSV infections progress to pneumonia, generally after 2–7 days of upper respiratory symptoms, which despite therapy carries a 50–100% mortality (12,84,94–96, 244). The risk of fatal RSV pneumonia is greatest prior to engraftment of the transplanted marrow. Wheezing is common, along with rales and rhonchi when pneumonia occurs. Notably, half of these patients have radiographic evidence of sinusitis even in the absence of symptoms (12). Chest radiographs show bilateral infiltrates in 78% and pleural effusions in 20% (12,94). Similar to infants, bacterial superinfection in RSV-infected immunosuppressed adults is uncommon in contrast to influenza-infected patients in whom bacterial superinfection develops in half of them (96). Autopsy findings are consistent with RSV pneumonia with multinucleated giant cells and syncytia in addition to organizing diffuse alveolar damage (94,96).

VIII. Diagnosis

Diagnostic methods include (1) detection of viral antigen by enzyme immunoassay (EIA), indirect and direct immunofluorescence (IFA, DFA), (2) detection of virus by culture, (3) detection of viral RNA by reverse transcriptase–polymerase chain reaction (RT-PCR), and (4) serological detection of RSV-specific IgM in acute serum or demonstration of a rise in RSV-specific IgG by EIA or neutralization assays (see Chap. 12). The first two methods are commercially available and are most commonly employed, whereas the latter two techniques are principally used in research laboratories. The advantages, disadvantages, and utility of rapid tests and culture are discussed in an excellent review by Kellogg (245). Several parameters influence sensitivity and specificity. The highest viral titers are found in secretions from the youngest infants, those with primary infection, and early in the course of illness. In addition, the type of specimen collected (nasal swab, nasal aspirate, nasal wash, endotracheal aspirate, or bronchoalveolar lavage [BAL]), and transport conditions and processing methods all effect results (245).

Identification of RSV infection by culture remains the cornerstone of diagnosis, and by definition is 100% specific. A nasal wash specimen is considered to be optimal for culture and is easily obtained from infants by rinsing each nasal cavity with 5 mL of saline using a suction bulb (246). BAL and tracheal aspirates also have high yield but are uncommonly obtained in young infants (245,247). Nasal swabs are the least desirable specimens with a sensitivity of 57% (245). Because RSV is thermolabile, it is important to place the sample quickly on cell culture. Optimal results are obtained by using several cell lines (i.e., HEp-2, MRC-5, WI38) and by assaying for RSV antigen by immunofluorescence at termination of each culture to identify nonsyncytial strains. A major drawback to culture is the 3–14 days required for results, since antiviral therapy or institution of infection control procedures may depend on timely diagnosis. The use of shell vials, in which viral antigen is detected by immunofluorescence after 2–4 days in culture, can speed diagnosis without sacrificing sensitivity (248–250). Overall, culture of nasal aspirates or washes has a sensitivity of about 85% in primary infection when rapid antigen detection tests are used as the reference test (245). Culture also allows detection of other or coinfecting viruses.

Culture is less sensitive in the diagnosis of repeat infection, especially in the elderly. This is presumably due to the lower viral titers in secretions and the shorter duration of shedding (72,77,80). In prospective studies of RSV infection in nursing home patients, culture identifies less than half of serologically confirmed infections despite meticulous surveillance and culture of all respiratory illnesses (10). In a prospective analysis of 54 illnesses in frail elderly, RSV infection was documented by serology in 11 patients, of which only 5 were identified by culture (251). The sensitivity of culture in immunocompromised adults is unknown, but the low viral titers in secretions may reduce yields (81). Nevertheless, virus can generally be recovered by the use of optimal sampling (nasal wash or BAL) and rapid placement on cell culture (12,95,96).

Rapid tests for detection of viral antigen in respiratory secretions have become commonplace and clearly supplement viral culture in the diagnosis of RSV. IFA or DFA can provide results in 3–6 hr, but they are labor intensive and depend on experienced interpreters. Although specimen handling and transport time are less important than for culture, samples must contain adequate numbers of columnar epithelial cells or sensitivity is lost (245). Sensitivity and specificity for these tests are >90% when culture is used as the standard (245,250). Specificity is enhanced when the typical inclusion body fluorescent pattern is noted. In elderly persons, DFA has poor sensitivity; detecting only 1 of 11 serologically confirmed illnesses in one series (251). In immunocompromised adults, DFA of nasal wash specimens was positive in 81% of culture-positive patients (94).

Commercial EIA are rapid, easily performed tests which require minimal technical skill (252). Sensitivity ranges from 52 to 98% compared with culture, but in infants, it was above 85% in most series (245). Specificity is generally greater than 90%. However, EIA has poor sensitivity in elderly or immunocompromised adults. In one study in the elderly, only 23 of 159 (14%) serologically confirmed RSV infections were detected by EIA of nasal swab specimens, and in another study, 0 of 11 were identified (11,251). In bone marrow transplant recipients, the utility of EIA varies markedly with the specimen tested. Sensitivity for nasal wash, endotracheal aspirate, and BAL are 17, 57, and 100%, respectively (81).

RT-PCR is reasonably sensitive, but preliminary information does not indicate substantial advantages over other rapid tests for diagnosis of primary infection (253,254). However, it may ultimately prove to be useful in persons shedding low quantities of virus or from whom inadequate samples are obtained, such as the elderly or immunosuppressed adult.

Serological diagnosis of RSV is principally used for research purposes, since diagnosis is retrospective. Repeat infections in children, adults, and the elderly generally result in diagnostic IgG antibody rises to F and G proteins (10,11). In primary infection in very young infants, results are less reliable because of the interference of high levels of maternally derived antibody or an immature immune system (148a,255). There are no data on the utility of serological diagnosis in immunocompromised adults.

In selecting diagnostic tests, the clinical situation must be considered. Culture and rapid tests complement each other and, optimally, both should be available. Many laboratories use rapid tests (IFA, DFA, or EIA) initially, and if they are negative, standard or shell vial culture is performed (257).

IX. Therapy

Treatment of RSV infection is directed at reversing the physiological and inflammatory effects of infection (e.g., hypoxia, hypercarbia, wheezing) and reducing viral shedding. In most infants, hypoxia is readily relieved by low concentrations of oxygen. Dehydration should be treated and dangerous hypercarbia and acidosis may require ventilatory support. The benefits of bronchodilators for acute bronchiolitis remain controversial (258–260). Although many studies which quantify the physiological benefit of bronchodilators demonstrate little objective change in airway flow or in oxygenation, most practitioners consider that a subset of infants with bronchiolitis clearly benefit (86). Thus, a brief trial of an inhaled bronchodilator is reasonable, and if improvement in clinical parameters or oxygenation occurs, an oral or inhaled bronchodilator should be continued. Corticosteroids have not been proven to alter the course of bronchiolitis in primary RSV infection (261).

Specific antiviral therapy for RSV infection is limited to a single agent despite the in vitro and in vivo activity of a wide range of compounds (262–265) (see Chap. 13). Ribavirin, a synthetic nucleoside with a broad antiviral activity, is approved for treatment of RSV infection by administration as a small-particle aerosol into a tent, mask, or ventilator (262). The drug is given for a total of 12–20 hr per day for 2–5 days at a reservoir concentration of 20 mg/mL. Ribavirin levels in respiratory secretions, but not in blood, exceed the inhibitory concentration for RSV by several hundredfold (266). Despite concerns about potential teratogenicity and the effects of drug accumulation in red blood cells, short-term toxicity has been negligible (266,267). Recently, high-dose, short-duration therapy (6 hr/day at 60 mg/mL) has been suggested as an alternative to standard therapy (268). Ribavirin was approved for use in the treatment of acute RSV infection in hospitalized infants in 1986 after three placebo-controlled double-blind randomized trials demonstrated improvement in clinical illness and decreased viral shedding in treated infants (262,269,270). Subsequent studies of ribavirin therapy in infants with bronchopulmonary dysplasia and congenital heart disease and in infants requiring mechanical ventilation supported the original findings (271). However, some investigators have questioned the practical relevance of the observed improvements in clinical illness, since mortality, duration of hospitalization, and long-term outcome were unaffected (266). In addition, other investigators have been unable to duplicate the findings of the original studies which contained small numbers of subjects (272). The high cost of therapy (>$3000 per infant treated) increases these concerns. Current recommendations by the Academy of Pediatrics Committee on Infectious Diseases conclude that ribavirin *may* be considered for use in selected infants at high risk of serious RSV disease (18). These include (1) those with complicated congenital heart disease, bronchopulmonary dysplasia or cystic fibrosis, or underlying medical conditions such as severe neurologic diseases; (2) healthy premature infants or those less than 6 weeks of age; (3) those with underlying immunosuppressive disorders; and (4) any infected infant with severe illness (generally judged by the degree of hypoxia).

The concept of immunoglobulin therapy for RSV infection is based on animal studies demonstrating substantial reduction in viral replication (156, 159–162,273,274). Published data on intravenous immunoglobulin for treatment of RSV-infected infants are limited to a single study of 35 infants which found a reduction in viral shedding and improved oxygenation compared with placebo-treated controls (275). Currently, multicenter studies are in progress to further evaluate this approach. Future therapeutic approaches may include aerosol or topical administration of IgG or IgA monoclonal antibodies (276, 277a,b).

Treatment of adults with severe RSV disease has not been well studied, and thus general recommendations are unavailable. Information on the benefit of ribavirin treatment of frail elderly with severe RSV pneumonia is limited to anecdotal experience and conclusions on efficacy cannot be made (A.R. Falsey, personal communication). However, if therapy is to be given to an agitated or uncooperative adult, high-dose short-course ribavirin therapy may be more acceptable to patients and staff. Results from treatment of bone marrow transplant recipients, although uncontrolled, suggest that early therapy before respiratory failure develops may be of benefit (94,96). Whimby reported that patients treated at least 1 day prior to the onset of respiratory failure had a 33% mortality (4 of 12) in contrast to 100% mortality (8 of 8) in patients untreated or treated after respiratory failure was evident (96). Another unproved approach, which also draws support from animal studies, combines treatment with aerosolized ribavirin and intravenous immunoglobulin (164, 278). The high mortality of RSV pneumonia in severely immunocompromised adults provides justification for recommended ribavirin therapy despite unproved benefit.

X. Prevention

Approaches to the prevention of RSV infection are prophylactic administration of immunoglobulin and vaccination; the former currently approved for clinical use, whereas the latter remains in development.

A. Immunoglobulin Prophylaxis

Encouraged by the results of experimental animal studies in which parenteral injection of neutralizing immunoglobulin protected animals from challenge with RSV, investigators pursued the concept of prophylactic immunoglobulin therapy for infants at high risk of severe RSV infection (274,279,280). In a multicenter placebo-controlled study in 249 high-risk infants less than 4 years of age, monthly administration of high-titered RSV-neutralizing immunoglobulin (RSVIG) was beneficial (279). The majority (75%) of infants were less than 1 year of age and 76% had underlying cardiopulmonary disease. Infants treated with RSVIG at 750 mg IgG/kg had a 62% reduction in lower respiratory tract RSV infections, lower illness severity scores, and reductions in ICU admissions and total ICU days in comparison with the control group. There was no effect on mortality rates, which were low in all groups (range 0–4%). Adverse events were infrequent, although five infants developed fluid overload during drug administration. A separate analysis of 162 preterm infants (with or without bronchopulmonary dysplasia [BPD]) found similar improvements in RSV lower respiratory tract disease, rates of hospitalization (4 of 58 vs 14 of 58), and reduced ICU days in the RSVIG group (280). However, the large volume of IgG which requires intravenous administration and expense are two significant drawbacks to this prophylactic approach. The latter concern may be resolved if high-potency neutralizing human monoclonal antibodies, which are currently in clinical trials, prove to be efficacious.

B. Vaccination: The Past

Despite 3 decades of effort, a successful RSV vaccine had not been developed. Prior vaccine candidates have included, in chronological order, a formalin-inactivated whole virus preparation, several intranasally administered live attenuated vaccines, and a parenterally administered live virus vaccine (19–22, 190,281–283). The failure and subsequent complications of the FI-RSV vaccine are described in the section on pathogenesis (Sec. VI). The youngest infants (less than 6 months of age at the time of immunization) developed more severe disease than controls who received a formalin-inactivated parainfluenza virus vaccine. At one of the vaccination sites, 14% required hospitalization compared with less than 1% of controls, whereas at another site, 69% of the vaccinees developed RSV pneumonia compared with 9% of controls (19,20).

Evidence that mucosal immunity plays a role in immunity to RSV prompted development of live attenuated viruses, principally temperature-sensitive (ts) or cold-adapted (ca) mutants (281–283). Although initial results were encouraging, this approach was abandoned, as the vaccines were either poorly immunogenic, excessively virulent, or genetically unstable. Finally, a large field trial used intramuscular vaccination with a nonattenuated RSV strain (190). Although enhanced illness was not evident, protective efficacy was lacking; perhaps due to the failure to induce sufficient systemic or local antibody (284).

C. Experimental Vaccines: The Future

Incorporation of various RSV genes, most notably the F gene, into viral vectors such as vaccinia virus and adenovirus have been successfully completed. Although promising in rodents, these vaccines did not reach clinical trials because of the lack of immunogenicity and efficacy in subhuman primates (285–288).

Currently, several experimental approaches to immunization are in clinical evaluation. Genetically stable, attenuated virus vaccines have been produced from previously tested ca/ts mutants by further chemical mutagenesis, and the precise genetic alterations defined by sequence analysis of viral RNA

(289,290). Introduction of multiple ca and ts mutations into the same virus should prevent wild-type reversion. Prototype vaccines of group A and B RSV strains have been characterized and results in preclinical primate studies are promising (159,289,291). The recent development by Collins of full-length infectious cDNA clones of RSV, which produce live virus on transfection of cells in tissue culture, offers the potential of a limitless supply of specifically tailored vaccine candidates (61). Preliminary experiments suggest that entire genes can be inserted into the RSV genome without affecting replication. Thus it may be possible to insert the G gene from group A virus into a group B virus parent, producing a chimeric virus expressing G proteins from both major virus groups.

Another approach to vaccination has been use of purified subunit vaccines composed of the RSV F protein which carries neutralizing, fusion-inhibiting epitopes which are conserved among most RSV strains. Preliminary results in previously infected children, 1–4 years of age, demonstrated stimulation of neutralizing antibody to both group A and B strains (292,293). Analogous to results with inactivated influenza vaccines, RSV-specific IgA is stimulated in only 15% of previously infected infants. Although there has been no evidence of enhanced disease when vaccinees have experienced RSV infection, trepidation concerning the use of an inactivated vaccine in young immunologically naive infants has slowed evaluation of subunit vaccines in the group at highest risk of severe disease. However, this vaccine approach may provide a practical means of boosting protective immunity in previously infected high-risk children (i.e., those with cystic fibrosis, bronchopulmonary dysplasia) and in the elderly (294). When administered to both healthy and frail elderly, purified F protein is safe and reasonably immunogenic resulting in fourfold neutralizing antibody responses in 60 and 47% of subjects, respectively (295,296). Efficacy studies in the elderly have not been performed. Another potential use of subunit vaccines is for immunization during the third trimester of pregnancy, in which enhanced placental transfer of protective neutralizing antibody may provide benefit during the early months of life (297). This approach has proved to be extremely successful in preventing neonatal tetanus in developing countries.

References

1. Morris JA, Blount RE Jr, Savage RE. Recovery of cytopathogenic agent from chimpanzees with coryza. Proc Soc Exp Biol Med 1956; 92:544–594.
2. Chanock R, Roizman B, Myers R. Recovery from infants with respiratory illness of a virus related to Chimpanzee Coryza Agent (CCA). Am J Hyg 1957; 66:281–290.
3. Glezen WP, Loda FA, Clyde WA Jr, Senior RJ, Chaeffer CI, Conley WG, et al. Epidemiologic patterns of acute lower respiratory disease of children in a pediatric group practice. J Pediatr 1971; 78:397–406.

4. Parrott RH, Kim HW, Arrobio JO, Hodes DS, Murphy BR, Brandt CD, et al. Epidemiology of respiratory syncytial virus infection in Washington, D.C. Am J Epidemiol 1973; 98:289–300.
5. Mufson MA, Levine HD, Wasil RE, Mocega-Gonzalez HE, Krause HE. Epidemiology of respiratory syncytial virus infection among infants and children in Chicago. Am J Epidemiol 1973; 1973; 98:88–95.
6. Brandt CD, Kim HW, Arrobio JO, Jeffries BC, Wood SC, Chanock R, et al. Epidemiology of respiratory syncytial virus infection in Washington, D.C. Am J Epidemiol 1973; 98:355–364.
7. Anonymous. Prospects for immunizing against respiratory syncytial virus. In: Katz SL, ed. New Vaccine Development: Establishing Priorities. Vol 1. Diseases of Importance in the United States. Washington, DC: National Academy Press, 1985: 397–409.
8. McIntosh K. Pathogenesis of severe acute respiratory infections in the developing world: respiratory syncytial virus and parainfluenza viruses. Rev Infect Dis 1991; 13:492–500.
9. Anderson LJ, Parker RA, Strikas RL. Association between respiratory syncytial virus outbreaks and lower respiratory tract deaths of infants and young children. J Infect Dis 1990; 161:640–646.
10. Falsey AR, Treanor JJ, Betts RF, Walsh EE. Viral respiratory infections in the institutionalized elderly: clinical and epidemiologic findings. J Am Geriatr Soc 1992; 40;115–119.
11. Falsey AR, Cunningham CK, Barker WH, Kouides RW, Yuen JB, Menegus M, et al. Respiratory syncytial virus and Influenza A infections in the hospitalized elderly. J Infect Dis 1995; 172:389–394.
12. Englund JA, Sullivan CJ, Jordan MC, Dehner LP, Vercellotti GM, Balfour HH. Respiratory syncytial virus infection in immunocompromised adults. Ann Intern Med 1988; 109:203–208.
13. McConnochie KM, Roghmann KJ. Bronchiolitis as a possible cause of wheezing in childhood: new evidence. Pediatrics 1984; 74:1–10.
14. Morgan WJ, Martinez FD. Risk factors for developing wheezing and asthma in childhood. Pediatr Clin North Am 1992; 39:1185–1203.
15. Hall CB, Hall WJ, Gala CL, MaGill FB, Leddy JP. Long-term prospective study in children after respiratory syncytial virus infection. J Pediatr 1984; 105:358–364.
16. Shaheen SO, Barker DJP, Shiell A, Crocker RJ, Wield G, Holgate ST. The relationship between pneumonia in early childhood and impaired lung function in late adult life. Am J Respir Crit Care Med 1994; 149:616–619.
17. Pullan CR. Wheezing, asthma and pulmonary dysfunction 10 years after infection with respiratory syncytial virus in infancy. Br Med J 1982; 284:1665–1669.
18. Committee on Infectious Diseases. Reassessment of the indications for Ribavirin therapy in respiratory syncytial virus infections. Pediatrics 1996; 97:137–140.
19. Kim HW, Canchola JG, Brandt CD, Pyles G, Chanock RM, Jensen K, et al. Respiratory syncytial virus disease in infants despite prior administration of antigenic inactivated vaccine. Am J Epidemiol 1969; 89:422–434.

20. Chin J, Magoffin RL, Shearer LA, Schieble JH, Lennette EH. Field evaluation of a respiratory syncytial virus vaccine and a trivalent parainfluenza virus vaccine in a pediatric population. AM J Epidemiol 1969; 89:449–463.
21. Kapikian AZ, Mitchell RH, Chanock RM, Shvedoff RA, Stewart CE. An epidemiologic study of altered clinical reactivity to respiratory syncytial (RS) virus infection in children previously vaccinated with an inactivated RS virus vaccine. Am J Epidemiol 1969; 89:405–421.
22. Fulginiti VA, Eller JJ, Sieber OF, Joyner JW, Minamitani M, Meiklejohn G. Respiratory virus immunization. I. A field trial of two inactivated respiratory virus vaccines; an aqueous trivalent parainfluenza virus vaccine and an alum-precipitated respiratory syncytial virus vaccine. Am J Epidemiol 1969; 89:435–448.
23. Collins P. The Molecular Biology of Human Respiratory Syncytial Viruses (RSV) of the Genus *Pneumovirus*. In: Kingsbury DW, ed. The Paramyxoviruses. New York: Plenum Press, 1991:103–162.
24. Bachi T. Direct observation of the budding and fusion of an enveloped virus by video microscopy. J Cell Biol 1988; 107:1689–1695.
25. Hendricks DA, Baradaran K, McIntosh K, Patterson JL. Appearance of a soluble form of the G protein of respiratory syncytial virus in fluids of infected cells. J Gen Virol 1987; 68:1705–1714.
26. Roberts SR, Lichtenstein D, Ball LA, Wertz GW. The membrane-associated and secreted forms of the respiratory syncytial virus attachment glycoprotein G are synthesized from alternative initiation codons. J Virol 1994; 68:4538–4546.
27. Huang YT, Collins PL, Wertz GW. Characterization of the 10 proteins of human respiratory syncytial virus: Identification of a fourth envelope-associated protein. Virus Res 1985; 2:157–173.
28. Walsh EE, Schlesinger JJ, Brandriss M. Purification and characterization of GP90, one of the envelope glycoproteins of respiratory syncytial virus. J Gen Virol 1986; 65:761–767.
29a. Langedijk JPM, Schaaper WMM, Meloen RH, van Oirschot JT. Proposed three-dimensional model for the attachment protein G of respiratory syncytial virus. J Gen Virol 1996; 77:1249–1257.
29b. Levine S, Klaiber-Franco R, Paradiso PR. Demonstration that glycoprotein G is the attachment protein of respiratory syncytial virus. J Gen Virol 1987; 68: 2521–2524.
30. Wertz GW, Collins PL, Huang Y, Gruber C, Levine S, Ball LA. Nucleotide sequence of the G protein gene of human respiratory syncytial virus reveals an unusual type of viral membrane protein. Proc Natl Acad Sci USA 1985; 82: 4075–4079.
31. Collins PL. O glycosylation of glycoprotein G of human respiratory syncytial virus is specified within the divergent ectodomain. J Virol 1990; 64:4007–4012.
32. Wertz GW, Krieger M, Ball LA. Structure and cell surface maturation of the attachment glycoprotein of human respiratory syncytial virus in a cell line deficient in O glycosylation. J Virol 1989; 63:4767–4776.
33. Collins PL, Mottet G. Oligomerization and post translation processing of glycoprotein G of human respiratory syncytial virus: altered O-glycosylation in the presence of brefeldin A. J Gen Virol 1992; 73:849–863.

34. Olmsted RA, Murphy BR, Lawrence LA, Elango N, Moss B, Collins PL. Processing, surface expression, and immunogenicity of carboxy-terminally truncated mutants of G protein of human respiratory syncytial virus. J Virol 1989; 63:411–420.
35. Palomo C, Garcia-Barreno B, Penas C, Melero JA. The G protein of human respiratory syncytial virus: significance of carbohydrate side-chains and the C-terminal end to its antigenicity. J Gen Virol 1991; 72:669–675.
36. Lambert DM. Role of oligosaccharides in the structure and function of respiratory syncytial virus glycoproteins. Virology 1988; 164:458–466.
37. Anderson LJ, Hierholzer JC, Tsou C, Hendry RM, Fernie BF, Stone Y, et al. Antigenic characterization of respiratory syncytial virus strains with monoclonal antibodies. J Infect Dis 1985; 151:626–633.
38. Johnson PR, Spriggs MK, Olmsted RA, Collins PL. The G glycoprotein of human respiratory syncytial viruses of subgroups A and B: extensive sequence divergence between antigenically related proteins. Proc Natl Acad Sci USA 1987; 84:5625–5629.
39. Sullender WM, Mufson MA, Anderson LJ, Wertz GW. Genetic diversity of the attachment protein of subgroup B respiratory syncytial viruses. J Virol 1991; 65:5425–5434.
40. Gottschalk J, Zbinden R, Kaempf L, Heinzer I. Discrimination of respiratory syncytial virus subgroups A and B by reverse transcription-PCR. J Clin Microbiol 1996; 34:41–43.
41. Walsh EE, Brandriss M, Schlesinger JJ. Immunological differences between the envelope glycoproteins of two strains of human respiratory syncytial virus. J Gen Virol 1987; 68:2169–2176.
42a. Johnson PR, Olmsted RA, Prince GA, Murphy BR, Alling DW, Walsh EE, et al. Antigenic relatedness between glycoproteins of human respiratory syncytial virus subgroups A and B: evaluation of the contributions of F and G glycoproteins to immunity. J Virol 1987; 61:3163–3166.
42b. Johnson TR, Johnson JE, Roberts SR, Wertz EW, Parker RA, Graham BS. Priming with secreted glycoprotein G of respiratory syncytial virus (RSV) augments interleukin-5 production and tissue eosinophilia after RSV challenge. J Virol 1998; 72:2871–2880.
42c. Karron RA, Buonaguria DA, Georgiu AF, Whitehead SS, Adamus JE, Clements-Mann ML, Harris DO, Randolph VB, Udem SA, Murphy BR, Sidhu MS. Respiratory syncytial virus (RSV) SH and G proteins are not essential for viral replication in vitro: clinical evaluation and molecular characterization of a cold-passaged, attenuated RSV subgroup B mutant. Proc Natl Acad Sci USA 1997; 94:13961–13966.
43. Walsh EE, Hruska J. Monoclonal antibodies to respiratory syncytial virus proteins: Identification of the fusion protein. J Virol 1983; 47:171–177.
44. Srinivasakumar N, Ogra PL, Flanagan TD. Characteristics of fusion of respiratory syncytial virus with HEp-2 cells as measured by R18 fluorescence dequenching assay. J Virol 1991; 65:4063–4069.
45. Collins PL, Huang YT, Wertz GW. Nucleotide sequence of the gene encoding the fusion (F) glycoprotein of human respiratory syncytial virus. Proc Natl Acad Sci USA 1984; 81:7683–7687.

46. Walsh EE, Brandriss MW, Schlesinger JJ. Purification and characterization of the respiratory syncytial virus fusion protein. J Gen Virol 1985; 66:409–415.
47. Walsh EE, Cote PJ, Fernie BF, Schlesinger JJ, Brandriss MW. Analysis of the respiratory syncytial virus fusion protein using monoclonal and polyclonal antibodies. J Gen Virol 1986; 67:505–513.
48. Beeler JA, vanWyke Coelingh K. Neutralization epitopes of the F glycoprotein of respiratory syncytial virus: effect of mutation upon fusion function. J Virol 1989; 63:2941–2950.
49. Cannon MJ, Bangham CRM. Recognition of respiratory syncytial virus fusion protein by mouse cytotoxic T cell clones and a human cytotoxic T cell line. J Gen Virol 1989; 70:79–87.
50. Pemberton RM, Cannon MJ, Openshaw PJM, Ball LA, Wertz GW, Askonas BA. Cytotoxic T cell specificity for respiratory syncytial virus proteins: fusion protein is an important target antigen. J Gen Virol 1987; 68:2177–2182.
51. Nicholas JA, Rubino KL, Levely ME, Adams EG, Collins PL. Cytolytic T-lymphocyte responses to respiratory syncytial virus: effector cell phenotype and target proteins. J Virol 1990; 64:4232–4241.
52. Cherrie AH, Anderson K, Wertz GW, Openshaw PJM. Human cytotoxic T cells stimulated by antigen on dendritic cells recognize the N, SH, F, M, 22K, and 1b proteins of respiratory syncytial virus. J Virol 1992; 66:2102–2110.
53. Walsh EE, Hall CB, Briselli M, Brandriss MW, Schlesinger JJ. Immunization with glycoprotein subunits of respiratory syncytial virus to protect cotton rats against viral infection. J Infect Dis 1987; 155:1198–1204.
54. Walsh EE. Humoral, mucosal and cellular immune response to topical immunization with a subunit respiratory syncytial virus vaccine. J Infect Dis 1994; 170:345–350.
55. Olmsted RA, Collins PL. The 1A protein of respiratory syncytial virus is an integral membrane protein present as multiple, structurally distinct species. J Virol 1989; 63:2019–2029.
56. Anderson K, King AMQ, Lerch RA, Wertz GW. Polylactosaminoglycan modification of the respiratory syncytial virus small hydrophobic (SH) protein: a conserved feature among human and bovine respiratory syncytial viruses. Virology 1992; 191:417–430.
57. Heminway BR, Yu Y, Perrine KG, Gustafson E, Bernstein JM, Galinski MS, et al. Analysis of respiratory syncytial virus F, G, and SH proteins in cell fusion. Virology 1994; 200:801–805.
58. Peeples ME. Paramyxovirus M Proteins. Pulling It All Together and Taking It on the Road. In: Kingsbury DW, ed. The Paramyxoviruses. New York: Plenum Press, 1991:427–456.
59. Grosfeld H, Hill MG, Collins PL. RNA replication by respiratory syncytial virus (RSV) is directed by the N, P, and L proteins; transcription also occurs under these conditions but requires RSV superinfection for efficient synthesis of full-length mRNA. J Virol 1995; 69:5677–5686.
60. Collins PL, Hill MG, Camargo E, Grosfeld H, Chanock RM, Murphy BR. Production of infectious human respiratory syncytial virus from cloned cDNA confirms an essential role for the transcription elongation factor from the 5′ proximal open

reading frame of the M2 mRNA in gene expression and provides a capability for vaccine development. Proc Natl Acad Sci USA 1995; 92:11563–11567.
61. Burkreyev AA, Camargo E, Collins PL. Recovery of infectious respiratory syncytial virus expressing an additional, foreign gene. J Virol 1996; 70:6634–6641.
62. Openshaw PJM, Anderson K, Wertz GW, Askonas BA. The 22,000-kilodalton protein of respiratory syncytial virus is a major target for K^d-restricted cytotoxic T lymphocytes from mice primed by infection. J Virol 1990; 64:1683–1689.
63. Nicholas JA, Rubino KL, Levely ME, Meyer AL, Collins PL. Cytotoxic T cell activity against the 22-kDa protein of human respiratory syncytial virus (RSV) is associated with a significant reduction in pulmonary RSV replication. Virology 191; 182:664–672.
64. Connors M, Collins PL, Firestone C, Murphy BR. Respiratory syncytial virus (RSV) F, G, M2 (22K), and N proteins each induced resistance to RSV challenge, but resistance induced by M2 and N proteins is relatively short-lived. J Virol 1991; 65:1634–1637.
65. Kulkarni AB, Collins PL, Bacik I, Yewdell JW, Bennink JR, Crowe JHE Jr, et al. Cytotoxic T cells specific for a single peptide on the M2 protein of respiratory syncytial virus are the sole mediators of resistance induced by immunization with M2 encoded by a recombinant vaccinia virus. J Virol 1995; 69:1261–1264.
66. Garcia-Barreno B, Delgado T, Melero JA. Identification of protein regions involved in the interaction of human respiratory syncytial virus phosphoprotein and nucleoprotein: significance for nucleocapsid assembly and formation of cytoplasmic inclusions. J Virol 1996; 70:801–808.
67. Garcia J, Garcia-Barreno B, Vivo A, Melero JA. Cytoplasmic inclusions of respiratory syncytial virus-infected cells: formation of inclusion bodies in transfected cells that coexpress the nucleoprotein, the phosphoprotein, and the 22K protein. Virology 1993; 195:243–247.
68. Walsh EE, Hall CB. Respiratory Syncytial Virus. In: Schmidt NJ, Emmons RW, eds. Diagnostic Procedures for Viral, Rickettsial and Chlamydial Infections. 6th ed. American Public Health Association, 1989:693–712.
69. Becker S, Soukup J, Yankaskas JR. Respiratory syncytial virus infection of human primary nasal and bronchial epithelial cell cultures and bronchoalveolar macrophages. Am J Respir Cell Mol Biol 1992; 6:369–374.
70. Gupta CK, Leszczynski J, Gupta KK, Siber GR. Stabilization of respiratory syncytial virus (RSV) against thermal inactivation and freeze-thaw cycles for development and control of RSV vaccines and immune globulin. Vaccine 1996; 14:1417–1420.
71. Verhoff J, Vander Ban M, Van Niewstadt AI. Bovine respiratory syncytial virus infection in young dairy cattle: clinical and hematological findings. Vet Rec 1984; 114:9–12.
72. Hall CB, Geiman JM, Biggar R, Kotok DI, Hogan PM, Douglas RG. Respiratory syncytial virus infections within families. N Engl J Med 1976; 294:414–419.
73. Hall CB, Douglas RG. Modes of transmission of respiratory syncytial virus. J Pediatr 1981; 99:100–103.
74. Hall CB, Douglas RG, Geiman JM. Possible transmission by fomites of respiratory syncytial virus. J Infect Dis 1980; 141:98–101.

75. Gala CL, Hall CB, Schnabel KC, Pincus PH, Blossom P, Hildreth SW, et al. The use of eye-nose goggles to control nosocomial respiratory syncytial virus infection. JAMA 1986; 256:2706–2708.
76. Hall CB, Schnabel KC, Gieman JM, Douglas RG. Infectivity of respiratory syncytial virus by various routes of inoculation. Infect Immun 1981; 33:779–783.
77. Hall CB, Douglas RG, Geiman JM. Respiratory syncytial virus infections in infants: quantitation and duration of shedding. J Pediatr 1976; 131:1–5.
78. Hall CB, Powell KR, MacDonald NE, Gala CL, Menegus ME, Suffin SC, et al. Respiratory syncytial viral infection in children with compromised immune function. N Engl J Med 1986; 315:77–81.
79. Hall CB, Walsh EE, Long CE, Schnabel KC. Immunity to and frequency of reinfection with respiratory syncytial virus. J Infect Dis 1991; 163:693–698.
80. Hall WJ, Hall CB, Speers DM. Respiratory syncytial virus infection in adults. Ann Intern Med 1978; 88:203–205.
81. Englund JA, Piedra P, Jewell A, Baxter BB, Whimbey E. Rapid diagnosis of respiratory syncytial virus (RSV) infection in immunocompromised adults (abstr). 34th Interscience Conference on Antimicrobial Agents and Chemotherapy, Orlando, FL, 1994.
82. Kim HW, Arrobio JO, Brandt CD, Jeffries BC, Pyles G, Reid JL, et al. Epidemiology of respiratory syncytial virus infection in Washington, D.C.: importance of the virus in different respiratory tract syndrome and temporal distribution of infection. Am J Epidemiol 1973; 98:216–225.
83. Washburne JF, Bocchini JA, Jamison RM. Summertime respiratory syncytial virus infection: epidemiology and clinical manifestations. South Med J 1992; 85:579–583.
84. Martin MA, Block MJ, Peallen MA, Wenzel RP. Respiratory syncytial virus infections in adult bone marrow transplant recipients. Lancet 1988; 1:1341–1343.
85. Clarke SKR, Gardner PS, Poole PM, Simpson H, Tobin JO. Respiratory syncytial virus infection: admissions to hospital in industrial, urban, and rural areas. Br Med J 1978; 2:796–798.
86. Hall CB, McCarthy CA. Respiratory Syncytial Virus. In: Mandell G, Bennett J, Dolin R, eds. Mandell, Douglas and Bennett's Principles and Practice of Infectious Disease. New York: Churchill Livingstone, 1996:1501–1519.
87. Denny FW, Clyde WA. Acute lower respiratory tract infections in nonhospitalized children. J Pediatr 1986; 108:635–646.
88. MacDonald NE, Hall CB, Suffin SC, Alexson C, Harris PJ, Manning JA. Respiratory syncytial viral infection in infants with congenital heart disease. N Engl J Med 1982; 307:397–400.
89. Navas L, Wang E, DeCarvalho V, Robinson J. Improved outcome of respiratory syncytial virus infection in a high risk hospitalized population of Canadian children. J Pediatr 1992; 121:348–354.
90. Henderson FW, Collier AM, Clyde WA, Denny FW. Respiratory syncytial-virus infections, reinfections and immunity. N Engl J Med 1979; 300:530–534.
91. Groothuis JR, Salbenblatt CK, Lauer BA. Severe respiratory syncytial virus infection in older children. Am J Dis Child 1990; 144:346–348.
92. Hall CB, Geiman JM, Douglas RG, Meagher MP. Control of nosocomial respiratory syncytial viral infections. Pediatrics 1978; 62:728–732.

93. Englund JA, Anderson LJ, Rhame FS. Nosocomial transmission of respiratory syncytial virus in immunocompromised adults. J Clin Microbiol 1991; 29:115–119.
94. Harrington RD, Hooton RM, Hackman RC, Storch GA, Osborne B, Gleaves CA, et al. An outbreak of respiratory syncytial virus in a bone marrow transplant center. J Infect Dis 1992; 165:987–993.
95. Hertz MI, Englund JA, Snover D, Bitterman PB, McGlave P. Respiratory syncytial virus-induced acute lung injury in adult patients with bone marrow transplants: a clinical approach and review of the literature. Medicine 1989; 68:269–281.
96. Whimbey E, Champlin RE, Couch RB, Englund JA, Goodrick JM, Raad I, et al. Community respiratory virus infections among hospitalized adult bone marrow transplant recipients. Clin Infect Dis 1996; 22:778–782.
97. Nicholson KG. Impact of influenza and respiratory syncytial virus on mortality in England and Wales from January 1975 to December 1990. Epidemiol Infect 1996; 116:51–63.
98. Fleming DM, Cross KW. Respiratory syncytial virus or influenza. Lancet 1993; 342:1507–1510.
99. Mathur U, Bentley DW, Hall CB. Concurrent respiratory syncytial virus and Influenza A infections in the institutionalized elderly and chronically ill. Ann Intern Med 1980; 93:49–52.
100. Sorvillo FJ, Huie SF, Strassburg MA, Butsumyo A, Shandera WX, Fannin SL. An outbreak of respiratory syncytial virus pneumonia in a nursing home for the elderly. J Infect Dis 1984; 9:252–256.
101. Dowell SF, Anderson LJ, Gary HEJ, Erdman DD, Plouffe JF, File TMJ, et al. Respiratory syncytial virus is an important cause of community-acquired lower respiratory infection among hospitalized adults. J Infect Dis 1996; 174:456–462.
102. Hall CB, Douglas RG, Geiman JM, Messner MK. Nosocomial respiratory syncytial virus infections. N Engl J Med 1975; 293:1343–1346.
103. Hendry RM, Fernie BF, Anderson LJ, McIntosh K. Antigenic and epidemiologic analysis of distinct strains of respiratory syncytial virus from two successive community outbreaks (1983–85). In: Mahy B, Kolakofsky D, eds. Biology of Negative Strand Viruses. Elsevier, 1987:397–403.
104. Hendry RM, Talis AL, Godfrey E, Anderson LJ, Fernie BF, McIntosh K. Concurrent circulation of antigenically distinct strains of respiratory syncytial virus during community outbreaks. J Infect Dis 1986; 153:291–297.
105. Waris M. Pattern of respiratory syncytial virus epidemics in Finland: two-year cycles with alternating prevalence of groups A and B. J Infect Dis 1991; 163:464–469.
106. Akerlind B, Norrby E. Occurrence of respiratory syncytial virus subtypes A and B strains in Sweden. J Med Virol 1986; 19:241–247.
107. Tsutsumi H, Onuma M, Suga K, Honjo T, Chiba Y, Chiba S, et al. Occurrence of respiratory syncytial virus subgroups A and B strains in Japan, 1980 to 1987. J Clin Microbiol 1988; 26:1171–1174.
108. Hall CB, Walsh EE, Schnabel KC, Long CE, McConnochie KM, Hildreth SW, et al. Occurrence of groups A and B of respiratory syncytial virus over 15 years: associated epidemiologic and clinical characteristics in hospitalized and ambulatory children. J Infect Dis 1990; 192:1283–1290.
109. Cane PA, Matthews DA, Pringle CR. Analysis of respiratory syncytial virus strain variation in successive epidemics in one city. J Clin Microbiol 1994; 32:1–4.

110. Anderson LJ, Hendry RM, Pierik LT, Tsou C, McIntosh K. Multicenter study of strains of respiratory syncytial virus. J Infect Dis 1991; 163:687–692.
111. McConnochie KM, Hall CB, Walsh EE, Roghmann KJ. Variation in severity of respiratory syncytial virus infections with subtype. J Pediatr 1990; 117:52–62.
112. Mufson MA, Belshe RB, Orvell C, Norrby E. Respiratory syncytial virus epidemics: variable dominance of subgroups A and B strains among children, 1981–1986. J Infect Dis 1988; 157:143–148.
113. Walsh EE, McConnochie KM, Long CE, Hall CB. Severity of respiratory syncytial virus infection is related to virus strain. J Infect Dis 1997; 175:814–820.
114. Mufson MA. Subgroup characteristics of respiratory syncytial virus strains recovered from children with two consecutive infections. J Clin Microbiol 1987; 25:1535–1539.
115. Becker S, Koren H, Henke D. Interleukin-8 expression in normal nasal epithelium and its modulation by infection with respiratory syncytial virus and cytokines tumor necrosis factor, interleukin-1, and interleukin-6. Am J Respir Cell Mol Biol 1993; 8:20–27.
116. Becker S, Quay J, Soukup J. Cytokine (tumor necrosis factor, IL-6 and IL-8) production by respiratory syncytial virus-infected human alveolar macrophages. J Immunol 1991; 147:4307–4312.
117. Noah T, Becker S. Respiratory syncytial-virus-induced cytokine production by a human bronchial epithelial cell line. Am J Physiol 1993; 265:L472–L478.
118. Arnold R, Humbert B, Werchau H, Gallati H, Konig W. Interleukin-8, interleukin-6, and soluble tumour necrosis factor receptor type I release from a human pulmonary epithelial cell line (A549) exposed to respiratory syncytial virus. Immunology 1994; 82:126–133.
119. Elias JA, Zheng T, Einarsson O, Landry M, Trow T, Rebert NA, et al. Epithelial interleukin-11. Regulation by cytokines, respiratory syncytial virus, and retinoic acid. J Biol Chem 1994; 269:22261–22268.
120. Mastronarde J, He B, Monick M, Mukaika N, Matsushima K, Hunninghake G. Induction of interleukin-8 (IL-8) gene expression by respiratory syncytial virus involves activation of nuclear factor (NF)-kB and NF-IL6. J Infect Dis 1996; 174:262–267.
121. Garafalo R, Sabry M, Jamaluddin M, Yu R, Casola A, Ogra PL, et al. Transcriptional activation of the interleukin-8 gene by respiratory syncytial virus infection in alveolar epithelial cells: nuclear translocation of the RelA transcription factor as a mechanism producing airway mucosal inflammation. J Virol 1996; 70:8773–8781.
122. Jamaluddin M, Garafalo R, Ogra PL, Brasier A. Inducible translational regulation of the NF-IL6 transcription factor by respiratory syncytial virus infection in pulmonary epithelial cells. J Virol 1996; 70:1554–1563.
123. Noah T, Henderson FW, Wortman I, Devlin R, Handy J, Koren H, et al. Nasal cytokine production in viral acute upper respiratory infection of childhood. J Infect Dis 1995; 171:584–592.
124. Okamoto Y, Kudo K, Ishikawa K, Ito E, Togawa K, Saito I, et al. Presence of respiratory syncytial virus genomic sequences in middle ear fluid and its relationship to expression of cytokines and cell adhesions molecules. J Infect Dis 1993; 168:1277–1288.

125. Neuzil K, Tang Y, Graham BS. Protective effects of TNF-a on respiratory syncytial virus infection in vitro and in vivo. Am J Med Sci 1996; 311:201–204.
126. Nakayama T, Sonoda S, Urano T, Saski K, Maehara N, Makino S. Detection of alpha-interferon in nasopharyngeal secretions and sera in children infected with respiratory syncytial virus. Pediatr Infect Dis J 1993; 12:925–929.
127. Midulla F, Villani A, Panuskas J, Dab I, Kolls J, Merolla R, et al. Respiratory syncytial virus lung infection in infants: immunoregulatory role of infected alveolar macrophages. J Infect Dis 1993; 168:1515–1519.
128. Hall CB, Douglas RG, Simons R, Geiman JM. Interferon production in children with respiratory syncytial, influenza and parainfluenza virus infections. J Pediatr 1978; 93:28–32.
129. Chonmaitree T, Roberts N, Douglas RG, Hall CB, Simons R. Interferon production by human mononuclear leukocytes: differences between respiratory syncytial virus and influenza viruses. Infect Immun 1981; 32:300–303.
130. McIntosh K. Interferon in nasal secretions from infants with viral respiratory tract infections. J Pediatr 1978; 93:33–36.
131. Preston F, Beier P, Popc J. Identification of the respiratory syncytial virus–induced immunosuppressive factor produced by human peripheral blood mononuclear cells in vitro as interferon-α. J Infect Dis 1995; 72:919–926.
132. Anderson J, Norden J, Saunders D, Toms G, Scott R. Analysis of the local and systemic immune responses induced in BALB/c mice by experimental respiratory syncytial virus infection. J Gen Virol 1990; 71:1561–1570.
133. Beem M. Repeated infection with respiratory syncytial virus. J Immunol 1967; 98:1115–1122.
134. Panuska J, Midulla F, Cirino N, Villani A, Gilbert I, McFadden J, et al. Virus induced alterations in macrophage production of tumor necrosis factor and prostaglandin E2. J Physiol 1990; 259:L396–L402.
135. Panuska J, Hertz MI, Taraf H, Villani A, Cirino N. Respiratory syncytial virus infection of alveolar macrophages in adult transplant patients. Am Rev Respir Dis 1992; 145:934–939.
136. Panuska J, Merolla R, Rebert N, Hoffman S, Tsivitse P, Cirino N. Respiratory syncytial virus induces interleukin-10 by human alveolar macrophages. J Clin Invest 1995; 96:2445–2453.
137. Fiorentino D, Zlotnik A, Mosmann T, Howard M, O'Garra A. IL-10 inhibits cytokine production by activated macrophages. J Immunol 1991; 147:3815–3822.
138. Moore K, O'Garra A, Malefyt R, Vieira P, Mosmann T. Interleukin-10. Ann Rev Immunol 1993; 11:165–190.
139a. Roberts N, Prill A, Mann T. Interleukin 1 and interleukin 1 inhibitor production by human macrophages exposed to influenza virus or respiratory syncytial virus. J Exp Med 1986; 163:511–519.
139b. Garofalo R, Kimpen JLL, Welliver RC, Ogra PL. Eosinophil degranulation in the respiratory tract during naturally acquired respiratory syncytial virus infection. J Pediatr 1992; 120:28–32.
139c. Sigurs N, Bjarnason R, Sigurbergsson F. Eosinophil cationic protein in nasal secretion and in serum and myeloperoxidase in serum in respiratory syncytial virus bronchiolitis: relation to asthma and atopy. Acta Paediatrica 1994; 83:1151–1155.

139d. Ingram JM, Rakes GP, Hoover GE, Platts-Mills TA, Heymann PW. Eosinophil cationic protein in serum and nasal washes from wheezing infants and children. J Pediatr 1995; 127:558–564.

139e. Simard C, Nadon F, Seguin C, Trudel M. Evidence that the amino acid region 124-203 of glycoprotein G from the respiratory syncytial virus (RSV) constitutes a major part of the polypeptide domain that is involved in the protection against RSV infection. Antiviral Research 1995; 28:303–315.

139f. Sparer TE, Matthews S, Hussell T, Rae AJ, Garcia-Barreno B, Melero JA, Openshaw PJM. Eliminating a region of respiratory syncytial virus attachment protein allows induction of protective immunity without vaccine-enhanced lung eosinophilia. J Exp Med 1998; 187:1921–1926.

139g. Simard C, Nadon F, Seguin C, Thien NN, Binz H, Basso J, Laliberte JF, Trudel M. Subgroup specific protection of mice from respiratory syncytial virus infection with peptides encompassing the amino acid region 174-187 from the G glycoprotein: the role of cysteinyl residues in protection. Vaccine 1997; 15:423–432.

139h. Srikiatkhachorn A, Braciale TJ. Virus-specific CD8$^+$ T lymphocytes downregulate T helper cell type 2 cytokine secretion and pulmonary eosinophilia during experimental murine respiratory syncytial virus infection. J Exp Med 1997; 186:421–432.

139i. Hancock GE, Speelman DJ, Heers K, Bortell E, Smith J, Cosco C. Generation of atypical pulmonary inflammatory responses in BALB/c mice after immunization with the native attachment (G) glycoprotein of respiratory syncytial virus. J Virol 1996; 70:7783–7791.

140. Glezen WP, Taber LH, Frank A, Kasel J. Risk of primary infection and reinfection with respiratory syncytial virus. Am J Dis Child 1986; 140:543–546.

141. Kasel J, Walsh EE, Frank A, Baxter BB, Taber LH, Glezen WP. Relation of serum antibody to glycoproteins of respiratory syncytial virus with immunity to infection in children. Viral Immunol 1987; 1:199–205.

142. Murphy BR, Graham BS, Prince GA, Walsh EE, Chanock RM, Karzon DT, et al. Serum and nasal-wash immunoglobulin G and A antibody response of infants and children to respiratory syncytial virus F and G glycoproteins following primary infection. J Clin Microbiol 1986; 23:1009–1014.

143. Ward K, Lambden P, Ogilvie M, Watt P. Antibodies to respiratory syncytial virus polypeptides and their significance in human infection. J Gen Virol 1983; 64:1867–1876.

144. Vianiopaa R, Meurman O, Sarkkinen H. Antibody response to respiratory syncytial virus structural proteins in children with acute respiratory syncytial virus infection. J Virol 1985; 53:976–979.

145. Gimenez H, Keir H, Cash P. Immunoblot analysis of the human antibody response to respiratory syncytial virus infection. J Gen Virol 1987; 68:1267–1275.

146. Watt P, Zardiz M, Lambden P. Age related IgG subclass response to respiratory syncytial virus fusion protein in infected infants. Clin Exp Immunol 1986; 64:503–509.

147. Wagner DK, Nelson DL, Walsh EE, Reimer CB, Henderson FW, Murphy BR. Differential immunoglobulin G subclass antibody titers to respiratory syncytial virus F and G glycoproteins in adults. J Clin Microbiol 1987; 25:748–750.

148. Wong D, Ogra PL. Neonatal respiratory syncytial virus infection: role of transplacentally and breast milk-acquired antibodies. J Virol 1986; 57:1203–1206.

148a. Murphy BR, Alling DW, Snyder MH, Walsh EE, Prince GA, Chanock RM, et al. Effect of age and preexisting antibody on serum antibody response of infants and children to the F and G glycoproteins during respiratory syncytial virus infection. J Clin Microbiol 1986; 24:894–898.
149. Kravetz H, Knight V, Chanock RM, Morris JA, Johnson K, Rifkind D, et al. Respiratory syncytial virus: III. Production of illness and clinical observations in adult volunteers. JAMA 1961; 176:657–663.
150. Johnson K, Chanock RM, Rifkind D, Kravetz H, Knight V. Respiratory syncytial virus: IV. Correlation of virus shedding serologic response and illness in adult volunteers. JAMA 1961; 176:663–667.
151. Johnson K, Bloom H, Mufson MA, Chanock RM. Natural reinfection of adults by respiratory syncytial virus. N Engl J Med 1962; 267:68–72.
152. Mills J, Van Kirk J, Wright PF, Chanock RM. Experimental respiratory syncytial virus infection of adults. Possible mechanisms of resistance to infection and illness. J Immunol 1971; 107:123–130.
153. Scott R, Kaul A, Scott M, Chiba Y, Ogra PL. Development of in vitro correlates of cell-mediated immunity to respiratory syncytial virus infection in humans. J Infect Dis 1978; 137:810–817.
154. Graham BS, Bunton L, Wright PF, Karzon DT. Respiratory syncytial virus in anti-u treated mice. J Virol 1991; 65:4936–4942.
155. Graham BS, Bunton L, Wright PF, Karzon DT. The role of T cell subsets in the pathogenesis of primary infection and reinfection with respiratory syncytial virus in mice. J Clin Invest 1991; 88:1026–1033.
156. Prince GA, Horswood RL, Chanock RM. Quantitative aspects of passive immunity to respiratory syncytial virus infection in infant cotton rats. J Virol 1985; 55:517–520.
157. Hill MG, Collins PL. Further studies of the transcriptional elongation factor M2 (ORF1) of respiratory syncytial virus (RSV) (abstr). Am Soc Virol 1996.
158. Crowe JE Jr, Collins PL, London WT, Chanock RM, Murphy BR. A comparison in chimpanzees of the immunogenicity and efficacy of live attenuated respiratory syncytial virus (RSV) temperature-sensitive mutant vaccines and vaccinia virus recombinants that express the surface glycoproteins of RSV. Vaccine 1993; 11: 1395–1404.
159. Crowe JE Jr, Bui PT, Sibert GR, Elkins WR, Chanock RM, Murphy BR. Cold-passaged temperature-sensitive mutants of human respiratory syncytial virus (RSV) are highly attenuated, immunogenic, and protective in seronegative chimpanzees, even when RSV antibodies are infused shortly before immunization. Vaccine 1995; 13L847–855.
160. Prince GA, Hemming VG, Horswood RL, Chanock RM. Immunoprophylaxis and immunotherapy of respiratory syncytial virus infection in the cotton rat. Virus Res 1985; 3:93–96.
161. Prince GA, Hemming VG, Horswood RL, Baron P, Chanock RM. Effectiveness of topical administered neutralizing antibodies in experimental immunotherapy of respiratory syncytial virus infection in cotton rats. J Virol 1987; 61:1851–1854.
162. Walsh EE, Schlesinger JJ, Brandriss M. Protection from respiratory syncytial virus infection in cotton rats by passive transfer of monoclonal antibodies. Infect Immun 1984; 43:756–758.

163. Taylor G, Stott EJ, Bew M, Fernie BF, Cote PJ, Collins A, et al. Monoclonal antibodies protect against respiratory syncytial virus infection in mice. Immunology 1984; 52:137–141.
164. Gruber W, Wilson S, Throop B, Wyde P. Immunoglobulin administration and Ribavirin therapy and efficacy in respiratory syncytial virus infection of the cotton rat. Pediatrics 1987; 21:270–274.
165. Graham BS, Davis T, Tang Y, Bunton L, Gruber W. Immunoprophylaxis and immunotherapy of respiratory syncytial virus-infected mice with RSV-specific immune serum. Pediatr Res 1993; 34:167–172.
166. Bangham CRM, Openshaw P, Ball LA, King AMQ, Wertz GW, Askonas BA. Human and murine cytotoxic T cells specific to respiratory syncytial virus recognize the viral nucleoprotein (N), but not the major glycoprotein (G), expressed by vaccinia virus recombinants. J Immunol 1986; 137:3973–3977.
167. Bangham CRM, McMichael A. Specific human cytotoxic T cells recognize B-cell lines persistently infected with respiratory syncytial virus. Proc Natl Acad Sci USA 1986; 83:9183–9187.
168. Isaacs D, Bangham C, McMichael A. Cell-mediated cytotoxic response to respiratory syncytial virus in infants with bronchiolitis. Lancet 1987; 2:769–771.
169. Chiba S, Higashidate Y, Suga K, Honjo K, Tsutsumi H, Ogra PL. Development of cell-mediated cytotoxic immunity to respiratory syncytial virus in human infants following naturally acquired infection. J Med Virol 1989; 28:133–139.
170. Taylor G, Stott EJ, Hayle A. Cytotoxic lymphocytes in the lungs of mice infected with respiratory syncytial virus. J Gen Virol 1985; 66:2533–2538.
171. Taylor G, Thomas L, Wyld S, Furze J, Sopp P, Howard C. Roles of T-lymphocyte subsets in recovery from respiratory syncytial virus infection in calves. J Virol 1995; 69:6658–6664.
172. Zinkernagel R, Hengartner H. T-cell mediated immunopathology versus direct cytolysis by virus: implication for HIV and AIDS. Immunol Today 1994; 15:262–268.
173. Cannon MJ, Stott EJ, Taylor G, Askonas BA. Clearance of persistent respiratory syncytial virus infections in immunodeficient mice following transfer of primed T cells. Immunology 1987; 62:133–138.
174. Askonas BA, Taylor P. T cell mediated immunity in virus infection. Immunol Lett 1987; 16:337–342.
175. Cannon MJ, Openshaw P, Askonas BA. Cytotoxic T cells clear virus but augment lung pathology in mice infected with respiratory syncytial virus. J Exp Med 1988; 168:1163–1168.
176. Muñoz J, McCarthy CA, Clark M, Hall CB. Respiratory syncytial virus infection in C57BL/6 mice: clearance of virus from the lungs with virus-specific cytotoxic T cells. J Virol 1991; 65:4494–4497.
177. Nicholas JA, Mitchell M, Levely ME, Rubino KL, Kinner J, Harn N, et al. Mapping an antibody-binding site and a T-cell–stimulating site on the 1A protein of respiratory syncytial virus. J Virol 1988; 62:4465–4473.
178. Bangham CRM, Cannon MJ, Karzon DT, Askonas BA. Cytotoxic T-cell response to respiratory syncytial virus in mice. J Virol 1985; 56:55–59.

179. Kim HW, Leikin S, Arrobio JO, Brandt CD, Chanock RM, Parrott RH. Cell-mediated immunity to respiratory syncytial virus induced by inactivated vaccine or by infection. Pediatr Res 1976; 10:75–78.
180. Stott EJ, Taylor G, Ball LA, Anderson K, Young KKY, King AMQ, et al. Immune and histologic responses in animals vaccinated with recombinant vaccinia viruses that express individual genes of respiratory syncytial virus. J Virol 1987; 61:3855–3861.
181. Scott R, Pullan CR, McQuillin J. Cell-mediated immunity in respiratory syncytial virus disease. J Med Virol 1984; 13:105–114.
182. Welliver RC, Kaul A, Ogra PL. Cell-mediated response to respiratory syncytial virus infection: relationship to the development of reactive airway disease. J Pediatr 1979; 94:370–375.
183. Alwan W, Record F, Openshaw P. $CD4^+$ T cells clear virus but augment disease in mice infected with respiratory syncytial virus. Comparison with the effects of $CD8^+$ T cells. Clin Exp Immunol 1992; 88:527–536.
184. Connors M, Kulkarni AB, Firestone C, Holmes K, Morse IH, Sotnikov A, et al. Pulmonary histopathology induced by respiratory syncytial virus (RSV) challenge of formalin-inactivated RSV-immunized BALB/c mice is abrogated by depletion of CD4+ T cells. J Virol 1992; 66:7444–7451.
185. Ahern W, Bird T, Court S, Gardner P, McQuillin J. Pathological changes in virus infections of the lower respiratory tract in children. J Clin Pathol 1970; 23:7–18.
186. Downham MAPS, Gardner PS, McQuillin J, Ferris JAJ. Role of respiratory viruses in childhood mortality. Br Med J 1975; 1:235–239.
187. King J, Burke A, Clemens J, Nair P, Farley J, Vink P, et al. Respiratory syncytial viral illnesses in HIV-infected and noninfected children. Pediatr Infect Dis J 1993; 12:733–778.
188. Fishaut M, Tubergen D, McIntosh K. Cellular response to respiratory viruses with particular reference to children with disorders of cell-mediated immunity. J Pediatr 1980; 96:179–186.
189. Milner M, Monte S, Hutchins G. Fatal respiratory syncytial virus infection in severe combined immunodeficiency syndrome. Am J Dis Child 1985; 139:1111–1114.
190. Belshe RB, VanVoris LP, Mufson MA. Parenteral administration of live respiratory syncytial virus vaccine: results of a field trial. J Infect Dis 1982; 145:311–319.
191. Merz D, Scheid A, Choppin P. Importance of antibodies to the fusion glycoprotein of paramyxoviruses in the prevention of spread of infection. J Exp Med 1980; 151:275–288.
192. Murphy BR, Prince GA, Walsh EE, Kim HW, Parrott RH, Hemming VG, et al. Dissociation between serum neutralizing and glycoprotein antibody responses of infants and children who received inactivated respiratory syncytial virus vaccine. J Clin Microbiol 1986; 24:197–202.
193. Murphy BR, Walsh EE. Formalin-inactivated respiratory syncytial virus vaccine induces antibodies to the fusion glycoprotein that are deficient in fusion-inhibiting activity. J Clin Microbiol 1988; 26:1595–1597.
194. Karzon DT. The immune basis for hypersensitivity to viral vaccines. Hum Immun Viruses 1983; 111–130.

195. Lennon R, Isacson P, Rosales T, Elsea W, Karzon DT, Winkelstein W. Skin tests with measles and poliomyelitis vaccines in recipients of inactivated measles virus vaccine. J Am Med Assoc 1976; 100:275.
196. Prince GA, Jenson A, Hemming VG, Murphy BR, Walsh EE, Horswood RL, et al. Enhancement of respiratory syncytial virus pulmonary pathology in cotton rats by prior intramuscular inoculation of formalin-inactivated virus. J Virol 1986; 57: 721–728.
197. Graham BS, Henderson G, Tang Y, Lu X, Neuzil K, Colley D. Priming immunization determines T helper cytokine mRNA expression patterns in lungs of mice challenged with respiratory syncytial virus. J Immunol 1993; 151:2032–2040.
198. Openshaw P, Clarke S, Record F. Pulmonary eosinophilic response to respiratory syncytial virus infection in mice sensitized to the major surface glycoprotein G. Int Immunol 1992; 4:493–500.
199. Volovitz B, Welliver R, DeCastro G, Krystofik D, Ogra PL. The release of leukotrienes in the respiratory tract during infection with respiratory syncytial virus: role in obstructive airway disease. Pediatr Res 1988; 24:504–507.
200. Gruber C, Levin S. Respiratory syncytial virus polypeptides. IV. The oligosaccharides of the glycoproteins. J Gen Virol 1985; 66:417–432.
201. Alwan W, Record F, Openshaw P. Phenotypic and functional characterization of T cell lines specific for individual respiratory syncytial virus proteins. J Immunol 1993; 150:5211–5218.
202. Alwan W, Openshaw P. Distinct patterns of T- and B-cell immunity to respiratory syncytial virus induced by individual viral proteins. Vaccine 1993; 11: 431–437.
203. Alwan W, Kozlowska W, Openshaw P. Distinct types of lung disease caused by functional subsets of antiviral T cells. J Exp Med 1994; 179:81–89.
204. Graham BS. Immunologic determinants of RSV-induced disease. Trends Microbiol 1996; 4:290–293.
205. Tang Y, Graham BS. Anti-IL-4 treatment at immunization modulates cytokine expression, reduces illness, and increased cytotoxic T lymphocyte activity in mice challenged with respiratory syncytial virus. J Clin Invest 1994; 94:1953–1958.
206a. Tang Y, Graham BS. Interleukin 12 treatment during immunization elicits a Th1-like immune response in mice challenged with respiratory syncytial virus and improves vaccine immunogenicity. J Infect Dis 1995; 172:734–738.
206b. Hussell T, Khan U. Openshaw PJM. IL-12 treatment attenuates T helper cell type 2 and B cell responses but does not improve vaccine-enhanced lung illness. J Immunol 1997; 159:328–334.
207. An S, Gould S, Keeling J, Fleming K. Role of respiratory viral infection in SIDS: detection of viral nucleic acid by in situ hybridization. J Pathol 1993; 171:271–278.
208. Lindgren C, Jing L, Graham BS, Grogard J, Sundell H. Respiratory syncytial virus infection reinforces reflex apnea in young lambs. Pediatr Res 1992; 31:381–385.
209. Neuzil K, Gruber WC, Chytil F, Stahlman M, Graham BS. Serum vitamin A levels in respiratory syncytial virus infection. J Pediatr 1994; 124:433–436.
210. Lindgren C, Grogaard J. Reflex apnoea response and inflammatory mediators in infants with respiratory tract infection. Acta Paediatr 1996; 85:798–803.

211. Lindgren C, Lin J, Graham BS, Gray M, Parker RA, Sundell H. Respiratory syncytial virus infection enhances the response to laryngeal chemostimulation and inhibits arousal from sleep in young lambs. Acta Pediatr Scand 1996; 85: 789–797.
212. Pickens D, Schefft G, Storch GA, Thach B. Characterization of prolonged apneic episodes associated with respiratory syncytial virus infection. Pediatr Pulmonol 1989; 6:195–201.
213. Bruhn F, Mokrohisky S, McIntosh K. Apnea associated with respiratory syncytial virus infection in young infants. J Pediatr 1977; 90:382–386.
214. Neuzil K, Gruber WC, Chytil F, Stahlman M, Graham BS. Safety of vitamin A therapy for infants with respiratory syncytial virus infection. Antimicrobial Agents and Chemotherapy 1995; 39:1191–1193.
215. Quinlan K, Hayani K. Vitamin A and respiratory syncytial virus infection. Serum levels and supplementation trial. Arch Pediatr Adolesc Med 1996; 150:25–30.
216. Sigurs N, Bjarnason R, Sigurbergsson F, Kjellman B, Bjorksten B. Asthma and immunoglobulin E antibodies after respiratory syncytial virus bronchiolitis: a prospective cohort study with matched controls. Pediatrics 1995; 95:500–505.
217. Welliver RC, Duffy L. The relationship of RSV-specific immunoglobulin E antibody response in infancy, recurrent wheezing, and pulmonary function at age 7–8 years. Pediatr Pulmonol 1993; 15:19–27.
218. Bui PT. Virus-specific IgE and IgG4 antibodies in serum of children infected with respiratory syncytial virus. J Pediatr 1987; 110:87–90.
219. Welliver RC, Kaul T, Ogra PL. The appearance of cell-bound IgE in respiratory-tract epithelium after respiratory syncytial virus infection. N Engl J Med 1980; 3:1198–1202.
220. Gerswhin L, Dungworth D, Himes S, Friebertshauser K. Immunoglobulin E responses and lung pathology resulting from aerosol exposure to calves to respiratory syncytial virus and *Micropolyspora faeni*. Int Arch Allergy Appl Immunol 1990; 92:293–300.
221. Leibovitz E, Freihorst J, Piedra P, Ogra PL. Modulation of systemic and mucosal immune responses to inhaled ragweed antigen in experimentally induced infection with respiratory syncytial virus: implications in virally induced allergy. Int Arch Allergy Appl Immunol 1988; 86:112–116.
222. Freihorst J, Piedra P, Okamoto Y, Ogra PL. Effect of respiratory syncytial virus infection on the uptake of and immune response to other inhaled antigens. Proc Soc Exp Biol Med 1988; 188:191–197.
223. Garafalo R, Kimpen J, Welliver RC, Ogra PL. Eosinophil degranulation in the respiratory tract during naturally acquired respiratory syncytial virus infection. J Pediatr 1992; 120:28–32.
224. Sigurs N, Bjarnason R, Sigurbergsson F. Eosinophil cationic protein in nasal secretion and in serum and myeloperoxidase in serum in respiratory syncytial virus bronchiolitis: relation to asthma and atopy. Acta Pediatr 1994; 83:1151–1155.
225a. Ingram J, Rakes G, Hoover G, Platts-Mills T, Heyman P. Eosinophil cationic protein in serum and nasal washes from wheezing infants and children. J Pediatr 1995; 127:558–564.

225b. Schwarze J, Hamelmann E, Bradley KL, Takeda K, Gelfand EW. Respiratory syncytial virus infection results in airway hyperresponsiveness and enhanced airway sensitization to allergen. J Clin Invest 1997; 100:226–233.
225c. Peebles RS, Jr, Sheller JR, Johnson JE, Mitchell DB, Graham BS. Respiratory syncytial virus infection prolonged methacholine-induced airway hyperresponsiveness in ovalbumin sensitized mice. Submitted.
225d. Van Schaik SM, Enhorning G, Vargas I, Welliver RC. Respiratory syncytial virus affects pulmonary function in BALB/c mice. J Infect Dis 1998; 177:269–276.
225e. Robinson PJ, Hegele RG, Schellenberg RR. Allergic sensitization increases airway reactivity in guinea pigs with respiratory syncytial virus bronchiolitis. J All Clin Immunol 1997; 100:492–498.
226. Sarkkinen H, Ruuskanen O, Meurman O, Puhakka H, Virolainen E, Eskola J. Identification of respiratory virus antigens in middle ear fluids of children with acute otitis media. J Infect Dis 1985; 151:444–448.
227. Henderson FW, Collier AM, Sanyal MA, Watkins JM, Fairclough DL, Clyde WA, et al. A longitudinal study of respiratory viruses and bacteria in the etiology of acute otitis media with effusion. N Engl J Med 1982; 306:1377–1383.
228. Chonmaitree T, Owen MJ, Patel JA, Hedgpeth D, Horlick D. Effect of viral respiratory tract infection on outcome of acute otitis media. J Pediatr 1992; 120: 856–862.
229. Hall CB, Hall WJ, Speers DM. Clinical and physiological manifestations of bronchiolitis and pneumonia. Am J Dis Child 1979; 133:798–802.
230. Wang EEL, Milner RA, Navas L, Maj H. Observer agreement for respiratory signs and oximetry in infants hospitalized with lower respiratory infections. Am Rev Respir Dis 1992; 145:106–109.
231. Shaw KN, Bell LM, Sherman NH. Outpatient assessment of infants with bronchiolitis. Am J Dis Child 1991; 145:151–155.
232. Church NR, Anas NG, Hall CB, Brooks JG. Respiratory syncytial virus–related apnea in infants. Am J Dis Child 1984; 138:247–250.
233. Wildin SR, Chonmaitree T, Swischuk LE. Roentgenographic features of common pediatric viral respiratory tract infections. Am J Dis Child 1988; 142:43–46.
234. Hall CB, Kopelman AE, Douglas RG, Geiman JM, Meagher MP. Neonatal respiratory syncytial virus infection. N Engl J Med 1979; 300:393–396.
235. Groothuis JR, Gutierrez KM, Lauer BA. Respiratory syncytial virus infection in children with bronchopulmonary dysplasia. Pediatrics 1988; 82:199–203.
236. Chandwani S, Borkowsky W, Krasinski K, Lawrence R, Welliver R. Respiratory syncytial virus infection in human immunodeficiency virus–infected children. J Pediatr 1990; 117:251–254.
237. Tristram DA, Miller RW, McMillan JA, Weiner LB. Simultaneous infection with respiratory syncytial virus and other respiratory pathogens. Am J Dis Child 1988; 142:834–836.
238. Hall CB, Powell KR, Schnabel KC, Gala CL, Pincus PH. Risk of secondary bacterial infection in infants hospitalized with respiratory syncytial viral infection. J Pediatr 1988; 113:266–271.
239. Pohl C, Green M, Wald ER, Ledesma-Medina J. Respiratory syncytial virus infections in pediatric liver transplant recipients. J Infect Dis 1992; 165:166–169.

240. Agius G, Dindinaud G, Biggar RJ, Peyre R, Vaillant V, Ranger S, et al. An epidemic of respiratory syncytial virus in elderly people: clinical and serological findings. J Med Virol 1990; 30:117–127.
241. Carilla A, Gohd R, Gordon W. A virologic study of chronic bronchitis. N Engl J Med 1964; 170:123–127.
242. Gump D, Phillips C, Forsyth B. Role of infection in chronic bronchitis. Amer Rev Respir Dis 1976; 113:465–474.
243. Fagon J, Chastre J. Severe exacerbations of COPD patients: the role of pulmonary infections. Sem Respir Infect 1996; 11:109–118.
244. Fouillard L, Mouthon L, Isnard LF, Strachowiak J, Aoudjhane M, Lucet JC, et al. Severe respiratory syncytial virus pneumonia after autologous bone marrow transplantation: a report of three cases and review. Bone Marrow Transpl 1992; 9:97–100.
245. Kellogg JA. Culture vs direct antigen assays for detection of microbial pathogens from lower respiratory tract specimens suspected of containing the respiratory syncytial virus. Arch Pathol Lab Med 1991; 115:451–458.
246. Hall CB. Clinically useful method for the isolation of respiratory syncytial virus. J Infect Dis 1975; 131:1–5.
247. Derish MT, Kulhanjian JA, Frankel LR, Smith DW. Value of bronchoalveolar lavage in diagnosing severe respiratory syncytial virus infections in infants. J Pediatr 1991; 119:761–763.
248. Meziere A, Mollat C, Lapied R, Billaudel S, Courtieu A. Detection of respiratory syncytial virus antigen after seventy-two hours of culture. J Med Virol 1990; 31:241–244.
249. Olsen MA, Schuck KM, Sambol AR, Flor SM, O'Brien J, Cabrera B. Isolation of seven respiratory viruses in shell vials: a practical and highly sensitive method. J Clin Microbiol 1993; 31:422–425.
250. Johnston SLG, Siegel CS. Evaluation of direct immunofluorescence, enzyme immunoassay, centrifugation culture, and conventional culture for the detection of respiratory syncytial virus. J Clin Microbiol 1990; 28:2394–2397.
251. Falsey AR, McCann RM, Hall WJ, Criddle MM. Evaluation of four methods for the diagnosis of respiratory syncytial virus infection in older adults. J Am Geriatr Soc 1996; 44:71–73.
252. Olsen MA, Shuck KM, Sambol AR. Evaluation of Abbott Test Pack RSV for the diagnosis of respiratory syncytial virus infections. Diagn Microbiol Infect Dis 1993; 16:105–109.
253. vanMilaan AJ, Sprenger MJW, Rothbarth PH, Brandenburg AH, Masurel N, Claas ECJ. Detection of respiratory syncytial virus by RNA-polymerase chain reaction and differentiation of subgroups with oligonucleotide probes. J Med Virol 1994; 44:80–87.
254. Freymuth F, Eugene C, Petitjean J, Gennetay E, Brouard J, Duhamel JF, et al. Detection of respiratory syncytial virus by reverse transcription–PCR and hybridization with a DNA enzyme immunoassay. J Clin Microbiol 1995; 33:3352–3355.
255. Wagner DK, Graham BS, Wright PF, Walsh EE, Kim HW, Reimer CB, et al. Serum immunoglobulin G antibody subclass responses to respiratory syncytial

virus F and G glycoproteins after primary infection. J Clin Microbiol 1986; 24: 304–306.
257. Treuhaft MW, Soukup JM, Sullivan BJ. Practical recommendations for the detection of pediatric respiratory syncytial virus infections. J Clin Microbiol 1985; 22:270–273.
258. Schuh S, Canny G, Reisman JJ, Kerem E, Bentur L, Petric M, et al. Nebulized albuterol in acute bronchiolitis. J Pediatr 1990; 117:633–637.
259. Wang EEL, Milner RA, Allen U, Maj H. Bronchodilators for treatment of mild bronchiolitis: a factorial randomised trial. Arch Dis Child 1992; 67:289–293.
260. Sly PD, Lanteri CJ, Raven JM. Do wheezy infants recovering from bronchiolitis respond to inhaled salbutamol? Pediatr Pulmonol 1991; 10:36–39.
261. Springer C, Bar-Yishay E, Uwayyed K. Corticosteroids do not affect the clinical or physiological status of infants with bronchiolitis. Pediatr Pulmonol 1990; 9: 181–185.
262. Hall CB, McBride JT, Walsh EE, Bell DM, Gala CL, Hildreth SW, et al. Aerosolized ribavirin treatment of infants with respiratory syncytial viral infection. N Engl J Med 1983; 308:1443–1447.
263. Wyde PR, Ambrose MW, Meyer HL, Gilbert BE. Toxicity and antiviral activity of LY253963 against respiratory syncytial and parainfluenza type 3 viruses in tissue culture and in cotton rats. Antiviral Res 1990; 14:237–248.
264. Tidwell RR, Geratz JD, Clyde WA, Rosenthal KU, Dubovi EJ. Suppression of respiratory syncytial virus infection in cotton rats by bis(5-amidino-2-benzimidazolyl)methane. Antimicrob Agents Chemother 1984; 26:591–593.
265. Wyde PR, Ambrose MW, Meyerson LR, Gilbert BE. The antiviral activity of SP-303, a natural polyphenolic polymer, against respiratory syncytial and parainfluenza type 3 viruses in cotton rats. Antiviral Res 1993; 20:145–154.
266. Carmack MA, Prober CG. Respiratory syncytial virus and ribavirin: quo vadis? Infect Agents Dis 1992; 1:99–107.
267. Committee on Infectious Diseases. Use of ribavirin in the treatment of respiratory syncytial virus infection. Pediatrics 1993; 92:501–504.
268. Englund JA, Piedra P, Jefferson LS, Wilson SZ, Taber LH, Gilbert BE. High-dose, short duration ribavirin aerosol therapy in children with suspected respiratory syncytial virus infection. J Pediatr 1990; 117:313–320.
269. Taber LH, Knight V, Gilbert BE. Ribavirin aerosol treatment of bronchiolitis associated with respiratory syncytial virus infection in infants. Pediatrics 1983; 72:613–618.
270. Hall CB, McBride JT, Gala CL, Hildreth SW, Schnabel KC. Ribavirin treatment of respiratory syncytial viral infection in infants with underlying cardiopulmonary disease. JAMA 1985; 254:3047–3051.
271. Meert KL, Sarnaik AP, Gelmini MJ, Lieb T, M.W. Aerosolized ribavirin in mechanically ventilated children with respiratory syncytial virus lower respiratory tract disease: a prospective, double-blind, randomized trial. Crit Care Med 1994; 22:566–572.
272. Wheeler JC, Wofford J, Turner RB. Historical cohort evaluation of Ribavirin efficacy in respiratory syncytial virus. Pediatr Infect Dis J 1993; 12:209–213.
273. Hemming VG, Prince GA, London WT, Baron P, Brown R, Chanock RM. Topically administered immunoglobulin reduces pulmonary respiratory syncytial virus shedding in owl monkeys. Antimicrob Agents Chemother 1988; 32:1269–1270.

274. Siber GR, Leszczynski J, Pena-Cruz V, Ferren-Gardner C, Anderson R, Hemming VG, et al. Protective activity of a human respiratory syncytial virus immune globulin prepared from donors screened by microneutralization assay. J Infect Dis 1992; 165:456–463.
275. Hemming VG, Rodriguez WJ, Kim HW, Brandt CD, Parrott RH, Burch B, et al. Intravenous immunoglobulin treatment of respiratory syncytial virus infections in infants and young children. Antimicrob Agents Chemother 1987; 31:1882–1886.
276. Weltzin R, Hsu SA, Mittler S, Georgakopoulos K, Monath TP. Intranasal monoclonal immunoglobulin A against respiratory syncytial virus protects against upper and lower respiratory tract infections in mice. Antimicrob Agents Chemother 1994; 38:2785–2791.
277a. Barbas CF, Crowe JE Jr, Caba D, Jones TM, Zebedee SL, Murphy BR, et al. Human monoclonal Fab fragments derived from combinatorial library bind to respiratory syncytial virus F glycoprotein and neutralize infectivity. Proc Natl Acad Sci USA 1992; 89:10164–10168.
277b. Graham BS, Tang YW, Gruber WC. Topical immunoprophylaxis of respiratory syncytial virus (RSV)-challenged mice with RSV-specific immune globulin. J Infect Dis 1995; 171:1468–1474.
278. Whimbey E, Champlin RE, Englund JA, Mirza N, Piedra P, Goodrich JM, et al. Combination therapy with aerosolized ribavirin and intravenous immunoglobulin for respiratory syncytial virus disease in adult bone marrow transplant recipients. Bone Marrow Transplant 1995; 16:393–399.
279. Groothuis JR, Simoes EAF, Levin MJ, Hall CB, Long CE, Rodriguez WJ, et al. Prophylactic administration of respiratory syncytial virus immune globulin to high-risk infants and young children. N Engl J Med 1993; 329:1524–1530.
280. Groothuis JR, Simoes EAF, Hemming VG, Respiratory Syncytial Virus Immune Globulin Study Group. Respiratory syncytial virus (RSV) infection in preterm infants and the protective effects of RSV immune globulin (RSVIG). Pediatrics 1995; 95:463–467.
281. Wright PF, Belshe RB, Kim HW, VanVoris LP, Chanock RM. Administration of a highly attenuated, live respiratory syncytial virus vaccine to adults and children. Infect Immun 1982; 37:397–400.
282. Wright PF, Shinozaki T, Fleet W, Sell SH, Thompson J, Karzon DT. Evaluation of a live, attenuated respiratory syncytial virus vaccine in infants. J Pediatr 1976; 88:931–936.
283. Kim HW, Arrobio JO, Pyles G, Brandt CD, Camargo E, Chanock RM, et al. Clinical and immunological response of infants and children to administration of low-temperature adapted respiratory syncytial virus. Pediatrics 1971; 48:745–755.
284. Prince GA, Horswood RL, Camargo E, Suffin SC, Chanock RM. Parenteral immunization with live respiratory syncytial virus is blocked in seropositive cotton rats. Infect Immun 1982; 37:1074–1078.
285. Hsu KL, Lubeck MD, Bhat BM, Bhat RA, Kostek B, Selling BH, et al. Efficacy of adenovirus-vectored respiratory syncytial virus vaccines in a new ferret model. Vaccine 1994; 12:607–612.

286. Hsu KL, Lubeck MD, Davis AR, Bhat RA, Selling BH, Bhat BM, et al. Immunogenicity of recombinant adenovirus-respiratory syncytial virus vaccines with adenovirus types 4, 5, and 7 vectors in dogs and a chimpanzee. J Infect Dis 1992; 166:769–775.
287. Elango N, Prince GA, Murphy BR, Venkatesan S, Chanock RM, Moss B. Resistance to human respiratory syncytial virus (RSV) infection induced by immunization of cotton rats with a recombinant vaccinia virus expressing the RSV G glycoprotein. Proc Natl Acad Sci USA 1986; 83:1906–1910.
288. Wertz GW, Stott EJ, Young KKY, Anderson K, Ball LA. Expression of the fusion protein of human respiratory syncytial virus from recombinant vaccinia virus vectors and protection of vaccinated mice. J Virol 1987; 61:293–301.
289. Crowe JE Jr, Bui PT, London WT, Davis AR, Hung PP, Chanock RM, et al. Satisfactorily attenuated and protective mutants derived from a partially attenuated cold-passaged respiratory syncytial virus mutant by introduction of additional attenuating mutations during chemical mutagenesis. Vaccine 1994; 12: 691–699.
290. Firestone C, Whitehead S, Collins PL, Murphy BR, Crowe JE Jr. Nucleotide sequence analysis of the respiratory syncytial virus (RSV) subgroup A cold-passaged (*cpts*-248/404) candidate live attenuated virus vaccine (abstr). Am Soc Virol, 1996.
291. Crowe JE Jr, Bui PT, Firestone C, Connors M, Elkins WR, Chanock RM, et al. Live subgroup B respiratory syncytial virus vaccines that are attenuated, genetically stable, and immunogenic in rodents and nonhuman primates. J Infect Dis 1996; 173:829–839.
292. Tristram DA, Welliver R, Mohar CK, Hogerman DA, Hildreth SW, Paradiso P. Immunogenicity and safety of respiratory syncytial virus subunit vaccine in seropositive children 18–36 months old. J Infect Dis 1993; 167:191–195.
293. Belshe RB, Anderson EL, Walsh EE. Immunogenicity of purified F glycoprotein of respiratory syncytial virus: clinical and immune responses to subsequent natural infection in children. J Infect Dis 1993; 168:1024–1029.
294. Piedra P, Grace S, Jewell A, Spinelli S, Bunting D, Hogerman D, et al. Purified fusion protein vaccine protects against lower respiratory tract illness during respiratory syncytial virus season in children with cystic fibrosis. Pediatr Infect Dis J 1996; 15:23–31.
295. Falsey AR, Walsh EE. Safety and immunogenicity of a respiratory syncytial virus subunit vaccine (PFP-2) in ambulatory adults over age 60. Vaccine 1996; 14: 1214–1218.
296. Falsey AR, Walsh EE. Safety and immunogenicity of a respiratory syncytial virus subunit vaccine (PFP-2) in the institutionalized elderly. Vaccine 1997; 15:1130–1132.
297. Englund JA. Passive protection against respiratory syncytial virus disease in infants: the role of maternal antibody. Pediatr Infect Dis J 1994; 13:449–453.

8

Parainfluenza Viruses

PETER F. WRIGHT

Vanderbilt University School of Medicine
Nashville, Tennessee

I. Introduction

Parainfluenza viruses (PIV) were discovered in a flurry of identification of new respiratory viruses that occurred in the late 1950s (1–3). Four separate serotypes which cause human respiratory disease were subsequently distinguished (4–6). Types 1, 2, and 3 are the most clinically important of the serotypes. Type 4 has been implicated only in upper respiratory tract disease. The three major strains can be distinguished on epidemiological grounds and to a lesser extent by the nature of the clinical illness they cause. Related human pathogens within the family *Paramyxoviridae* include respiratory syncytial virus (RSV) and the viruses causing measles and mumps. As a group, the PIV are second only to RSV as a cause of serious lower respiratory disease in infants and children. Clinically, the PIV have a particular propensity to cause laryngotracheobronchitis or croup in young children (7). However, parainfluenza virus type 3 (PIV3) has a broader tropism and can cause bronchiolitis and pneumonia in young infants. In this respect, and others, PIV3 is most like RSV. PIV's most striking impact in the adult population is in individuals who are medically immunosuppressed in conjunction with organ transplantation or are otherwise immunocompromised. In such patients, PIV can cause progressive pneumonitis. Experimental infection of healthy adults with PIV1 or PIV3 leads to a mild to moderate upper respiratory infection with symptoms of nasal discharge, obstruction, and sneezing and clinical evidence of erythema of the nasal passages and throat—in short, a "cold." Many infections in children are also confined to the upper respiratory tract, but PIV infection in this setting is often accompanied by otitis media.

Questions we will try to address here for PIV are (1) why there is a localization of pathology and clinical symptomatology to the laryngeal and tracheal area; (2) why infection is confined to the epithelial layer of the respiratory tract in contrast to other structurally related viruses such as mumps that have such a different pathogenesis with viremia and localization in acinar tissue; (3) what may be learned about human disease from the pathogenesis of related animal viruses; (4) how can we put PIV in perspective with other causes of infectious pulmonary disease; and (5) what the prospects are for prevention and therapy of disease caused by PIV.

II. Similarity to Other Respiratory Viruses

Parainfluenza viruses share a number of structural, replicative, pathogenic, and clinical properties with the influenza virus and RSV (Table 1). The paramyxovirus and orthomyxovirus families to which these viruses belong have devised a number of ways of thwarting the usual protective immune responses, allowing reinfection throughout life. The influenza virus exhibits progressive antigenic variation and occasional emergence of a new strain through reassortment with surface proteins from animal reservoirs of influenza A strains. RSV infects very young infants in the face of maternal antibody and induces transient immunity, with reinfection of adults possible at 3- to 6-month intervals. PIV1 is the prototype virus for which mucosal IgA antibody, a relatively transient form of immunity, has been demonstrated to be important. PIV3 causes persistent and severe infection in immunocompromised patients and has been demonstrated in remote environments such as Antarctica in closed populations over prolonged periods of time. The latter observation suggests that this normally self-limited infection may be persistent in otherwise healthy individuals or that reinfection occurs with great frequency.

A number of animal counterparts exist to the human PIV strains that have provided models of infection and understanding of immunity to PIV. These include Newcastle disease virus (NDV) in chickens and Sendai virus in mice. However, no animal model short of the chimpanzee is fully permissive for human PIV strains. There is no animal that experiences a croup-like illness with PIV. Bovine and murine PIV are animal counterparts of human PIV that

Table 1 Comparison of Parainfluenza Viruses with Influenza Virus and Respiratory Syncytial Virus

	Parainfluenza	Influenza	RSV
Structure			
Size	150–200 nm	80–120 nm	150–300 nm
Enveloped	Yes	Yes	Yes
Genetic material	Single-stranded Nonsegmented Negative-sense RNA	Single-stranded 8-Segmented Negative-sense RNA	Single-stranded Nonsegmented Negative-sense RNA
Surface glycoproteins	HN hemagglutinin neuraminidase F-fusion	H hemagglutinin N neuraminidase	G attachment F fusion
Total proteins coded	6 + Accessory proteins	10	10
Replication	Cytoplasmic	Cytoplasmic/nuclear	Cytoplasmic
Receptor	Sialic acid	Sialic acid	Unknown
Cell entry	Plasma membrane	Endosomal	Plasmic membrane
Proteolytic activation of surface glycoprotein	Yes	Yes	Yes
Syncytial formation	Varying	No	Yes
Pathogenesis			
Localization	Respiratory tract	Respiratory tract	Respiratory tract
Spread	Small droplet	Aerosol	Small droplet
Epidemiology	Fall season PIV 1, 2 Endemic PIV3	Yearly Winter epidemic	Yearly Winter epidemic

are antigenically so closely related that they are being evaluated as vaccine candidates in humans.

III. Replicative Strategy

PIV attachment to sialic acid receptors on cells occurs via the hemagglutinin component of the hemagglutinin-neuraminidase (HN) surface glycoprotein protein (8,9). Hemagglutinin binds red blood cells, providing a ready marker for infection in tissue culture and a rapid way of quantitating virus and detecting an immune response (see further discussion in Section VII). Neuraminidase in the bifunctional HN protein may facilitate viral exit from the cell by cleaving the virus from sialic acid on the cell surface. The other surface protein, the fusion protein (F), facilitates penetration of the host cell. These surface proteins require cleavage by a host protease for successful viral replication and amplification of titer (see further discussion in Sec. IV).

Once within the cytoplasm, the RNA genome unfolds from a helical configuration to assume a flexible strand of approximately 1000 nm in length that is still bound to the nucleocapsid binding protein (N). The negative-sense genomic RNA must first be copied to positive-strand replicative intermediate RNA and mRNA before additional negative-strand RNA copies and translation of viral proteins can occur. Replication and transcription are facilitated by copies of the nucleocapsid phosphoprotein (P) and polymerase protein (L) that enter into the cell with the virus. Six nonoverlapping mRNA encode for individual proteins. The earliest mRNA transcribed, the internal proteins N and L, generate the most protein copies. Viral replication occurs entirely within the cytoplasm of the cell. The other major structural protein of PIV is the matrix protein (M), which is located between the nucleocapsid and the envelope. M protein binds nucleocapsid rendering the protein-RNA complex transcriptionally inactive and interacts with the surface proteins to facilitate viral packaging. A number of partially characterized nonstructural proteins have roles in the regulation of viral replication.

PIV are released from the cell by budding at the cell membrane. PIV buds from polarized cells, such as those of respiratory epithelium, from the apical surface of the cell (10). Another function of the fusion protein, in conjunction with HN, is to mediate cell fusion or syncytium formation (11). Syncytium formation is seen in tissue culture cells to a varying degree with different PIV. Theoretically, cell fusion allows spread of virus from cell-to-cell without release into the extracellular environment and hence could spare PIV from the neutralizing effect of antibody (12).

IV. Pathogenesis of Parainfluenza Virus Infections

A. Receptor Specificity

The receptor for the parainfluenza viruses, sialic acid, is widespread (13). However, viral replication is confined to respiratory epithelial cells, dendritic cells, and macrophages lining the respiratory tract. Therefore, receptor availability alone does not account for the limited distribution of infection in the respiratory tract. In the mouse, Sendai virus, a murine virus closely resembling PIV1, replicates in ciliated and secretory cells but not in basal epithelial cells even when the basal cells are directly exposed to the viral inoculum (14). We do not know why PIV causes localized laryngotracheal symptoms in humans.

B. Immune Response

The first line of defense against PIV comprises nonspecific defense mechanisms including ciliary motility, respiratory protease inhibitors that may block activation of PIV surface proteins, and a mucous blanket that is difficult to penetrate. Other relevant innate defense mechanisms may include local antiviral cytokine production and natural killer cells.

In young children undergoing primary infection, PIV replication in the upper respiratory tract can be documented for 10–12 days (15). The dendritic cells and perhaps macrophages play a key role in antigen presentation to the immune system and initiation of the cognate response. Infection of epithelial cells, the primary site of productive infection, may also play a role in immunity by cytokine expression that amplifies and directs the lymphocyte response toward the Th1 response that characterizes natural infection.

Polar budding of newly formed virus from the apical surface of infected epithelial cells makes it difficult to conceptualize how antigen presentation occurs directly from such cells (see further discussion below). One would have to assume that there were immunocompetent cells within the external respiratory environment. In fact, in animals, cytotoxic lymphocytes (CTL) recognizing the nucleoprotein of Sendai virus can be found in bronchoalveolar lavage fluid of mice at the time of viral clearance (16). The role of specialized microfold (M) cells in antigen uptake in the respiratory tract is less defined than it is for certain viruses (e.g., reoviruses) in the murine enteric tract (17).

Another mechanism for termination of viral infection may be the appearance of IgA in the respiratory tract. With RSV, it has been shown that there may be a period of antigen-antibody complex equilibrium with antibody bound to infected cells before free antibody appears (18). In addition to neutralization of free virus in the respiratory cavity, IgA has the capability of intracellular neutralization of virus during transcytosis across epithelial cells in vitro (19). This recently described method for viral neutralization not only gives IgA the ability to neutralize intracellular virus but also might allow internal proteins to become targets for neutralization; for example, by interfering with binding of nucleocapsid protein to RNA. It is not yet entirely clear what the patterns of intracellular trafficking are within the epithelial cell that might allow antibody and viral protein to contact each other. Certain bacteria produce IgA proteases that presumably can inactivate the neutralizing potential of IgA (20). Finally, serum IgG antibodies can enter the respiratory tract particularly with inflammation and to a greater extent in the lower than upper respiratory tract at which point viral shedding in the immunocompetent host terminates quite rapidly. Passive antibody of either the IgA (21) or IgG (22, 23) class delivered topically to the respiratory tract can limit viral shedding. IgE has also been implicated in the pathogenesis of bronchiolitis associated with PIV3 (24).

Although reinfection can be readily demonstrated with PIV (25), there is resistance to experimental challenge with live, attenuated intranasal vaccines and with wild-type virus in those who have previously experienced infection. The peak titer of vaccine virus in nasal wash specimens after vaccination will be 3–4 $\log_{10}$ pfu/mL secretion of virus for 8–10 days duration in the naive child but only 1–2 logs for 2–4 days in the child who has been previously infected. In adults, the prime determinant of resistance to PIV1 was shown to be the presence of IgA in the nasal wash prior to administration of wild-type experimental infection (26). This study is by far the clearest demonstration that IgA antibody has a critical role in protection against reinfection with respiratory viruses.

In animal models utilizing vaccinia virus recombinants expressing individual PIV proteins, the major contribution to resistance to challenge comes from the surface proteins, HN and F (27). The major CTL peptide determinants for PIV1 in humans were shown to be on the HN, P, and N proteins (28). This immune arm, as discussed below, is probably central to viral clearance during infection, but the debate over which defense mechanism to tailor vaccines toward continues.

In animal models, and presumably in humans, the induction of the immune response may differ considerably between the upper and lower respiratory tracts (29). The upper respiratory tract is continuously exposed to diverse antigenic stimulation and responses are directed toward IgA differentiation. The role of CTL or the IgG serum antibody in clearance of virus from the upper respiratory tract may be limited. The termination of viral replication in the lower respiratory tract can be linked temporarily to the appearance of CTL that have the capability of lysing virally infected cells (30). In particular, $CD8^+$ cells recognize foreign peptides expressed in the context of class I major histocompatibility complex (MHC) receptors. In addition to the virus-specific lymphocyte response there is a marked increase in the numbers of total lymphocytes in mediastinal lymph nodes and in peribronchial and perivascular regions as a bystander effect (31). It is not known whether this lymphocytic infiltration may in itself lead to diminution in pulmonary function.

C. Viral Persistence

In tissue culture, cell lines persistently infected with PIV3 can be readily established (32). As previously mentioned, in Antarctica, PIV1 and PIV3 were grown repeatedly for up to 7 months from an isolated population living at the South Pole station (33). The virus survived on inanimate objects for only 2 weeks, indicating that repeated viral recovery indicated persistent infection or repeated transmission within the small cohort at this station (34). Finally, these viruses can persistently infect immunocompromised patients (see Sec. VI).

D. Surface Protein Cleavage as a Determinant of Virulence

A major determinant of PIV virulence in animal models appears to be the cleavability of FO, the fusion precursor protein. If the fusion protein of Sendai virus is modified so that it is cleaved by ubiquitous intracellular proteases, as in a mutant called F1-R, Sendai will cause systemic disease (35). A single round of viral growth in organ cultures representing lung, brain, heart, liver, pancreas, spleen, kidney, and testis is possible with wild-type virus and with the F1-R mutant with the modified fusion protein, but only the F1-R virus with the more readily cleaved fusion protein will continue to grow in organs other than the lung (36). In this respect, PIV F protein cleavage role in virulence is similar to that of the influenza hemagglutinin. In certain avian influenza strains with a readily cleaved hemagglutinin, there is disseminated influenzal infection in birds. NDV is a PIV counterpart of the avian flu strains. NDV virulence in chickens depends on fusion cleavage. Sendai virus variants differ in virulence depending on mutations in the F protein that alter the proteolytic enzyme site in FO, allowing cleavage by elastase or chymotrypsin instead of the enzymes usually used: trypsin and a protein called tryptase Clara (37).

Work with Sendai virus in the mouse has suggested that the proteolytic activity resulting in cleavage of FO may be mediated by extracellular serine proteases produced in specialized secretory, nonciliated respiratory tract epithelial cells in the mouse called Clara cells (38). The production of tryptase Clara has been localized to Clara cells, a secretory nonciliated epithelial cell subset, by immunohistochemistry, and it may be secreted into the lumen of the respiratory tract (39). A Clara cell counterpart exists in both the upper and lower respiratory tract of humans, but the role of human Clara cells in the pathogenesis of respiratory viruses is not known. Proteins can be found within human respiratory secretions that mediate the proteolytic activation of influenza (40), and serine protease inhibitors such as aprotinin limit infection in the murine model. Endogenous inhibitors of this protease activity may include surfactin and secretory leukocyte protease inhibitor (41). The story is made more interesting by the fact that certain bacteria (e.g., *Staphylococcus aureus*) can produce proteases that effectively cleave the hemagglutinin of influenza viruses increasing virulence and providing a model of viral bacterial synergy (42).

E. Polarity of Viral Release

Another factor implicated in the systemic spread versus localized respiratory infection with PIV has been the polarity of viral budding from the infected polarized cell. The Sendai virus mutant with the readily cleaved fusion protein, F1-R, has amino acid changes in the M protein that allow viral transport and expression on the basolateral surface of Madin-Darby canine kidney (MDCK) cells in culture. This basolateral expression of F protein is essential for the ability of Sendai to cause fusion of cells in vitro (43). Furthermore, when a virus was derived that had the readily cleaved F protein but did not bud from the basolateral surface of polarized cells, it would not cause systemic illness on inoculation into the murine respiratory tract (44). If inoculated systemically, the new mutants would cause illness. Thus, Sendai virus requires both a readily cleaved F protein and basolateral budding to be fully pathogenic when given by the natural route of acquisition, the respiratory tract.

V. Epidemiology

Epidemics of influenza and RSV spread rapidly through a community in the winter or rainy months. PIV by contrast can be endemic in a community (PIV3) or cause fall epidemics (PIV1 or PIV2). Nucleotide sequence and resultant antigenic differences are seen among PIV field strains, as with all single-stranded negative-sense RNA viruses. However, antigenic changes in PIV do not appear to be progressive over time (45). This is in contrast to influenza where progressive antigenic drift is one of the ways the differences are seen among PIV field strains, as with all single-stranded negative-sense RNA viruses; antigenic changes in PIV do not appear to be progressive over time (45). This is in contrast to influenza where progressive antigenic drift is one of the ways the virus escapes from immune surveillance. In spite of the difficulty in routinely identifying PIV, a number of centers have done longitudinal studies of outpatient pediatric populations and hospitalized patients that have defined the impact of PIV (46,47). These studies are extremely informative. At Vanderbilt University Medical Center, approximately 1500 children have been followed longitudinally with viral cultures done on all children with febrile upper respiratory tract disease, otitis media, or lower respiratory tract signs (48). Seventeen percent of children under age 2 years had a PIV isolated; 9% PIV3, 5% PIV1, 2% PIV, and 1% other PIV strains. Of the 293 PIV isolates, 16% were associated with lower respiratory tract disease. PIV1 caused croup almost exclusively, whereas PIV2 and PIV3 caused pneumonia and bronchiolitis as well. In studies from North Carolina, 3 cases of croup per 100 children occurred in the first 5 years of life. When a virus is identified in croup, 65% of the time it is a PIV. An older estimate is that 1.3% of cases of croup are hospitalized. This hospitalization rate may have changed with different approaches to therapy (see below). In the past, as many children were intubated for respiratory distress due to croup as were for epiglottitis. Now the latter disease has virtually disappeared with immunization for *Haemophilus influenzae*.

There was a recent estimate of the cost of a PIV1 and PIV2 outbreak based on pediatric emergency room visits. PIV was recovered from 49% of children with croup, 10% of those with bronchiolitis, and 12% of those with pneumonia (49). Based on extrapolation to national figures, the investigators estimated that these two viruses during this epidemic accounted for 250,000 emergency room visits and 70,000 hospitalizations per year with a total health cost of $190 million for the United States.

VI. Infections in Immunocompromised Hosts

Reviews of the role of PIV infections have been published from the Pulmonary Division of the University of Minnesota in patients receiving bone marrow transplants or lung transplants. In 1253 patients receiving bone marrow transplants, 27 patients were documented to have PIV infection. Although 8 of these infections were confined to the upper respiratory tract, the other 19 had lower respiratory tract disease, and 6 of the 19 patients died (50). Nineteen of the 27 infections were caused by PIV3, and they occurred throughout the year, as would be predicted by the endemic behavior of this virus. In most cases, the virus was isolated from the upper respiratory tract, but in four cases, it was identified only from bronchoalveolar lavage fluid. Severity of disease did not correlate with the degree of immunosuppression, age of patient, or reason for transplantation. The series of lung transplant patients is obviously smaller, but the risk of PIV infection was higher, with 12% (10) of the total transplanted patients experiencing infection (51). In these patients, the diagnosis was more likely to be established by bronchoalveolar lavage (9 of 10). Eight of 10 virus isolates were PIV3. In this group, ribavirin was widely used. In that study, viral cultures were slow to be identified as positive; at a median of 5 days after inoculation. Of all the organisms identified in this population, RSV (nine isolates) and PIV were the most common. By contrast, only two patients with cytomegalovirus (CMV) were identified. In the lung transplant patients, younger age appeared to be a risk factor of more frequent disease. In a pediatric series of 500 transplant patients, 45 viral respiratory infections were documented (52). Thirty-two of these were PIV. Nine cases required supplemental oxygen, eight required intubation, and eight died. Five of the latter patients had PIV (four PIV3 and one PIV1).

An instructive case record of the Massachusetts General Hospital presents an immunodeficient male child who had received extensive chemotherapy for neuroblastoma and was hypogammaglobulinemic and lymphopenic with a single lymphocyte in his admission differential (53). PIV3 was cultured from his respiratory tract over a 14-week period. An open lung biopsy showed giant cell formation in the lung and PIV recovery in viral cultures from lung tissue. He slowly improved with intravenous ribavirin. Persistent PIV infection has been reported with primary immunodeficiencies but not with human immunodeficiency virus (HIV) infection. The pattern of infection seen in the immunocompromised is different than that seen in the normal host but does not appear to give strong clues as to what the protective components of immunity are either for clearance of infection or the prevention of subsequent infection (54). Many patients with primary immunodeficiency exhibit both abnormal cellular and humoral responses to specific pathogens (see also Chap. 5).

VII. Viral Diagnosis

The PIV are optimally grown in primary rhesus monkey or cynomolgus kidney cells or in the continuous cell line LLCMK2 (55). The viruses cause varying degrees of cytopathology. The growth of some strains of PIV3 is accompanied by large multinucleated syncytia. All of the PIV exhibit hemadsorption when guinea pig red cells are added to an infected monolayer. Influenza is the major confounding virus exhibiting a similar hemadsorption pattern. Once a hemadsorping virus is identified, further speciation can be accomplished by immunofluroescent staining of infected cells or by inhibition of the hemadsorption by preincubation with virus-specific antibodies. All of this takes a considerable period of time (1–3 weeks), which is not helpful in terms of the immediate management or diagnosis in the individual patient. Fluorescence assays utilizing virus-specific antibodies can identify individual infected cells obtained directly from nasal secretions. These methods vary in sensitivity depending on the adequacy of collection and skill of the microscopist. The polymerase chain reaction (PCR) has been used to characterize PIV isolates and may represent the future of diagnostic virology (56). Antibody response can be measured by microneutralization assays or hemagglutination inhibition assays. A serum antibody response is quite routinely seen following primary infection. The IgA mucosal response appears to be more variable with primary infection, particularly in the very young child (see also Chap. 12).

VIII. Therapy

The therapy of childhood croup has been empiric with several areas of controversy. The use of humidified air was based on the common observation that exposure to mist in the shower or to cold air during the trip to the emergency room improved the clinical symptoms. However, recent controlled trials of mist have indicated no improvement. Racemic epinephrine offers transitory improvement, but close observation of the child must continue. The use of glucocorticoids represents the greatest area of controversy (57). A recent study of a nebulized steroid suggested a more rapid improvement in the respiratory embarrassment of mild to moderate croup under observation in the emergency room (58). Part of the controversy is generated out of a clinical impression that these are two kinds of croup: (1) spasmodic croup, which can be recurrent and has an association with atopic disease and perhaps asthma; and (2) infectious croup. The former is considered more responsive to alpha-adrenergic agents and steroids. However, unless there is a clear history of recurrent croup, it is difficult to differentiate between spasmodic and infectious croup in the individual child. There does not appear to be any adult equivalent of croup either because of the larger diameter of the adult airway or accumulated immunity to PIV, the viruses primarily implicated in this disease. In severe PIV infection, ribavirin has been used, including intravenously, in persistent infection in immunocompromised patients. However, the clinical benefit of ribavirin in this setting, if any, remains unestablished.

In animal models, aprotinin, a serine protease inhibitor, has decreased viral shedding and improved clinical outcome in paramyxovirus pneumonia (59). This is an attractive future approach to therapy.

IX. Prevention

The initial approach to development of a vaccine for PIV was by formalin-inactivation of whole virus. This PIV vaccine, given as a control arm in trials of a formalin-inactivated RSV vaccine candidate, did not protect against PIV reinfection (60,61). On the other hand, previous immunization with inactivated PIV did not cause the enhanced illness seen with inactivated RSV vaccine (see Chap. 7), although the number of PIV recovered were less than with RSV. Subsequently, more recent work has focused on two approaches, both of which have utilized live attenuated vaccines (62). The first involved the sequential passage of a human PIV strain isolated from a child with respiratory illness at progressively lower temperatures to derive a vaccine that was cold adapted (i.e., would grow below its normal temperature range of replication, 25°C) and temperature sensitive (i.e., was limited in growth at the upper end of its range, 38–39°C) (63). The second approach involved the utilization of a wild-type bovine PIV3 strain as an attenuated candidate for humans (64). Both vaccine candidates exhibit a comparable degree of attenuation and appear safe and immunogenic in young seronegative children (65–67). Both are advancing through phase 1 and 2 trials with the expectation that they may be widely used to prevent illness in children and potentially in the elderly or those who are immunocompromised.

Approaches in earlier stages of vaccine development include the following. Sendai virus, a murine PIV strain which is similar to PIV1, is being considered in animal models as a vaccine candidate against human PIV1 (68). Subunit vaccines continue to be considered as potential vaccine candidates (69). Reverse genetic techniques may soon allow the introduction of specific attenuating mutations into the PIV as is being done with RSV and measles virus (70,71).

Other components for the prevention of nosocomial spread of PIV infection are careful handwashing by health-care personnel and cohorting of hospitalized patients with documented PIV infection (72). Nosocomial spread has been documented in an intermediate care pediatric ward (73) and in a neonatal nursery (74).

X. Summary

In the context of this chapter, we have tried to answer the questions posed in the introduction, although understanding of the pathogenesis of parainfluenza remains speculative and incomplete. PIV represent a well-understood group of viruses in terms of epidemiology and clinical manifestations of respiratory illness, particularly croup. They have proven to be valuable models for understanding the role of proteolytic cleavage of surface proteins in the systemic spread of viruses and in dissecting the local immune response to respiratory pathogens. Efforts at immunization are directed toward an easily administered vaccine that could be given universally early in life to prevent the more severe manifestations of PIV disease associated with primary infection.

References

1. Beale AJ, McLeod DL, Stackiw W, Rhodes AJ. Isolation of cytopathogenic agents from the respiratory tract in acute laryngotracheobronchitis. Br Med J 1958; 1: 302–303.
2. Chanock RM. Association of a new type of cytopathogenic myxovirus with infantile croup. J Exp Med 1956; 104:555–576.
3. Chanock RM, Parrott RH, Cook K, et al. Newly recognized myxoviruses from children with respiratory disease. N Engl J Med 1958; 258:207–213.
4. Chanock RM, Vargosko A, Luckey A, et al. Association of hemadsorption viruses with respiratory illness in childhood. JAMA 1959; 169:548–553.
5. Johnson KM, Chanock RM, Cook MK, Huebner RJ. Studies of a new human hemadsorption virus I isolation, properties and characterization. Am J Hyg 1960; 71:81–92.

6. Kapikian AZ, Bell JA, Mastrota FM, Huebner RJ, Wong DC, Chanock RM. An outbreak of parainfluenza 2 (croup-associated) virus infection. JAMA 1963; 183: 324–330.
7. Denny FW, Murphy TF, Clyde WA Jr, Collier AM, Henderson FW. Croup: an 11 year study in a pediatric practice. Pediatrics 1983; 71:871–876.
8. Colman PM, Hoyne PA, Lawrence MC. Sequence and structure alignment of *Paramyxovirus* hemagglutinin-neuraminidase with influenza virus neuraminidase. J Virol 1993; 67:2972–2980.
9. Coelingh KLVW, Winter CC, Jorgensen ED, Murphy BR. Antigenic and structural properties of the hemagglutinin-neuraminidase glycoprotein of human parainfluenza virus type 3: sequence analysis of variants selected with monoclonal antibodies which inhibit infectivity, hemagglutination, and neuraminidase activities. J Virol 1987; 61:1473–1477.
10. Blau DM, Compans RM. Polarization of viral entry and release in epithelial cells. Sem Virol 1996; 7:245–253.
11. Lamb RA. Paramyxovirus fusion: a hypothesis for changes. Virology 1993; 197: 1–11.
12. Moscona A, Peluso RW. Fusion properties of cells infected with human parainfluenza virus type 3: receptor requirements for viral spread and virus-mediated membrane fusion. J Virol 1992; 66:6280–6287.
13. Markwell MAK. New frontiers opened by the exploration of host cell receptors. In: Kingsbury DW, ed. The Paramyxoviruses. New York: Plenum Press, 1991: 407.
14. Massion PP, Funari P, Ueki I, Ikeda S, McDonald DM, Nadel JA. Parainfluenza (Sendai) virus infects ciliated cells and secretory cells but not basal cells of rat tracheal epithelium. Am J Respir Cell Mol Biol 1993; 9:361–370.
15. Frank AL, Taber LH, Wells CR, Wells JM, Glezen WP, Paredes A. Patterns of shedding of myxo-viruses and paramyxoviruses in children. J Infect Dis 1981; 144: 433–441.
16. Hou S, Doherty PC. Clearance of Sendai virus by CD8+ T cells requires direct targeting to virus-infected epithelium. Eur J Immunol 1995; 25:111–116.
17. Wolf JL, Rubin DH, Finberg R, et al. Intestinal M cells: a pathway for entry of reovirus into the host. Science 1981; 212:471–472.
18. McIntosh K, McQuillin J, Gardner PS. Cell-free and cell-bound antibody in nasal secretions from infants with respiratory syncytial virus infection. Infect Immun 1979; 23:276–281.
19. Mazanec MB, Huang YT, Pimplikar SW, Lamm ME. Mechanisms of inactivation of respiratory viruses by IgA, including intraepithelial neutralization. Semin Virol 1996; 7:285–292.
20. Kornfeld SJ, Plaut AG. Secretory immunity and the bacterial IgA proteases. Rev Infect Dis 1981; 3:521–534.
21. Manzanec MB, Nedrud JG, Lamm ME. Immunoglobulin A monoclonal antibodies protect against Sendai virus. J Virol 1987; 61:2624–2626.
22. Manzanec MB, Lamm ME, Lyn D, Portner A, Nedrud JG. Comparison of IgA versus IgG monoclonal antibodies for passive immunization of the murine respiratory tract. Virus Res 1992; 23:1–12.

23. Prince GA, Porter DD. Treatment of parainfluenza virus type 3 bronchiolitis and pneumonia in a cotton rat model using topical antibody and glucocorticosteroid. J Infect Dis 1996; 173:598–608.
24. Welliver RC, Wong DT, Middleton E Jr, Sun M, McCarthy N, Ogra PL. Role of parainfluenza virus–specific IgE in pathogenesis of croup and wheezing subsequent to infection. J Pediatr 1982; 101:889–896.
25. Glezen WP, Frank AL, Taber LH, Kasel JA. Parainfluenza virus type 3: seasonality and risk of infection and reinfection in young children. J Infect Dis 1984; 150: 851–857.
26. Smith CB, Purcell RH, Bellanti JA, Chanock RM. Protective effect of antibody to parainfluenza type 1 virus. N Engl J Med 1966; 275:1145–1153.
27. Spriggs MK, Murphy BR, Prince GA, Olmsted RA, Collins PL. Expression of the F and HN glycoproteins of human parainfluenza virus type 3 recombinant vaccinia viruses: contributions of the individual proteins to host immunity. J Virol 1987; 61:3416–3423.
28. Dave VP, Allan JE, Slobod KS, Smith FS, Ryan KW, Takimoti T, Power UF, Portner A, Hurwitz JL. Viral cross-reactivity and antigenic determinants recognized by human parainfluenza virus type 1-specific cytotoxic T-cells. Virology 1994; 199:376–383.
29. Doherty PC. Anatomical environment as a determinant in viral immunity (review). J Immunol 1995; 155:1023–1027.
30. Hou S, Doherty PC, Zijlstra M, Jaenisch R, Latz JM. Delayed clearance of Sendai virus in mice lacking class I MHC–restricted CD-T cells. J Immunol 1992; 149: 1319–1325.
31. Tripp RA, Hou S, McMickle A, Houston J, Doherty PC. Recruitment and proliferation of $CD8^+$ T cells in respiratory virus infections. J Immunol 1995; 154:6013–6021.
32. Moscona A, Galinski MS. Characterization of human parainfluenza virus type 3 persistent infection in cell culture. J Virol 1990; 64:3212–3218.
33. Muchmore HG, Parkinson AJ, Humphries JE, et al. Persistent parainfluenza virus shedding during isolation at the South Pole. Nature 1981; 289:187–189.
34. Parkinson AJ, Muchmore HG, Scott EN, Scot LV. Survival of parainfluenza viruses in the South Pole environment. Appl Environ Microbiol 1983; 46:901–905.
35. Tashiro M, Yokogoshi Y, Tobita K, Seto JT, Rott RR, Kido H. Tryptase Clara, an activating protease for Sendai virus in rat lungs, is involved in pneumopathogenicity. J Virol 1992; 66:7211–7216.
36. Tashiro M, Yamakawa M, Tobita K, Klenk H-D, Rott R, Seto JT. Organ tropism of Sendai virus in mice: proteolytic activation of the fusion glycoprotein in mouse organs and budding site at the bronchial epithelium. J Virol 1990; 64:3627–3634.
37. Scheid A, Choppin PW. Protease activation mutants of Sendai virus: activation of biological properties by specific proteases. Virology 1976; 69:265–277.
38. Kido H, Yokogoshi Y, Sakai K, Tashiro M, Kishino Y, Fukutomi A, Katunuma N. Isolation and characterization of a novel trypsin-like protease found in rat bronchiolar Clara cells. J Biol Chem 1992; 267:13573–13579.
39. Sakai K, Kawaguchi Y, Kishino Y, Kido H. Electron immunohistochemical localization in rat bronchiolar cells of tryptase Clara, which determines the pneu-

motropism and pathogenesis of Sendai virus and influenza virus. J Histol Cytol 1993; 41:89–93.
40. Morel-Barbey CL, Oeltmann TN, Edwards KM, Wright PF. Role of respiratory tract proteases in infectivity of influenza A viruses. J Infect Dis 1987; 155:667–672.
41. Kido H, Sakai K, Hishino Y, Tashiro M. Pulmonary surfactant is a potential endogenous inhibitor of proteolytic activation of Sendai virus and influenza A virus. FEBS Lett 1993; 322:115–119.
42. Scheiblauer H, Reinacher M, Tashiro M, Rott R. Interactions between bacteria and influenza A virus in the development of influenza pneumonia. J Infect Dis 1992; 166:783–791.
43. Tashiro M, Yamakawa M, Tobita K, Klenk H-D, Seto JT, Rott R. Significance of basolateral domain of polarized MDCK cells for Sendai virus-induced cell fusion. Arch Virol 1992; 125:129–139.
44. Tashiro M, Seto JT, Choosakul S, Yamakawa M, Klenk H-D, Rott R. Budding site of Sendai virus in polarized epithelium cells is one of the determinants for tropism and pathogenicity in mice. Virology 1992; 187:413–422.
45. Coelingh KLVW, Winter CC, Murphy BR. Antigenic variation in the hemagglutinin-neuraminidase protein of human parainfluenza type 3 virus. Virology 1985; 143:569–582.
46. Glezen WP, Loda FSA, Clyde WA Jr, et al. Epidemiologic patterns of acute lower respiratory disease of children in a pediatric group practice. J Pediatr 1971; 78: 397–406.
47. Knott AM, Long CE, Hall CB. Parainfluenza viral infections in pediatric outpatients: seasonal patterns and clinical characteristics. Pediatr Infect Dis J 1994; 13: 269–273.
48. Reed G, Jewett PH, Thompson J, Tollefson S, Wright PF. Epidemiology and clinical impact of parainfluenza virus infections in otherwise healthy infants and young children <5 years old. J Infect Dis 1996; 175:807–813.
49. Henrickson KJ, Kuhn SM, Savatski LL. Epidemiology and cost of infection with human parainfluenza virus types 1 and 2 in young children. Clin Infect Dis 1994; 18:770–779.
50. Wendt CH, Weisdorf DJ, Jordan MC, Balfour HH Jr, Hertz MI. Parainfluenza virus respiratory infection after bone marrow transplantation. N Engl J Med 1992; 326:921–926.
51. Wendt CH, Fox JM, Hertz MI. Paramyxovirus infection in lung transplant recipients. J Heart Lung Trans 1995; 14:479–485.
52. Apalsch AM, Green M, Ledesma-Medina J, Nour B, Wald ER. Parainfluenza and influenza infections in pediatric organ transplant recipients. Clin Infect Dis 1995; 20:394–399.
53. Case 31-1996, Weekly Clinicopathological Exercises, Case Records of the Mass. Gen. Hosp. N Engl J Med 1996; 335:1133–1140.
54. Jarvis WR, Middleton PJ, Gelfand EW. Parainfluenza pneumonia in severe combined immunodeficiency disease. J Pediatr 1979; 94:423–425.
55. Frank AL, Couch RB, Griffis CA, Baxter BD. Comparison of different tissue cultures for isolation and quantitation of influenza and parainfluenza viruses. J Clin Microbiol 1979; 10:32–36.

56. Karron RA, Froelich JL, Bobo L, Belshe RB, Yolken RH. Rapid detection of parainfluenza virus type 3 RNA in respiratory specimens: use of reverse transcription-PCR-enzyme immunoassay. J Clin Microbiol 1994; 32:484–488.
57. Kairys SW, Olmstead EM, O'Connor FT. Steroid treatment of laryngotracheitis; a meta-analysis of the evidence of randomized trials. Pediatrics 1989; 83:683–693.
58. Klassen TP, Feldman ME, Watters LK, Sutcliffe T, Rowe PC. Nebulized budesonide for children with mild-to-moderate croup. N Engl J Med 1994; 331:285–289.
59. Ovcharenko AV, Zhirnov OP. Aprotinin aerosol treatment of influenza and paramyxovirus bronchopneumonia of mice. Antivir Res 1994; 23:107–118.
60. Fulginiti VA, Eller JJ, Sieber OF, Joyner JW, Minamitani M, Meiklejohn G. Respiratory virus immunization I A field trial of two inactivated respiratory virus vaccines; and aqueous trivalent parainfluenza virus vaccine and an alum-precipitated respiratory syncytial virus vaccine. Am J Epidemiol 1969; 89:435–448.
61. Chin J, Magoffin RL, Shearer LA, Schieble JH, Lennette EH. Field evaluation of a respiratory syncytial virus vaccine and a trivalent parainfluenza virus vaccine in a pediatric population. Am J Epidemiol 1989; 89:449–463.
62. Murphy BR, Hall SL, Kulkarni AB, Crowe JE Jr, et al. An update on approaches to the development of respiratory syncytial virus (RSV) and parainfluenza type 1 (PIV3) vaccines. Virus Res 1994; 32:13–36.
63. Belshe RB, Hissom FK. Cold adaptation of parainfluenza virus type 3: induction of three phenotypic markers. J Med Virol 1982; 10:235–242.
64. Coelingh KLVW, Winter CC, Tierney EL, London WT, Murphy BR. Attenuation of bovine parainfluenza virus type 3 in nonhuman primates and its ability to confer immunity to human parainfluenza virus type 3 challenge. J Infect Dis 1988; 157:655–662.
65. Belshe RB, Karron RA, Newman FK, Anderson EL, Nugent SL, Steinhoff M, Clements ML, Wilson MH, Hall SL, Thierney EL, Murphy BR. Evaluation of a live attenuated, cold-adapted parainfluenza virus type 3 vaccine in children. J Clin Microbiol 1992; 30:2064–2070.
66. Karron RA, Wright PF, Newman FK, Makene M, et al. A live human parainfluenza type 3 vaccine is attenuated and immunogenic in healthy infants and children. J Infect Dis 1995; 172:1445–1450.
67. Karron RA, Wright PF, Hall SL, Makhene M, Thompson J, Burns BA, Tollefson S, Steinhoff MC, Wilson MH, Harris DO, et al. A live attenuated bovine parainfluenza virus type 3 vaccine is safe, immunogenic, and phenotypically stable in infants and children. J Infect Dis 1995; 171:1107–1114.
68. Sangster M, Smith FS, Coleclough C, Hurwitz JL. Human parainfluenza virus type 1 immunization of infant mice protects from subsequent Sendai virus infection. Virology 1996; 212:13–19.
69. Homa FL, Brideau RJ, Lehman DJ, Thomsen DR, Olmsted RA, Wathen MSW. Development of a novel subunit vaccine that protects cotton rats against both human respiratory syncytial virus and human parainfluenza virus type 3. J Gen Virol 1993; 74:1995–1999.
70. Grosfeld H, Hill MG, Collins PL. RNA replication by respiratory syncytial virus (RSV) is directed by the N, P, and L proteins; transcription also occurs under these

conditions but requires RSV superinfection for efficient synthesis of full-length mRNA. J Virol 1995; 69:5677–5686.
71. Radecke F, Speilhofer P, Kaelin K, Huber M, Dotsch C, Christiansen G, Billeter MA. Rescue of measles virus from cloned DNA. EMBO J 1995; 14:5773–5784.
72. Ansari SA, Springthorpe VS, Sattar SA, Rivard S, Rahman M. Potential role of hands in the spread of respiratory viral infections: studies with human parainfluenza virus 3 and rhinovirus 14. J Clin Microbiol 1991; 29:2115–2119.
73. Karron RA, O'Brien KL, Froehlich JL, Brown VA. Molecular epidemiology of a parainfluenza type 3 virus outbreak on a pediatric ward. J Infect Dis 1993; 167:1441–1445.
74. Singh-Naz N, Willy M, Riggs N. Outbreak of parainfluenza virus type 3 in a neonatal nursery. Pediatr Infect Dis 1990; 9:31–33.

9

Adenoviruses

SHAW-GUANG LEE
Wyeth–Lederle Vaccines and Pediatrics
Pearl River, New York

WILLIAM C. GRUBER
Vanderbilt University School of Medicine
Nashville, Tennessee

I. Introduction

In 1953, Rowe first described a filterable agent which disrupted surgically removed adenoidal tissue of children in culture (1). Adenoviruses were soon established as a cause of acute respiratory disease (ARD) in military personnel (2–4) and later in open populations of children and adults. The name *adenovirus* was adopted in 1956 based on the frequent isolation of adenoviruses from adenoids. Subsequently, adenoviruses were found in a large variety of animal species, including frogs, mammals of various kinds, and birds. To date, 49 different serotypes of adenoviruses have been isolated from humans. Human adenoviruses are most commonly recognized as respiratory pathogens. However, adenoviruses are also implicated in other clinical syndromes involving the gastrointestinal tract, urinary bladder, and occasionally the liver, pancreas, and central nervous system.

The adenovirus genome consists of a linear, double-stranded DNA molecule of 32–36 kb that is packaged into a protein shell (capsid) of 70–100 nm diameter (6). Adenoviruses have been exploited effectively for studies of DNA replication, gene expression, and cell transformation. In the past decade, remarkable viral schemes to counteract host defense mechanisms have also been revealed. More recently, adenoviral genes and virion components have been dissected and reassembled in different ways for ferrying foreign DNA into cells; the resulting formulations have been tested as vectors for vaccine delivery and gene therapy. These applications have provided additional insights into the biology and pathophysiology of adenoviral infection and disease.

In this chapter, the general properties of adenoviruses will be introduced and respiratory diseases caused by adenoviruses will be described. Viral and cellular factors related to the pathogenesis of adenoviral pulmonary disorders will be reviewed and the use of adenoviruses for gene delivery will be discussed.

II. Classification and Morphology of Adenoviruses

A. Classification

The 49 serotypes of human adenoviruses are divided into 6 subgenera, A–F, according to their structural, biochemical, and immunological characteristics and oncogenic potential (5). Each subgenera contains one or more serotypes separated on the basis of neutralization with type-specific antisera. Table 1 summarizes the six subgenera, serotypes, disease pattern, hemagglutination characteristics, and oncogenic properties. The following briefly lists adenoviral serotypes and the organ targets for diseases (7–9).

Subgenera A: The members usually cause cryptic infections but are classified as highly oncogenic in the hamster. Adenoviral serotypes 12 (AD12), Ad18, and Ad31 have been isolated from stools and may cause diarrhea.

Subgenera B: Subgenera B.1 viruses, Ad3, Ad7, and Ad21 appear in epidemic outbreaks of respiratory disease among military recruits and at times cause fatal infections in infants. A new isolate of Ad11, Ad11a, is associated with outbreaks of pneumonia, whereas another closely related genome, Ad11p, causes hemorrhagic cystitis (10,11). Subgenera B.2, Ad34, and Ad35 were originally isolated from renal transplant recipients. Subgenera B adenoviruses are moderately oncogenic in the mouse (12).

Subgenera C: These adenoviruses have been the most common causes of upper and lower respiratory tract diseases and gastrointestinal illnesses in small children. Ad1, Ad2, and Ad5 can infect adenoids and tonsils persistently and are shed in stools for years.

Subgenera D: This is the largest adenovirus subgenera, including more than half of all recognized human adenoviruses. This group appears to be labile, with the appearance of multiple intermediate

Table 1 Human Adenoviruses: Classification and Common Diseases

Subgenera	Hemagglutination groups	Serotypes (common diseases)[a]	Oncogenic potential	
			tumors in animals	transformation in tissue culture
A	IV (Little or no agglutination)	12, 18, 31	High	+
B	I (Complete agglutination of monkey erythrocytes)	3 and 7 (P, PCF, ARD, PN), 11 (P, EC, HC), 14 (PCF, ARD), 16, 21 (P, HC), 34 and 35 (ID)	Moderate	+
C	III (Partial agglutination of rat erythrocytes)	1 and 2 (P, PN, Hep), 5 (P, PT, Hep), 6	Low or none	+
D	II (Complete agglutination of rat erythrocytes)	8 (EC), 9, 10, 13, 15, 17, 19 (EC), 20, 22–20, 32, 33, 36, 37 (EC), 38–39, 42, 43–49 (AIDS)	Low or none (mammary tumors)	+
E	III	4 (PCF, ARD, PN)	Low or none	
F	III	40, 41 (GI)	Unknown	+

[a]P, pharyngitis; PCF, pharyngoconjunctival fever; ARD, acute respiratory disease of military recruits; PN, pneumonia; EC, epidemic keratoconjunctivitis; PT, pertussis-like syndrome; HC, acute hemorrhagic cystitis; GI, gastroenteritis; ID, disease in patients with immunodeficiency AIDS, recovery from patients with HIV infection.

and intertypic strains. Curiously, most members of this subgenera have not been associated with significant human pathology. However, there are exceptions. Ad8, Ad19, and Ad37 are the predominant pathogens of epidemic adenovirus-associated keratoconjunctivitis in the United States. Several subgenera D serotypes are also characterized by prolonged shedding in stools. Many new isolates of this group are found in acquired immunodeficiency syndrome (AIDS) patients (10).

Subgenera E: Ad4 is the only human member of this subgenera and has been a significant cause of outbreaks of respiratory infections among military recruits and children (2).

Subgenera F: Ad40 and Ad41 cause diarrhea.

The array of disorders listed above indicates the varied tissue tropism and pathogenic potential of different adenoviral serotypes. Although the basic molecular determinants underlying this phenomena are not well understood, some important clues have been found in the adenoviral early gene products and in the fiber molecule. These will be discussed in later sections.

B. Morphology

The adenovirus is a nonenveloped DNA virus with an icosahedral capsid composed of 252 capsomeres composed of 240 nonvertex hexon capsomeres and 12 vertex pentons. Protruding from each of the penton bases is an antenna-like structure called the fiber (6) (Fig. 1). The hexon, penton, and fiber constitute the major adenoviral antigens important in viral classification and diagnosis. Inside the capsid is a nuclear core containing the viral DNA and at least three viral proteins. Despite the large variety of serotypes and recovery from many hosts, the overall genomic organization and viral morphology of different adenoviruses is strikingly similar. Ad2 and Ad5 of subgenera C, which are completely sequenced, have been the prototypes for comparison with other viruses. The actual DNA sequence coding for proteins with common functions among adenoviral serotypes can be quite divergent. This divergence can be exploited for examination of adenoviral phylogeny and genetic diversity (15).

III. Life Cycle and Replication

A. Cell Entry

Adenoviruses are commonly transmitted by the fecal/oral route, contaminated water, or aerosol. Sexual activity and organ transplantation may be responsible for viral transmission of the newly identified group D serotypes. Infections may begin in the eyes, nasopharynx, or lung and spread to other organs by viremia.

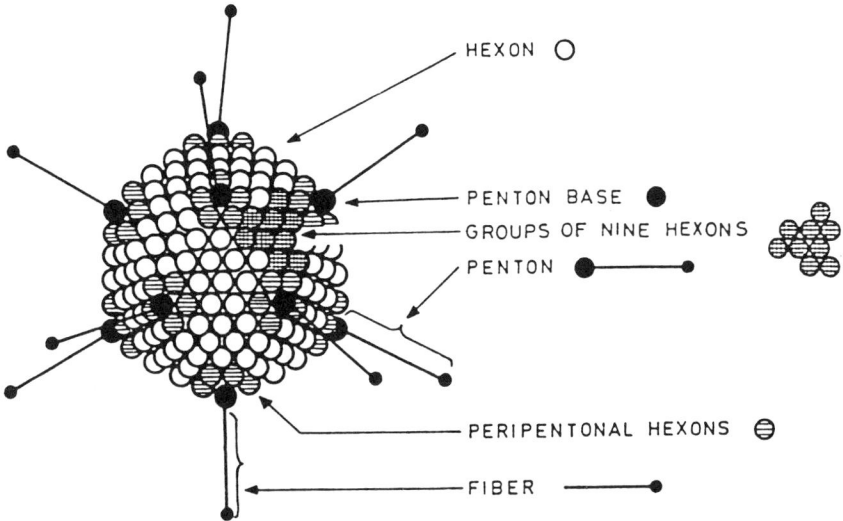

Figure 1 External structure of adenovirus. (From Ref. 6.)

Human and animal adenoviruses appear to be species restricted in nature. However, human adenoviruses adsorb, penetrate, and make early proteins in a variety of animal cells, indicating that receptors for this virus are rather ubiquitous. Monkey and rodent cells can be infected, but intracellular blocks to interaction between cellular and viral components prevent or limit production of progeny virus (16–18). Recently, the cotton rat has been exploited as an animal model to study lung pathology and the pathogenesis of adenoviral infection, but titers of recoverable virus are generally low (19,20). This model has also been used to evaluate the safety and potential efficacy of repetitive adenovirus-mediated delivery of the cystic fibrosis transmembrane conductance regulator (CFTR) gene to airway epithelial cells (21).

The adenovirus attaches target cells through the capsid fiber protein (22) and is then internalized through receptor-mediated endocytosis (23). A putative primary receptor for the fiber has been identified which also appears to be a receptor for Coxsackie B viruses (24). The host cell adhesion molecule integrins α-V-beta-3 and α-V-beta-5 have been identified as secondary receptors (25–27). These integrin molecules interact with the arginine-glycine-aspartic acid (RGD) sequences on the adenoviral penton base. After internalization, the penton base induces the disruption of the endosomal membrane resulting in the release of adenoviruses from the endosomes (27). Uncoating then commences and adenoviral DNA enters the nucleus where replication takes place.

The process of adsorption and internalization of adenovirus into target cells is remarkably efficient, and it has become possible to modify adenoviral cell tropism by engineering the fiber and penton proteins (28,29). Understandably, adenoviruses have become attractive candidates for the delivery of macromolecules into cells.

B. Gene Expression

Viral gene expression can be grossly divided into early and late phases demarcated by the onset of viral DNA replication. Early genes are clustered in groups, E1 through E4, and they are transcribed from individual promoters. Late genes are generated by the alternative splicing of a single, polycistronic mRNA that is transcribed from a single promoter, the powerful major late promoter. In general, the early genes function in cell transformation, in viral DNA transcription and replication, and in opposing host antiviral defenses. The late genes function in the synthesis of structural proteins and the assembly of progeny viruses.

Early Genes

The E1A gene regions are the first to be expressed after infection. E1A proteins are the vanguards for transcription of other viral genes and can recondition the cellular environment for optimal viral gene expression (30). They are potent regulators which activate or repress transcription, and they can force infected cells to reenter the S phase of the cell cycle, which is optimal for viral DNA replication. E1A proteins can immortalize primary rodent cells and transform them in cooperation with a second oncogene such as E1B. In contrast to rodent cells, no evidence has been found to suggest a role for E1A in any human cancers. The E1B region functions in the protection of DNA sequences during viral infection. E1B proteins can also block apoptosis, or programmed cell death, which infected cells sometimes employ as a sacrifice to limit viral spread (31).

E1-deleted adenoviruses are defective in DNA replication but can be rescued from a human cell line (293 cells) that constitutively expresses E1 proteins. E1-deleted adenoviruses are being used widely in current adenovirus-mediated gene transfer, because they are incapable of replication in recipient cells but allow expression of inserted genes.

The E2 region encodes genes whose functions are directly involved in viral DNA synthesis, including a DNA polymerase, a DNA binding protein, and a preterminal protein that is covalently bound to the 5' termini of the viral genome. The terminal protein serves as a primer in viral DNA replication.

The E3 region was originally viewed as being "nonessential," because it was found to be dispensable for adenoviral growth in tissue culture. Yet, it is now known that several E3 proteins can act as immune modulators that modify host antiviral immune responses (32). The role of these proteins in pathogenesis will be discussed below.

The proteins encoded by the E4 region play a role in the shutoff of host gene expression and the assembly of the virion. They also regulate the transition from early to late gene expression.

DNA Replication and Late Gene Expression

Adenoviral DNA synthesis begins at approximately 5–7 hr postinfection. An origin of replication is embedded within two terminal inverted repeat sequences, which are 100–150 base pairs long. The covalently bound preterminal protein contains a serine residue which forms an ester bond with the deoxycytidine monophosphate (dCMP) at the end of the adenoviral genome. The 3'-OH group of the complex then serves as the primer for nascent DNA synthesis. The adenovirus encodes its own DNA polymerase and a DNA binding protein that mediates chain elongation. A small number of nuclear factors also aid in viral DNA replication (33).

Adenoviral late gene region transcription occurs under the control of the major late promoter. A large transcript terminating near the right end of the genome is processed to yield five families of the late mRNA (L1–L5) that encode structural virion proteins, including hexon, penton, and fiber. Historically, it was the studies with the adenovirus late mRNA that led to the landmark discovery that eukaryotic mRNA are not always colinear with their genes but are spliced products of separated coding regions ("exons") intervened by noncoding regions ("introns") in the genomic DNA (34,35). All the adenoviral late mRNA contain three common exons, the tripartite leader, which enhance their translation (36). Another set of viral transcripts, the virus-associated RNA (VA RNA) produced by viral RNA polymerase III can block interferon-induced antiviral effects (37,38).

Adenoviral DNA replication is gradually accompanied by an inhibition of cellular DNA and protein synthesis. Thus, during the late stages of viral infection, proteins and DNA synthesis in the infected cell are exclusively virus directed. In permissive cells, the viral infection cycle lasts about 32–48 hr and approximately 10^4 infectious virions per cell are produced (16).

IV. Unique Role of Specific Viral Proteins

A. E1 Genes

The use of a variety of adenoviral mutants has facilitated the determination of which viral gene or genes are required to produce lesions. E1B 55-K, which shuts off host protein synthesis during adenoviral replication, has been found to play a pathogenic function in pneumonia. The E1B 19 kDa protein, on the other hand, blocks the onset of apoptosis and protects against the induction of cytolysis (31).

B. E3 Genes

The E3 region genes deserve special mention. Messenger RNA from the E3 gene region are made from complicated splicing events resulting in nine different messages, six of which have been identified at the protein level. It seems illogical for adenoviruses to maintain this complexity over the course of evolution if the expressed genes conferred no benefit for viral replication. In fact, adenoviral E3 genes are well conserved in all serotypes and appear to play important immunomodulatory roles.

The best-characterized E3 protein is known as gp19K. The E3 gp19K protein, anchored in the endoplasmic reticulum, binds directly to the peptide-binding domain of major histocompatibility complex (MHC) class I, abrogates MHC class I glycosylation, and retains MHC class I viral peptide antigen complex in the reticulum membrane (57). Specific lysis of a virus-infected cell is typically performed by cytotoxic T lymphocytes (CTL) which recognize infected cells through the surface display of viral peptide antigens in complex with MHC class I that is transported from inside the cells. By intercepting the transport of the MHC class I to the surface, gp19K allows adenovirus-infected cells to evade immune recognition and consequent killing by adenovirus-specific CTL. In the cotton rat model, E3 gp19K seems to serve an ameliorative role in reducing the response to infection (20,58).

The mechanism by which the adenovirus persists in tonsillar cells and escapes host immunological destruction may be due to E3 gp19K. Additionally, the E3 promoter is unique among adenoviral promoters in that it can be activated in lymphoid cells (59), resulting in sustained and preferential expression of E3 proteins in lymphocytes and viral persistence. Interestingly, this ability of E3 gp19K to mask infected cells from recognition by CTL can be harnessed as a novel therapeutic strategy in controlling transplant rejection. In a recent transgenic animal study, the adenoviral E3 region was found to prolong the survival of a pancreatic islet allograft (60).

Although there is an overall high degree of conservation in the organization of the E3 region among the adenoviruses, there are distinctive features among different serotypes. For instance, when comparing the E3 regions of subgenera B virus Ad35 and subgenera C Ad5, substantial differences in gene splicing, polyadenylation, and the abundance of E3 mRNA and glycoprotein product were found (61). Such subtle differences in E3 gene expression can potentially influence the pathological outcome.

During adenoviral infection, E1A induces susceptibility to tumor necrosis factor-α (TNF-α), which mediates the lysis of susceptible tumor cells as well as some virus-infected cells (62). During cell lysis, TNF-α activates cytosolic phospholipase A-2, which releases arachidonic acid that is crucial for cell death. Since arachidonic acid serves as the substrate for potent inflammatory mediators such as leukotrienes, prostaglandins, and platelet-activating factor, TNF-α not only induces cell lysis but also generates strong inflammatory signals. However, this sensitizing action of E1A is countered by a number of E3 proteins (14.7 K and a 10.4 K/14.5 K dimer) (63,64). The E3 anti-TNF proteins protect cells from the cytolytic effect of TNF-α and also diminish the inflammatory response to adenoviral infection by preventing the activation of the phospholipase A-2 by TNF-α (65).

The E3-10.4 K/14.5 K dimer can downregulate the epidermal growth factor receptor of adenovirus-infected cells and thus affect signal transduction. Recently, another E3 protein, the 11.6 K protein, has been shown to function in the efficient death or lysis of adenovirus-infected cells and has been termed the "adenovirus death protein." This may represent a new class of proteins that promote cell death, since it is not related in sequence to other apoptosis-inducing proteins (66).

In making adenovirus gene–delivery vectors, E3 regions are usually deleted to "make room" for the insertion of foreign DNA. Although E3 regions are nonessential for viral growth in vitro, their important immune-modulating functions warrant thorough understanding when constructing safe and efficient recombinant adenoviral vectors.

In analyzing adenoviral DNA in the lungs of chronic obstructive pulmonary disease (COPD) patients, the E1A region is preferentially found more often in the epithelium of resected pulmonary nodules from patients with COPD than from patients without obstruction (47). In a later study, the E1A DNA was shown to be expressed at the protein level in lung tissues. Since the adenoviral E1A protein is a promiscuous transactivator for a large number of host genes, the expression of the E1A protein has the potential of influencing the inflammatory processes and stimulating tissue growth in the repair process. In lungs in which E1A but not E3 is expressed, airway cells could have been sensitized to cell lysis by TNF-α without benefiting from the counterbalance exerted by the E3 14.7 K protein. The combination of smoking and E1A activities could amplify the inflammatory response and produce COPD.

C. Fiber

The attachment of adenoviruses to specific cell receptors is a key determinant of host cell tropism. The distal, C-terminal domain of the fiber terminates in a knob that projects from the virion and presumably contains the cell binding domain. This region also functions as a hemagglutination determinant. Variability in the knob region can account for the serological differences among serotypes and can alter the receptor recognition profile of the virus. Such a difference was found in two closely related Ad11 subtypes; Ad11p causes persistent urinary tract infection, whereas Ad11a causes acute respiratory tract infection (67).

Fiber-mediated attachment is followed by a subsequent interaction of the RGD motif on the penton base with the host cell integrin molecules. The abundance of integrin expression may be a limiting factor in viral internalization and susceptibility to viral infection (25–27).

V. Viral Pathogenesis

In human infection, adenovirus-infected cells may become damaged and die, producing disease of various severity. Cells may become persistently infected, in which case there are long periods of low-level replication and shedding of the virus. Alternatively, portions of viral DNA may persist by integrating into the host genome. The latent infection may not yield whole virus, but certain viral DNA are expressed intermittently, which may become important in maintaining latency and influence the pathophysiological state of the infected sites. The extent of genome remaining latent and molecular mechanisms to maintain this state are unknown.

A. Acute Infection

Human adenoviruses most commonly infect cells of the respiratory tract, but the virus can be recovered from cells of other organs. Controlled studies demonstrated that the viral inoculum required to produce ARD is significantly smaller when delivered by aerosol than when delivered to the nasal mucosa (39,40). Human and animal adenoviruses appear to be species restricted in nature. Human adenoviruses can adsorb, penetrate, and make early proteins in animal cells, indicating that the receptor or receptors for this virus are rather ubiquitous. Monkey and rodent cells can be infected, but intracellular blocks to interaction between cellular and viral components prevent or limit production of progeny virus (17–19). Hence, there is no ideal animal model in which to study human adenoviral pathogenesis.

In 1984, it was discovered that the cotton rat (*Sigmadon hispidus*) can develop a type of pneumonia that is pathologically similar to that seen in humans when administered genera C virus by the intranasal route despite low titers of recoverable virus (41). The cotton rat has been effectively exploited as an animal model to study lung pathology and effects of the E3 gene region on the pathogenesis of adenoviral infection (20). This model has also been used to evaluate the safety and potential efficacy of repetitive adenovirus-mediated delivery of the CFTR gene to airway epithelial cells (21). Adenoviruses defective in DNA replication and late gene expression produce lung pathology similar to that induced by wild-type adenovirus in the cotton rat (42). The mouse is not permissive for human adenoviral replication but allows early gene expression. Intranasally administered Ad5 also can induce a pulmonary infiltrate in the mouse (19). Hence, abortive adenoviral infections can still lead to tissue injury and early gene expression can contribute to the development of pulmonary inflammatory response. Penton is directly toxic to cells in tissue culture independent of viral replication (43). These adenoviral properties may help to explain adverse pulmonary reactions seen after administration of replication-deficient adenoviral vectors as gene therapy (44).

Acute adenoviral infection quickly leads to a shutdown of host protein synthesis and cell death. Histopathological evaluation of acute fatal adenoviral respiratory tract infection can reveal extensive destruction of bronchial epithelium and bronchial glands (Fig. 2a). Infected respiratory epithelial cells, called "smudge" cells, often contain enlarged nuclei with loss of nuclear membrane integrity (Fig. 2b). Two types of nuclear changes are described: discrete Feulgen-negative, amphophilic, or eosinophilic intracellular inclusions early in infection or a diffuse accumulation of strongly Feulgen-positive basophilic or amphophilic material later in infection. Similar patterns of tissue necrosis, mononuclear infiltration, and irregular amphophilic or basophilic inclusions can be observed in an acutely infected liver. Electron microscopic studies of tissues from fatal infections demonstrate numerous intranuclear Feulgen-positive inclusion bodies, which consist of 75–80 viral particles in a crystalline array that is typical of adenoviral particles (Fig. 2c).

B. Chronic Persistent Infection and Latency

Human adenoviruses can produce persistent infection in which viral shedding can be observed years after the clinical symptoms subside. Members of group C (serotype 1, 2, 5, and 6) are most frequently found in such circumstances. The persistence of adenoviruses in tonsillar tissue has been reconfirmed by a number of investigators since their original isolation from this source. They may be isolated months to years after initial infection, or they may remain latent with identifiable DNA in tonsils in the absence of recoverable virus (45).

Adenoviral DNA may be identified for prolonged periods from the lung. Some observers have reported recovery of adenovirus or identified capsid proteins from bronchoalveolar washes of children with asthma for over 12 months after infection (46). Latent adenovirus may contribute to chronic

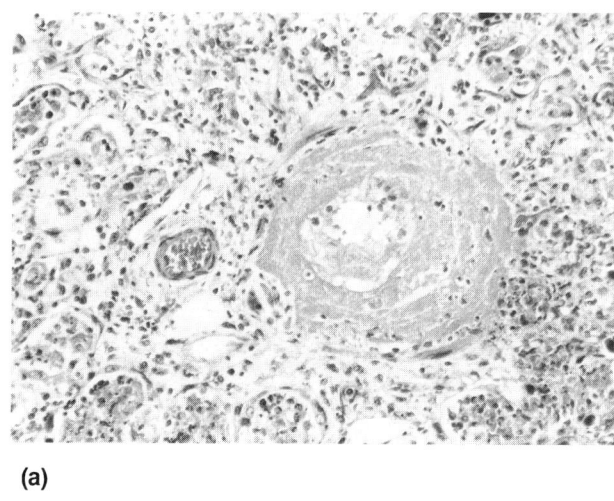

(a)

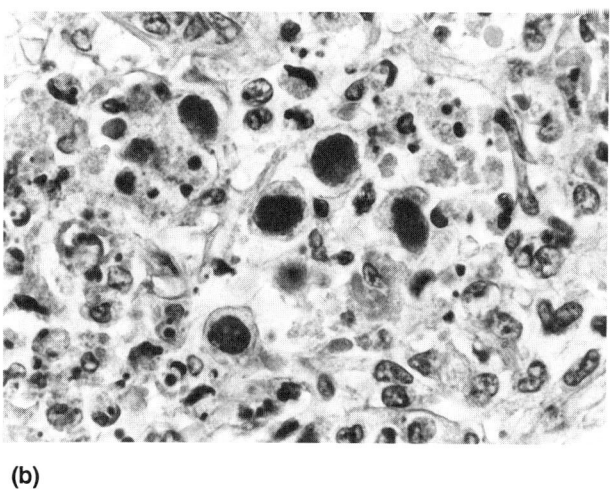

(b)

Figure 2 Histopathology of adenoviral infection of the respiratory tract. (a) Intraluminal fibrin marks the location of a bronchiole; the epithelium is completely ulcerated, although the mural smooth muscle remains. The corresponding artery is at left (magnification, 62.5×). (b) Infected epithelial cells contain characteristic "smudge"-type inclusions (magnification, 250×). (c) Ultrastructural appearance of inclusions is characterized by orderly crystalline arrays of virus. (Photographs courtesy of Joyce Johnson, Department of Pathology, Vanderbilt University.)

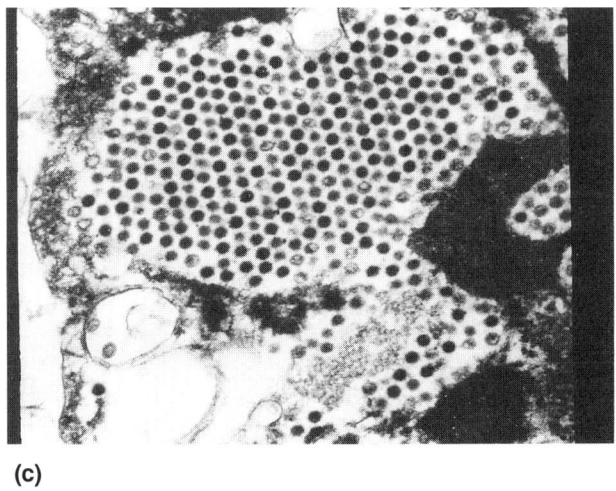
(c)

Figure 2 Continued.

airways obstruction. Matsuse et al. reported identification of adenovirus E1A DNA more commonly in lung airway epithelium of patients with COPD than in subjects without COPD; E3 gene region DNA was recovered with equal frequency in both groups (47). It has been speculated that expressed E1A proteins acting as transcription factors augment an inflammatory response to lung epithelial cells containing adenoviral E1A DNA; this inflammatory response then promotes airway obstruction. E1A proteins have been identified in human lung epithelial cells by immunohistochemistry (48), and a guinea pig animal model has been developed in which E1A DNA and protein expression have been identified at 47 days following Ad5 infection in the absence of recoverable adenovirus (49). The investigators noted evidence of increased airway inflammation at the day 47 time point, suggesting the possible utility of the model in exploring the relationship of adenovirus to chronic airway disease.

Reactivation of latent adenoviral infection may be important in the occurrence of new isolates of adenoviruses and disease in immunocompromised patients (50–53). The seven most recent human adenoviruses to be characterized (Ad 43–49) are all subgenera D serotypes isolated primarily from AIDS patients (10,53). The immunocompromised host may provide an ideal environment for genetic recombinations among adenoviruses associated with persistent infection and for allowing normally innocuous adenoviruses to cause disease.

C. Mechanisms for Terminating Infection and Preventing Reinfection

After adenoviral infection, most patients develop both group-specific and type-specific antibodies to the infecting adenovirus strain. Neutralization is serotype specific and is directed against epitopes predominantly on the hexon protein and the terminal knob region of fiber protein. Some epitopes on the penton can also be recognized by neutralizing antibodies (54,55). Patients may continue to shed adenoviruses intermittently, especially in their stool, for many months after a successful humoral immune response has occurred. Immune clearance of infecting viruses presumably requires successful interactions among macrophages, lymphocytes, natural killer cells, and humoral factors, including antibody, complement, interferon, and cytokines. Although there is some evidence that humoral responses modify the course of adenoviral infections, cell-mediated immune mechanisms are responsible for the containment and resolution of adenoviral infections. This conclusion is corroborated by recent studies in gene therapy using replication-defective adenoviral vectors. In normal mouse liver, when E1-deleted adenoviral vectors were inoculated, a strong inflammatory reaction was stimulated and transgene expression declined dramatically over the initial few weeks (56). Hence, a cell-directed inflammatory response was generated in the absence of release of progeny virus. This study suggests that T-cell–mediated immune response directed against adenoviral proteins eliminates the adenoviral vector and damages local tissues.

VI. Epidemiology

Human adenoviral infections occur throughout life, and adenoviruses account for approximately 5–10% of febrile acute respiratory disease. The serotypes associated with common clinical syndromes are shown in Table 1. Infections with adenoviral serotypes 1, 2, and 5 occur early in life. Hence, adults uncommonly experience illness due to these serotypes, yet they often remain susceptible to serotypes 3, 4, 7, and 21. Epidemics caused by respiratory adenoviruses commonly have occurred in institutional settings or circumstances associated with crowding. Of special interest are the epidemic infections of military recruits by adenovirus in the 1950s and 1960s (4,68). Adenoviral attack rates reached 90% in barracks of susceptible military recruits. In the United States, adenoviruses types 4 and 7 were the major causes, whereas types 3, 14, and 21 have been responsible in other geographical areas. These serotypes are uncommon in the general population and do not give prolonged carriage after the acute infection (69). In the crowded environment of training camps, the viral spread appears to have been via respiratory droplets. Diseases were acute with febrile respiratory and constitutional syndromes, accounted for 80–90%

of hospital admissions, and were uniquely confined to newly inducted men. Epidemics reached peak incidence at 4–6 weeks after beginning military training. Epidemics of pharyngoconjunctival fever or febrile sore throat quickly involved up to 70% of such groups. Regular, repeated intakes of fresh recruits maintained epidemics over long periods of time. Although only a few instances of fatalities were reported, 20–40% of these patients required hospitalization, which resulted in costly interruption of military training (70). The impact of acute respiratory distress in military troops propelled the development of an effective enterically administered live adenovirus vaccine that is now widely utilized in the military (71,72).

Young children in crowded environments also favor adenoviral spread. Nearly 67% of well children exposed in a day-care setting to children with symptomatic adenoviral infection developed febrile adenoviral respiratory illness within 2 weeks of exposure (73).

Immunocompromised patients are not only at risk for infection due to serotypes commonly associated with respiratory disease in healthy age-matched populations, but they also seem to be at risk for "opportunistic" adenoviral disease. Pulmonary disease, including pneumonia and bronchial necrosis, due to serotypes 1, 2, 5, and 6 have been reported in patients with humoral and cellular immunodeficiency. Cases of adenoviral pneumonia have been reported in the kidney and lung transplant recipients (50,51), and increasingly instances of disseminated adenoviral infection occurring in bone marrow transplant patients are being reported (52,53). Disease is often severe with high mortality due to lung and liver involvement. The otherwise uncommon Group B serotypes 34, 35, and D serotypes 42–47 have been associated with life-threatening pneumonia in human immunodeficiency virus (HIV)–infected patients (53), and have accounted for one third of isolates from bone marrow transplant patients (74). Up to 20% of bone marrow transplant patients have been shown to shed adenovirus, and disease rates have exceeded 6% with 54% mortality (75). Graft-versus-host disease is an apparent risk factor (74).

VII. Clinical Manifestations

Adenoviruses induce clinical manifestations ranging from an apparent infection or benign upper respiratory tract infection to necrotizing bronchitis or even disseminated fatal disease. Adenoviruses most commonly infect the respiratory tract, causing mild and self-limited nasal congestion, coryza, and cough. However, fatal pneumonia and disseminated disease have been reported in infants, in young adults, and especially in immunocompromised patients. Adenoviruses account for at least 7% of childhood acute respiratory infections and 17% of all infant diarrhea (5,7).

A significant portion of the serious respiratory diseases found in young children appears to be associated with the pediatric adenoviruses types 1, 2, 5, 6, and 8. One of the more common manifestations of adenoviral infection is acute follicular conjunctivitis, or "pink eye." This illness is accompanied by lacrimation, itching, burning, and conjunctival injection. This relatively mild disease is caused by a variety of adenoviral serotypes and should be distinguished from epidemic keratoconjunctivitis caused by serotypes 8 and 37. The latter highly contagious condition is characterized by early symptoms of follicular conjunctivitis but often progresses to include chronic, painful, superficial, epithelial opacities of the cornea that can lead to prolonged visual impairment.

Although adenoviruses may cause isolated symptoms of coryza, they more often produce illness including pharyngitis and tonsillitis. Adenoviruses account for up to 25% of exudative pharyngitis in pediatric patients and 75% of nonstreptococcal pharyngitis in military recruits (76–78). These illnesses are generally associated with malaise, fever, chills, myalgia, and headache. In some instances, pharyngitis is combined with conjunctivitis and fever in a distinctive syndrome called pharyngoconjunctival fever. This condition has been described frequently since Beal's original description in France in 1907 (79). Outbreaks have been linked to inadequately chlorinated swimming pool water, and attack rates often exceed 60% in exposed persons. Serotypes 3, 4, and 7 account for most cases. Adenovirus along with influenza virus and respiratory syncytial virus are the most common viral agents associated with the complication of otitis media in children, appearing to confer a greater risk than pneumococcal colonization (38).

Adenoviruses are a significant cause of lower respiratory tract disease. Serotypes 3, 4, 7, and 21 are most commonly implicated as causes of laryngotracheobronchitis or pneumonia. Occasionally, a pertussis-like syndrome, clinically indistinguishable from that caused by *Bordetella pertussis*, results from adenoviral infection (7,81). One of the most feared complications of adenoviral lower respiratory disease is bronchiolitis obliterans. The pathophysiology of this disease is characterized by intraluminal fibrosis leading to irreversible narrowing of small airways (82–84). The final stage of this process is shown in Figure 3. Adenoviral infections in patients after solid organ or bone marrow transplantation are associated with a poor prognosis. Mortality rates range from approximately 18% in renal transplant patients to nearly 60% in bone marrow transplant patients (85). It has also been estimated that up to 45% of AIDS patients with adenoviral infection die within 2 months of the diagnosis of adenoviral infection (85). Disease in immunocompromised patients often involves not only the lung but also the liver, kidney, and central nervous system. Infection in otherwise healthy newborns can mimic manifestations seen in older immunocompromised patients, and adenoviral infection

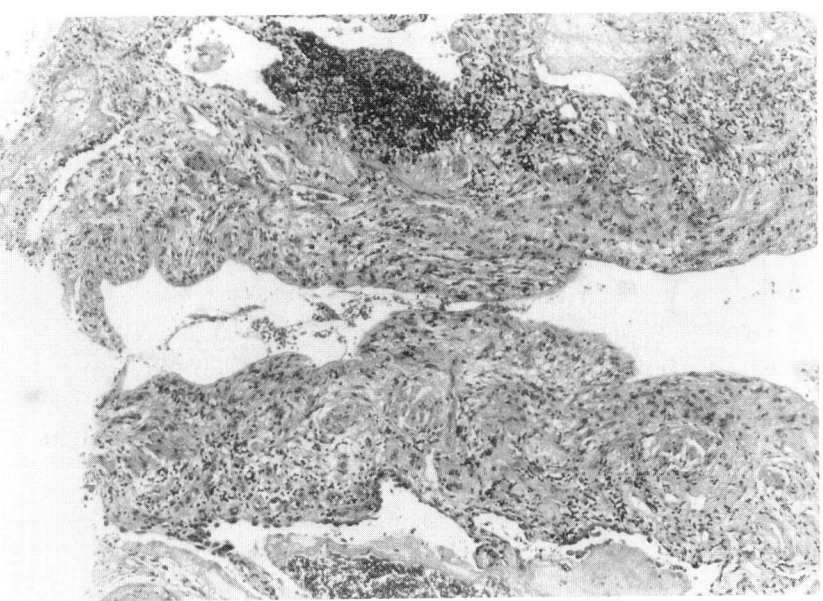

Figure 3 A longitudinal section along a bronchiole shows luminal aggregates of granulation tissue which virtually totally obstruct the airway. (Photographs courtesy of Joyce Johnson, Department of Pathology, Vanderbilt University.)

should be included in the differential diagnosis of newborn pneumonia and sepsis (86).

Adenoviral infection cannot usually be distinguished on clinical grounds alone. Often multiple diagnoses are entertained, and antibiotic therapy is begun for presumptive bacterial illness. Radiographic findings may reveal peribronchial, lobar, or diffuse infiltrates. Since many of the clinical manifestations of adenoviral infection are shared by other pathogens, suspicion of this virus requires a discerning clinician. Attempts should be made to identify virus in respiratory secretions, cerebrospinal fluid (CSF), stool, or biopsy specimens. Immunofluorescence is of limited utility for reliable identification of respiratory adenoviruses directly from clinical specimens. Complement fixation and enzyme-linked immunosorbent assay (ELISA) antibody response to the cross-reactive adenoviral group antigen can be measured on acute and convalescent serum samples to diagnose infection, but these tests lack immediacy. Rapid antigen-detection methods generally lack sufficient sensitivity to be relied on routinely (87,88). DNA amplification and hybridization techniques offer the promise of increased sensitivity (89), and have been used for in situ diagnosis from paraffin-embedded lung tissue specimens (90).

Obstructive airway disease has been described as a complication of adenoviral infection, but findings vary. Military recruits were noted to have mild transient decreases in both vital capacity and maximal voluntary ventilation, with negligible alterations in flow parameters after adenovirus 4 infection (91). Other investigators have noted a restrictive lung disease in adults which resolves over several months after adenoviral pneumonia. Young children have been noted to have chronic cough and persistent radiographic and pulmonary function abnormalities consistent with obstructive airways disease 8–10 years after adenovirus 3 pneumonia in infancy. Native inhabitants of some parts of Canada seem particularly disposed to this poor outcome (92,93). Many of these children have been noted to have persistent obstructive and restrictive abnormalities on pulmonary function testing (92). Adenoviruses 3, 7, and 21 of subgenera B appear to be particularly disposed to induction of chronic airway obstruction in children experiencing pneumonia (94). Other investigators have suggested that adenoviral infection is less commonly a cause of prolonged ventilatory abnormalities than pathogens such as *Mycoplasma pneumoniae* (95).

VIII. Therapy: Antivirals and Passive Immunoglobulin Treatment

There are no antiviral treatments which have been proven effective for adenoviral infection. Potential antiviral agents have been tested in animal models. Successful therapy with vidarabine for adenovirus type 11–associated acute hemorrhagic cystitis after allogenic bone marrow transplantation has been reported (96). However, this drug is no longer on the market, having been replaced by acyclovir for treatment of herpes virus infections. Cidofovir (HPMPC, GS-504), a broad-spectrum, long-acting nucleoside monophosphate analogue was found to inhibit adenovirus type 5 in the New Zealand rabbit ocular replication model after topical application (97), and it may be promising in the treatment of epidemic keratoconjunctivitis. Patient survival after the use of intravenous ribavirin for disseminated adenovirus has been reported, but controlled trials have not been performed (98,99). The use of a polyclonal immunoglobulin product did not appear to modify the risk of disease in a neonatal intensive care adenovirus 8 outbreak (100).

IX. Prevention: Current and Potential Vaccine Strategies

The high morbidity rate of adenovirus respiratory disease in military recruit populations, with its attendant disruption of training and the cost of medical care, together with an appreciable incidence of pulmonary complications, initiated a search for effective vaccines. The first preparations consisted of formalin-inactivated virus grown in monkey kidney cell culture. These vaccines, containing adenoviruses types 3, 4, and 7, the types responsible for epidemic acute respiratory disease in these populations, were shown to be highly protective. However, when some of the vaccine viruses were found to produce tumors in hamsters and to be contaminated with simian vacuolating virus 40 (SV40) virus (101), the inactivated adenoviral vaccine was withdrawn from production. Subsequently, a bivalent live adenoviral vaccine with types 4 and 7 was developed (102). The adenoviruses were propagated in human cells (WI38) and were administered orally in enteric-coated gelatin capsules. After ingestion, the live viruses establish a silent infection in the intestinal tract without any symptoms or signs in the respiratory tract. Subsequently, serum antibodies develop and protection from infection occurs. The vaccine has been shown to be safe, immunogenic, and up to 80% effective in reducing type-specific adenoviral disease in military populations among whom disease had been prevalent at the training base (103).

Despite concern about the oncogenic potential of these viruses, no increased incidence of tumors in military recipients of these vaccines has been reported. Spread of the vaccine virus has not been encountered among recruits sharing barrack facilities. The vaccine was licensed in 1980 for use with the US and Canadian armed forces but has not been licensed for the civilian population.

In subjects receiving the adenoviral vaccine, neutralizing antibodies are detected. The antibody titer values are lower than those produced after acute respiratory distress caused by the same virus type. However, the induced level of serological antibodies is sufficient enough for protection. During the course of vaccination studies, it was discovered that the early administration of vaccine was critical. In the military, the current practice is to administer the vaccine tablet within the first 2 hr after arrival of new recruits. The vaccine does not seem to produce a local secretory response (IgA) that occurs in the respiratory tract after natural infections. Furthermore, reinfection of the respiratory tract may occur with viral shedding, although the reinfection is usually clinically mild or asymptomatic.

The adenovirus types 1, 2, and 5, which are associated with childhood illness, have been shown to be safe and immunogenic when administered to adult volunteers with the use of the same technique of enteric immunization. Nonetheless, the approach of enteric immunization was not pursued in children. Evidence is lacking that these adenovirus types are sufficiently important causes of severe pediatric disease to warrant development of vaccine, and some concern remains regarding potential oncogenesis of these viruses. In addition, it is known that adenoviral vaccines, although attenuated, can be spread to family contacts of vaccinated children (104).

X. Adenoviruses as Gene-Delivery Vectors

Adenoviruses have assumed prominence in the broader scientific literature, primarily due to their use as molecular tools. Indeed, adenoviral vectors containing foreign genes may prove to be useful for the treatment of genetic conditions (105) and malignancies (106), and they may be exploited as vaccines (107). The strong promoters of adenoviruses can be harnessed into producing high levels of recombinant proteins, and otherwise empty capsid structures can be employed as vehicles to transport macromolecules into cells (108). More recently, adenoviruses have been engineered to control transplant rejection and the generation of transgenic animals (109).

Detailed knowledge of the genetics and biochemistry of adenoviruses has facilitated the manipulation of the adenoviral genome. In contrast to retroviruses, adenoviruses can infect a large number of cells independent of the cell's mitotic stage, and integration of the adenoviral genomes into the chromosome rarely occurs. Recombinant adenoviruses are capable of efficient in situ gene transfer to various organs, including lung, brain, pancreas, gallbladder, and liver. The inserted genes are usually expressed at high levels with expected biological functions. Two general approaches are used for generation of adenoviral vectors.

For purposes of immunization, vectors are constructed which are replication competent to ensure high expression of the inserted immunogen. The cassette of foreign DNA coding for immunogen is typically inserted in the E3 or E4 region from which native adenoviral DNA is deleted. E3-deletion vectors expressing hepatitis B, herpes simplex, RSV, and HIV are under investigation (110–112).

For gene therapy, replication of the adenoviral "carrier" is an undesirable feature; the intent is to transmit a "corrected" gene insert into the cell while preserving cellular function. The first-generation adenoviral vectors of replication-deficient vectors were made from Ad2 or Ad5 lacking the E1A and E1B genes. This deletion not only removes the transformation genes in the E1 region but also renders the recombinant adenoviral replication defective. In terms of respiratory diseases, such adenoviral vectors have been the leading candidates for therapy of two common hereditary lung diseases: α_1-anti–trypsin deficiency (113) and cystic fibrosis (114). Clinical trials in the therapy of airway epithelial cells of the cystic fibrosis patients by the administration of adenoviruses carrying the CFTR gene are now underway, but early results are disappointing (115). There are problems associated with these first-generation adenoviral vectors: They evoke strong cellular immunity with inflammatory responses that rapidly eliminate infected cells in vivo and limit transgene expression (116). The presence of the capsid proteins in recombinant adenoviruses, usually administered at high dosages, also stimulates humoral responses that may eventually preclude repeated administration.

It is clear that leaky viral protein expression does take place in the current replication-deficient adenoviral vectors. Innovative, modified, and safer vehicles that are as efficient as adenoviral vectors, but lacking the extra baggage, are being designed. Considerable efforts are directed to make second-generation adenoviral vectors (117); more deletions have been made in the E3, E4, E2 or even the entire coding regions that results in a "gutless" adenoviral vector (118,119). An adenoviral dodecahedron has been assembled in vitro using only penton pentameric bases and the trimeric fiber. This dodecahedron can be taken up by HeLa cells, as demonstrated by immunofluorescence and electron microscopy. Furthermore, the carboxy-terminus of the fiber was extended with lysine residues to which polylysine-tagged DNA can be attached. The DNA was shown to get into the cell and be expressed. The lack of hexon in this formulation and early gene expression may reduce the impact of humoral and cellular immune response to vector administration. Efficacy of gene delivery and expression and lack of immunogenicity will be determining factors to assess the superiority of one vector to the other. Alternatively, targeting the early antigen-processing stages of immune response with specific antibody in combination with adenoviral vector–delivery is being explored. Targeting the CD40 ligand reduces humoral response to coadministered vector, allowing inserted gene expression (120). There are also attempts to narrow or broaden tissue tropism by modifying the fiber and penton molecules (121).

Exploitation of adenoviruses as vectors may contribute to the promise of gene therapy. These ubiquitous human pathogens may be harnessed to become widely used therapeutic tools.

XI. Summary

Adenoviruses of different serotypes demonstrate various tropisms, but the pulmonary tree is a major target with disease occurring in infants, in the immunosuppressed, and under conditions of crowding as seen in military training camps. In the latter setting, a live vaccine is used to good effect to prevent epidemic disease. Adenovirus has a complex set of genes which can potentially be manipulated, making the virus a rich source for vector development and for molecular investigation in gene regulation and immune modulation.

Acknowledgments

Thanks to Carol Walsh for assisting with manuscript preparation and Joyce Johnson, Department of Pathology, Vanderbilt University, for providing photographs of adenoviral pathology.

References

1. Rowe WP, Huebner RJ, Gillmore LK, Parrott RH, Ward TG. Isolation of a cytopathogenic agent from human adenoids undergoing spontaneous degeneration in tissue culture. Proc Soc Exp Biol Med 1953; 84:570–573.
2. Dingle J, Langmuir AD. Epidemiology of acute respiratory disease in military recruits. Am Rev Respir Dis 1968; 97:1–65.
3. Enders JF, Bell JA, Dingle JH, et al. "Adenoviruses": group name proposed for new respiratory tract viruses. Science 1956; 124:119–120.
4. Hilleman MR. Epidemiology of adenovirus respiratory infections in military recruit populations. Ann NY Acad Sci 1957; 67:262–272.
5. Wandell G. Molecular epidemiology of human adenoviruses. Curr Top Microbiol Immunol 1984; 110:191–217.
6. Philipson L. Structure and assembly of adenoviruses. Curr Top Microbiol Immunol 1983; 109:2–52.
7. Brandt CD, Kim HW, Vargosko AJ, Jeffries BC, Arrobio JO, Rindge B, Parrott RH, Chanock RM. Infections in 18,000 infants and children in a controlled study of respiratory tract disease: adenovirus pathogenicity in relation to serologic type and illness syndrome. Am J Epidemiol 1969; 90:484–500.
8. Straus SE. Adenovirus infections in humans. In: Gingsberg HS, ed. Adenoviruses. New York: Plenum Press, 1984:451–495.
9. Horwitz MS. Adenoviruses. In: Fields BN, Knipp DM, Howley PM, eds. Fields Virology. 3rd ed. Philadelphia: Lippincott-Raven, 1996:2149–2170.
10. Hierholzer JC, Wigand R, Anderson LJ, Adrian T, Gold JW. Adenoviruses from patients with AIDS: a plethora of serotypes and a description of five new serotypes of subgenus D (types 43–47). J Infect Dis 1988; 158:804–813.
11. Mei YF, Wadell G. Hemagglutination properties and nucleotide sequence analysis of the fiber gene of adenovirus genome types 11p and 11a. Virology 1993; 194:453–462.
12. Trentin JT, Yoshiro Y, Taylor G. The quest for human cancer viruses. Science 1962; 137:835–841.
13. Adrian T, Schafer G, Cooney MK, Fox JP, Wigand R. Persistent enteral infections with adenovirus types 1 and 2 in infants: no evidence of reinfection. Epidemiol Infect 1988; 101:503–509.
14. Fox JP, Hall CE, Cooney MK. The Seattle Virus Watch. VII. Observations of adenovirus infections. Am J Epidemiol 1977; 105:362–386.
15. Gruber WC, Russell DJ, Tibbetts C. Fiber gene and genomic origin of human adenovirus type 4. Virology 1993; 196:603–611.
16. Shenk T. Adeniviridae: The viruses and their replication. In: Fields BN, Knipe DM, Howley PM, eds. Fields Virology. 3rd ed. Philadelphia: Lippincott-Raven, 1996:2112–2148.
17. Klessig DF, Anderson CW. Block to multiplication of adenovirus serotype 2 in monkey cells. J Virol 1975; 16:1650–1668.
18. Duncan SJ, Gordon FCA, Gegory DW, McPhie JL, Postlethwaite R, White R, Wilcox HNA. Infection of mouse liver by human adenovirus type 5. J Gen Virol 1978; 40:45–51.

19. Ginsberg HS, Moldawer LL, Sehgal PB, Redington M, Kilian PL, Chanock RM, Prince GA. A mouse model for investigating the molecular pathogenesis of adenovirus pneumonia. Proc Natl Acad Sci USA 1991; 88:1651–1655.
20. Ginsberg HS, Horswood RL, Chanock RM, Prince GA. Role of early genes in pathogenesis of adenovirus pneumonia (published erratum appears in Proc Natl Acad Sci USA 1991; 15:88[2]:681). Proc Natl Acad Sci USA 1990; 87: 6191–6195.
21. Zabner J, Petersen DM, Puga AP, Graham SM, Couture LA, Keyes LD, Lukason MJ, St George JA, Gregory RJ, Smith AE, et al. Safety and efficacy of repetitive adenovirus-mediated transfer of CFTR cDNA to airway epithelia of primates and cotton rats. Nature Genet 1994; 6:75–83.
22. Varga MJ, Weibull C, Everitt E. Infectious entry pathway of adenovirus type 2. J Virol 1991; 65:6061–6070.
23. Wickham TJ, Mathias P, Cheresh DA, Nemerow GR. Integrins α-v-beta-3 and α-v-beta-5 promote adenovirus internization but not virus attachment. Cell 1993; 73:309–319.
24. Bergelson JM, Cunningham JA, Droguett G, Kurt-Jones EA, Krithivas A, Hong JS, Horwitz MS, Crowell RL, Finberg RW. Isolation of a common receptor for Coxsackie B viruses and adenoviruses 2 and 5. Science 1997; 275:1320–1323.
25. Goldman MJ, Wilson JM. Expression of α-v-beta-5 integrin is necessary for efficient adenovirus-mediated gene transfer in the human airway. J Virol 1995; 69: 5951–5958.
26. Mathias P, Wickham T, Moore M, Nemerow G. Multiple adenovirus serotypes use α-v integrins for infection. J Virol 1994; 68:6811–6814.
27. Wickham TJ, Mathias P, Cheresh DA, Nemerow GR. Integrins α-v-beta-3 and α-v-beta-5 promote adenovirus internalization but not virus attachment. Cell 1993; 73:309–319.
28. Krasnykh VN, Mikheeva GV, Douglas JT, Curiel DT. Generation of recombinant adenovirus vectors with modified fibers for altering viral tropism. J Virol 1996; 70:6839–6846.
29. Wickham TJ, Carrion ME, Kovesdi I. Targeting of adenovirus penton base to new receptors through replacement of its RGD motif with other receptor-specific peptide motifs. Gene Ther 1995; 2:750–756.
30. Nevins JR. Adenovirus E1A: Transcriptional regulation and alteration of cell growth control. Curr Top Microbiol Immunol 1995; 199:25–32.
31. Rao L, Debbas M, Sabbatini P, Hockenbery D, Korsmeyer S, White E. The adenovirus E1A proteins induce apoptosis, which is inhibited by the E1B 19-kDa and Bcl-2 proteins. Proc Natl Acad Sci USA 1992; 89:7742–7746.
32. Wold WM, Gooding LR. Region E3 of adenoviruses: a cassette of genes involved in host immunosurveillance and virus–cell interactions. Virology 1991; 184:1–8.
33. Bosher J, Dawson A, Hay RT. Nuclear factor I is specifically targeted to discrete subnuclear sites in adenovirus type 2–infected cells. J Virol 1992; 66:3140–3150.
34. Bergert SM, Moore C, Sharp PA. Spliced segments at the 5′ terminus of adenovirus 2 late mRNA. Proc Natl Acad Sci USA 1977; 74:3171–3175.
35. Chow LT, Gelinas RE, Broker TR, Roberts RJ. An amazing sequence arrangement at the 5′ ends of adenovirus 2 messenger RNA. Cell 1977; 12:1–8.

36. Dolph PJ, Huang J, Schneider RJ. Translation by the adenovirus tri-partite leader: elements which determine independence from cap binding protein complex. J Virol 1990; 64:2669–2677.
37. Ghadge GD, Swaminathan S, Katze MG, Thimmapaya B. Binding of the adenovirus VAI RNA to the interferon-induced 68-kDa protein kinase correlates with function. Proc Natl Acad Sci USA 1991; 88:7140–7144.
38. Ma Y, Mathews MB. Comparative analysis of the structure and function of adenovirus virus–associated RNAs. J Virol 1993; 67:6605–6617.
39. Couch RB, Cate TR, Douglas GJ, Gerone PJ, Knight V. Effect of route of inoculation on experimental respiratory viral disease in volunteers and evidence for airborne transmission. Bacteriol Rev 1966; 30:517–529.
40. Couch RB, Knight V, Douglas RGJ, Black SH, Hamory BH. The minimal infectious dose of adenovirus type 4; the case for natural transmission by viral aerosol. Trans Am Clin Climatol Assoc 1969; 80:205–211.
41. Pacini DL, Dubovi EJ, Clyde WA Jr. A new animal model for human respiratory tract disease due to adenovirus. J Infect Dis 1984; 150:92–97.
42. Prince GA, Porter DA, Jenson AB, Horswood RL, Chanock RM, Ginsberg HS. The pathogenesis of type 5 adenovirus in the cotton rat (*Sigmodon hispidus*). J Virol 1993; 67:101–111.
43. Pettersson U, Hoglund S. Structural proteins of adenoviruses. Virology 1969; 39:90–106.
44. Crystal RG, Mastrangeli A, Sanders A, Cooke J, King T, Gilbert F, Henschke C, Pascal W, Herena J, Harvey BG, et al. Evaluation of repeat administration of a replication deficient, recombinant adenovirus containing the normal cystic fibrosis transmembrane conductance regulator cDNA to the airways of individuals with cystic fibrosis. Hum Gene Ther 1995; 6:667–703.
45. Hu Y, Sperber K, Mayer L, Hsu MT. Persistent infection of human adenovirus type-5 in human monocyte cell lines. Virology 1992; 188:793–800.
46. Macek V, Sorli J, Kopriva S, Marin J. Persistent adenoviral infection and chronic airway obstruction in children. Am J Respir Crit Care Med 1994; 150:7–10.
47. Matsuse T, Hayashi S, Kuwano K, Keunecke H, Jeffries WA, Hogg JC. Latent adenoviral infection in the pathogenesis of chronic airway obstruction. Am Rev Respir Dis 1992; 146:177–184.
48. Elliott WM, Hayashi S, Hogg JC. Immunodetection of adenoviral E1A proteins in human lung tissue. Am J Respir Cell Mol Biol 1995; 12:642–648.
49. Vitalis TZ, Keicho N, Itabashi S, Hayashi S, Hogg JC. A model of latent adenovirus 5 infection in the guinea pig (*Cavia porcellus*). Am J Respir Cell Mol Biol 1996; 14:225–231.
50. Myerowitz RL, Stalder H, Oxman MN, Levin MJ, Moore M, Leith JD, Gantz NM, Pellegrini J, Hierholzer JC. Fatal disseminated adenovirus infection in a renal transplant recipient. Am J Med 1975; 58:591–598.
51. Ohori NP, Michaels MG, Jaffe R, Williams P, Yousem SA. Adenovirus pneumonia in lung transplant recipients. Hum Pathol 1995; 26:1073–1079.
52. Flomenberg P, Babbitt J, Drobyski WR, Ash RC, Carrigan DR, Sedmak GV, McAuliffe T, Camitta B, Horowitz MM, Bunin N, Casper JT. Increasing incidence of

adenovirus disease in bone marrow transplant recipients. J Infect Dis 1994; 169:775–781.
53. Crawford-Miksza L, Schnurr DP. Seroepidemiology of new AIDS-associated adenoviruses among the San Francisco Men's Health Study. J Med Virol 1996; 50:230–236.
54. Bellanti JA, Artenstein BC, Brandt BS, Klutinis BS, Buescher EL. Immunoglobin responses in serum and nasal secretions after natural adenovirus infection. J Immunol 1969; 103:891–898.
55. Toogood CI, Crompton J, Hay RT. Antipeptide antisera define neutralizing epitopes on the adenovirus hexon. J Gen Virol 1992; 73:1429–1435.
56. Yang Y, Nunes FA, Berencsi K, Furth EE, Gonczol E, Wilson JM. Cellular immunity to viral antigens limits E1-deleted adenoviruses for gene therapy. Proc Natl Acad Sci USA 1994; 91:4407–4411.
57. Burgert HG, Kvist S. The E3/19K protein of adenovirus type 2 binds to the domains of histocompatibility antigens required for CTL recognition. EMBO J 1987; 6: 2019–2026.
58. Gingsberg HS, Lundholm-Beuchamp U, Horswood RL, Pernis B, Wold WSM, Chanock RM, Prince GA. Role of early region 3 (E3) in pathogenesis of adenovirus disease. Proc Natl Acad Sci USA 1989; 86:3823–3827.
59. Williams JL, Garcia J, Harrich D, Pearson L, Wu F, Gaynor R. Lymphoid specific gene expression of the adenovirus early region 3 promoter is mediated by NF-k B binding motifs. EMBO J 1990; 9:4435–4442.
60. Horwitz MS, Fejer G, Gyory I, Tufariello J, Efrat S. Multiple functions of adenovirus E3 immunoregulatory genes: effects on acute viral pathogenesis and prolongation of survival of pancreatic islet allografts-allograft. J Cell Biochem 1995; 199(suppl):279.
61. Balser CF, Horwitz MS. Subgenera B adenovirus type early region 3 mRNA differ from those of the subgenera C adenoviruses. Virology 1996; 215:165–177.
62. Tracey KJ, Cerami A. Tumor necrosis factor, other cytokines and siease. Annu Rev Cell Biol 1993; 9:317–343.
63. Sparer TE, Tripp RA, Dillehay DL, Hermiston TW, Wold WSM, Gooding LR. The role of human adenovirus early region 3 proteins (gp19K, 10.4K, 14.5K, and 14.7K) in a murine pneumonia model. J Virol 1996; 70:2431–2439.
64. Goodings LR, Elmore LW, Tollefson AE, Brady HA, Wold WSM. A 14,700 mw protein from the E3 region of adenovirus inhibits cytolysis by tumor necrosis factor. Cell 1988; 53:341–346.
65. Thorne TE, Voelkel-Johnson C, Casey WM, Parks LW, Laster S. The activity of cytosolic phospholipase A2 is required for the lysis of adenovirus-infected cells by tumor necrosis factor. J Virol 1996; 70:8502–8507.
66. Tollefson AE, Scaria A, Hermiston TW, Ryerse JS, Wold LJ, Wold WM. The adenovirus death protein (E3-11.6K) is required at very late stages of infection for efficient cell lysis and release of adenovirus from infected cells. J Virol 1996; 70: 2296–2306.
67. Mei YF, Wadell G. Hemagglutination properties and nucleotide sequence analysis of the fiber gene of adenovirus genome types 11p and 11a. Virology 1993; 194:453–462.
68. Grayston JT, Woolridge RL, Loosli CG, Gundelfinger BF, Johnson PB, Pierce WE. Adenovirus infection in naval recruits. J Infect Dis 1959; 104:61–70.

69. Schmitz H, Wigand R, Heinrich W. Worldwide epidemiology of human adenovirus infection. Am J Epidemiol 1983; 117:455–466.
70. Resenbaum MJ, Edwards EA, Frank PF. Epidemiology and prevention of acute respiratory disease in naval recruits: I. Ten years of experience with microbial agents isolated from naval recruits with acute respiratory disease. Am J Public Health 1965; 55:38–46.
71. Rubin RA, Rorke LB. Adenovirus vaccines. In: Plotkin SA, Mortimer EA Jr, eds. Vaccines. Philadelphia: Saunders, 1988:492–512.
72. Lee SG, Hung PP. Vaccines for control of respiratory disease caused by adenoviruses. Rev Med Virol 1993; 3:209–216.
73. Edwards KM, Thompson J, Paolini J, Wright PF. Adenovirus infections in young children. Pediatrics 1985; 76:420–424.
74. Shields AF, Hackman RC, Fife KH, Corey L, Meyers JD. Adenovirus infections in patients undergoing bone-marrow transplantation. N Engl J Med 1985; 312: 529–533.
75. Flomenberg P, Babbitt J, Drobyski WR, Ash RC, Carrigan DR, Sedmak GV, McAuliffe T, Camitta B, Horowitz MM, Bunin N, et al. Increasing incidence of adenovirus disease in bone marrow transplant recipients. J Infect Dis 1994; 169: 775–781.
76. Moffet HL, Siegel AC, Doyle HK. Nonstreptococal pharyngitis. J Pediatr 1968; 73:51–60.
77. Chanock RM. Impact of adenoviruses in human disease. Prevent Med 1974; 3: 466–472.
78. Dudding BA, Top FHJ, Winter PE, Buescher EL, Lamson TH, Leibovitz A. Acute respiratory disease in military trainees: the Adenovirus Surveillance Program, 1966–1971. Am J Epidemiol 1973; 97:187–198.
79. Beal R. Sur une forme particuliere de conjonctivite aigue ave flooicules. Annales D'oculistique 1907; Jan:1–33.
80. Henderson FW, Collier AM, Sanyal MA, Watkins JM, Fairclough DL, Clyde WAJ, Denny FW. A longitudinal study of respiratory viruses and bacteria in the etiology of acute otitis media with effusion. N Engl J Med 1982; 306:1377–1383.
81. Collier AM, Connor JD, Irving WR. Generalized type 5 adenovirus infection associated with the pertussis syndrome. J Pediatr 1966; 69:1073–1078.
82. Myers JL, Colby TV. Pathologic manifestations of bronchiolitis, constrictive bronchiolitis, cryptogenic organizing pneumonia, and diffuse panbronchiolitis (review). Clin Chest Med 1993; 14:611–622.
83. Penn CC, Liu C. Bronchiolitis following infection in adults and children (review). Clin Chest Med 1993; 14:645–654.
84. Becroft DM. Bronchiolitis obliterans, bronchiectasis, and other sequelae of adenovirus type 21 infection in young children. J Clin Pathol 1971; 24:72–82.
85. Hierholzer JC. Adenoviruses in the immunocompromised host (review). Clin Microbiol Rev 1992; 5:262–274.
86. Abzug MJ, Levin MJ. Neonatal adenovirus infection: four patients and review of the literature (review). Pediatrics 1991; 87:890–896.
87. August MJ, Warford AL. Evaluation of a commercial monoclonal antibody for detection of adenovirus antigen. J Clin Microbiol 1987; 25:2233–2235.

88. Hierholzer JC, Johansson KH, Anderson LJ, Tsou CJ, Halonen PE. Comparison of monoclonal time-resolved fluorimmunoassay with monoclonal capture-biotinylated detector enzyme immunoassay for adenovirus antigen detection. J Clin Microbiol 1987; 25:1662–1667.
89. Kinchington PR, Turse SE, Kowalski RP, Gordon YJ. Use of polymerase chain amplification reaction for the detection of adenoviruses in ocular swab specimens. Invest Ophthalmol Vis Sci 1994; 35:4126–4134.
90. Matsuse T, Matsui H, Shu CY, Nagase T, Wakabayashi T, Mori S, Inoue S, Fukuchi Y, Orimo H. Adenovirus pulmonary infections identified by PCR and in situ hubridization in bone marrow transplant recipients. J Clin Pathol 1994; 47:973–977.
91. Klocke RA, Artenstein MS, Green RW, Dennehy JJ, Richert JH. The effect of acute respiratory infection on pulmonary function in military recruits. Am Rev Respir Dis 1966; 93:549–555.
92. Herbert FA, Wilkinson D, Burchak E, Morgante O. Adenovirus type 3 pneumonia causing lung damage in childhood. Can Med Assoc J 1977; 116:274–276.
93. Wenman WM, Pagtakhan RD, Reed MH, Chernick V, Albritton W. Adenovirus bronchiolitis in Manitoba: epidemiologic, clinical, and radiologic features. Chest 1982; 81:605–609.
94. Sly PD, Soto-Quiros ME, Landau LI, Hudson I, Newton-John H. Factors predisposing to abnormal pulmonary function after adenovirus type 7 pneumonia. Arch Dis Child 1984; 59:935–939.
95. Laitinen LA, Miettinen AK, Kuosma E, Huhtala L, Lehtomaki K. Lung function impairment following mycoplasmal and other acute pneumonias. Eur Respir J 1992; 5:670–674.
96. Kitabayashi A, Hirokawa M, Kuroki J, Nishinari T, Niitsu H, Miura AB. Successful vidarabine therapy for adenovirus type 11-associated acute hemorrhagic cystitis after allogenic bone marrow transplantation. Bone Marrow Transplant 1992; 14:853–854.
97. de Oliveira CB, Stevenson D, LaBree L, McDonnell PJ, Trousdale MD. Evaluation of Cidovovir (HPMPC, GS-504) against adenovirus type 5 infection in vitro and in a New Zealand rabbit ocular model. Antiviral Res 1996; 31:165–172.
98. McCarthy AJ, Bergin M, De Silva LM, Stevens M. Intravenous ribavirin therapy for disseminated adenovirus infection. Pediatr Infect Dis 1995; 14:1003–1004.
99. Wulffraat N, Geelan S, van Dijken P, De Graff-Meeder B, Kuis W, Boven K. Recovery from adenovirus pneumonia in a severe combined immunodeficiency patients treated with intravenous ribavirin. Transplantation 1995; 59:927.
100. Piedra PA, Kasel JA, Norton HJ, Gruber WC, Garcia-Prats JA, Baker CJ. Evaluation of an intravenous immunoglobulin preparation for the prevention of viral infection among hospitalized low birth weight infants. Pediatr Infect Dis 1990; 9:470–475.
101. Rowe WP, Baum SG. Evidence for a possible genetic hybrid between adenovirus type 7 and SV 40 viruses. Proc Natl Acad Sci USA 1964; 52:1340–1344.
102. Couch RB, Chanock RM, Cate TR, Lang DJ, Knight V, Huebner RJ. Immunization with type 4 and 7 adenovirus by selective infection of the intestinal tract. Am Rev Respir Dis 1963; 88(suppl):394–403.

103. Peckinpaugh RO, Pierce WE, Rosenbaum MJ, Edwards EA, Jackson GG. Mass enteric live adenovirus vaccination during epidemic ARD. JAMA 1968; 205:75–80.
104. Mueller RE, Muldoon RL, Jackson GG. Communicability of enteric liver adenovirus type 4 vaccine in families. J Infect Dis 1969; 119:60–66.
105. Bramson JL, Graham FL, Gauldie J. The use of adenoviral vectors for gene therapy and gene transfer in vivo. Curr Opin Biother 1995; 6:590–595.
106. Descamps V, Duffour MT, Mathieu MC, Fernandez N, Cordier L, Abina MA, Kremer E, Perricaudet M, Haddada H. Strategies for cancer gene therapy using adenoviral vectors. J Mol Med 1996; 74:183–189.
107. Randrianarison-Jewtoukoff, Perricaudet M. Recombinant adenoviruses as vaccines. Biologicals 1995; 23:145–157.
108. Cotten M. Adenovirus-augmented, receptor-mediated gene delivery and some solutions to the common toxicity problems. Curr Topics Microbiol Immunol 1995; 199(pt 3):283–295.
109. Tsukui T, Kanegae Y, Saito I, Toyoda Y. Transgenesis by adenovirus-mediated gene transfer into mouse zona-free eggs. Nature Biotechnol 1996; 14:982–985.
110. Chengalvala MV, Bhat BM, Bhat R, Lubeck MD, Mizutani S, Davis AR, Hung PP. Immunogenicity of high expression adenovirus-hepatitis B virus recombinant vaccines in dogs. J Gen Virol 1994; 75(pt 1):125–131.
111. Gallichan WS, Rosenthal KL. Specific secretory immune responses in the female genital tract following intranasal immunization with a recombinant adenovirus expressing glycoprotein B of herpes simplex virus. Vaccine 1995; 13:1589–1595.
112. Lubeck MD, Natuk RJ, Chengalvala M, Chanda PK, Murthy KK, Murthy S, Mizutani S, Lee SG, Wade MS, Bhat BM, et al. Immunogenicity of recombinant adenovirus-human immunodeficiency virus vaccines in chimpanzees following intranasal administration (published erratum appears in AIDS Res Hum Retroviruses 1995; 11[1]:189). AIDS Res Hum Retroviruses 1994; 10:1443–1449.
113. Rosenfeld MA, Siegfried W, Yoshimura K, Yoneyama K, Fukayama M, Stier LE, Paakko PK, Gilardi P, Stratford-Perricaudet L, Perricaudet M, Jallat S, Parvirani A, Lecocq LP, Crystal RG. Adenovirus-mediated transfer of a recombinant a-1-antitrypsin gene to the lung epithelium in vivo. Science 1991; 252:431–434.
114. Zabner J, Couture LA, Gregory RJ, Graham SM, Smith AE, Welsh MJ. Adenovirus-mediated gene transfer transiently corrects the chloride transport defect in nasal epithelial of patients with cystic fibrosis. Cell 1993; 75:207–216.
115. Crystal RG, McElvaney NG, Rosenfeld MA, Chu CS, Mastrangeli A, Hay JG, Brody SL, Jaffe HA, Eissa NT, Danel C. Administration of an adenovirus containing the human CFTR cDNA to the respiratory tract of individuals with cystic fibrosis. Nature Genet 1994; 8:42–51.
116. Yang Y, Su Q, Wilson JM. Role of viral antigens in destructive cellular immune responses to adenovirus vector-transduced cells in mouse lungs. J Virol 1996; 70:7209–7212.
117. Wang Q, Finer MH. Second-generation adenovirus vectors. Nature Med 1996; 2:714–716.
118. Kochanek S, Clemens PR, Mitani K, Chen HH, Chan S, Caskey CT. A new adenoviral vector: Replacement of all viral coding sequences with 28 kb of DNA

independently expressing both full length dystrophin and b-galactosidase. Proc Natl Acad Sci USA 1996; 93:5731–5736.
119. Fisher KJ, Choi H, Burda J, Chen SJ, Wilson JM. Recombinant adenovirus deleted of all viral genes for gene therapy of cystic fibrosis. Virology 1996; 217: 11–22.
120. Yang Y, Su Q, Grewal IS, Schilz R, Flavell RA, Wilson JM. Transient subversion of CD40 ligand function diminishes immune responses to adenovirus vectors in mouse liver and lung tissues. J Virol 1996; 70:6370–6377.
121. Krasnykh VN, Mikheeva GV, Douglas JT, Curiel DT. Generation of recombinant adenovirus vectors with modified fibers for altering viral tropism. J Virol 1996; 70:6839–6846.

10

The Common Cold
Rhinoviruses and Coronaviruses

MARK R. DENISON

Vanderbilt University School of Medicine
Nashville, Tennessee

I. Introduction

By definition, "common colds" are just that—the most frequent infectious illness of humans. With from four to six colds per year in young children and two to four colds per year in adults, colds are an important cause of discomfort, occasional complications, and economic loss worldwide. Thus there are compelling reasons to understand the replication and pathogenesis of viruses that cause common colds. The enthusiasm to study common colds resulted in the establishment of common cold units in the United Kingdom and similar groups in the United States during the 1960s and 1970s (1). Early studies identified the principal viral etiologies of colds, notably rhinoviruses and coronaviruses, and much progress was made in understanding the transmission, pathology, and clinical illness of common cold viruses. Subsequently, in the 1980s and 1990s, more emphasis was placed on the structure and replication of rhinoviruses and coronaviruses. Most recently, the ability to define immune responses to common cold viruses has led to an increased understanding of the important role of host response during acute colds. In addition, detailed understanding of the molecular biology and structure of rhinoviruses and coronaviruses has allowed development of an increasing number of agents with antiviral activities against the common cold viruses.

The initial enthusiasm directed toward diagnosis, treatment, and prevention of common colds has been tempered for several reasons: (1) It is now known that there are over 100 serotypes of rhinoviruses that cause colds, in addition to the several strains of coronaviruses, and thus the likelihood of any successful vaccine substantially reducing the burden of common colds is less; (2) homotypic and heterotypic antibodies may not protect from reinfection; and (3) available antiviral agents have not resulted in clinically important lessening of cold severity or duration during natural colds. The "success" of common cold viruses in human populations reflects the multitude of approaches used by the rhinoviruses and coronaviruses to infect their host, replicate, and spread prior to elimination by host defenses.

Nonetheless, important advances have occurred in our understanding of viral replication, transmission, cold pathogenesis, pulmonary physiology, and viral interference. We are entering yet another chapter of the study of common cold viruses in which it is being recognized that these viruses have a much more complex interaction with the host than previously thought, and they are important in causing or exacerbating other illnesses such as allergic responses or asthma. It is not the purpose of this chapter to delineate the entire history of cold virus research; that is much better accomplished in excellent reviews by other experts in the field (1–5). Rather this chapter will highlight the advances in the understanding of rhinoviral and coronaviral replication, pathogenesis, prevention, and treatment that have been occurring in recent years.

II. Rhinoviruses

A. Viral Replication

The rhinoviruses have become more of a model for the study of picornaviruses over the last several years. Many aspects of their structure, replication, and effect on host cells has been investigated in great detail, rivaling that of the best studied of the picornaviruses, the polioviruses. Human rhinoviruses (RV) have been used to determine the detailed structure of the virus-delivery system (virion), the structure and function of viral enzymes such as the virus-encoded proteinases, and the viral and host factors required for viral replication. In addition, knowledge of the molecular structure of the viral capsid has led to rational design of antiviral agents that might be active against rhinoviruses.

The human RV (HRV) belong to the picornavirus family (*pico* lt. small + *RNA virus*) of which the enteroviruses (poliovirus, echoviruses, coxsackieviruses) and hepatitis A virus are also members (5). The genome of the rhinoviruses is a single-stranded positive-sense (mRNA-sense) RNA molecule approximately 7.2 kb in length (6). The RNA genome is infectious when transfected into permissive cells, and "infectious" cDNA copies of the rhinoviral genome have been used to determine the genetics of many aspects of rhinoviral replication (7). Different RV subsets have been shown to bind to cells using either intracellular adhesion molecule-1 (ICAM-1) or low-density lipoprotein (LDL). RV14 is the type virus of those binding to ICAM-1; also known as the major group rhinoviruses (8). RV1a is the type virus of those binding to LDL; also referred to as the minor group rhinoviruses (9).

Expression of cell surface receptors has been shown to be required for viral replication, both by blockade of viral receptors using antireceptor monoclonal antibodies and by studies rendering RV-resistant cells permissive after transfection of receptor-expressing plasmids (8). In addition, it appears that receptor/virus interactions may be required for later expression of soluble mediators from virus-infected cells (10). The site for viral binding to receptor has been identified as the region surrounding the apex of a viral pentamer of the protein icosohedral capsid. Binding of virus occurs in the "canyon," or depression, surrounding the vertex (11). This binding is specific and results in internalization of the viral particle into cellular endosomes. In addition, it initiates a series of capsid structural changes that culminates in release (or injection) of the genome RNA into the cell cytoplasm. Because the virus/receptor interaction is required for viral infection, and because this interaction is so specific, the structure of the viral capsid has become a focus of much attention in regard to viral replication, host immune response, and as a possible target for prophylactic or therapeutic drugs. The availability of the complete three-dimensional (3D) structure of the rhinoviral capsid has made it possible to perform studies of viral interactions with monoclonal antibodies, soluble receptor or receptor fragments, and potential chemotherapeutic agents (12).

Following uncoating of the rhinoviral genome RNA, replication is initiated by translation of the genome RNA into a single 250-kDa polyprotein that contains all of the structural and nonstructural proteins encoded by the virus (13). The expression and processing of this viral polyprotein has been characterized in great detail (6,14). The intact polyprotein is never seen in natural conditions, because the polyprotein contains two proteinases (2A and 3C) that immediately process the nascent polyprotein into intermediate precursors and mature proteins. The 2A and 3C proteinases also have profound effects on the host cell; 2A initiates a cascade of cleavages that results in cleavage of p220, a critical component of the complex that allows translation of capped message (15,16). Thus translation of the cellular capped message is abolished, allowing the uncapped RV genome RNA to be exclusively translated by a novel mechanism involving internal initiation of translation.

The crystallographic structure of the RV14 3C proteinase has been determined and the location of catalytic and substrate binding residues precisely defined (17). These studies have confirmed predictions that the rhinoviral 3C proteinases are members of an unusual family of viral proteinases that have the structure of cellular serine proteinases such as chymotrypisin but replace the catalytic serine with a cysteine residue. The rhinoviral 3C proteinases have a unique cleavage site specifically that makes them attractive targets for antiviral agents. The 3D structure of RV 3C proteinase has provided a basis for searches for drugs that might inhibit all rhinoviral serotypes based on conservation of proteinase structure and activity even among serologically distinct rhinoviruses (17).

Following translation of the nonstructural and structural proteins, the viral RNA genome is replicated. Rhinoviral replication is an entirely cytoplasmic process. Replication of rhinoviruses in the cytoplasm involves assembly of 60 subunits (protomers) consisting of VP1, VP0, and VP3 into 12 pentamers. The inside of the capsid consists of the RNA core including the covalently bound VPg molecule. During the final maturation of the provirion particles, VP0 is cleaved to yield VP2 and VP4, resulting in infectious viral particles that are then released from the cell by cell lysis. The entire life cycle requires from 5 to 10 hr (5).

B. Pathogenesis

Transmission of rhinoviruses has been studied in both experimental and natural conditions. Transmission by direct contact such as hand-to-hand, hand-to-nose, and hand-to-eye has been readily demonstrated in experimental settings (18–20). Rhinoviruses are relatively stable on environmental surfaces and on skin. Certainly inoculation into the anterior nares is effective, and it is used as the route of experimental infection in volunteer studies. Transmission of rhinoviruses also occurs by the respiratory route alone, as elegantly demonstrated in a series of studies using shields designed to eliminate hand-to-nose or hand-to-eye contact (21,22). It is interesting that it has been more difficult to demonstrate routes of transmission in natural settings. The factors thought to be most important for transmission include viral titer, the presence of symptomatic illness, and duration of exposure (2). One study by Meschievitz (23) demonstrated that among couples without children present, 200 hr of contact was required for 50% transmission of rhinovirus from an experimentally infected partner to the uninfected partner. Thus although transmission can clearly occur by both direct contact and respiratory routes, it may not be as efficient as expected in natural settings (24) and there may be many other factors involved in the acquisition of infection and the development of symptomatic colds.

Inoculation of rhinoviruses is thought to occur primarily in the anterior nose, whereas replication has been demonstrated to occur initially in the posterior nasopharynx. Viral replication occurs in the epithelium of the nasal mucosa (25,26). Following primary replication and shedding of virus, transmission occurs to the anterior nasopharynx and nares and possibly to the lower respiratory tract. There has been one report of viremia in infants (27), but there have been no other experimental data supporting viremia or systemic replication of rhinoviruses. Initial replication has been demonstrated to occur in the nasopharynx, probably in M cells within adenoid tissues. Virus may reach these tissues by normal mucociliary transport (28). The peak of viral replication occurs from 24 to 48 hr after infection.

During initial viral replication in the nasopharyngeal epithelium, it does not appear that a large proportion of epithelial cells are infected, nor that there is significant demonstrable cytopathic effect in infected cells. This has been demonstrated both by in cyto infection of explanted respiratory epithelium (29) and in biopsies of different regions of the upper respiratory tract during experimental rhinoviral infections in volunteers (30). Infection can be readily identified by viral culture of secretions and by immunofluorescence and electron microscopic studies of biopsied tissues: however, sloughing of the epithelial layer and disruption of function of ciliated cells is uncommon. Although epithelial cells are shed during infection, the amount of shedding does not correlate with severity of infection (31). This has been somewhat of a mystery to investigators, since rhinoviruses are efficient agents during infection of cultured cells, result in shutoff of host cell translation and transcription, and result in demonstrable cytopathic effect and cell death within 12–24 hr (5). Finally, computed tomographic (CT) studies of the sinuses of 31 naturally infected individuals has shown that inflammation and edema of the sinus mucosa is the rule rather than the exception—occurring in 87% of maxillary sinuses, 65% of ethmoid sinuses, and 32% of frontal sinuses and 39% of sphenoid sinuses (32). The investigators concluded that rhinoviral colds normally are associated with rhinosinusitis rather than just rhinitis.

Viral replication increases for 2–3 days, as measured by titer of virus in nasal secretions. The duration of viral shedding may vary from several days to up to 28 days (33). The maximum degree of shedding correlates with the number of cells infected in biopsy specimens and also is associated with the occurrence and severity of clinical illness (34).

The pathophysiology of colds still has not been adequately explained. However, many different proposed mechanisms have been investigated and much about humoral, cytokine, and cellular responses to rhinoviral infection has been learned. The first observed process during infection is an increase in nasal secretions. Igarashi et al. performed a careful analysis of nasal secretions during experimental infections with HRV 39. They demonstrated that early in infection the proteins found in nasal secretions were predominantly plasma proteins, specifically IgG and albumin, and that at later times proteins such as lactoferrin, lysozyme, and secretory IgA predominated. They concluded that early secretions resulted from increased vascular leakage of plasma and there was a transition at later times to predominant glandular secretions.

There have been a number of studies performed to look at the histology of the nasal mucosa during experimental rhinoviral colds. Winther described evidence for an increase in neutrophils in the epithelium and subepithelial layers by day 2 of symptomatic colds but no increase in lymphocytes in the nasal mucosa or the mucosa of the inferior turbinates (35). Neutrophils have been detected in nasal secretions during rhinoviral infection, and it has been proposed that rhinovirus-infected cells may express neutrophil chemoattractants (36). However, a more recent study of the immunohistochemistry of nasal mucosal biopsies has not confirmed these findings. Fraenkel et al. performed biopsies on experimentally infected volunteers with and without allergic rhinitis (37). They found no increases in mucosal mast cells, eosinophils, lymphocytes, or neutrophils in either patient population. They concluded that these findings, together with evidence of increased neutrophils in nasal secretions, may be a result of increased vascular permeability and rapid transit from the blood stream into the nasal mucus. In their population, there was a subset of individuals with increased mucosal neutrophils by immunohistochemical analyses. Thus it remains to be determined what role, if any, neutrophils play in the immunopathogenesis of colds or in clearance of viral infection.

B. Rhinoviral Infections and Inflammatory Mediators

In part due to the lack of direct cytopathology related to rhinoviral infections, as well as the lack of a dramatic local cellular response to infection, it has long been proposed that inflammatory mediators must be responsible for the local and systemic manifestations of rhinoviral colds. Two studies from the same laboratory measured levels of kinins, esterase activity, albumin, neutrophils, and histamine in nasal secretions during experimental and natural colds (38,39). Similar results were obtained in both studies; specifically, it was demonstrated that infected, symptomatic individuals had increased levels of kinins, TAME esterase, and albumin and increased numbers of neutrophils in nasal secretions. Further, the degree of symptomatology was correlated with increases in all of these factors. In contrast, histamine levels in nasal secretions did not change during either experimental or natural colds. In a separate study, Proud et al. showed that nasal instillation of bradykinin reproduced the upper respiratory symptomatology associated with common colds, including rhinorrhea, nasal obstruction, and persistent sore throat (40). Interestingly, nasal obstruction was unilateral on the side of bradykinin administration. They also noted increased albumin and TAME esterase in nasal secretions. Again, no increases in histamine were noted, and the investigators concluded that the nasal instillation of bradykinin likely does not result in mast cell activation, and that many of the upper respiratory findings of colds may be mediated by secreted kinins. These studies also supported the conclusion that histamine is not a mediator of upper respiratory tract symptoms associated with rhinoviral infection.

It is likely that other mediators play a role in the rest of the spectrum of illness associated with colds, as well as with the lower respiratory tract findings and induction of immune response to the viral infection. Recently, other cytokines and presumed inflammatory mediators have been measured in nasal secretions. Concentrations of immunoreactive interleukin-1b (IL-1b) were shown by Proud et al. to be elevated during experimental rhinovirus 39 and HH (not neutralized by antisera to 89 numbered rhinoviral serotypes) (41). Levels of IL-1 had the same temporal pattern as observed in the studies of kinins and, in fact, correlated with increases in albumin and kinins in nasal secretions. This analysis was performed as part of a study to assess the effect of glucocorticoid prophylaxis of rhinoviral colds (42). Although the numbers in each group were small, there was evidence to suggest that glucocorticoids have no effect on the elaboration of IL-1b in nasal secretions. The source of the IL-1b was not determined, but based on the known functions of IL-1b, it was proposed that IL-1b may play a role in antigen presentation and the induction of specific lymphocytes against the infecting rhinovirus.

Both IL-8 and IL-6 have also been detected in increased levels in nasal secretions of persons with symptomatic rhinoviral infections (43,44). Zhu et al. investigated the role of HRV induction of IL-6 in rhinoviral pathogenesis (10). Study patients were challenged with HRV39 and levels of IL-6 in nasal secretions were measured at baseline and throughout infection. No IL-6 was detected at baseline, but high levels were detected in volunteers who developed colds, and the levels of IL-6 correlated with the levels of symptomatic cold scores. The IL-6 was biologically active as measured by inducing [^{3}H]thymidine incorporation in B9.11 cells. These results were correlated with in vitro studies demonstrating that RV infection of pulmonary-derived MRC-5 and A549 cells in culture resulted in upregulation of IL-6 production, principally through stimulation of IL-6 mRNA synthesis. Both major (RV14) and minor (RV1a) group rhinoviruses were able to stimulate IL-6 production. Further, IL-6 was not induced by ultraviolet-inactivated virus. Finally, the study demonstrated that specific regions of the IL-6 promoter were required for the rhinoviral response, and that the NF-κB site was critical.

This study is the first to draw a strong correlation between the nasal secretion of a cytokine, possible sites of induction and synthesis, and possible pathogenic roles. IL-6 is known to stimulate acute phase responses, to activate

T lymphocytes, to play a role in differentiation of immunoglobulin, and to function as an endogenous pyrogen. It is also a regulator of pulmonary inflammation and plays a role in mucosal IgA responses. Thus it may not only play a role locally in the upper respiratory tract but also distally in the lungs.

C. Rhinoviral Infections and Cellular Immune Responses

A variety of cellular immune responses have also been characterized during rhinoviral infections. Decreases in total circulating lymphocyte counts have been demonstrated during experimental infection with HRV25 (45,46). The amount of decrease in $CD4^+$ lymphocytes correlated with severity of cold symptoms, as well as with amount of viral shedding. In contrast, $CD8^+$ cells and B cells were unaffected. The investigators suggested selective migration of $CD4^+$ cells to the mucosal epithelium as an explanation for this selective decrease, but this was not demonstrated.

Activation of peripheral blood mononuclear cells during rhinoviral infection has also been proposed to be involved in pathogenesis of upper respiratory findings, as well as the exacerbations of asthma that have been observed with rhinoviral infections. Hsia et al. measured several indices of cellular immune response during experimental infections with an unnumbered rhinovirus (47). They demonstrated that peripheral blood mononuclear cells (PBMC) are activated during rhinoviral infection, with increases in natural killer (NK) cell activity and with increased mitogen-stimulated generation of interferon-γ (IFN-γ) and IL-2. However, there was no increased IFN-γ noted in the bloodstream.

The mechanism of lymphocyte activation was addressed by Gern et al. in a study of patients with allergic rhinitis (AR) (48). They were able to demonstrate specific binding of HRV16 to PBMC isolated from patients with AR. Specifically, they reported binding of rhinovirus to $CD54^+$ (ICAM-1^+) lymphocytes and monocytes, and binding was enhanced fourfold in PBMC populations enriched for monocytes but not lymphocytes. Within the PBMC population, activation of 30–70% of T cells occurred as defined by expression of the early activation marker CD69. Activation of lymphocytes occurred only when monocytes were present in the PBMC population, was blocked by antibody against ICAM-1, and could not be induced by UV-inactivated virus. The implications of this latter finding were not addressed, but it was concluded that a monocyte-dependent mechanism was required for T-cell activation, possibly through soluble factors.

D. Rhinoviral Infections, Lower Respiratory Tract Infection, Allergic Rhinitis, and Asthma

Although much has been learned about the rhinoviral immune response and immunopathogenesis, it is still difficult to develop a model that accounts for the local and systemic findings of rhinoviral colds. Clearly, secreted cytokines are likely to determine much of the symptomatology observed in upper respiratory infections. Just as clearly, systemic cellular immune responses are activated. It is presumed that these play a role in local viral clearance and also in the pathogenesis of local illness. However, other investigators have been more interested in the associations of infections with rhinoviruses and other "common cold" pathogens with lower respiratory tract disease and with precipitation or exacerbation of asthma. It has long been recognized that episodes of wheezing are common in children with asthma during upper respiratory infections, but the mechanism by which this occurs has been unclear.

Improvement in rhinoviral diagnostic methods has allowed estimates that viral infections can be detected in up to 85% of asthma exacerbations, with more severe exacerbations improving the detection rate (44). These asthma episodes resulted in a median fall in peak flow of 80 L/min (35% reduction). Cold symptoms preceded the lower respiratory tract findings by 1–2 days. Hospital admissions for asthma also had a strong statistical association with rates of upper respiratory infections in a sentinel cohort of children and adults. Similar findings were obtained in a study of 138 adults with asthma; specifically, colds were reported in 80% of episodes of asthma and 89% of colds were associated with asthma symptoms (49). Isolates viruses included rhinoviruses and coronaviruses, as well as parainfluenza, influenza B, and respiratory syncytial virus. Rhinoviruses have been isolated from sputum of children with bronchitis and from secretions obtained by bronchoscopy during experimental infections (50,51). Rhinoviral infection has also been associated with significant lower respiratory tract disease in children and adults (52–54). Despite all of this information, no unequivocal data for lower respiratory tract replication of rhinoviruses in natural infections have been obtained. Rhinoviruses can bind and enter monocytes, but replication has not been shown to occur (48,55).

Based on these observations, several important questions can be raised. First, are individuals with a history of asthma, allergic rhinitis, or atopy more likely to become infected with rhinoviruses? Second, if such individuals become infected with rhinoviruses, are they more likely to experience symptomatic colds? Third, do colds exacerbate responses to environmental allergens in atopic or asthmatic individuals? Fourth, what is the mechanism by which rhinoviral infection results in asthma in such persons? The first two questions have been addressed in two studies of experimental rhinoviral infections in volunteers with and without a history of allergic rhinitis. Bardin et al. inoculated 22 volunteers (11 nonatopic, 5 atopic, and 6 atopic and asthmatic) with HRV16 and measured clinical scores, nasal wash albumin, viral shedding, and serum IgE (56). All 22 volunteers became infected and 17 developed clinical colds. There was no difference in the incidence of clinical colds in the atopic and nonatopic populations, although the numbers may have been too small to detect a difference. However, there was a significant increase in the severity of colds in the atopic group; measured by clinical scores and nasal wash albumin. Some of the volunteers were found to have preexisting levels of neutralizing antibody but atopic individuals developed severe colds independent of the presence of neutralizing antibody. In contrast, levels of IgE, which were generally higher in the atopic population, did not correlate with severity of illness or viral shedding.

A separate volunteer study of 20 "allergic" and 18 nonallergic adults was performed by Doyle et al. in which participants were inoculated with HRV39 and a battery of clinical and physiological measurements were obtained, including nasal patency, nasal secretion weights, rhinomanometry, spirometry, and tympanometry (57). All 38 patients were infected, and there was no difference between groups in the number of persons that developed clinical colds. There was also no difference in the clinical severity of colds, degree of nasal secretion, or outcome. There was earlier onset of decreased mucus clearance, nasal obstruction, and eustachian tube dysfunction in the allergic group, but the severity and temporal pattern of response was the same as the nonallergic group. Additional studies by the same group demonstrated that there were increased nasal responses to histamine provocation after RV infection in both allergic and nonallergic patients but no differences between the groups. The investigators noted that this study was intentionally performed during nonallergy season to avoid confounding factors. This condition was not established in the study by Bardin et al., but they did not believe that preexisting allergic rhinitis might have influenced the observed results. It can be stated that under experimental conditions, allergic and nonallergic patients can be equivalently infected, that a majority will develop colds, and that preexisting neutralizing antibodies will not prevent development of cold symptoms.

The question of response to allergens was investigated by Calhoun et al. using local allergen provocation in experimentally infected volunteers (58). Seven AR patients and 5 non-AR controls were infected with RV16, and all 12 patients became infected and developed colds of similar clinical severity and with similar respiratory physiology by spirometry. All patients then underwent bronchoscopy with segmental antigen provocation and bronchoalveolar lavage before, during, and 1 month after infection. Lavage fluid was analyzed for histamine, tumor necrosis factor-α (TNF-α), eosinophils, and viral culture. RV16 alone did not induce changes in the airway either in normal subjects or AR patients. TNF-α levels were increased in both patient groups by infection alone. Antigen challenge resulted in increased histamine release and eosinophils in the AR group but not in the normal controls, and these effects were present up to 1 month after RV16 infection. There was no evidence of lower respiratory tract infection in any patients. Thus it appeared that both RV infection and antigen challenge were necessary for a potentiated response, but that inflammatory cytokines, rather than direct viral infection, were responsible for the potentiation of response to antigen.

E. Epidemiology

Immunity to rhinoviruses has been detected whenever it has been looked for even in remote or isolated populations (59,60). Many factors have been implicated as being important in the susceptibility to infection and the development of colds. Fox has reported data from Seattle Watch, a longitudinal study from 1965 to 1969 and again from 1975 to 1979 (33,61). Both studies demonstrated two peaks of rhinoviral infections—in the spring and again in the fall. Young children were the most susceptible to rhinoviral infection, with increasing susceptibility being associated with decreasing age. In the initial study, rates were lowest among mothers, probably due to repeated exposure and high levels of antibody. The second study confirmed this, indicating that stable immunity to homotypic viruses did not emerge until after 10 years of age. It also appeared that in the interval, no new dominant infecting viral serotypes had emerged. Rhinoviruses were the most common (56%) viruses isolated during the latter study. In separate studies, stress has been shown to be associated with increased rates of symptomatic colds in a dose–response manner (62,63). The possible mechanism for this finding has not been addressed. Chilling, long proposed to increase the risk for colds, has been clearly shown not to contribute to the risk for upper respiratory infection (64).

F. Clinical Illness

The lack of evidence for significant destruction of respiratory epithelium or transmission or replication to the lower respiratory tract has always been somewhat surprising given the significant symptomatology that may be associated with the common cold. Following a 1- to 4-day incubation period, typical symptoms of pharyngitis, sneezing, nasal obstruction, and rhinorrhea appear and predominate, with a mean duration of 7 days, but lasting for up to 2 weeks in 25% of patients (2,28). Although symptoms referrable to the upper respiratory tract are most common, generalized complaints of chills, fever, headache, myalgia, chest pain, and anorexia are defined in 22–76% of patients.

The complications of colds are many and varied. Rhinoviruses have been associated with the subsequent onset of otitis media in children and with sinusitis at all ages. Some of this may be related to obstruction of sinus ostia or eustachian tubes leading to bacterial infection from prior colonization. However, there is also evidence that inflammation of the sinus mucosa is part of the primary presentation of rhinoviral infection.

G. Antivirals and Symptomatic Treatment of Rhinoviral Colds

Alas, it still remains true that we cannot cure the common cold. Although analysis of the capsid structure of the rhinoviruses has been accomplished, and much is known about the local response to infection and the presenting findings of the common cold, it has been difficult to intervene successfully. Many of the features described in the previous sections of this chapter make it clear why this has been so difficult. Replication of virus may occur only in small amounts in local areas of the nasopharynx and nasal mucosa; symptoms of colds may principally result from neurogenic reflexes and inflammatory cytokines that may be elaborated even after viral replication has ceased; inflammation, edema, and obstruction may involve not only the nasal passage but also multiple sinuses; distal effects on the lower respiratory tract may be prominent in some individuals; different viruses (coronaviruses) and different rhinoviruses may elicit different patterns of response; and infections may occur even in the presence of homotypic neutralizing antibodies. Thus it is becoming clear the therapy of colds may require multiple modalities.

Efforts at a rational design of antivirals have hinged on understanding the structure of the viral capsid. Agents that bind to the pocket in the floor of the canyon at the icosohedral five-fold vertex include pyridazines, flavones, and isoxazode derivatives (1). All of these agents exhibit activity in vitro against rhinoviral infection, but they have been disappointing in clinical trials of common colds whether administered orally or by topical sprays. Although there are concerns with resistance developing in vitro (65), the principal concerns are adequate delivery and maintenance during the brief period of viral replication preceding symptomatic colds.

Interferon does not appear to be induced to any significant levels during rhinoviral colds in contrast to the high levels seen in association with clearance of influenza virus infections. Nonetheless, intranasal recombinant IFN-α has been effective in prophylaxis against experimentally induced colds (66,67) and for prevention of transmission to contacts of a family member with a cold (68). Interferon does not appear to be effective for the treatment of established colds, but in one study, it did reduce the frequency of eustachian tube dysfunction (69). Unfortunately, administration of high doses of IFN-α is also associated with the onset of symptoms of nasal stuffiness and blood-tinged secretions (67).

Two different approaches to the prevention of rhinoviral binding have been via antireceptor antibodies and soluble ICAM-1 (sICAM-1). Monoclonal antibodies against ICAM-1 block infection by major group rhinoviruses in vitro (70,71) and have protected chimpanzees from seroconversion to HRV15 (70). In studies with human volunteer experimental infections, high doses (100 mg) and multiple doses (ten) were required to reduce viral titer and delay the onset of symptoms (72). sICAM-1 also blocks binding of major group rhinoviruses in vitro but has not yet been tested in humans (73,74).

Other approaches not based on "rational" design or steps in viral replication have also been assessed. Because of the low-temperature requirements (33°C) for optimal rhinoviral replication, it has been postulated that increasing the ambient temperature in the nasal passages might block or abort viral replication. A summary of multiple studies suggested that warm inhaled air would be of no reproducible clinical benefit and had no effect on viral replication or shedding (75). Zinc gluconate lozenges dissolved in the mouth have also been suggested to cause significant reductions in cold symptoms when administered shortly after the onset of symptoms, but two randomized controlled trials indicated that it was of no benefit (76). Trials of corticosteroids have been attempted based on the hypothesis that blocking of cytokine release might ameliorate cold symptoms. Gustafson et al. tested oral steroids against placebo in 47 men before and during experimental infection with HRV39 (77). The frequency of viral shedding did not differ between the groups, but the mean titer was higher in the steroid group than the placebo group. Kinin levels in nasal secretions were reduced in the steroid group, but there was no difference in respiratory or systemic symptoms in the two groups. A similar study of nasally administered beclamethasone combined with oral prednisone showed an initial reduction in nasal obstruction, secretion, and kinin concentrations but overall no significant difference with placebo (42). Thus steroids do not appear to play a role in the reduction in the severity of clinical colds and may increase or prolong viral shedding.

III. Coronaviruses

Coronaviruses (CV) cause a wide range of infections in humans and other animals, including gastroenteritis, hepatitis, encephalomyelitis, and tracheobronchitis (3). Coronaviral infections of humans have been implicated in upper respiratory infections, gastroenteritis, lower respiratory infections, and rare cases of meningitis/encephalitis. The only consistent documented associations with human illness have been with upper respiratory infections. Studies of respiratory infections caused by human CV have always been provocative, indicating that from 10 to 30% of upper respiratory infections at all ages may be caused by these viruses, and that they may be implicated in more serious respiratory illnesses than rhinoviruses (4). However, CV have languished at the bottom of many lists of human pathogens because of the difficulty in isolating and characterizing the agents during outbreaks of illness. It has not been possible to identify directly coronaviral growth without sometimes extensive passage. In the case of the human CV OC43, isolation has required passage in primary fetal organ culture. Thus, historical diagnostic studies were for the most part limited to use of paired sera to detect the two main CV causing colds, 229E and OC43. This in turn limited the ability of investigators to define serological variants or determinants of infection, reinfection, host response, and pathogenesis. It is only recently that the advent of improved diagnostic methods such as enzyme-linked immunosorbent assay (ELISA) using nasal secretions, oligonucleotide probes, and reverse transcriptase–polymerase chain reaction (RT-PCR) have made it possible to revisit studies last performed in the 1960s or 1970s.

Another challenge has been provided by the immense size (in RNA terms) of the coronaviral genome. The coronavirus genome is 27–32 kb in length, four times as large as the rhinovirus genome (approximately 7.5 kb) (78,79). The entire genome of 229E has been sequenced and the predicted functional domains have been determined. Until the advent of methods for stably cloning such a large RNA molecule into a complementary DNA (cDNA), it has been difficult to study the genetics of viral replication or define the determinants of host immune response. Nevertheless, significant progress has been made in defining the mechanisms of viral replication and identifying potential targets for therapeutic intervention.

A. Viral Replication

Coronaviruses are named for their distinctive ultrastructure consisting of spherical pleomorphic particles containing a halo of glycoproteins which give the virions the appearance of a "corona" of spikes. The virions are 100- to 120-nm particles consisting of a lipid bilayer incorporating several proteins: the spike (S), matrix (M), small membrane (E), and nucleocapsid (N) proteins are the known structural proteins of HCV 229E. The RNA is organized as a helical nucleocapsid, possibly within a separate capsid-like structure formed by the N protein. The S protein is responsible for binding to cellular receptors, and it is the protein against which neutralizing antibodies are induced during infection.

Tropism for 229E is likely determined by virus/receptor interactions. The receptor for 229E has been identified as human aminopeptidase N (hAPN) (80–83). This is a cell surface glycoprotein expressed on human lung, kidney, and intestinal cells, as well as fibroblasts and nerve synapses. Human aminopeptidase N is an exopeptidase that functions in the gut to digest short peptides and in the brain to break down neurotransmitter peptides. The location of hAPN on lung cells is consistent with the established role of 229E in upper respiratory infections and occasionally with lower respiratory tract infections. Just as clearly, tropism and viral replication must be affected by factors in addition to virus/receptor interactions. The studies identifying hAPN as the receptor for 229E also showed that OC43 does not use the hAPN molecule as a receptor. The receptor for OC43 remains unknown, but based on the relatedness of OC43 to the murine coronavirus, mouse hepatitis virus (MHV), it is likely that the receptor will be a member of the chorioembryonic antigen (CEA) family of molecules (3).

Replication of coronaviruses is initiated by translation of the input genome RNA, which also functions as an intact mRNA molecule, resulting in expression of a 750-kDa polyprotein from the 5'-most region, gene 1. At least two virus-encoded proteinase domains have been identified within the gene 1 polyprotein, and they have been shown to be responsible for cleavage of the polyprotein into the individual proteins that are likely to be involved in replication of the viral RNA genome (78,79,84,85). Available results along with predictions based on the genome sequence indicate that there are more than 15 distinct proteins within the polyprotein, and that many of these have no known homology to identified cellular or viral proteins; thus it is possible that the proteins may mediate unique functions in coronaviral replication that might be targets for antiviral approaches.

The two 229E proteinases (PLP-1 and 3Clpro) share similarities to papain and to the 3C proteinases of the picornaviruses, respectively (86). There are significant similarities in the organization, conserved domains, and putative enzymes encoded by 229E and MHV, and thus parallel studies of MHV are likely to yield information critical to understanding mechanisms for interfering with coronaviral replication. The coronavirus 3C-like proteinase (3Clpro), like the rhinovirus 3C proteinase, is predicted to have a structure analogous to cellular serine proteinases but with a catalytic cysteine substituted for the serine of the cellular enzymes (87,88). 3Clpro is likely to mediate the majority of cleavages within the gene 1 polyprotein, and thus it will likely be a critical target for any future efforts at intervention. So far, only one study has demonstrated that an inhibitor of 3Clpro in vitro that rapidly blocks polyprotein processing also eliminates viral replication in tissue culture (89).

Following synthesis of nonstructural (replicase) proteins, transcription and replication of the RNA genome occurs (90). Synthesis of structural proteins requires transcription of a nested set of subgenomic mRNA via a novel leader-primed transcription mechanism. Coronaviral replication is thought to occur largely in membrane-bound complexes. Localization of many proteins, specifically the structural S, N, M, and E proteins, occurs in endoplasmic reticulum. Assembly of coronaviral particles occurs in the Golgi and trans-Golgi regions with budding into smooth-walled vesicles and release of virus from the cell surface via the cell secretory apparatus. In tissue culture, expression of the S glycoprotein on cell surfaces can result in dramatic cell-cell fusion with syncytia formation. It is not known if this plays a role in the cytopathology during natural infections in humans and animals.

B. Pathogenesis of Infections Caused by Human Coronaviruses

Human coronaviruses can replicate in a number of cell lines, but cultivation is usually to low titer and requires several days. Conditions similar to those used for rhinovirus (33°C) have been used to grow 229E to higher titers. OC43 has also been adapted for growth in tissue culture, but primary isolates cannot be grown in cell culture. The pathogenesis of coronaviral respiratory infection has not been as well studied as that of the rhinoviruses. Transmission of coronaviruses occurs well in environments such as schools, among siblings of coronavirus-infected children (91), and military bases (92). Transmission probably occurs in a manner similar to that of rhinoviruses. A study of airborne survival of 229E concluded that stability was maximal at 6°C and 50% relative humidity (93). Coronaviruses, notably 229E, are also able to infect efficiently individuals during volunteer studies (94,95). The precise cells initially infected are not known, but a wide variety of cells in the respiratory tract contain the hAPN receptor for 229E on their apical surfaces (80). Thus it is possible that many cells in the upper respiratory tract are infected, and it is postulated that direct viral damage may contribute to the clinical presentation. 229E can cause syncytia formation in tissue culture; however, one study by Winther et al. of 229E infection of explanted nasal epithelial cells in culture showed clear evidence for infection but no cytopathology (29). Rhinoviruses and coronaviruses demonstrated similar patterns of replication without gross cytopathic effect in contrast to a clear cytopathic effect with influenza and adenovirus. In contrast, infection of macrophages with 229E results in syncytia formation and cell death within 24 hr (96). No studies have been reported for localization of 229E or OC43 replication during natural or experimental infections. Thus it remains to be determined how much destruction of which cells is mediated by viral replication during initial stages of infection.

The host factors involved in the pathogenesis of coronaviral respiratory illness have not been completely defined. The incubation period of coronaviral infection is longer than that of rhinoviruses; 4–5 days for coronaviruses versus 1–2 days for rhinovirus colds (97). Greiff et al. assessed the response of the nasal mucosa to coronavirus 229E infection in volunteers (95). Nine of 19 subjects developed colds 4–5 days after inoculation with virus. Men who experienced colds had increased nasal secretion that was characterized by an albumin content consistent with plasma exudation. Patients with colds also demonstrated increased sensitivity to histamine induction of plasma exudation. Thus it was concluded that microvascular exudation and mucosal hyperresponsiveness were hallmarks of the response to coronaviral infection and might also be involved in asthma exacerbation by coronaviruses (95). A different study compared the cytokine profile of nasal secretions in 229E-infected volunteers with control patients with allergic rhinitis subjected to allergen challenge (AR) (98). The AR patients had increased IL-1b and granulocyte-macrophage colony-stimulating factor (GM-CSF) levels but no increase in IFN-α. In contrast, the inoculated patients who developed colds had increased IL-1b and increased IFN-α. The levels of IFN-α correlated with symptoms scores and nasal secretion. This pattern of response was most consistent with a TH1 subset response. The source of the cytokines was not identified.

The role of antibodies in protection from infection or modification of illness is also not completely understood. In a volunteer study designed to look at prophylactic recombinant interferon, it was noted that preexisting antibody titers of >1:32 did not prevent infection or illness in subjects but did lessen the probability of seroconversion during infection (99). A study by Callow more completely assessed antibody response, symptomatology, and viral excretion in order to define factors important in coronaviral infection, development of colds, and recovery from infection (100). Volunteers were inoculated intranasally with human CV (HCV) 229E. Some of the volunteers had preexisting mucosal IgA and circulating IgG against 229E. In this study, the presence of antibody was associated with decreased infection after experimental inoculation, but even high titers were not entirely protective from infection in all subjects. Similar to the study by Turner et al., the presence of high-titer antibodies did correlate with decreased severity of infection. Total nasal protein and specific local IgA following inoculation correlated more strongly with protection from infection with 229E and with decreased severity of illness than did circulating IgG or neutralizing antibody. A subsequent study by the same group involved longitudinal follow-up of a panel of participants for a year and experimental reinoculation after 1 year to assess protection from reinfection (101). It was noted that acute and transient decreases in circulating lymphocytes occurred in infected individuals compared with those who did not become infected. The noninfected volunteers also had immediate significant increases in local nasal antibodies compared with infected persons whose local and circulating antibody responses were delayed then slowly declined over a 3-month period. A year later all of the originally uninfected volunteers became infected after reinoculation, whereas those who were infected in the original inoculation had variable rates of infection and uniformly less symptomatic illness. Thus it appeared that some protection is provided by preexisting antibody, but it is not complete, wanes over time, and leaves persons vulnerable to reinfection after a variable period.

Thus results of experimental infections in volunteers suggest that susceptibility to infection and clinical illness, severity of illness, and recovery are influenced by strain variants (102), length of time since a previous upper respiratory infection (100), and the presence of specific antibodies.

C. Epidemiology

The incidence and severity of disease caused by the two main groups of HCV, 229E and OC43 has probably been underestimated in the past owing to difficulty in diagnosis. However, in spite of these challenges, coronaviruses have been identified wherever they have been looked for, including North and South America, Europe, and Asia (103–106). Most of the surveys performed used serological assays based on ELISA and immunofluorescence. Children begin to acquire antibodies to both 229E-like strains and OC43-like strains at an early age and prevalence of antibodies increases rapidly. By adulthood, between 85 and 100% of adults will have antibodies to both OC43 and 229E (104,107). Wide variance has been found in the incidence of respiratory infections caused by 229E and OC43. Both viruses have been reported to have a late fall to early spring peak, with well-defined peaks of activity; however, one study of adults in London reported most seroconversions during the summer, with two peaks from June to September and again from December to February (108). HCV 229E has been suggested to cause outbreaks on an every-other-year basis, and OC43 with some periodicity but less regularity (4). However, Macnaughton et al. suggested a frequency of HCV infection of 1 per 7.8 months per person. Carefully done studies in adults (103) and children (91, 109) indicate that HCV accounts for 18–35% of respiratory infections that have a definite diagnosis (between 50 and 70%). Studies using hemagglutination inhibition (HAI) and CF assays have found 229E to have a higher incidence than OC43. A study by McGill et al. used ELISA to OC43 in a population of patients with chronic obstructive pulmonary disease and found an overall incidence of 4.4% (110). A 3-year study of military recruits found 52% of 75 men hospitalized for serious respiratory illness had seroconversion to OC43 (92).

Coronaviruses appear to be likely to cause respiratory infections at extremes of age as well as in patients predisposed to illness such as those with COPD and military recruits. A prospective study of 40 premature infants followed for respiratory illness described clinical presentations with coronaviral infections that were typical for lower respiratory infection with other pathogens (111). At the other end of the age spectrum, coronaviruses may contribute to acute illness and pulmonary complications in long-term care facilities (112,113). A study by Falsey et al. in a day-care center for older persons concluded that coronaviral infection was an equally important cause of acute respiratory illness as respiratory syncytial virus (RSV) and influenza (114). Coronavirus 229E readily cocirculated with RSV and influenza in this environment and was just as likely to cause serious illness requiring hospitalization as the other agents. In this setting, the clinical illnesses associated with 229E, RSV, and influenza could not be discerned by symptoms or examination.

As diagnostic tests evolve, it is likely that we will discover that CV play a larger role in respiratory infections than previously predicted. Certainly, important questions remain to be addressed: How do CV with only two identified major types (OC43 and 229E) continue to infect people, likely on a regular basis, throughout life? It is known that coronaviruses have high levels both of polymerase error and mutation during replication, and also undergo significant copy-choice homologous recombination; it may be that rapid selection of variants accounts for escape from homotypic immunity. One study by Reed indicates that this may be the case in isolates from volunteer studies over a 2-year period (102).

D. Clinical Presentation

Clinical illness associated with human coronaviral infection is most typically an upper respiratory infection. Symptoms of pharyngitis, rhinorrhea, headache, malaise, and cough are common. A recent study (97) confirmed the results of previous studies in that the etiology of viral upper respiratory cannot be determined based on severity of colds or other clinical findings. It also confirmed that colds caused by coronaviruses have a longer mean incubation period prior to illness compared with rhinoviruses.

Lower respiratory tract infection may be more common with coronaviral infection than with rhinoviruses. Infections in young infants may be more common than previously thought. Nosocomial infection of premature neonates and young infants suggests that coronaviruses may act in a fashion similar to respiratory syncytial virus and cause first infections at a young age (111). Of 13 specimens from the premature infants that were positive for viruses, 10 were positive for coronaviruses. The children could not be differentiated based on clinical presentation or management. Findings in confirmed coronaviral infections included bradycardia, apnea, hypoxemia, fever, and abdominal distention. Diffuse pulmonary infiltrates were seen in two cases.

Coronaviral respiratory infection has been associated with symptoms of asthma in both children and adults. A longitudinal study of children with recurrent upper and lower respiratory infections (index) and their siblings (control) demonstrated that in the children who were diagnosed with coronaviral infections, the index patients were more likely (8 of 33) to have wheezing than their control siblings (0 of 15) (91). It was not determined if this wheezing was from lower respiratory tract infection. In a study designed to determine the relationship of viral infections to asthma episodes, it was concluded that viral upper respiratory infections are associated with 80–85% of asthma exacerbations in school-age children. Coronaviruses (OC43 and 229E) were identified in 16% of the viral infections compared with 35% caused by rhinoviruses (115). A study of adults with asthma yielded surprisingly similar results, with 80% of episodes of asthma being associated with colds and with rhinoviruses and coronaviruses emerging as the two most frequently identified viral infections (49).

E. Diagnosis

It has been difficult to determine the true incidence of respiratory and other infections caused by human coronaviruses, because diagnostic methods have in the past been slow, insensitive, or both. Primarily, diagnosis has relied on evidence of seroconversion in paired serum samples (49,109,110). However, many infections that occur in the setting of preexisting antibody may not result in seroconversion (101). Culture of clinical specimens has been difficult for 229E and especially for OC43, resulting in a large number of false negative diagnoses. Other diagnostic methods, such as RNA-RNA hybridization, Western blot, and RT-PCR have only been recently attempted and only in isolated cases (116,117,118). In one study of adult and pediatric sera, Western blot using recombinant expressed coronaviral nucleocapsid (N) and/or spike (S) protein was more sensitive (55%) than immunofluorescence (16%) in a pediatric population (117). Direct RNA hybridization using nasal secretions from volunteers suggested that this method might be adaptable for screening for 229E (119). Although the numbers were too small for statistical evaluation, RNA hybridization results matched the results of viral culture for detecting viral shedding. RT-PCR was used in one large clinical study of viral infections and asthma, and it detected a number of infections not identified by culture or serology (115).

F. Treatment

There have been few trials of specific antiviral agents or of nonspecific agents against coronaviruses, most likely because of the challenges of tracking viral titers during natural or experimental infections. Interferons have been most investigated because of their known effects in the prophylaxis of rhinoviral colds. Both IFN-α2b and IFN-β serine inhibit 229E replication more than 90% in plaque reduction assays (120) but appeared to be ineffective in the prophylaxis of natural colds (121). Higgins et al. reported that administration of intranasal IFN-α before and after experimental coronaviral inoculation resulted in decreased incidence of infection, as well as decreased severity of colds and decreased viral shedding in those who did become infected (122). Another study using recombinant IFN of unknown type reported that intranasal treatment starting 1 week before inoculation and continuing for 1 week after inoculation did not reduce the incidence of infection, but the duration and severity of colds experienced by volunteers was lessened (99).

Specific antiviral agents have not been tested against coronaviruses in natural or experimentally induced colds. However, several proteinase inhibitors with low toxicity, including leupeptin, cystatin C, and E64, have been shown to inhibit coronaviral replication in cyto (89,123,124). As more is discovered concerning the molecular biology of coronaviral replication, it is likely that new agents will be identified that specifically inhibit viral functions. Because coronaviruses cause a significant number of human infections and likely on a recurring basis, they remain attractive targets for development of antiviral agents. There are a limited number of coronaviral strains, and the known coronaviruses have significant conservation of demonstrated or putative functional proteins. Thus animal coronaviruses such as mouse hepatitis virus may be good models for development of antivirals for testing and use in humans.

IV. Summary

Rhinoviruses and coronaviruses are most classically associated with upper respiratory infection. Coronaviruses remain much less definable because of the difficulty in their isolation. However, there is now increasing evidence that both viruses may be triggers for reactive airway disease. The implications of this for future research on asthma and its potential control are significant.

References

1. Tyrrell DA. A view from the Common Cold Unit. Antiviral Res 1992; 18:105–125.
2. Couch RB. Rhinoviruses. In: Fields BN, Knipe DM, Howley PM, Chanock RM, Monath TP, Melnick JL, Roizman B, eds. Fields Virology. 3rd ed. Philadelphia: Lippincott-Raven, 1996:713–734.
3. Holmes KV, Lai MMC. Coronaviridae: the viruses and their replication. In: Fields BN, Knipe DM, Howley PM, Chanock RM, Monath TP, Melnick JL, Roizman B, eds. Fields Virology. 3rd ed. Philadelphia: Lippincott-Raven, 1996:1075–1093.
4. McIntosh K. Coronaviruses. In: Fields BN, Knipe DM, Howley PM, Chanock RM, Monath TP, Melnick JL, Roizman B, eds. Fields Virology. 3rd ed. Philadelphia: Lippincott-Raven, 1996:1095–1103.
5. Reuckert RR. Picornaviridae: the viruses and their replication. In: Fields BN, Knipe DM, Howley PM, Chanock RM, Monath TP, Melnick JL, Roizman B, eds. Fields Virology. 3rd ed. Philadelphia: Lippincott-Raven, 1996:609–654.
6. Callahan PL, Mizutani S, Colonno RJ. Molecular cloning and complete sequence determination of RNA genome of human rhinovirus type 14. Proc Natl Acad Sci USA 1985; 82:732–736.
7. Mizutani S, Colonno RJ. In vitro synthesis of an infectious RNA from cDNA clones of human rhinovirus type 14. J Virol 1985; 56:628–632.

8. Staunton DE, Merluzzi VJ, Rothlein R, Barton R, Marlin SD, Springer TA. A cell adhesion molecule, ICAM-1, is the major surface receptor for rhinoviruses. Cell 1989; 56:849–853.
9. Hofer F, Gruenberger M, Kowalski H, Machat H, Huettinger M, Kuechler E, Blass D. Members of the low density lipoprotein receptor family mediate cell entry of a minor-group common cold virus. Proc Natl Acad Sci USA 1994; 91:1839–1842.
10. Zhu Z, Tang W, Ray A, Wu Y, Einarsson O, Landry ML, Gwaltney JJ, Elias JA. Rhinovirus stimulation of interleukin-6 in vivo and in vitro. Evidence for nuclear factor kappa B-dependent transcriptional activation. J Clin Invest 1996; 97:421–430.
11. Rossmann MG, Arnold E, Erickson JW, Frankenberger EA, Griffith JP, Hecht HH, Johnson JE, Kamer G, Luo M, Mosser AG, et al. Structure of a human common cold virus and functional relationship to other picornaviruses. Nature 1985; 317:145–153.
12. Rossmann MG, McKinlay MA. Application of crystallography to the design of antiviral agents. Infect Agents Dis 1992; 1:3–10.
13. Skern T, Sommergruber W, Blaas D, Gruendler P, Fraundorfer F, Pieler C, Fogy I, Kuechler E. Human rhinovirus 2: complete nucleotide sequence and proteolytic processing signals in the capsid protein region. Nucleic Acids Res 1985; 13:2111–2126.
14. Stanway G, Hughes PJ, Mountford RC, Minor PD, Almond JW. The complete nucleotide sequence of a common cold virus: human rhinovirus 14. Nucleic Acids Res 1984; 12:7859–7875.
15. Lamphear BJ, Kirchweger R, Skern T, Rhoads RE. Mapping of functional domains in eukaryotic protein synthesis initiation factor 4G (eIF4G) with picornaviral proteases. Implications for cap-dependent and cap-independent translational initiation. J Biol Chem 1995; 270:21975–21983.
16. Haghighat A, Svitkin Y, Novoa I, Kuechler E, Skern T, Sonenberg N. The eIF4G-eIF4E complex is the target for direct cleavage by the rhinovirus 2A proteinase. J Virol 1996; 70:8444–8450.
17. Matthews DA, Smith WW, Ferre RA, Condon B, Budahazi G, Sisson W, Villafranca JE, Janson CA, McElroy HE, Gribskov CL, et al. Structure of human rhinovirus 3C protease reveals a trypsin-like polypeptide fold, RNA-binding site, and means for cleaving precursor polyprotein. Cell 1994; 77:761–771.
18. Gwaltney JM Jr, Hendley JO. Rhinovirus transmission: one if by air, two if by hand. Am J Epidemiol 1978; 107:357–361.
19. Gwaltney JM Jr, Moskalski PB, Hendley JO. Hand-to-hand transmission of rhinovirus colds. Ann Intern Med 1978; 88:463–467.
20. Gwaltney JM Jr, Hendley JO. Transmission of experimental rhinovirus infection by contaminated surfaces. Am J Epidemiol 1982; 116:828–833.
21. Dick EC, Hossain SU, Mink KA, Meschievitz CK, Schultz SB, Raynor WJ, Inhorn SL. Interruption of transmission of rhinovirus colds among human volunteers using virucidal paper handkerchiefs. J Infect Dis 1986; 153:352–356.
22. Dick EC, Jennings LC, Mink KA, Wartgow CD, Inhorn SL. Aerosol transmission of rhinovirus colds. J Infect Dis 1987; 156:442–448.
23. Meschievitz CK, Schultz SB, Dick EC. A model for obtaining predictable natural transmission of rhinoviruses in human volunteers. J Infect Dis 1984; 150:195–201.

24. D'Alessio DJ, Meschievitz CK, Peterson JA, Dick CR, Dick EC. Short-duration exposure and the transmission of rhinoviral colds. J Infect Dis 1984; 150:189–194.
25. Winther B, Gwaltney JM Jr, Mygind N, Turner RB, Hendley JO. Sites of rhinovirus recovery after point inoculation of the upper airway. JAMA 1986; 256:1763–1767.
26. Winther B. Effects on the nasal mucosa of upper respiratory viruses (common cold). Dan Med Bull 1994; 41:193–204.
27. Urquhart GE, Grist NR. Virological studies of sudden, unexplained infant deaths in Glasgow 1967–70. J Clin Pathol 1972; 25:443–446.
28. Gwaltney JM Jr. Rhinovirus infection of the normal human airway. Am J Respir Crit Care Med 1995; 152:S36–S39.
29. Winther B, Gwaltney JM, Hendley JO. Respiratory virus infection of monolayer cultures of human nasal epithelial cells. Am Rev Respir Dis 1990; 14:839–845.
30. Arruda E, Boyle TR, Winther B, Pevear DC, Gwaltney JM Jr, Hayden FG. Localization of human rhinovirus replication in the upper respiratory tract by in situ hybridization. J Infect Dis 1995; 171:1329–1333.
31. Turner RB, Hendley JO, Gwaltney JM Jr. Shedding of infected ciliated epithelial cells in rhinovirus colds. J Infect Dis 1982; 145:849–853.
32. Gwaltney JM Jr, Phillips CD, Miller RD, Riker DK. Computed tomographic study of the common cold. N Engl J Med 1994; 330:25–30.
33. Fox JP, Cooney MK, Hall CE. The Seattle virus watch. V. Epidemiologic observations of rhinovirus infections, 1965–1969, in families with young children. Am J Epidemiol 1975; 101:122–143.
34. Douglas RGJ, Cate TR, Gerone JP, Couch RB. Quantitative rhinovirus shedding patterns in volunteers. Am Rev Respir Dis 1966; 94:159–167.
35. Winther B, Farr B, Turner RB, Hendley JO, Gwaltney JM Jr, Mygind N. Histopathologic examination and enumeration of polymorphonuclear leukocytes in the nasal mucosa during experimental rhinovirus colds. Acta Otolaryngol Suppl (Stockh) 1984; 413:19–24.
36. Turner RB. The role of neutrophils in the pathogenesis of rhinovirus infections. Pediatr Infect Dis J 1990; 9:832–835.
37. Fraenkel DJ, Bardin PG, Sanderson G, Lampe F, Johnston SL, Holgate ST. Immunohistochemical analysis of nasal biopsies during rhinovirus experimental colds. Am J Respir Crit Care Med 1994; 150:1130–1136.
38. Naclerio RM, Proud D, Lichtenstein LM, Kagey SA, Hendley JO, Sorrentino J, Gwaltney JM Jr. Kinins are generated during experimental rhinovirus colds. J Infect Dis 1988; 157:133–142.
39. Proud D, Naclerio RM, Gwaltney JM Jr, Hendley JO. Kinins are generated in nasal secretions during natural rhinovirus colds. J Infect Dis 1990; 161:120–123.
40. Proud D, Reynolds CJ, Lacapra S, Kagey-Sobotka A, Lichtenstein LM, Naclerio RM. Nasal provocation with bradykinin induces symptoms of rhinitis and a sore throat. Am Rev Respir Dis 1988; 137:613–616.
41. Proud D, Gwaltney JM Jr, Hendley JO, Dinarello CA, Gillis S, Schleimer RP. Increased levels of interleukin-1 are detected in nasal secretions of volunteers during experimental rhinovirus colds. J Infect Dis 1994; 169:1007–1013.
42. Farr BM, Gwaltney JM Jr, Hendley JO, Hayden FG, Naclerio RM, McBride T, Doyle WJ, Sorrentino JV, Riker DK, Proud D. A randomized controlled trial of

glucocorticoid prophylaxis against experimental rhinovirus infection. J Infect Dis 1990; 162:1173–1177.
43. Teran LM, Johnston SL, Shute JK, Church MK, Holgate ST. Increased levels of interleukin-8 in the nasal aspirates of children with virus-associated asthma. J Allergy Clin Immunol 1994; 93:272.
44. Johnston SL. Natural and experimental rhinovirus infections of the lower respiratory tract. Am J Respir Crit Care Med 1995; 152(suppl):46–52.
45. Levandowski RA, Pachucki CT, Rubenis M. Specific mononuclear cell response to rhinovirus. J Infect Dis 1983; 148:1125.
46. Lavandowski RA, Ou DW, Jackson GG. Acute-phase decrease of T lymphocyte subsets in rhinovirus infection. J Infect Dis 1986; 153:743–748.
47. Hsia J, Goldstein AL, Simon GL, Sztein M, Hayden FG. Peripheral blood mononuclear cell interleukin-2 and interferon-gamma production, cytotoxicity, and antigen-stimulated blastogenesis during experimental rhinovirus infection. J Infect Dis 1990; 162:591–597.
48. Gern JE, Vrtis R, Kelly EA, Dick EC, Busse WW. Rhinovirus produces nonspecific activation of lymphocytes through a monocyte-dependent mechanism. J Immunol 1996; 157:1605–1612.
49. Nicholson KG, Kent J, Ireland DC. Respiratory viruses and exacerbations of asthma in adults. Br Med J 1993; 307:982–986.
50. Horn ME, Brain EA, Gregg I, Inglis JM, Yealland SJ, Taylor P. Respiratory viral infection and wheezy bronchitis in childhood. Thorax 1979; 34:23–28.
51. Halperin SA, Eggleston PA, Beasley P, Suratt P, Hendley JO, Groschel DH, Gwaltney JM Jr. Exacerbations of asthma in adults during experimental rhinovirus infection. Am Rev Respir Dis 1985; 132:976–980.
52. Kellner G, Popow KT, Kundi M, Binder C, Kunz C. Clinical manifestations of respiratory tract infections due to respiratory syncytial virus and rhinoviruses in hospitalized children. Acta Paediatr Scand 1989; 78:390–394.
53. Krilov L, Pierik L, Keller E, Mahan K, Watson D, Hirsch M, Hamparian V, McIntosh K. The association of rhinoviruses with lower respiratory tract disease in hospitalized patients. J Med Virol 1986; 19:345–352.
54. McMillan JA, Weiner LB, Higgins AM, Macknight K. Rhinovirus infection associated with serious illness among pediatric patients. Pediatr Infect Dis J 1993; 12:321–325.
55. Gern JE, Dick EC, Lee WM, Murray S, Meyer K, Handzel ZT, Busse WW. Rhinovirus enters but does not replicate inside monocytes and airway macrophages. J Immunol 1996; 156:621–627.
56. Bardin PG, Fraenkel DJ, Sanderson G, Dorward M, Lau LC, Johnston SL, Holgate ST. Amplified rhinovirus colds in atopic subjects. Clin Exp Allergy 1994; 24:457–464.
57. Doyle WJ, Skoner DP, Fireman P, Seroky JT, Green I, Ruben F, Kardatzke DR, Gwaltney JM Jr. Rhinovirus 39 infection in allergic and nonallergic subjects. J Allergy Clin Immunol 1992; 89:968–978.
58. Calhoun WJ, Dick EC, Schwartz LB, Busse WW. A common cold virus, rhinovirus 16, potentiates airway inflammation after segmental antigen bronchoprovocation in allergic subjects. J Clin Invest 1994; 94:2200–2208.

59. Brown PK, Taylor-Robinson D. Respiratory virus antibodies in sera of persons living in isolated communities. Bull WHO 1966; 34:895–900.
60. Hamre D. Rhinoviruses. Mongr Virol 1967; 1:1–85.
61. Fox JP, Cooney MK, Hall CE, Foy HM. Rhinoviruses in Seattle families, 1975–1979. Am J Epidemiol 1985; 122:830–846.
62. Cohen S, Tyrrell DA, Smith AP. Psychological stress and susceptibility to the common cold. N Engl J Med 1991; 325:606–612.
63. Stone AA, Bovbjerg DH, Neale JM, Napoli A, Valdimarsdottir H, Cox D, Hayden FG, Gwaltney JJ. Development of common cold symptoms following experimental rhinovirus infection is related to prior stressful life events. Behav Med 1992; 18:115–120.
64. Douglas RG Jr, Lindgren KM, Couch RB. Exposure to cold environment and rhinovirus common cold. Failure to demonstrate effect. N Engl J Med 1968; 279:742–747.
65. Dearden C, Al NW, Andries K, Woestenborghs R, Tyrrell DA. Drug resistant rhinoviruses from the nose of experimentally treated volunteers. Arch Virol 1989; 109:71–81.
66. Hayden FG, Gwaltney JM Jr. Intranasal interferon-alpha 2 treatment of experimental rhinoviral colds. J Infect Dis 1984; 150:174–180.
67. Samo TC, Greenberg SB, Palmer JM, Couch RB, Harmon MW, Johnson PE. Intranasally applied recombinant leukocyte A interferon in normal volunteers. II. Determination of minimal effective and tolerable dose. J Infect Dis 1984; 150:181–188.
68. Hayden FG, Albrecht JK, Kaiser DL, Gwaltney JM Jr. Prevention of natural colds by contact prophylaxis with intranasal alpha 2-interferon. N Engl J Med 1986; 314:71–75.
69. Sperber SJ, Doyle WJ, McBride TP, Sorrentino JV, Riker DK, Hayden FG. Otologic effects of interferon beta serine in esperimental rhinovirus colds. Arch Otolaryngol Head Neck Surg 1992; 118:933–936.
70. Colonno RJ, Callahan PL, Long WJ. Isolation of a monoclonal antibody that blocks attachment of the major group of human rhinoviruses. J Virol 1986; 57:7–12.
71. Sperber SJ, Hayden FG. Protective effect of rhinovirus receptor blocking antibody in human fibroblast cells. Antiviral Res 1989; 12:231–238.
72. Hayden FG, Gwaltney JM Jr, Colonno RJ. Modification of experimental rhinovirus colds by receptor blockade. Antiviral Res 1988; 9:233–247.
73. Marlin SD, Staunton DE, Springer TA, Stratowa C, Sommergruber W, Merluzzi VJ. A soluble form of intercellular adhesion molecule-1 inhibits rhinovirus infection. Nature 1990; 344:70–72.
74. Greve JM, Forte CP, Marlor CW, Meyer AM, Hoover LH, Wunderlich D, McClelland A. Mechanisms of receptor-meidated rhinovirus neutralization defined by two soluble forms of ICAM-1. J Virol 1991; 65:6015–6023.
75. Hendley JO, Abbott RD, Beasley PP, Gwaltney JM Jr. Effect of inhalation of hot humidified air on experimental rhinovirus infection. JAMA 1994; 271:1112–1113.

76. Farr BM, Conner EM, Betts RF, Oleske J, Minnefor A, Gwaltney JM Jr. Two randomized controlled trials of zinc gluconate lozenge therapy of experimentally induced rhinovirus colds. Antimicrobial Agents Chemother 1987; 31:1183–1187.
77. Gustafson LM, Proud D, Hendley JO, Hayden FG, Gwaltney JM Jr. Oral prednisone therapy in experimental rhinovirus infections. J Allergy Clin Immunol 1996; 97: 1009–1014.
78. Herold J, Raabe T, Schelle PB, Siddell SG. Nucleotide sequence of the human coronavirus 229E RNA polymerase locus. Virology 1993; 195:680–691.
79. Lee H-J, Shieh C-K, Gorbalenya AE, Koonin EV, LaMonica N, Tuler J, Bagdzhadhzyan A, Lai MMC. The complete sequence (22 kilobases) of murine coronavirus gene 1 encoding the putative proteases and RNA polymerase. Virology 1991; 180: 567–582.
80. Yeager CL, Ashmun RA, Williams RK, Cardellichio CB, Shapiro LH, Look AT, Holmes KV. Human aminopeptidase N is a receptor for human coronavirus 229E. Nature 1992; 357:420–422.
81. Levis R, Cardellichio CB, Scanga CA, Compton SR, Holmes KV. Multiple receptor-dependent steps determine the species specificity of HCV-229E infection. Adv Exp Med Biol 1995; 380:337–343.
82. Kolb AF, Maile J, Heister A, Siddell SG. Characterization of functional domains in the human coronavirus HCV 229E receptor. J Gen Virol 1996; 77:2515–2521.
83. Tresnan DB, Levis R, Holmes KV. Feline aminopeptidase N serves as a receptor for feline, canine, porcine, and human coronaviruses in serogroup I. J Virol 1996; 70:8669–8674.
84. Denison MR, Perlman S. Translation and processing of mouse hepatitis virus virion RNA in a cell-free system. J Virol 1986; 60:12–18.
85. Denison MR, Zoltick PW, Hughes SA, Giangreco B, Olson AL, Perlman S, Leibowitz JL, Weiss SR. Intracellular processing of the N-terminal ORF 1a proteins of the coronavirus MHV-A59 requires multiple proteolytic events. Virology 1992; 189:274–284.
86. Gorbalenya A, Koonin E. Comparative analysis of amino-acid sequences of key enzymes of replication and expression of positive-strand RNA viruses: validity of approach and functional and evolutionary implications. Sov Sci Rev D Physiochem Biol 1993; 11:1–81.
87. Lu Y, Lu X, Denison MR. Identification and characterization of a serine-like proteinase of the murine coronavirus MHV-A59. J Virol 1995; 69:3554–3559.
88. Ziebuhr J, Herold J, Siddell SG. Characterization of a human coronavirus (strain 229E) 3C-like proteinase activity. J Virol 1995; 69:4331–4338.
89. Kim JC, Spence RA, Currier PF, Lu X, Denison MR. Coronavirus protein processing and RNA synthesis is inhibited by the cysteine proteinase inhibitor, E64d. Virology 1995; 208:1–8.
90. Lai MMC. Coronavirus: organization, replication, and expression of genome. Annu Rev Microbiol 1990; 44:303–333.
91. Isaacs D. Flowers D, Clarke JR, Valman HB, MacNaughton MR. Epidemiology of coronavirus respiratory infections. Arch Dis Child 1983; 58:500–503.
92. Wenzel RP, Hendley JO, Davies JA, Gwaltney JM Jr. Coronavirus infections in military recruits. Three-year study with coronavirus strains OC43 and 229E. Am Rev Respir Dis 1974; 109:621–624.

93. Ijaz MK, Brunner AH, Sattar SA, Nair RC, Johnson-Lussenburg CM. Survival characteristics of airborne human coronavirus 229E. J Gen Virol 1985; 66:2743–2748.
94. Callow KA, Tyrrell DA, Shaw RJ, Fitzharris P, Wardlaw AJ, Kay AB. Influence of atopy on the clinical manifestations of coronavirus infection in adult volunteers. Clin Allergy 1988; 18:119–129.
95. Greiff L, Andersson M, Akerlund A, Wollmer P, Svensson C, Alkner U, Persson CG. Microvascular exudative hyperresponsiveness in human coronavirus-induced common cold. Thorax 1994; 49:121–127.
96. Patterson S, Macnaughton MR. Replication of human respiratory coronavirus strain 229E in human macrophages. J Gen Virol 1982; 60:307–314.
97. Tyrrell DA, Cohen S, Schlarb JE. Signs and symptoms in common colds. Epidemiol Infect 1993; 111:143–156.
98. Linden M, Greiff L, Andersson M, Svensson C, Akerlund A, Bende M, Andersson E, Persson CG. Nasal cytokines in common cold and allergic rhinitis. Clin Exp Allergy 1995; 25:166–172.
99. Turner RB, Felton A, Kosak K, Kelsey DK, Meschievitz CK. Prevention of experimental coronavirus colds with intranasal alpha-2b interferon. J Infect Dis 1986; 154:443–447.
100. Callow KA. Effect of specific humoral immunity and some non-specific factors on resistance of volunteers to respiratory coronavirus infection. J Hyg (Lond) 1985; 95:173–189.
101. Callow KA, Parry HF, Sergeant M, Tyrrell DA. The time course of the immune response to experimental coronavirus infection of man. Epidemiol Infect 1990; 105:435–446.
102. Reed SE. The behaviour of recent isolates of human respiratory coronavirus in vitro and in volunteers: evidence of heterogeneity among 229E-related strains. J Med Virol 1984; 13:179–192.
103. Larson HE, Reed SE, Tyrrell DA. Isolation of rhinoviruses and coronaviruses from 38 colds in adults. J Med Virol 1980; 5:221–229.
104. Hasony HJ, Macnaughton MR. Prevalence of human coronavirus antibody in the population of southern Iraq. J Med Virol 1982; 9:209–216.
105. Schmidt OW, Allan ID, Cooney MK, Foy HM, Fox JP. Rises in titers of antibody to human coronaviruses OC43 and 229E in Seattle families during 1975–1979. Am J Epidemiol 1986; 123:862–868.
106. Matsumoto I, Yoshida S, Takahashi K, Kawana R. Virological surveillance of acute respiratory tract illnesses of children in Morioka, Japan. I. Epidemiological patterns of infection with respiratory viruses over a 10-year period. Kansenshogaku Zasshi 1991; 65:423–432.
107. McIntosh K, Kapikian AZ, Turner HC, Hartley JW, Parrott RH, Chanock RM. Seroepidemiologic studies of coronavirus infection in adults and children. Am J Epidemiol 1970; 91:585–592.
108. Macnaughton MR. Occurrence and frequency of coronavirus infections in humans as determined by enzyme-linked immunosorbent assay. Infect Immun 1982; 38:419–423.

109. Macnaughton MR, Flowers D, Isaacs D. Diagnosis of human coronavirus infections in children using enzyme-linked immunosorbent assay. J Med Virol 1983; 11:319–325.
110. Gill EP, Dominguez EA, Greenberg SB, Atmar RL, Hogue BG, Baxter BD, Couch RB. Development and application of an enzyme immunoassay for coronavirus OC43 antibody in acute respiratory illness. J Clin Microbiol 1994; 32:2372–2376.
111. Sizun J, Soupre D, Legrand MC, Giroux JD, Rubio S, Cauvin JM, Chastel C, Alix D, de PL. Neonatal nosocomial respiratory infection with coronavirus: a prospective study in a neonatal intensive care unit. Acta Paediatr 1995; 84:617–620.
112. Nicholson KG, Baker DJ, Farquhar A, Hurd D, Kent J, Smith SH. Acute upper respiratory tract viral illness and influenza immunization in homes for the elderly. Epidemiol Infect 1990; 105:609–618.
113. Falsey AR. Noninfluenza respiratory virus infection in long-term care facilities. Infect Control Hosp Epidemiol 1991; 12:602–608.
114. Falsey AR, McCann RM, Hall WJ, Tanner MA, Criddle MM, Formica MA, Irvine CS, Kolassa JE, Barker WH, Treanor JJ. Acute respiratory tract infection in daycare centers for older persons. J Am Geriatr Soc 1995; 43:30–36.
115. Johnston SL, Pattemore PK, Sanderson G, Smith S, Lampe F, Josephs L, P. S, O'Toole S, Myint SH, Tyrrell DA, Holgate ST. Community study of role of viral infections in exacerbations of asthma in 9–1 year old children. Br Med J 1995; 310:1225–1229.
116. Myint S, Siddell S, Tyrrell D. The use of nucleic acid hybridization to detect human coronaviruses. Arch Virol 1989; 104:335–337.
117. Pohl KA, Raabe T, Siddell SG, ter Meulen V. Detection of human coronavirus 229E-specific antibodies using recombinant fusion proteins. J Virol Methods 1995; 55: 175–183.
118. Myint S, Johnston S, Sanderson G, Simpson H. Evaluation of nested polymerase chain methods for the detection of human coronaviruses 229E and OC43. Mol Cell Probes 1994; 8:357–364.
119. Myint S, Siddell S, Tyrrell D. Detection of human coronavirus 229E in nasal washings using RNA:RNA hybridisation. J Med Virol 1989; 29:70–73.
120. Sperber SJ, Hayden FG. Comparative susceptibility of respiratory viruses to recombinant interferons-alpha 2b and -beta. J Interferon Res 1989; 9:285–293.
121. Sperber SJ, Levine PA, Sorrentino JV, Riker DK, Hayden FG. Ineffectiveness of recombinant interferon-beta serine nasal drops for prophylaxis of natural colds. J Infect Dis 1989; 160:700–705.
122. Higgins PG, Phillpotts RJ, Scott GM, Wallace J, Bernhardt LL, Tyrrell DA. Intranasal interferon as protection against experimental respiratory coronavirus infection in volunteers. Antimicrob Agents Chemother 1983; 24:713–715.
123. Appleyard G, Tisdale M. Inhibition of the growth of human coronavirus 229E by leupeptin. J Gen Virol 1985; 66:363–366.
124. Collins AR, Grubb A. Inhibitory effects of recombinant human cystatin C on human coronaviruses. Antimicrob Agents Chemother 1991; 35:2444–2446.

11

Hantaviruses

STEPHEN Q. SIMPSON
University of Kansas Medical Center
Kansas City, Kansas

HOWARD LEVY
University of New Mexico Health Sciences Center
Albuquerque, New Mexico

I. Introduction

Hantavirus pulmonary syndrome (HPS) is a systemic disease that is caused by a newly discovered and characterized virus of the *Hantavirus* genus in the *Bunyaviridae* family. The recognition of this syndrome in 1993 by physicians in the Four Corners area of the southwestern United States, the boundary common to the states of New Mexico, Arizona, Utah, and Colorado, led to the discovery of a previously unrecognized virus. The virus has not been officially named by the International Committee on Taxonomy of Viruses. It has been called Four Corners virus (FCV), Muerto Canyon virus, and Convict Creek virus, but it is most frequently referred to as the sin nombre virus (SNV). Until the recognition of HPS and SNV, no indigenous hantaviruses were known to cause human disease in North America. The clinical syndrome induced by SNV infection resembles other hantaviral syndromes except that it principally affects the cardiac and pulmonary systems rather than primarily causing hemorrhagic fever and renal dysfunction. In addition, SNV is more lethal than any previously recognized hantaviral infection. This chapter discusses the characteristics of hantaviruses with emphasis on the unique characteristics of HPS.

Table 1 The Hantaviruses

Virus	Host rodent (species)	Geographical range of host	Syndrome in humans	Mortality rate	Reference
Hantaan	Striped field mouse (*Apodemus agrarius*)	Central Asia, China, Korea, southern Siberia, Europe	HFRS	5%	—
Seoul	Norway (common) rat (*Rattus norvegicus*)	Urban-worldwide	HFRS	1–2%	—
Puumala	Bank vole (*Clethrionomys glareolus*)	Russia, northern Europe, Asia Minor, Korea	Nephropathia epidemica	0.1–1.0%	—
Dobrava/ Belgrade	Yellow-necked field mouse (*Apodemus falvicollis*)	Europe, Balkans	HFRS	15%	—
Thailand	Bandicoot rat (*Bandicota indicia*)	Southeastern China, India, northern Malay Peninsula	None known	—	—
Thottopalayam	Shrew (*Suncus murinus*)	India	None known	—	—
Tobetsu	Grey sided vole (*Clethrionomys rubocanus*)	Hokkaido, Japan	Preliminary information only	—	4
Tula	European common vole (*Microtus arvalis*)	Russia, Asia, Europe	None known	—	—
Khabarovsk	Reed vole (*Microtus fortis*)	East Russia	None known	—	—
Topografov	Lemming (*Lemmus sibericus*)	Siberia	None known	—	5

Virus	Rodent host	Geographic distribution	Disease	Mortality	Ref
Sin Nombre/ Muerto Canyon/ Convict Creek/ Four Corners	Deer mouse (*Peromyscus maniculatus*)	Western North America, Mexico, Canada	HPS	50%	6
New York-1/ Shelter Island/ Rhode Island	White-footed mouse (*Peromyscus leucopus*)	Eastern North America, Canada	HPS	1 fatal case	7,44
Black Creek Canal	Cotton rat (*Sigmodon hispidus*)	USA, Venezuela, Peru	HPS with hemorrhage	1 case	8
Muleshoe	Cotton rat (*Sigmodon hispidus*)	West Texas	None known	—	9
Bayou	Rice rat (*Oryzomys palustris*)	Louisiana	HPS with hemorrhage	1 fatal case	10,38
Prospect Hill	Meadow vole (*Microtus pennsylvanicus*)	Eastern North America, Canada	None known	—	—
Bloodland Lake	Prairie vole (*Microtus ochrogaster*)	Southern Canada, Midwestern USA	None known	—	—
Isla Vista	California meadow mouse (*Microtus californicus*)	California, Oregon, Baja California, Mexico	None known	—	11
El Moro Canyon	Western harvest mouse (*Reithrodontomys megalotis*)	Western states of USA, Central Mexico, Canada	None known	—	12
Rio Segundo	Mexican harvest mouse (*Reithrodontomys mexicanus*)	Mexico, Costa Rica, South America	None known	—	—
Delgadito	*Sigmodon alstoni*	Venezuela	None known	—	—
Rio Mamoré	*Oligoryzomys microtis*	Bolivia	None known	—	13
Andes	*Oligoryzomys longicaudatis*	Argentina, Chile	HPS	70%	14

The hantaviruses constitute a genus of enveloped, negative sense RNA viruses belonging to the family *Bunyaviridae* (Table 1) (1–3). California encephalitis was the only bunyavirus-induced disease in North America prior to the HPS outbreak, although this family of viruses causes hemorrhagic fevers throughout the world. Early in the investigation of the initial HPS outbreak, researchers at the University of New Mexico and the Centers for Disease Control and Prevention (CDC) were able to clone large segments of the SNV genome by using consensus oligonucleotide sequences (genome sequences that are common to multiple species) from other hantaviral species as amplimers for reverse transcription–polymerase chain reaction (RT-PCR) (15–17). The amplified DNA sequences were cloned in *Escherichia coli* and nucleotide sequence analysis of these cloned segments confirmed that this virus was indeed a novel hantavirus that was most closely related to Prospect Hill and Puumala viruses (18).

Forty-eight cases of HPS were reported in the United States during 1993, with an overall case fatality rate of 56%, the majority of which occurred in the region known as the Four Corners area. As of August 7, 1996, 143 cases have been identified in 25 states in the United States with a mortality of 50%, and additional cases have been found in Canada and South America.

II. Viral Replication

HPS is caused by tripartite, negative-sense RNA-enveloped hantavirus members of the family *Bunyaviridae*. There is some variation in the morphology of bunyaviruses, but most are spherical, 80–120 nm in diameter, and have a lipid bilayer envelope with glycoprotein projections (Fig. 1) (19). The viral genome is encased within a nucleocapsid protein shell and consists of three segments: the S, or small, segment which codes for the nucleocapsid protein (N protein); the M, or medium, segment which codes for the viral envelope glycoproteins (two proteins: G1 and G2); and the L, or large, segment which codes for viral transcriptase and possibly other proteins. The envelope glycoproteins may mediate attachment of the virus to mammalian cell surface receptors.

The replication strategy of the SNV has not been reported and must be inferred from the replication strategies of other hantaviruses, specifically Hantaan virus, and of other bunyaviruses. Viral replication begins with host cell attachment and entry. The envelope glycoproteins G1 and G2 mediate attachment, presumably by interaction with host cell receptors, although the specific receptors have not been isolated (20). Neutralizing and hemagglutination-inhibiting sites were found on both G1 and G2 of Hantaan virus, suggesting that both proteins are important to cellular attachment (21). Electron microscopy of cells infected with the Rift Valley fever virus (genus *Phlebovirus*)

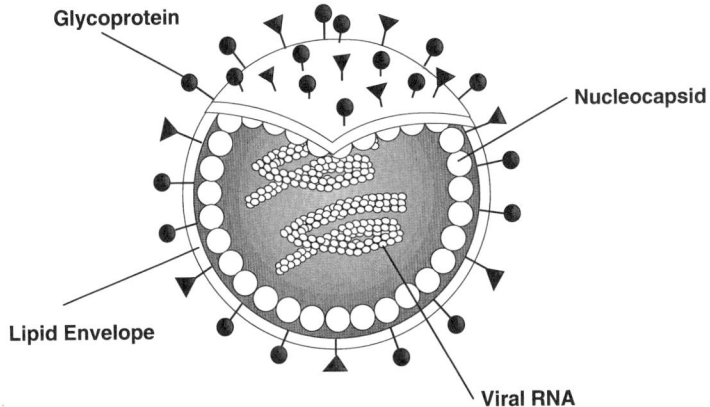

Figure 1 Schematic diagram showing the structure of viruses of the family *Bunyaviridae*. The glycoprotein "spikes" mediate attachment to as yet uncharacterized target cell receptors. Sin Nombre virus conforms to this structural pattern. (Courtesy of Charlotte Hill, *The Albuquerque Tribune*.)

demonstrate viral particles within phagocytic vacuoles (22). This finding suggests a mechanism for cell entry that could involve acidification of vacuoles with subsequent endosomal fusion and release of nucleocapsid/genomic material into the cellular cytoplasm, as has been demonstrated in alphaviruses (23). However, no direct evidence of this mechanism for cell entry has been documented for any member of the *Bunyaviridae*, including the hantaviruses.

All members of the *Bunyaviridae* follow a simple negative-sense scheme for protein synthesis in which complementary mRNA is directly transcribed from the viral genome (20). Transcription of the L segment has not been studied in detail for any of these viruses. For the Hantaan virus, the S segment and the M segment are transcribed in single open reading frames, which encode only N and G1 and G2, respectively (24,25). Some members of the family encode nonstructural proteins in the M segment, the S segment, or both segments, but the function of these proteins has not been determined (20). Certain members of the *Phlebovirus* genus use an ambisense strategy for synthesizing these nonstructural proteins, in which both the virus-sense RNA and the complementary-sense RNA encode proteins (26,27). It is likely that the SNV transcription strategy most closely resembles that of the Hantaan virus. Mechanisms for the switch from protein synthesis to genome replication are not well studied for any of the *Bunyaviridae*.

The envelope proteins of *Bunyaviridae* contain signals that localize budding virions to smooth-surface vesicles in the host cell Golgi area, a distinguishing feature among negative-sense RNA viruses (28,29,30). The predicted amino acid sequences of the Hantaan virus and other *Bunyaviridae* indicate a hydrophobic anchor region in the carboxy-terminal region (31). In contrast, electron microscopy of SNV-infected cells shows that the virions bud predominantly from the plasma membrane (32). Following budding into the Golgi cisternae, virions of other *Bunyaviridae* are thought to be released from the host cell by exocytosis. The mechanism for release of SNV virions has not been reported.

III. Epidemiology

A. Reservoir

Each hantavirus is predominantly associated with a specific rodent reservoir, usually rural field mice, voles, or rats. Unlike other genuses of *Bunyaviridae* which are transmitted to human hosts by arthropod vectors, hantaviruses appear to be spread directly via aerosolization of rodent urine and feces that contain shed viral particles. Ingestion of contaminated food is also a postulated route of transmission.

Since human disease is acquired directly or indirectly from rodents, knowledge of the ecology and biology of these small mammals has great importance in understanding human diseases caused by the *Bunyaviridae*. During the initial rodent infection, the virus disseminates throughout the rodent's body during a several-day period of viremia. After this viremic period, hantaviral antigens are detectable in lungs, kidneys, and other organs, and these tissues appear to remain antigen positive for the duration of the rodent's life. The rodents remain healthy but shed virus in urine, feces, and saliva in spite of developing neutralizing IgM and IgG antibodies.

The primary host for SNV is the deer mouse, *Peromyscus maniculatus*, as was demonstrated by homology of viral sequences from patients and from rodents trapped in and around patient homes. Smaller numbers of ground squirrels, prairie dogs, and pack rats are also infected (33,34). The deer mouse is found in rural locales throughout the continental United States except in areas of the Eastern Seaboard and the Gulf Coast. It is a small (11–20 cm nose to tail) brown rodent with a white underbelly and white paws. It has large ears and a prominently bicolored tail of brown and white. A dramatic increase in the rodent population in the Four Corners area occurred just prior to the initial outbreak of HPS, providing increased human-rodent contact and leading to the initial outbreak and recognition of the disease (34). Genetic linkage analysis suggests that SNV is not a recent variant of the genus but has existed in its present form for many years (18). Since each hantavirus survives in its own, unique rodent reservoir, it is possible that SNV and other recently

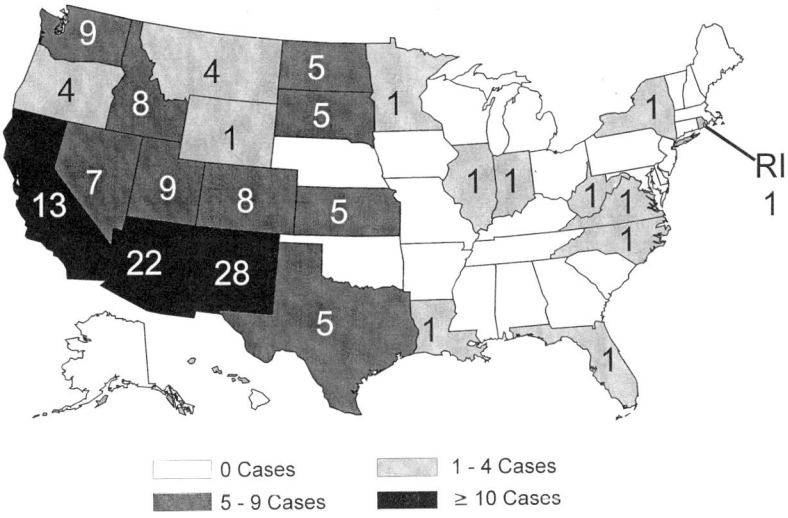

Figure 2 Hantavirus pulmonary syndrome cases by U.S. state of residence as of August 7, 1996. Total cases (n = 143 in 25 states). (Courtesy of the Centers for Disease Control and Prevention, Southwest Field Office, Albuquerque, New Mexico.)

discovered North American hantaviruses coevolved with their respective hosts. Multiple cases of HPS due to SNV infection as long ago as 1959 have been retrospectively diagnosed by high titers of anti-SNV IgG in serum collected since the recognition of the disease in 1993, demonstrating that the disease itself has existed unrecognized for years (35,36).

B. Strain Variation

At this writing, all but five cases of HPS within the United States have occurred within the geographical range of the deer mouse (Fig. 2). These five cases demonstrate that at least three other genetically distinct hantaviruses are capable of causing HPS. A nonfatal case of HPS in south Florida was attributed to Black Creek Canal virus, whose rodent host is the cotton rat, *Sigmodon hispidus* (37). "Bayou virus" caused a fatal case of HPS in Louisiana with the rice rat, *Oryzomys palustris*, as the reservoir (38,39). An SNV-like virus (New York-1) with *Peromyscus leucopus* as the reservoir caused two fatal cases of HPS, one in Rhode Island and the other on Long Island, New York (40,41). Hantaviruses have caused HPS in eastern Texas, Uruguay, and in São Paulo, Brazil; the serologically detected viruses have not been characterized and may be distinct from SNV (37–39,42–44). Some nucleotide sequence variations occur regionally, but amino acid sequences are highly conserved among the genetic variants. Isolates from throughout North America show saturation for synonymous nucleotide substitutions (nucleotide substitutions that do not result in a change in amino acid sequence) but a very low frequency of nonsynonymous substitutions (45).

In 1996, a closely related hantavirus was isolated from the long-tailed rice rat ("colilargo") of Argentina and was named the Andes virus (46). During November of that year, an outbreak of HPS, presumed but not proven to be caused by Andes virus, occurred in the Neuquen region of the Patagonian Andes (47). This outbreak, with a mortality rate of 70%, was characterized by human-to-human transmission of the virus, a finding never before documented for any hantaviral infection (48).

C. Other Factors

HPS has a remarkable predilection for affecting healthy adults; the median age of patients confirmed to have HPS is 35 years, with a range of 11–69 years. Remarkably, preadolescent children have suffered only mild illnesses and have not required mechanical ventilation. The overall case fatality rate stands at 51%. There does not appear to be a seasonal effect for SNV in contrast to hemorrhagic fever with renal syndrome, which is more common in the spring and autumn, but a geographical effect is evident. HPS is contracted in rural locales in parallel with the distribution of the rodent reservoir.

IV. Clinical Manifestations

A. Disease Course

The prototype of the *Hantavirus* genus is the Hantaan virus (49). The Hantaan virus causes a life-threatening illness, hemorrhagic fever with renal syndrome (HFRS). The clinical manifestations of HFRS are classically described in five phases that are germane to this discussion because of their similarity to the clinical phases of HPS. A *febrile* phase is marked by the sudden onset of fevers accompanied by myalgias, malaise, and headache. Within 1–3 days, large amounts of plasma extravasate into the peritoneum and retroperitoneum and lead to intense back and abdominal pain. By the end of the febrile phase, massive proteinuria is present. The second, or *shock*, phase begins abruptly and lasts from several hours to several days. Vascular leakage leads to depletion of blood volume and a rise in hematocrit to as high as 70%. Disseminated intravascular coagulation (DIC) associated with thrombocytopenia is common, and patients die from bleeding. Proteinuria persists and azotemia that eventually leads to *renal failure* begins. Approximately one third of all deaths from the infection occur during this phase of the illness. During the second week of the illness, oliguric renal failure develops (phase 3). Pulmonary edema is common at this point. During the fourth phase, patients have an extremely large-volume *diuresis*. Complete recovery is typical in a prolonged *convalescent* phase. Other hantaviruses cause similar illnesses with varying degress of severity (see Table 1).

The syndrome induced by SNV infection is characterized by four clinical phases: prodrome, pulmonary edema and shock, diuresis, and convalescence. During the initial *prodrome* phase, typically lasting 3–6 days, symptoms are virtually identical to the febrile phase of HFRS (50). The onset of respiratory symptoms and shock is abrupt. Mortality is greatest in the first 24 hr of the *pulmonary edema and shock* phase of the illness, which characteristically lasts 3–6 days. Patients who survive the shock phase enter the diuretic phase of the illness. During this diuretic phase, patients may have urine flow rates of 300–500 mL/hr, and rapid resolution of respiratory and hemodynamic abnormalities. Following *diuresis* and extubation, patients enter the *convalescent* phase of the illness, which may last as long as 6 months.

These phases of HPS are strikingly similar to the clinical phases of HFRS except that vascular permeability is largely limited to the pulmonary capillaries in HPS rather than peritoneal and renal capillaries. Additionally, HPS has not been associated with renal failure or severe DIC. Currently, there are no known cases of asymptomatic SNV infection or of SNV infection that does not cause pulmonary edema, although such infections may exist.

Early diagnosis of HPS is often difficult, because the most common signs and symptoms are the same as those of other viral prodromes (50,51). Nearly all patients complain of fever or chills and most have myalgias or headache. Nausea, vomiting, and diarrhea are prominent symptoms (51). Cough is a common complaint late in the prodrome and is nonproductive; however, with the onset of pulmonary edema, patients expectorate amber-colored pulmonary secretions. Despite the central role that pulmonary problems play in the syndrome, dyspnea is not a frequent presenting complaint. Dyspnea is associated with advanced disease and often signals impending respiratory failure. Conjunctivitis, odynophagia, meningismus, rash, sinusitis, otalgia, and pleuritic pain are usually absent as presenting complaints.

Examination of the lungs is normal during the prodromal phase of HPS. After the onset of pulmonary edema, examination reveals either rales or diminished breath sounds, and percussion dullness may be present in the lung bases. An S3 gallop may be present. Severe abdominal tenderness is present in about 10% of patients. Although hypotension is an unusual finding on presentation, it indicates advanced disease and requires aggressive resuscitation. Petechiae are not seen in spite of thrombocytopenia. Peripheral edema is absent early in the illness, developing only with volume administration during the shock phase of the illness.

B. Respiratory Pathophysiology

HPS most profoundly affects respiratory and cardiac physiology, and the disease characteristically progresses very rapidly after the onset of respiratory symptoms (51). Patients who present with dyspnea typically require intubation and mechanical ventilation within 1–6 hr. All patients with HPS have pulmonary edema. The severity varies, ranging from interstitial edema in relatively mild cases to diffuse alveolar flooding with profound hypoxemia (51,52). Pulmonary edema is manifested by PaO_2/FIO_2 ratios as low as 55 (during mechanical ventilation with positive end-expiratory pressure [PEEP]), diffuse interstitial or alveolar infiltrates on chest radiograph, and low respiratory system compliance. The capillary leak can be so severe that several liters of amber-colored edema fluid resembling plasma may be suctioned from the trachea.

We demonstrated two lines of evidence that support increased pulmonary capillary permeability as the etiology of pulmonary edema in HPS (51). Only patients who are premorbid and who receive intensive volume resuscitation prior to insertion of a flow-directed pulmonary artery catheter have an initial pulmonary artery occlusion (PAOP) pressure >15 mmHg. The PAOP is characteristically <8 mmHg prior to volume resuscitation. Second, edema fluid reveals ratios of edema fluid total protein to serum total protein <0.6, a ratio which is characteristic of increased permeability pulmonary edema (Table 2) (53).

Respiratory system compliance is decreased owing to a combination of interstitial and alveolar edema and pleural effusion. Chest wall edema may also contribute to the decrease in respiratory system compliance, but this contribution has not been documented by measurement of transpulmonary pressures. Surviving patients recover to near-normal respiratory functioning quite rapidly and are usually extubated in less than a week. Pulmonary function tests after recovery may show mild air trapping or diminished diffusing capacity which resolve in 3–6 months.

C. Cardiovascular Derangements

Nearly all patients with HPS fit the accepted criteria for diagnosis of the sepsis syndrome. All HPS patients have fever, tachypnea, and tachycardia, and many have lactic acidosis as evidence of organ hypoperfusion (54). However, the hemodynamic parameters in HPS are unique. Most patients with bacteremic and viremic shock have an elevated cardiac output and low systemic vascular

Table 2 Comparison of Protein Concentrations in Serum and Tracheal Aspirate Fluid in Three Fatal Sin Nombre Virus Infections

	Total protein (g/dL)	Ratio[a]	Albumin (g/dL)	LDH (IU/L)
Patient A				
trachea	5.1	0.98	2.6	4191
serum	5.2	—	2.5	1498
Patient B				
trachea	4.3	1.19	2.1	3469
serum	3.6	—	1.6	4104
Patient C				
trachea	2.8	0.82	1.8	2934
serum	3.4	—	1.5	2810

[a]Total protein in tracheal fluid/total protein in serum.
Source: Ref. 37.

resistance, whereas patients with HPS have a diminished cardiac output and normal or elevated systemic vascular resistance (Table 3) (55–58). The cardiac output reductions in HPS are due to reductions in myocardial contractility (51). Echocardiography in patients with severe disease shows markedly decreased left ventricular ejection fractions without evidence of local or diffuse ischemia.

Table 3 Hemodynamic Summary Data at Clinical Nadir of Eight Patients with Sin Nombre Virus Infection

Patient	Cardiac index (L/min/m^2)	PAOP (mmHg)	SVRI (dyne·sec·cm^{-5}/m^2)	Mean PA (mmHg)	Stroke volume index (mL/beat/m^2)
1	3.0	8	1653	23	29.0
2[a]	1.6	11	2951	48	12.5
3[a]	1.8	28	2997	NA	10.5
4	2.6	11	2097	26	29.0
5	1.0	24	NA	20	7.1
6	2.8	10	1828	28	25.0
7[a]	2.7	13	2154	28	21.9
8[a]	3.2	20	1110	35	23.8
Mean	2.4	15	2112	30	19.8

PAOP, pulmonary artery occlusion pressure (wedge pressure); SVRI, systemic vascular resistance index; PA, pulmonary artery pressure; NA, not available.
[a]Patients who died.
Source: Simpson SQ. Hantavirus pulmonary syndrome. Curr Pulmonol 1996; 17:155–180.

Patients with HPS often present with intravascular volume depletion, as evidenced by increased hematocrit and decreased PAOP (50,51). This decrease in intravascular volume results from a decrease in oral fluid intake due to the patient's gastrointestinal symptoms and from extravasation of plasma across leaking capillary beds. When a flow-directed pulmonary artery catheter is placed at this stage, hypotensive patients typically have low cardiac stroke volume and low cardiac output in addition to low PAOP. The hemodynamic profile is that of hypovolemic shock, and the loss of adequate preload to the left ventricle may contribute significantly to early hypotension. However, intravascular volume repletion fails to significantly improve stroke volume or cardiac output, as evidence that myocardial contractility is also decreased. The cardiac output is maintained by a marked increase in the pulse rate (51). Death is due to progressive myocardial insufficiency and shock. The terminal event is, almost uniformly, the progressive development of pulseless electrical activity.

A number of factors could impair left ventricular functioning in HPS. Acidosis and high levels of PEEP both have detrimental effects on cardiac output (52,59). High pulmonary artery pressures, as are seen in patients with severe HPS, may directly impair right ventricular functioning and impair left ventricular performance through the phenomenon of ventricular interdependence (36,58,60–65). Autopsy studies reveal normal myocardial tissue excluding infarction or myocarditis. In other forms of sepsis, left and right ventricular functioning are impaired by a circulating myocardial depressant factor or factors (56,57,68). It appears likely that a myocardial depressant factor is also responsible for the reduced cardiac output of HPS.

D. Laboratory Findings

A triad of hematological findings that includes thrombocytopenia, left-shifted neutrophilic leukocytosis, and circulating immunoblasts is characteristic of HPS. The white blood cell count is usually increased, and neutrophilia with immature forms, including myelocytes and promyelocytes, is present. All patients have a lymphocyte population that includes at least 10% immunoblasts, a finding not seen in similar disorders such as acute respiratory distress syndrome (ARDS). The immunoblasts contain deeply basophilic cytoplasm, enlarged nuclei, and variably prominent nucleoli and vary in size with mature circulating plasma cells at the upper extreme of size (66,67). Thrombocytopenia is found in 79% of cases at presentation and in all patients during their hospital course, but the severity of thrombocytopenia does not correlate with the prognosis (51). Hemoconcentration with hematocrits as high as 77% is common (67).

Most patients have elevated prothrombin times and partial thromboplastin times and levels of d-dimer may be increased, which are indicative of thrombolysis (66,67). These findings in combination with thrombocytopenia suggest that DIC may be present, but it is not associated with schistocytes or overt bleeding. Lactate dehydrogenase (LDH), 2,5-trichlorophenoxyacetic acid (2,5-T), alanine aminotransferase (ALT), are increased in all cases (51). Hypoalbuminemia is a common finding (66).

Arterial blood gases and lactate levels help to establish the severity of disease. Elevations of the alveolar–arterial oxygen gradient or frank hypoxemia are present in all cases. An increased serum lactate level identifies patients in whom poor tissue perfusion or metabolic derangement due to direct viral infection or effects of inflammatory mediators is present. In the University of New Mexico series of 24 patients, all with a serum lactate level of 4 mmol/L or greater died despite aggressive treatment except for two patients who were treated with extracorporeal membrane oxygenation (ECMO).

E. Radiographic Findings

All patients with HPS have abnormal chest radiographic findings; chest radiograph abnormalities were noted on admission in 13 of 16 cases of HPS (68). The other three patients developed similar abnormalities within 48 hr of presentation. Kerley B lines, hilar indistinctness, or peribronchial cuffing indicative of pulmonary interstitial edema are found. As hypoxemia worsens, many patients also develop air space flooding that begins in dependent regions and progresses to involve all lung fields. In severe cases, diffuse lung infiltrates develop within 2–6 hr. Air space opacification begins centrally and progresses outward unlike other forms of noncardiogenic pulmonary edema. Additionally, radiographically detectable pleural effusions develop in nearly all HPS patients (69).

F. Diagnosis

The diagnosis of HPS is confirmed by identification of antibodies to SNV antigens in serum or by detection of SNV genetic material in blood mononuclear cell preparations via RT-PCR (70,71). The diagnosis can also be confirmed at autopsy by immunohistochemical analysis of infected tissues using anti-SNV antibodies or by a positive RT-PCR of these tissues. PCR lacks the ability to diagnose remote infection, because SNV is cleared from the circulation within 2–4 weeks after the onset of clinical symptoms (70). At the University of New Mexico, a Western blot assay was developed based on recombinant N and G proteins expressed in *E. coli* (71). Patients who are acutely ill have both IgG and IgM antibodies to the viral nucleocapsid protein, as well as IgG antibodies to the glycoprotein-1 protein of the SNV. The laboratories of the Special Pathogens Branch of the Division of Viral and Rickettsial Diseases at the CDC have used two forms of enzyme-linked immunosorbent assay (ELISA) (67). An IgM-capture ELISA is used to quantitate acute antibodies to radiation-inactivated SNV. IgG antibodies are detected in a sandwich ELISA using recombinant SNV nucleocapsid protein. A recombinant immunoblot assay has been developed in the form of a test strip and uses nucleocapsid and G1 glycoprotein antigens.

Serological testing with a 24-hr turnaround can be obtained from the University of New Mexico by contacting the infectious diseases physician on call. One may obtain testing from the CDC by contacting the CDC directly or by contacting one's own state health department. The turnaround time of the CDC test is approximately 1 week depending on the day of the week that a specimen is received. Cases are recorded by the CDC if the serology is confirmed by the Special Pathogens Laboratory. Acute specimens are considered positive if they contain high titers of IgM antibody; patients may be diagnosed after recovering from a compatible illness if their serum contains elevated titers of IgG and if review of their medical records by CDC investigators demonstrates clinical features sufficiently characteristic of HPS. The diagnosis can also be confirmed by positive immunohistochemical staining of biopsy or autopsy tissues for SNV antigens or by RT-PCR of these tissues demonstrating the presence of viral RNA.

V. Pathology

A. Respiratory Tract

At autopsy, the lungs of patients with HPS are grossly edematous and have an average combined weight nearly twice normal (66). Pleural effusions are uniformly present, ranging in volume from 200 to 8400 mL. Histologically, variable amounts of alveolar and septal edema are found (66,67). Hyaline membranes with little cellular debris are usually present, the respiratory epithelium is intact, and type II pneumocytes appear to be nonactivated. An interstitial infiltration of mononuclear cells is present, and many of the mononuclear cells are enlarged and have the characteristics of immunoblasts. Intravascular neutrophils are common, but neutrophils are present only rarely in the interstitium, alveoli, and bronchioles. No vasculitis has been identified in pulmonary vessels, and no viral inclusions or cytopathic effects are seen on light microscopy, although immunological staining reveals viral antigens in the pulmonary endothelium. Electron microscopy reveals rare endothelial inclusions of 90- to 110-nm particles consistent in appearance with hantaviral virions. These histopathological findings distinguish HPS from diffuse alveolar damage or ARDS, in which the infiltrate is predominantly neutrophilic, type II pneumocytes are activated, and extensive cellular debris is present.

Immunohistochemistry of autopsy tissue using a monoclonal antibody to hantavirus antigens (GB04-BF07) and using polyclonal immune sera of SNV-infected *Peromyscus maniculatis* demonstrates abundant staining of pulmonary endothelial cells (67). A fine, granular-appearing stain localizes in the pulmonary microvascular endothelium and is only seen rarely in the endothelium of larger veins and arteries. When sections of multiple lung segments are available, the microvascular staining appears to be uniform throughout the lungs.

B. Cardiovascular System

The heart in all patients with fatal HPS is grossly and histologically normal with no evidence of significant coronary artery disease or recent myocardial infarction (66). Neither myocarditis nor cardiomyopathy is found. A small pericardial effusion was seen in one patient. These findings are striking, since mortality is most closely associated with myocardial dysfunction. Myocardial capillaries contain SNV antigens in most specimens, with antigen loads ranging from focal involvement to extensive, diffuse staining. The myocardium itself does not stain.

C. Other Organs

Examination of the liver shows a portal triaditis in about half of the cases, with expanded pools of lymphocytes, including large immunoblasts (66,67). No hepatic necrosis is seen. The spleen and lymph nodes typically contain an infiltrate of immunoblasts. No retroperitoneal fluid has been found in any case. The brain, kidneys, adrenals, pancreas, skeletal muscle, and skin are normal both macroscopically and histologically. SNV antigens are detected in the kidneys, with medullary endothelium staining most prominently, but viral antigens are also present within cortical and glomerular endothelium. Lymphocytes within splenic lymphoid follicles typically contain SNV antigens, and macrophages in a number of tissues, including the lungs, also stain positively. SNV antigens are seen in multiple other tissues, including skeletal muscle, adrenal glands, intestine, and brain, although these tissues stain less intensely and less consistently than the lungs.

VI. Viral Pathogenesis

Attempts to explain the pathogenesis of shock and lung injury in HPS have been hampered, as for other hantaviral diseases, by the lack of an animal model. Mice and other rodents develop infection but not illness and so are useless as models of human disease. Macaque monkeys may be a useful, but expensive, alternative. Any hypothesis regarding pathogenesis must tie together several important findings: (1) severe pulmonary capillary leak,

(2) hantaviral inclusions and positive immunohistochemical staining for SNV antigens in pulmonary capillary endothelium, (3) mononuclear cell infiltration of the lungs, (4) circulating immunoblasts, (5) mononuclear infection by SNV, and (6) progressive, severe myocardial depression. Several hypotheses have been advanced, although, at present, insufficient data exist to confirm or to rule out any of them.

A. Pulmonary Injury

The presence of pulmonary capillary leak in conjunction with endothelial invasion by virus suggests the possibility of direct injury to endothelial cells. Very little data are available regarding this hypothesis, although in vitro testing shows pulmonary vascular endothelial cells to be highly susceptible to infection by SNV (72). Light and electron microscopic sections do not demonstrate endothelial disruption or necrosis, although some edema of pulmonary endothelial cells is demonstrated by electron microscopy (66,67). However, viral infection could impair functioning of endothelial cells in the absence of overt cell death, altering their capacity to prevent fluid extravasation. Other negative-sense RNA viruses induce programmed cell death (apoptosis) in target cells in vitro (73). If such a mechanism were active in vivo, lung sections from patients who died rapidly may not yet demonstrate endothelial disruption.

A second hypothesis involves the potential for pulmonary injury mediated by specific antibodies to SNV either directed to antigens expressed in pulmonary endothelium or in the form of immune complex deposition within the lung. Immune complexes of SNV and anti-SNV are unlikely, since SNV antigens have not been detected in the serum of HPS patients, nor has antibody deposition been detected in lung tissue. Additionally, these mechanisms of lung injury involve neutrophil infiltration of the lungs and are ameliorated by inhibition of such infiltration (74,75). No serological evidence of immune complex activation has been found in HPS patients.

Given that HPS is a viral disease and that the lungs are infiltrated with mononuclear cells, an attractive hypothesis is that cell-mediated immunity directed toward antigen-expressing pulmonary capillary endothelial cells results in direct injury to these cells and in loss of structural integrity of the capillary. Cell-mediated immunity in this syndrome is possible by four potential mechanisms: (1) T-cytotoxic cell (CD8) recognition of FCV antigen expression by pulmonary endothelial cells in the context of class I major histocompatibility complex (MHC) recognition, resulting in direct lysis or injury of endothelium; (2) T-helper cell (CD4) recognition of SNV antigen in the context of class II MHC recognition, with interferon-γ (IFN-γ) and interleukin-2 (IL-2) activation of other lymphocyte subsets; (3) a pathway that is dominated by IL-2–activated natural killer (NK) cells; or (4) antibody-dependent, cell-mediated cytotoxicity (ADCC). Preliminary immunophenotyping studies of mononuclear cells infiltrating the lungs in fatal HPS demonstrate only rare cells staining positively for CD16, an NK cell marker (66). Among infiltrating T lymphocytes, the ratio of helper ($CD4^+$) to suppressor ($CD8^+$) cells is approximately 2:1. Additionally, double staining of peripheral blood leukocytes with CD8 and HLA-DR (a marker of mononuclear cell activation) by flow cytometry enhances for a population of cells of the approximate size of the lymphoblasts in peripheral blood (66). These results suggest that the lymphoblasts may be activated T lymphocytes and that activated T lymphocytes may play a role in the pathogenesis of HPS. There is little evidence regarding the possibility of ADCC in HPS, although it appears that patients simultaneously develop peripheral immunoblasts, develop a serum antibody response, and become critically ill. Serological surveys of populations at risk for deer mouse exposure and the development of HPS demonstrate antibodies to SNV in only 1% of those tested (76). This low rate of seroprevalence suggests that the possibility of two episodes of exposure, with severe illness developing during the second exposure (as is seen in dengue hemorrhagic fever), is unlikely. Nevertheless, mild disease in preadolescents suggests that this is a possible mechanism of severe disease.

All four of these mechanisms of cell-mediated immunity are likely to involve the secretion of cytokines that function either to injure virus-infected cells or to amplify the immune response. Serum cytokine profiles in patients with HPS also suggest that activated T cells are present during SNV infection (77). In a study comparing HPS nonsurvivors, HPS survivors, and control patients with ARDS, circulating levels of IFN-γ, soluble CD4, soluble IL-2 receptor, and IL-6 were highest in patients with fatal SNV infection. Levels of soluble CD8 were higher in patients with HPS than in patients with ARDS. Additional studies demonstrate that levels of soluble tumor necrosis factor (TNF) receptors are increased in HPS, although neither TNF-α nor TNF-β was increased over normal controls (78). Levels of TNF receptors correlate with mortality in HPS, and in surviving patients, convalescent levels are significantly lower than in sera collected on admission. These TNF receptor data may indicate that levels of TNF were elevated at some time prior to collection of the serum specimens and that target cells had bound TNF and released their cell surface receptors. In combination, the immunophenotyping data and the cytokine data support the hypothesis that cellular immunity mediated by activated T cells may result in lung injury in HPS.

B. Myocardial Injury

The cytokine and cytokine receptor data also suggest possible mechanisms for the severe myocardial depression in HPS. The effects of TNF-α on myocardial contractility have been studied extensively in vitro in myocyte models, ex vivo in isolated beating myocardia, and in vivo in animal models (79–84). The predominant finding of all of these studies is that of a profound negative inotropic effect of TNF on cardiac muscle, although kinetic studies indicate that contractility may temporarily increase on exposure of cardiac myocytes to TNF before diminishing to subnormal levels (85). IL-2 and IL-6 also produce reductions of myocardial contractility in vitro (86,87). The inotropic effects of all of these cytokines may be mediated through induction of nitric oxide synthesis by myocardial cells, as inhibition of inducible nitric oxide synthase abrogates the cytokine-induced reductions in contractility (88–90). Since each of these cytokines individually reduces myocardial contractility, simultaneously increased circulating levels of all three cytokines (which our data support) could result in profound reductions in cardiac output.

Chronic SNV infection has not been described and patients have a well-developed IgG response when they present with the clinical syndrome. Reinfection with another hantaviral strain, although clinically possible, has not been described.

C. Protective Mechanisms for Terminating Infection and Preventing Reinfection

Neutralizing antibodies in infected hosts are directed against envelope glycoproteins G1 and G2. However, it is not clear whether these antibodies are, in fact, protective. Rodents express these antibodies, yet viral infection is maintained throughout the animal's normal life cycle. Other factors that protect rodents from ill effects due to infection with any of the hantaviruses remain to be elucidated. Additionally, patients presenting with HPS have IgG antibodies at the time of diagnosis. Preadolescent humans have a flu-like syndrome but fail to become critically ill with SNV infection. The mechanism of protection is not known. Some investigators hypothesize that children sustain a lower infective load than adults, although others believe that the ratio of infective load to body size may in fact be greater in children.

VII. Therapy

A. General Treatment Measures

HPS confronts physicians with a central treatment dilemma: As patients develop a severe pulmonary capillary leak, they are simultaneously developing myocardial insufficiency and shock that demands increased cardiac filling pressures. There is no proven specific therapy for the treatment of SNV infection or HPS, and treatment measures are entirely supportive in nature. Adequate care requires advanced monitoring and life support techniques, so HPS patients should be cared for in a facility equipped for the treatment of severe shock. Until the diagnosis of HPS is confirmed by serology, patients should be treated empirically with appropriate antibiotics to cover infections that may initially resemble HPS, including pneumonic plague and legionellosis.

B. Antivirals

In general, viruses belonging to the family *Bunyaviridae* have been sensitive in vitro to the antiviral agent ribavirin (Virazole). Ribavirin inhibits the growth of SNV in vitro and has proven efficacy in the treatment of HFRS. Between June 8 and September 1, 1993, the case fatality rate for persons with confirmed hantaviral infection who received ribavirin was 6 of 14 (43%), as compared with 11 of 15 (73%) for patients with confirmed hantaviral infection who did not receive ribavirin ($P = .14$ Fisher's exact test, not significant) (91). Since the untreated patients were largely discovered during the early phase of the epidemic, direct comparison with the ribavirin-treated patients is not possible. The fulminant course of HPS by the time patients present to a medical center suggests that there is insufficient time for an antiviral agent to be effective. In addition, the low viral load implicates mechanisms such as immunological and cytokine mediators as the predominant factor in disease rather than overwhelming viremia. A National Institutes of Health (NIH)–sponsored, placebo-controlled, double-blind trial of ribavirin is now underway, with the goal of identifying and enrolling patients as early as possible in the course of disease. Patients who have a compatible illness and who meet the entry criteria of fever and thrombocytopenia may be enrolled at one of three centers (currently): University of Alabama at Birmingham, University of New Mexico, or University of Utah.

C. Passive Immunoglobulin

Passive immunoglobulin therapy has not been investigated in HPS but has been utilized with success in other hemorrhagic fevers. The survivor immunoglobulin donor pool is extremely small.

D. Salvage Therapy

ECMO provides assistance for both the failing heart and the failing lungs in HPS. We have used venoarterial ECMO to treat three patients with severe HPS (one following prolonged cardiopulmonary resuscitation). Two patients survived to leave the hospital and resume their normal activities. Further studies are necessary to determine the overall utility of this treatment modality in HPS.

Early in the initial outbreak of HPS in 1993, and before the causative agent was known, several patients who met criteria for the sepsis syndrome were enrolled in a multicenter trial of a bradykinin antagonist in sepsis. Too few patients were enrolled to analyze seriously, but this event raises the important issue of whether patients should be treated with any of the investigational therapeutic agents for sepsis syndrome that are available under protocol. Some of our findings suggest that modification of the immune response may be of benefit in the syndrome. Corticosteroids have been administered to some patients with HPS. However, since no attempts were made to systematically study their effects, their role in the treatment of HPS is not clear. We prefer ECMO as the salvage option at present.

VIII. Prevention

The key to HPS prevention is avoiding contact with rodents and their excreta (92). Houses should be kept clean and holes of entry sealed. Vegetation should be cleared from around the foundation. Pet food and water should be put away at night. Food and garbage must be stored in containers with tight lids. Natural predators should be encouraged. If rodents are being trapped, particle masks and rubber gloves must be worn. Traps and rodents must be thoroughly disinfected and they should be disposed of in sealed bags. Precautions must be taken to spray trapping areas with flea killers because of the coincident risk of plague.

Although programs for vaccination against HFRS have been initiated, immunity is not induced against Puumala virus, which is the closest antigenically to SNV (93). There are currently no plans for developing a vaccine for SNV given the very large population at risk but the rarity of disease.

Acknowledgments

This work is supported by a grant from the Centers for Disease Control and Prevention and the New Mexico Department of Health.

References

1. Peters CJ, Johnson KM. Viral hemorrhagic fevers. In: Hoeprich PD, Jordan MC, Ronald AR, eds. Infectious Diseases. 5th ed. Philadelphia: Lippincott, 1994:924–929.

2. Peters CJ, Johnson KM. California encephalitis viruses, hantaviruses, and other *Bunyaviridae*. In: Mandell GL, Bennett JE, Dolin R, eds. Principles and Practice of Infectious Disease. 4th ed. New York: Churchill Livingstone, 1995: 1567–1572.
3. McCormick JB. Crimean-Congo hemorrhagic fever (CCHF). In: Strickland GT, ed. Hunter's Tropical Medicine. 7th ed. Philadelphia: Saunders, 1991:248–254.
4. Clement J, Heyman P, McKenna P, Colson P, Avsi-Zupanc T. The hantaviruses of Europe: from the bedside to the bench. Emerg Infect Dis 1997; 3:205–211.
5. Plyusnin A, Vapalahti O, Lundkvist A, Henttonen H, Vaheri A. Newly recognised hantavirus in Siberian lemmings. Lancet 1996; 347:1835–1836.
6. Li D, Schmaljohn AL, Anderson K, Schmaljohn CS. Complete nucleotide sequences of the M and S segments of two hantavirus isolates from California: evidence for reassortment in nature among viruses related to hantavirus pulmonary syndrome. Virology 1995; 206:973–983.
7. Hjelle B, Lee SW, Song W, Torrez-Martinez N, Song JW, Yanagihara R, Gavrilovskaya I, Mackow ER. Molecular linkage of hantavirus pulmonary syndrome to the white-footed mouse, Peromyscus leucopus: genetic characterization of the M genome of New York virus. J Virol 1995; 69:8137–8141.
8. Khan AS, Gaviria M, Rollin PE, Hlady WG, Ksiazek TG, Armstrong LR, Greenman R, Ravkov E, Kolber M, Anapol H, Sfakianaki ED, Nichol ST, Peters CJ, Khabbaz RF. Hantavirus pulmonary syndrome in Florida: association with the newly identified Black Creek Canal virus. Am J Med 1996; 100:46–48.
9. Rawlings JA, Torrez-Martinez N, Neill SU, Moore GM, Hicks BN, Pichuantes S, Nguyen A, Bharadwaj M, Hjelle B. Cocirculation of multiple hantaviruses in Texas, with characterization of the small (S) genome of a previously undescribed virus of cotton rats (*Sigmodon hispidus*). Am J Trop Med Hyg 1996; 55:672–679.
10. Khan AS, Spiropoulou CF, Morunov S, Zaki SR, Kohn MA, Nawas SR, McFarland L, Nichol ST. Fatal illness associated with a new hantavirus in Louisiana. J Med Virol 1995; 46:281–286.
11. Song W, Torrez-Martinez N, Irwin W, Harrison FJ, Davis R, Ascher M, Jay M, Hjelle B. Isla Vista virus: a genetically novel hantavirus of the California vole Microtus californicus. J Gen Virol 1995; 76:3195–3199.
12. Torrez-Martinez N, Song W, Hjelle B. Nucleotide sequence anlaysis of the M genomic segment of El Moro Canyon hantavirus: antigenic distinction from four corners hantavirus. Virology 1995; 211:336–338.
13. Hjelle B, Torrez-Martinez N, Koster FT. Hantavirus pulmonary syndrome-related virus from Bolovia. Lancet 1996; 347:57.
14. Lopez N, Padula P, Rossi C, Lazaro ME, Franze-Fernandez MT. Genetic identification of a new hantavirus causing severe pulmonary syndrome in Argentina. Virology 1996; 220:223–226.
15. Elliott LH, Ksiazek TG, Rollin PE, Spiropoulou CF, Morzunov S, Monroe M, Goldsmith CS, Humphrey CD, Zaki SR, Krebs JW, Maupin G, Gage K, Childs JE, Nichol ST, Peters CJ. Isolation of the causative agent of hantavirus pulmonary syndrome. Am J Trop Med Hyg 1994; 51:102–108.
16. Feldmann H, Sanchez A, Morzunov S, Spiropoulou CF, Rollin PE, Ksiazek TG, Peters CJ, Nichol ST. Utilization of autopsy RNA for the synthesis of the nucleo-

capsid antigen of a newly recognized virus associated with hantaviral pulmonary syndrome. Virus Res 1993; 30:351–367.
17. Spiropoulou CF, Morzunov S, Feldmann H, Sanchez A, Peters CJ, Nichol ST. Genome structure and variability of a virus causing hantavirus pulmonary syndrome. Virol 1994; 200:715–723.
18. Hjelle B, Jenison S, Torrez-Martinez N, Yamada T, Nolte K, Zumwalt R, MacInnes K, Myers G. A novel hantavirus associated with an outbreak of fatal respiratory disease in the southwestern United States: evolutionary relationships to known hantaviruses. J Virol 1994; 68:592–596.
19. Butler JC, Peters CJ. Hantaviruses and hantavirus pulmonary syndrome. Clin Infect Dis 1994; 19:387–395.
20. Schmaljohn CS, Patterson JL. *Bunyaviridae* and their replication. In: Fields BN, Knipe DM, eds. Fundamental Virology. 2nd ed. New York: Raven Press, 1991: 545–564.
21. Arikawa J, Schmaljohn AL, Dalrymple JM, Schmaljohn CS. Characterization of Hantaan virus envelope glycoprotein antigenic determinants defined by monoclonal antibodies. J Gen Virol 1989; 70:615–624.
22. Ellis DS, Shirodaria PV, Fleming E, Simpson DIH. Morphology and development of Rift Valley fever virus in Vero cell cultures. J Med Virol 1988; 24:161–174.
23. Marsh M, Helenius A. Adsorptive endocytosis of Semliki Forest virus. J Mol Biol 1980; 142:439–454.
24. Schmaljohn CS, Jennings G, Hay J, Dalrymple JM. Coding strategy of the S genome segment of Hantaan virus. Virology 1986; 155:633–643.
25. Schmaljohn CS, Schmaljohn AL, Dalrymple JM. Hantaan virus M RNA: coding strategy, nucleotide sequence, and gene order. Virology 1987; 157:31–39.
26. Parker MD, Smith JF, Dalrymple JM. Rift Valley fever virus intracellular RNA: a functional analysis. In: Compans RW, Bishop DHL, eds. Segmented Negative Strand Viruses. Orlando, FL: Academic Press, 1984:21–28.
27. Suzich JQ, Collett MS. Rift Valley fever virus M segment: cell-free transcription and translation of virus-complementary RNA. Virology 1988; 164:478–486.
28. Lyons MJ, Heyduk J. Aspects of the developmental morphology of California encephalitis virus in cultured vertebrate and arthropod cells and in mouse brain. Virology 1973; 54:37–52.
29. Murphy FA, Harrison AK, Whitfield SG. Morphologic and morphogenetic similarities of Bunyamwera serological supergroup viruses and several other arthropod-borne viruses. Intervirology 1973; 297–316.
30. von Bonsdorff C-H, Saikku P, Oker-Blom N. Electron microscopy study on the development of Uukuniemi virus. Acta Virol 1970; 14:109–114.
31. Schmaljohn CS, Arikawa J, Hasty SE, Rasmussen L, Lee HW, Lee PW, Dalrymple JM. Conservation of antigenic properties and sequences encoding the envelope proteins of prototype Hantaan virus and two virus isolates from Korean haemorrhagic fever patients. J Gen Virol 1988; 69:1949–1955.
32. Goldsmith CS, Elliott LH, Peters CJ, Zaki SR. Ultrastructural characteristics of Sin Nombre virus, causative agent of hantavirus pulmonary syndrome. Arch Virol 1995; 140:2107–2122.

33. Childs JE, Ksiazek TG, Spiropoulou CF, Krebs JW. Serologic and genetic identification of Peromyscus maniculatus as the primary rodent reservoir for a new hantavirus in the southwestern United States. J Infect Dis 1994; 169:1271–1280.
34. Nichol ST, Spiropoulou CF, Morzunov S, Rollin PE, Ksiazek TG, Feldmann H, Sanchez A, Childs J, Zaki S, Peters CJ. Genetic identification of a hantavirus associated with an outbreak of acute respiratory illness. Science 1993; 262:914–916.
35. Yamada T, Hjelle B, Lanzi R, Morris C, Anderson B, Jenison S. Antibody responses to Four Corners hantavirus infections in the deer mouse (*Peromyscus maniculatus*): identification of an immunodominant region of the nucleocapsid protein. J Virol 1995; 69:1939–1943.
36. Zapol WM, Snider MT. Pulmonary hypertension in severe acute respiratory failure. N Engl J Med 1977; 296:476–480.
37. CDC. Newly identified hantavirus—Florida, 1994. MMWR 1994; 43:99–105.
38. Morzunov SP, Feldmann H, Spiropoulou CF, Semenova VA, Rollin PE, Ksiazek TG, Peters CJ, Nichol ST. A newly recognized virus associated with a fatal case hantavirus pulmonary syndrome in Louisiana. J Virol 1995; 69:1980–1983.
39. Torrez-Martinez N, Hjelle B. Enzootic of Bayou hantavirus in rice rats (*Oryzomys palustris*) in 1983. Lancet 1995; 346:780–781.
40. CDC. Hantavirus pulmonary syndrome—northeastern United States, 1994. MMWR 1994; 43:548–549.
41. Song JW, Baek LJ, Gajdusek DC, Yanagihara R, Gavrilovskaya I, Luft BJ, Mackow ER, Hjelle B. Isolation of a pathogenic hantavirus from the white footed mouse (*Peromyscus leucopus*). Lancet 1994; 344:1637.
42. CDC. Hantavirus pulmonary syndrome—Virginia, 1993. MMWR 1994; 43:876–877.
43. CDC. Update: hantavirus-associated illness—North Dakota, 1993. MMWR 1993; 42:707.
44. Hjelle B, Krolikowski J, Torrez-Martinez N, Chavez-Giles F, Vanner C, Laposata E. A phylogenetically distinct hantavirus implicated in a case of hantavirus pulmonary syndrome in the northeastern United States. J Med Virol 1995; 46:21–27.
45. Peters CJ, Khan 25, Zaki SR. Hantaviruses in the United States. Arch Intern Med 1996; 156:705–706.
46. Lopez N, Padula P, Rossi C, Lazaro ME, Franze-Fernandez MT. Genetic identification of a new hantavirus causing severe pulmonary syndrome in Argentina. Virology 1996; 220:223–226.
47. Enria D, Padula P, Segura EL, Pini N, Edelstein A, Riva Posse C, Weissenbacker MC. Hantavirus pulmonary syndrome in Argentina: possibility of person to person transmission. Medicina 1996; 56:709–711.
48. Wells RM, Estani SS, Yadon ZE, Enria D, Padula P, Pini N, Mills JN, Peters CJ, Segura EL, Hantavirus Pulmonary Syndrome Group for Patagonia. An unusual hantavirus outbreak in southern Argentina: person-to-person transmission? Emerg Infect Dis 1997; 3:171–174.
49. McKee KT Jr, LeDuk JW, Peteers CJ. Hantaviruses. In: Belshe RB, ed. Textbook of Human Virology, 2nd ed. St Louis: Mosby-Yearbook, 1991:615–632.
50. Duchin JS, Koster FT, Peters CJ, Simpson GL, Tempest B, Zaki SR, Ksiazek TG, Rollin PE, Nichol S, Umland ET, Moolenaar RL, Reef SE, Nolte KB, Gallaher

MM, Butler JC, Breiman RF, and the Hantavirus Study Group. Hantavirus pulmonary syndrome: a clinical description of 17 patients with a newly recognized disease. N Engl J Med 1994; 330:949–955.
51. Hallin GW, Simpson SQ, Crowell RE, James DS, Koster FT, Mertz GJ, Levy H. Cardiopulmonary manifestations of hantavirus pulmonary syndrome. Crit Care Med 1996; 24:252–258.
52. Dull SM, Brillman JC, Simpson SQ, Sklar DP. Hantavirus pulmonary syndrome: recognition and emergency department management. Ann Emerg Med 1994; 24: 530–536.
53. Fein A, Grossman RF, Jones JG, Overland E, Pitts L, Murray JF, Staub NC. The value of edema fluid protein measurement in patients with pulmonary edema. Am J Med 1979; 67:32–38.
54. Bone RC, Fisher CJ Jr, Clemmer TP, Slotman GJ, Metz CG, Balk RA, The Methylprednisolone Severe Sepsis Study group. Sepsis syndrome: a valid clinical entity. Crit Care Med 1989; 17:389–393.
55. Parker MM, Parrillo JE. Septic shock—hemodynamics and pathogenesis. JAMA 1983; 250:3324–3327.
56. Parrillo JE. Pathogenetic mechanisms of septic shock. N Engl J Med 1993; 328: 1471–1477.
57. Parrillo JE, Burch C, Shelhamer JH, Parker MM, Natanson C, Schuette W. A circulating myocardial depressant substance in humans with septic shock: septic shock patients with a reduced ejection fraction have a circulating factor that depresses in vitro myocardial cell performance. J Clin Invest 1985; 76:1539–1553.
58. Sibbald WJ, Driedger AA, Cunningham DG, Cheung H. Right and left ventricular performance in acute hypoxemic respiratory failure. Crit Care Med 1986; 14:852–857.
59. Dorinsky PM, Whitcomb ME. The effect of PEEP on cardiac output. Chest 1983; 84:210–216.
60. Calvin JE. Acute right heart failure. Pathophysiology, recognition, and pharmacological management. J Cardiothorac Vasc Anesth 1991; 5:507–513.
61. Dhainault JF, Brunet F. Right ventricular performance in adult respiratory distress syndrome. Eur Respir J 1990; 3:490s–495s.
62. Her C, Lees DE. Accurate assessment of right ventricular function in acute respiratory failure. Crit Care Med 1993; 21:1665–1672.
63. Sibbald WJ, Driedger AA, Myers ML, Short AIK, Wells GA. Biventricular function in the adult respiratory distress syndrome: hemodynamic and radionuclide assessment, with special emphasis on right ventricular function. Chest 1983; 84: 126–134.
64. Wiedemann HP, Matthay RA. Acute right heart failure. Crit Care Clin 1985; 1: 631–661.
65. Zimmerman GA, Morris AH, Cengiz M. Cardiovascular alterations in the adult respiratory distress syndrome. Am J Med 1982; 73:25–34.
66. Nolte KB, Feddersen RM, Foucar K, Zaki SR, Koster FT, Madar D, Merlin TL, McFeeley PJ, Umland ET, Zumwalt RE. Hantavirus pulmonary syndrome in the United States: a pathological description of a disease caused by a new agent. Hum Pathol 1995; 26:110–120.

67. Zaki SR, Greer PW, Coffield LM, Goldsmith CS, Nolte KB, Foucar K, Feddersen RM, Zumwalt RE, Miller GL, Khan AS. Hantavirus pulmonary syndrome: pathogenesis of an emerging infectious disease. Am J Pathol 1995; 146:552–579.
68. Ketai LH, Williamson MR, Telepak RJ, Levy H, Koster FT, Nolte KB, Allen SE. Hantavirus pulmonary syndrome: radiographic findings in 16 patients. Radiology 1994; 191:665–668.
69. Bustamante EA, Levy H, Simpson SQ. Pleural fluid characteristics in hantavirus pulmonary syndrome. Chest 1997; 112:1133–1136.
70. Hjelle B, Spiropoulou CF, Torrez-Martinez N, Morzunov S, Peters CJ, Nichol ST. Detection of Muerto Canyon virus RNA in peripheral blood mononuclear cells from patients with hantavirus pulmonary syndrome. J Infect Dis 1994b; 170:1013–1017.
71. Jenison S, Yamada T, Morris C, Anderson B, Torrez-Martinez N, Keller N, Hjelle B. Characterization of human antibody responses to Four Corners hantavirus infections among patients with hantavirus pulmonary syndrome. J Virol 1994; 68:3000–3006.
72. Voss TG, Rollin PE, Zaki S, Feldman H, Peters CJ. Susceptibility of human endothelial cells to infection by Sin Nombre virus. Proceedings of the 3rd International Congress on Hantaviral Infections. Helsinki, Finland, May 31–June 3, 1995.
73. Takizawa T, Matsukawa S, Higuchi Y, Nakamura S, Nakanishi Y, Fukuda R. Induction of programmed cell death (apoptosis) by influenza virus infection in tissue culture cells. J Gen Virol 1993; 74:2347–2355.
74. Mulligan MS, Smith CW, Anderson DC, Todd RF III, Miyasaka M, Tamatani T, Issekutz TB, Ward PA. Role of leukocyte adhesion molecules in complement-induced injury. J Immunol 1993; 150:2401–2406.
75. Mulligan MS, Wilson GP, Todd RF, Smith CW, Anderson DC, Varini J, Issekutz TB, Myasaka M, Tamatani T, Rusche JR, Vaporciyan AA, Ward PA. Role of β1 and β2 intergrins and ICAM-1 in lung injury following deposition of IgG and IgA immune complexes. J Immunol 1993; 150:2407–2417.
76. Simonsen L, Dalton MJ, Breiman RF, Hennessy T, Umland ET, Sewell CM, Rollin PE, Ksiazek TG, Peters CJ. Evaluation of the magnitude of the 1993 hantavirus outbreak in the southwestern United States. J Infect Dis 1995; 172:729–733.
77. Simpson SQ, Mapel V, Montoya J, Montoya J, Koster FT, Bice DE, Williams AJ. Evidence for T lymphocyte activation in the hantavirus pulmonary syndrome (abstr). Chest 1995; 108(suppl):97S.
78. Simpson SQ, Mapel V, Montoya J, Koster FT, Bice DE, Williams AJ. Evidence for tumor necrosis factor activation in the hantavirus pulmonary syndrome (abstr). Crit Care Med 1996; 24(suppl):A26.
79. Kapadia S, Torre-Amione G, Yokoyama T, Mann DL. Soluble TNF binding proteins modulate the negative inotropic properties of TNF-alpha in vitro. Am J Physiol 1995; 268(Pt 2):H517–525.
80. Yokoyama T, Vaca L, Rossen RD, Durante W, Hazarika P, Mann DL. Cellular basis for the negative inotropic effects of tumor necrosis factor-alpha in the adult mammalian heart. J Clin Inv 1993; 92:2303–2312.
81. Herbertson MJ, Werner HA, Goddard CM, Russel JA, Wheeler A, Coxon R, Walley KR. Anti-tumor necrosis factor-alpha prevents decreased ventricular contractility in endotoxemic pigs. Am J Res Crit Care Med 1995; 152:480–488.

82. Krosl P, Pretorius J, Redl H, Schlag G. Myocardial function in septic sheep. Shock 1994; 1:325–334.
83. Walley KR, Hebert PC, Wakai Y, Road JD, Cooper JD. Decrease in left ventricular contractility after tumor necrosis factor-alpha infusion in dogs. J Appl Physiol 1994; 76:1060–1067.
84. Reithmann C, Werdan K. Tumor necrosis factor alpha decreases inositol phosphate formation and phosphatidylinositol-bisphosphate (PIP2) synthesis in rat cardiomyocytes. Naunyn-Schmiedebergs Arch Pharmacol 1994; 349:175–182.
85. DeMeules JE, Pigula FA, Mueller M, Raymond SJ, Gamellie RL. Tumor necrosis factor and cardiac function. J Trauma 1992; 32(6):686–692.
86. Kunigawa K, Takahashi T, Kohmoto O, Yao A, Aoyagi T, Momomura S, Herata Y, Serizawa T. Nitric oxide-mediated effects of interleukin-6 on [Ca2+]i and cell contraction in cultured chick ventricular myocytes. Cir Res 1994; 75:285–295.
87. Weisensee D, Bereiter-Hahn J, Schoeppe W, Low-Friedrich I. Effects of cytokines on the contractility of cultured cardiac myocytes. Int J Immunopharmacol 1993; 15:581–587.
88. Finkel MS, Oddis CV, Jacob TD, Watkins SC, Hattler BG, Simmons RL. Negative inotropic effects of cytokines on the heart mediated by nitric oxide. Science 1992; 257:387–389.
89. Ungureanu-Longrois B, Balligand JL, Simmons WW, Okada I, Kobzik L, Lowenstein CJ, Kunkel SL, Kelly RA, Smith TW. Induction of nitric oxide synthase activity by cytokines in ventricular myocytes is necessary but not sufficient to decrease contractile responsiveness to beta-adrenergic agonists. Cir Res 1995; 77:494–502.
90. Schulz R, Panas DL, Catena R, Moncada S, Olley PM, Lopaschuk GD. The role of nitric oxide in cardiac depression induced by interleukin-1 beta and tumour necrosis factor-alpha. Br J Pharmacol 1995; 114:27–34.
91. Levy H, Simpson SQ. Hantavirus pulmonary syndrome. Am J Respir Crit Care Med 1994; 149:1710–1713.
92. CDC. Hantavirus infection—Southwestern United States: interim recommendations for risk reduction. MMWR 1993; 42(RR-11):1–13.
93. Chu YK, Jennings GB, Schmaljohn CS. A vaccinia virus–vectored Hantaan virus vaccine protects hamsters from challenge with Hantaan and Seoul viruses but not Puumala virus. J Virol 1995; 69:6417–6423.

Part Three

DIAGNOSIS

12

Laboratory Diagnosis of Infection with Respiratory Viruses

MARILYN A. MENEGUS

University of Rochester Medical Center
Rochester, New York

I. Introduction

The laboratory diagnosis of viral infections of the respiratory tract is complex because of the large number of viruses that cause respiratory disease and the many approaches that exist for their detection. In addition, there is also a subset of viral respiratory tract pathogens that are not detected by routine methods.

The laboratory methods most widely used to detect viruses that infect the respiratory tract include isolation in cell culture, immunofluorescent microscopy, enzyme-linked immunosorbent assay (ELISA), and, less frequently, the polymerase chain reaction (PCR). In addition, for some viruses, infection can be demonstrated by measuring the antibody response to the infecting pathogen. Depending on resources, staffing, specimen volume, and a variety of other factors, a laboratory may integrate these technologies to provide comprehensive coverage for a wide variety of respiratory tract pathogens. Other laboratories require selection of the particular virus or viruses to be sought.

II. Specimen Collection

The importance of collecting the appropriate clinical specimens for the laboratory diagnosis of viral respiratory disease cannot be overemphasized. The epithelium and lymphoid tissue of the upper respiratory tract is the primary site of replication for most of the viruses that cause upper as well as lower respiratory tract disease. Although virus is found in secretions as well as in the infected epithelium, the greatest concentration of virus and viral antigen is found intracellularly. Therefore, collection methods that maximize the recovery of epithelial cells as well as of secretions are the most desirable. This is particularly true for immunofluorescence methods, because demonstrating viral antigen in exfoliated cells forms the basis for this diagnostic approach.

Vigorously collected nasopharyngeal swabs and throat swabs are probably adequate for most diagnostic purposes, and they are the most convenient specimens to collect. However, substantial increases in sensitivity have been demonstrated in studies of more rigorously collected specimens such as nasal suctions and nasal washes (1). The tools of the diagnostic laboratory can also be applied to diagnostic specimens obtained at bronchoscopy, such as bronchoalveolar lavages (BALs), bronchial brushes, and transbronchial biopsies (2).

Specimens obtained for viral culture should be placed in specialized viral transport media (VTM). VTM are designed to maintain the stability of the virus during transport and to minimize the growth of bacteria and fungi by addition of antibiotics. Use of VTM is particularly important for the recovery of respiratory viruses, because many are sensitive to changes in pH, drying, and other adverse conditions encountered during transport. In addition, the respiratory viruses are among the most likely to be inactivated by freezing or by exposure to less than optimal temperatures. Ideally, specimens should be delivered to the laboratory within an hour or two of collection. Specimens that cannot be delivered immediately should be held at refrigerator temperature (4°C), because viruses, unlike bacteria that multiply at 22–36°C, are inactivated within this temperature range. The transport conditions recommended for viral isolation can also be used for specimens obtained for immunofluorescent microscopy, because those conditions maintain cellular integrity as well as virus viability. Specimens that cannot be delivered to the laboratory within 3 days of collection should be frozen at –70°C. Even when frozen under ideal conditions, loss in viability is inevitable, particularly for the more labile viruses such as cytomegalovirus and respiratory syncytial virus. Freezing at conventional freezer temperatures (–10–20°) will completely destroy the infectivity of most respiratory viruses (3).

III. Isolation of Viruses in Cell Culture

Viral isolation in cell culture remains the most widely used approach for the diagnosis of respiratory viral infections despite the many alternative diagnostic methods developed in recent years. The flexibility afforded by culture and its ability to detect a wide range of respiratory tract pathogens are the primary reasons that it remains the method of choice. However, respiratory virus cultures are the most complex and costly cultures performed in the virus laboratory. To provide comprehensive coverage for all respiratory tract pathogens, the laboratory must use several different types of cells, because no one cell culture supports the growth of all viruses. In addition, two temperatures of incubation (33 and 36°C) must be used to assure recovery of all respiratory viruses and to maximize the speed of such recovery. Laboratories that incubate cultures only at 36°C rarely recover rhinoviruses, and those that incubate cultures only at 33°C may delay the recovery of several other respiratory viruses. In some cases, the lower temperature of incubation may even compromise the recovery of certain viruses, particularly cytomegalovirus.

Viral replication in cell culture results in characteristic morphological changes in the cultured cells known as the cytopathic effect (CPE). Cell cultures are examined at regular intervals under low power (40–100×) for CPE. In some cases, CPE is characteristic and serves as the basis for a presumptive or even final identification of a virus isolate. For isolates that cannot be identified by CPE alone, definitive identification is accomplished using immunological tools such as immunofluorescence and ELISA.

Some viruses (influenza and parainfluenza) are better detected by hemadsorption than by CPE. During their replicative cycle, such viruses produce a glycoprotein, the hemagglutinin that is inserted into the cell membrane. Red blood cells (RBCs) added to the culture identify infected cells by adhering to the membrane bound hemagglutinin. This procedure, known as hemadsorption, is performed at periodic intervals during the incubation period.

The speed with which viruses are recovered depends on the nature of virus, the quantity of virus in the specimen, and the frequency with which cultures are read for CPE and hemadsorption. Some are recovered within the first few days of incubation, whereas others may take 10 or more days to recover. In most laboratories, the incubation period for comprehensive respiratory virus cultures ranges from 10 to 21 days (3).

IV. Antigen Detection

During the 70s and 80s, much work was done on the development and validation of methods for the detection of viral antigens in respiratory tract specimens.

Initial studies were based on the use of polyclonal antibodies raised in animals. Although results were promising, such assays were difficult to standardize because the supplies of antiserum were limited, and there was substantial lot-to-lot variation among the preparations. Fortunately, the development of monoclonal antibody–based assays resolved these difficulties and advanced the development of antigen-detection methods.

Using antigen detection, the etiology of respiratory tract infections can be established within a few hours of specimen collection and often the specialized transport conditions required for specimens intended for culture can be averted (3).

V. Immunofluorescent Antibody Staining

In the late 60s and early 70s, Gardner and McQuillan championed the use of fluorescent antibody staining (FA) for the diagnosis of respiratory tract disease (4). They demonstrated that the technology could be used to detect most respiratory viruses, and in some cases, notably in the case of respiratory syncytial virus (RSV), the sensitivity of FA approached that of culture.

Today, high-quality commercially prepared reagents are available for use in FA detection of influenza A and B, parainfluenza 1, 2, and 3, adenovirus, RSV and cytomegalovirus (CMV) (5–10). However, successful application of the technology still demands considerable technical skill and high-quality clinical specimens; that is, specimens with an ample number of well-preserved infected cells. Cells are recovered by low-speed centrifugation followed by several wash steps to remove mucous secretions. Spots of the washed cells are applied to microscope slides, air dried, and fixed with acetone. The spots are then stained either by the direct or indirect method with fluorescine conjugated antibodies. Some laboratories routinely apply a battery of antisera to the respiratory viruses, whereas others require identification of the virus or viruses sought. Stained cell spots are examined using a fluorescent microscope (3–5).

VI. Enzyme-Linked Immunosorbent Assays

The development of ELISAs for the diagnosis of respiratory virus infections paralleled the development of FA assays, and the evolution of ELISA assays was similarly advanced by monoclonal antibody technology. Initially, investigator-developed assays were done in microtiter plates, a format that restricted their use to the clinical laboratory. The microtiter assays were similar in sensitivity and specificity to FA assays, but manufacturing and regulatory complexities limited the commercial development of microtiter format ELISAs for comprehensive panels of respiratory tract pathogens. However, the clinical importance of RSV in children resulted in the development of several commercially produced laboratory-use immunoassays for this pathogen. More recently, single-test ELISA devices (STEDs), similar to those used in urine pregnancy testing, have been marketed. The U.S. Food and Drug Administration (FDA)–approved STEDs for influenza A and RSV are now available, and a STED for influenza B is now under development by at least one manufacturer. STEDs are convenient, include positive and controls, and, although originally developed for office use, they are now widely used for rapid diagnostic testing by clinical laboratories (11).

In contrast to FA, ELISAs detect soluble viral antigens in the clinical specimen. Therefore, specimens for ELISA testing are quite stable even under adverse transport conditions, since neither the integrity of cells in the specimen nor viral viability are necessary for ELISA reactivity (3).

VII. Polymerase Chain Reaction

Despite its relatively recent introduction, the PCR is already a widely used diagnostic tool. PCR is a complex reaction that results in the exponential amplification of target nucleic acid (e.g., a 100- to 500-bp fragment of viral nucleic acid) yielding approximately a billion copies of target DNA as the endproduct. Both DNA and RNA can be amplified, but to amplify RNA, a reverse transcriptase step that first creates a complementary copy of DNA must be included (RT-PCR). The product of a positive reaction, the amplified DNA, or amplicon, is then detected by any one of a number of methods. Demonstrating that the amplified product is the expected size using ethidium bromide–stained agarose gel electrophoresis is the simplest form of amplicon detection. However, most investigators prefer the added specificity that can be achieved by using DNA probes to detect the product DNA. Many probe hybridization formats are described, but to date, no single method has emerged as the method of choice (12).

Respiratory viruses are for the most part RNA viruses, therefore, RT-PCR assays must be used to detect them. Such assays now exist for almost all of the respiratory viruses, including rhinoviruses, influenza viruses, respiratory syncytial virus, parainfluenza viruses, and coronaviruses (13–18). In general, these assays appear to be more sensitive than traditional cell culture and antigen-detection methods for detecting virus in clinical specimens. However, the number of studies done to date is limited, and presently PCR detection of respiratory tract pathogens remains investigational.

Like antigen detection tests, application of PCR assays to the diagnosis of respiratory tract infections is limited by the fact that separate assays must be developed for each virus which is sought. However, in contrast to antigen-detection assays, reagents can be combined to allow detection of several pathogens in a single reaction (multiplex PCR). Thus far, there are no commercially developed PCR assays for any of the respiratory viruses, and even investigator-developed assays are only available through a limited number of research laboratories. Nevertheless, it seems likely that as PCR evolves and methods are simplified, PCR, like antigen detection, will find a place in the routine diagnosis of viral infections of the respiratory tract.

In addition to being used to detect viruses in clinical specimens, PCR is also being used as an alternative method for the identification of viral isolates. Methods for subtyping RSV, for distinguishing between rhinoviruses and enteroviruses, and for typing and subtyping influenza appear to be comparable to traditional methods and, in some cases, are more definitive (19–21). However, viral typing using PCR is presently performed only in laboratories doing research on respiratory pathogens.

VII. Serology

Traditionally, serodiagnosis is accomplished by demonstrating a fourfold or greater rise in antibody titer between serum specimens obtained during the acute and convalescent phases of a patient's illness. The greatest sensitivity is achieved when the acute phase serum is collected early during the course of the illness before the antibody response develops. Timing for collection of the convalescent serum is not as critical. Usually, a 2- to 4-week interval between the acute and convalescent phase serum specimens is recommended to assure sufficient time for an antibody titer rise to take place. However, titer rises can be demonstrated in serum specimens spaced only days apart, so if it seems unlikely that a patient will return for the convalescent phase serum, or if such a specimen cannot be obtained, testing more closely spaced serum specimens should be attempted. Serodiagnosis is by definition retrospective, but it can be useful for establishment of a diagnosis when viral isolation attempts are negative or to confirm the association of a viral isolate with disease. However, serology cannot be used to exclude a viral etiology, because, depending on the virus, the patient's age, and the serological test used, failure to detect an antibody response occurs in 30–50% of culture-documented cases of infection.

A variety of serological tests, including complement fixation (CF), hemagglutination inhibition (HI), serum neutralization (SN), indirect immunofluorescence (IF), and ELISA can be used to detect the antibody response to viral infections. However, for the diagnosis of the respiratory virus infections, there is greater experience with the complement fixation (CF) and hemagglutination (HI) tests than any others, and these tests remain the best standardized and the most widely used clinically. Crude lysates of infected cells serve as the antigen substrate for both the CF and HI tests. Antibody measured by CF tends to be broadly reactive or group specific. In contrast, HI antibody is type specific and correlates better with immunity than CF antibody. Antibody to most of the respiratory viruses can also be detected by ELISA. ELISA tests designed to measure virus-specific IgM, IgA, and IgG antibody responses, antibody to individual viral antigens, and even to synthetic peptides have been established. Although ELISA testing has refined the understanding of humoral and mucosal immunity to the respiratory viruses, criteria for interpretation of tests vary from laboratory to laboratory, limiting their diagnostic utility (3,6–10).

IX. Rhinoviruses

Rhinoviruses are a common cause of acute respiratory disease, and they cause approximately one third of all "common colds." Although most infections are relatively mild, more severe disease occasionally occurs in the elderly, possibly in immunocompromised hosts and in individuals with underlying pulmonary disease. Outbreaks tend to occur in the spring and fall (22–25) (see Chap. 10).

Currently, isolation of viruses in cell culture is the only widely available way to diagnose rhinovirus infections. Serological testing for diagnostic purposes is impractical, because there are over 1000 rhinovirus serotypes and the viruses do not hemagglutinate or share common antigens which can be detected in such tests. Unfortunately, lack of a common antigen makes the development of antigen-detection tests impossible as well (3,24). PCR tests that amplify conserved, group-specific nucleic acid sequences can be used to demonstrate rhinoviruses in clinical specimens, but their use is presently limited to research laboratories (16,19,26).

Rhinoviruses are fastidious in their growth requirements. They are best isolated in human diploid fibroblast cells incubated at 33°C. In addition, continuous rotation of infected cell cultures favors more rapid growth and development of cell rounding or typical rhinovirus CPE. In most cases, virus is isolated within 5–7 days of specimen inoculation. Rhinoviruses can also be isolated in primary monkey kidney cells and in certain strains of HeLa cells, but most laboratories rely on human diploid fibroblast cells for primary isolation (3).

The techniques used to identify viral isolates thought to be rhinoviruses differ from laboratory to laboratory. Some laboratories issue a final rhinovirus identification based solely on the typical CPE and on the growth requirements of the isolate, whereas others do additional testing. The testing required for more definitive identification includes acid lability testing (rhinoviruses are inactivated at pH 3) and lipid solubility (chloroform or ether) testing. Rhinoviruses, unlike most other respiratory viruses, do not have a lipid envelope and are stable when treated with lipid solvents. In experienced hands, identification based on CPE alone is sufficiently accurate in most cases. Specific serotyping of rhinovirus isolates can be accomplished by viral neutralization tests using intersecting pools of antisera, but such testing is rarely performed by clinical laboratories (3,24).

X. Respiratory Syncytial Virus

RSV is best known as the most important cause of bronchiolitis and pneumonia in infants and young children (27). Although RSV infection is also common in adults, it usually causes only mild upper respiratory disease. However, in certain populations, more severe disease occurs. RSV is now accepted as a common cause of upper and lower respiratory disease in the institutionalized elderly and as a cause of severe and even fatal pneumonia in immunocompromised hosts (27–31) (see Chap. 7).

Even though antigen-detection techniques play an important role in the diagnosis of RSV infections, cell culture methods are still widely used. RSV is effectively recovered in a variety of cells, including human diploid fibroblast cells, primary monkey kidney cells, and a variety of heteroploid cell lines. Among the heteroploid cells, Hep-2 cells are generally accepted as the most sensitive for viral recovery. In most cases, viral CPE in the form of large syncytial cells develops after 2 and 7 days of incubation at 36°C, but it is not unusual for it to take longer. The amount of viable virus in the specimen is an important determinant of how quickly positivity or CPE is recognized. RSV is the most labile of the respiratory viruses, so special care should be taken to assure that maximum viability is maintained during transport to the laboratory. Specimens should be inoculated into cell culture as soon as possible after collection for optimum virus recovery (27).

Rapid antigen-detection methods for the diagnosis of RSV are now provided by most large hospitals and medical centers. Several commercially developed FA and ELISA tests (STEDs and conventional) are available, and there are many published evaluations of these assays. Overall the performance characteristics of RSV antigen detection tests appear quite similar; sensitivity and specificity range from 70 to 95% and 90 to 100%, respectively (3,9,11, 32,33). However, to date, the number of studies done in adults is limited (34).

XI. Influenza Viruses

Among the respiratory viruses, the influenza viruses are recognized as the single most important cause of morbidity and mortality among adults, particularly the elderly (see Chap. 6). Secondary bacterial pneumonia is a common complication of acute infection with influenza, and this accounts for the majority of the lower respiratory tract disease associated with this virus. In comparison, primary influenza pneumonia is rare and occurs almost exclusively in young adults or children (35). Infection among the institutionalized elderly is a particular concern that often prompts diagnostic testing (36).

Isolation of influenza viruses in cell culture remains the standard against which all other diagnostic methods are measured. In the past, influenza isolation was accomplished by inoculating specimens into embryonated eggs. However, cell culture supplanted the use of eggs for diagnostic purposes when the two were found to be equally sensitive. Primary rhesus or cynomolgous monkey kidney cells are the most widely used cells for the diagnosis of influenza, because they also support the replication of a wide range of other viruses. Continuous cell lines, including LLC-MK2, GMK-AH-1, and BSC-1 cells, are equal in sensitivity to primary monkey kidney cells if trypsin is included in the culture media, and many laboratories that focus only on the recovery of influenza find these cells more convenient (3,35).

Influenza A and B both produce CPE (cell rounding) in cell culture after 2–5 days of incubation. However, hemadsorption can usually be demonstrated several days before the development of CPE. Therefore, most laboratories favor hemadsorption at regular intervals as a primary detection tool. In our laboratory, hemadsorption is performed routinely on days 3, 7, and 10 or if CPE is observed. Using this protocol, over 90% of all isolates are demonstrated by day 3. Isolates can be categorized as either influenza A or B by a variety of immunoassays. However, FA using monoclonal antibodies directed against one of the group-specific viral antigens (nucleocapsid or M protein) is the most widely used method. Identification of viral subtypes (e.g., H1N1) is based on demonstrating differences in the viral hemagglutinin using the hemagglutination-inhibition assay (35). Subtype identification is important epidemiologically but not for routine patient care purposes. Therefore, many laboratories limit viral identification to identification of isolates as A or B.

Strain-specific identification is also accomplished using the hemagglutination-inhibition assay. Isolates are tested using antisera with defined reactivity to known influenza strains. Minor differences in reactivity reflect mutations in the hemagglutinin and are called antigenic drifts. Antigenic shifts are characterized by a lack of reactivity to reagents from previously circulating strains and represent major changes in the antigenic properties of the hemagglutinin (35).

Influenza virus infections can also be detected by FA staining of exfoliated epithelial cells. Monoclonal antibodies specific for the group-specific antigens of both influenza A and B are commercially available and are widely used. A STED for influenza A is also used by many laboratories for the rapid diagnosis of infection. When compared with viral isolation, rapid tests for influenza A and B do not appear to be as sensitive as those for RSV assays. In reported studies, the sensitivity of immunoassays for influenza ranges from 50 to 90% (36–38).

XII. Parainfluenza Viruses

There are four serologically distinct human parainfluenza viruses (see Chap. 8). Parainfluenza 1 and 2 are the principal causes of laryngotracheobronchitis (croup) in infants and young children. Although parainfluenza 3 also causes croup, it is a more frequent cause of pneumonia and bronchiolitis when it infects the lower respiratory tract. Parainfluenza 4 is seldom encountered as a pathogen even in children (39). In contrast to infections in children, parainfluenza virus infections in adults are more likely to be asymptomatic or to result in only mild upper respiratory disease. However, like RSV, parainfluenza viruses are also a well-recognized cause of upper and lower respiratory tract infections in the institutionalized elderly and of severe and even fatal pneumonia in immunocompromised hosts (39–41).

Cell culture remains an important tool for the diagnosis of parainfluenza virus infections, because antigen-detection methods for parainfluenza viruses are not as well developed as they are for influenza and respiratory syncytial viruses. Primary rhesus or cynomolgus monkey kidney cells effectively recover all parainfluenza serotypes. Unfortunately, none of the more convenient, continuous cell lines that are useful for recovery of influenza viruses is effective for primary isolation of parainfluenza viruses. Replication of each parainfluenza viral serotype results in a different CPE: parainfluenza 1, cell rounding; parainfluenza 2, syncytial cell formation; parainfluenza 3, spindle cell formation; and parainfluenza 4, nonspecific degeneration. However, in most cases, viral replication is recognized earlier by hemadsorption than by CPE (3,39). In our experience, approximately 50% of parainfluenza viruses are recognized either by CPE, hemadsorption, or both within the first 5 days of incubation.

Specific viral identification must be performed after a virus is detected and cells are found to be hemadsorption positive. In the past, hemadsorption inhibition and hemagglutination inhibition tests were used to distinguish among the hemadsorbing viruses (influenza, parainfluenza, and mumps). Presently, most laboratories rely on FA using commercially prepared monoclonal antibody reagents. Cells are scraped from an infected tube and stained either with antibody to each serotype or with a pool of parainfluenza virus antibodies for type-specific and group-specific identification respectively (3,7,39).

In addition to being used for viral identification, FA is also used by some laboratories to detect virus-infected, exfoliated cells in patient specimens. In most studies, FA staining is 70–80% sensitive compared with cell culture isolation. Although investigator-developed ELISA assays for parainfluenza are described, commercial assays are not yet available (3,4,7,39,42).

XIII. Adenoviruses

Adenoviruses differ from the other respiratory viruses discussed thus far in several ways. In contrast to the other viruses, adenoviruses are unenveloped, double-stranded DNA (dsDNA) viruses that are relatively stable to environmental change. Consequently, unlike the other respiratory viruses, adenoviruses can be isolated from rectal swabs as well as respiratory tract specimens. The adenovirus group is also large, presently consisting of at least 49 distinct viral serotypes, and its disease spectrum is more diverse than that of the other respiratory viruses (see Chap. 9). As well as causing respiratory disease, adenoviruses also cause a variety of other disease syndromes, including exanthems, conjunctivitis cystitis, diarrheal disease, and even disseminated disease. Some serotypes are recognized causes of complex syndromes (e.g., respiratory disease accompanied by conjunctivitis and an exanthem), whereas others produce more restricted disease (e.g., only conjunctivitis or diarrheal disease). Although the disease spectrum of some serotypes is well characterized, others require additional definition (8).

Cell culture remains the primary means of establishing the laboratory diagnosis of adenovirus infection. Growth of adenoviruses associated with respiratory disease can be accomplished using a number of different cell types, including human embryonic kidney, HeLa, and A549. Adenovirus can also be recovered in the cells most commonly used for viral isolation, primary monkey kidney and human fibroblasts, but viral recovery in these cells is not as efficient (8,43). The CPE characteristic of adenoviruses consists of cell rounding and is often described as resembling grape-like clusters; it is generally recognized within 2–7 days of specimen inoculation. Group-specific identification of viral isolates is readily accomplished by IF using monoclonal antibody to the group-specific antigen (hexon) shared by all adenoviruses. However, serotype-specific identification is more complex. Serotyping is traditionally performed by viral neutralization or hemagglutination inhibition using type-specific antisera. Other strategies for specific typing, including genotyping, have been proposed, but none is routinely used by clinical laboratories. In fact, most laboratories provide specific serotyping of adenovirus isolates only in selected cases (8).

Like the other respiratory viruses, adenoviruses can be detected in respiratory secretions by immunodetection techniques. However, immunodetection is not as sensitive for demonstrating adenovirus infections as it is for detecting infection with the other respiratory viruses. Some laboratories offer routine testing for adenoviruses by IF on exfoliated epithelial cells, but most prefer culture for the diagnosis of adenovirus infections (3–4,8). Although commercial ELISAs are available for the diagnosis of enteric adenovirus infections, none is approved for use on respiratory tract specimens.

Adenoviruses can also be demonstrated in formalin-fixed paraffin-embedded lung specimens by conventional histology, in situ hybridization, and electron microscopy. Large basophilic inclusions known as smudge cells may be seen in infected lungs stained with hematoxylin and eosin. The characteristic morphology, size of the viral capsid, and, in some cases, the tendency of the capsids to aggregate in crystalline arrays makes adenoviruses easier to visualize by electron microscopy than many of the other respiratory viruses (44).

Type-specific as well as group-specific antibodies develop in response to adenovirus infections. Group-specific antibody tests are preferred for diagnostic purposes. Type-specific antibodies can also be detected (either by neutralization or hemagglutination inhibition assays) but require knowledge of the infecting serotype. Serological studies can be useful for establishing the diagnosis in the absence of a viral isolate and for confirming a temporal relationship between the viral infection and the patient's illness (8). This may be useful, because prolonged shedding of adenoviruses can occur.

XIV. Coronaviruses

Coronaviruses appear to account for a significant proportion of human respiratory disease (see Chap. 10). However, our understanding of this group of viruses is incomplete, because viral recovery in culture systems is extremely difficult. Some coronavirus strains can be isolated in cell culture, but others are cultivable only in organ cultures (tracheal rings or nasal epithelium). Coronaviruses can be recovered in human embryonic kidney cells and human fibroblasts, but these cells are not viewed as reliable for primary isolation of coronaviruses from clinical specimens. Viral replication in cell and organ cultures is detected by immunofluorescence and electron microscopy.

Because of the difficulties associated with viral isolation, most of the information we now have regarding the relationship between coronaviruses and respiratory disease comes from serological studies. Two serologically distinct, culture-adapted coronavirus strains, 229E and OC43, serve as the substrate for most serological assays for coronavirus. Complement fixation and hemagglutination inhibition assays are the most widely used serological tests (45). Diagnostic testing for respiratory viruses available through routine clinical laboratories does not include coronaviruses because of the difficulties involved in their cultivation and because commercial reagents are not available for serological studies.

XV. Cytomegalovirus

Cytomegalovirus pneumonia is common in the immunocompromised hosts and can occur among those experiencing recurrent infection as well as primary infection (see Chap. 5). However, those experiencing primary infection are at greatest risk for developing lower respiratory disease (10).

The diagnosis of CMV pneumonia is supported by establishing active viral infection in the host. Virus can be demonstrated in a variety of specimen types, including oral secretions, urine, sputum, BALs, and blood, but finding virus in BALs and blood is viewed as correlating best with CMV disease. However, the positive predictive value relative to disease ranges from poor to moderate depending on the patient population because of the large number of asymptomatic infections in immunocompromised hosts. In contrast, high negative predictive values can be achieved if very sensitive viral detection techniques are used. Much of the diagnostic uncertainty derives from the fact that the pathogenesis of CMV pneumonia remains poorly understood. Prophylactic therapy and preemptive therapy based on the demonstration of active infection in patients at risk for CMV pneumonia is now being advocated by many in recognition of the fact that an accurate diagnosis of CMV pneumonia cannot be achieved using currently available methods (46).

Active CMV infection can be demonstrated by a variety of methods. CMV replication in tissues and exfoliated cells is recognized by identification of the typical basophilic intranuclear and acidophilic intracytoplasmic inclusions. However, among the available methods, traditional pathological tools are by far the least sensitive. The sensitivity of tissue and cell examination for CMV can be significantly enhanced by immunostaining using monoclonal antibodies and by in situ hybridization techniques. The superiority of immunostaining and cell culture for demonstrating CMV in cells obtained by BAL and in fixed lung specimens has been demonstrated in a number of studies. Theoretically, sufficient CMV antigen is present in respiratory tract specimens to be detected by ELISA techniques as well, but technical difficulties have prevented the development of such assays (10).

Although threatened to be replaced by more rapid and sensitive methods, cell culture remains an important tool for demonstrating active infection with CMV. Specimens are inoculated into human diploid fibroblast cells (a variety of strains are used) and incubated at 36°C for 14–28 days depending on laboratory practice. In traditional tube cultures, viral replication is recognized by the development of focal cell rounding, the typical CPE of CMV.

CPE is generally recognized within 7–14 days postinoculation, but for specimens with small amounts of virus, the first observation of CPE at 21 days is not unusual. The long delays imposed by traditional culture methods led to development of a modified culture method, the shell vial assay. The shell vial assay combines cell culture with immunostaining to achieve a more rapid diagnosis. Vials containing human diploid fibroblast cells on coverslips are inoculated, centrifuged, and then incubated for 18–48 hr at 36°C. The coverslips are then removed and stained with a monoclonal antibody to CMV. Thus, results can be reported in 18–48 hr. In some laboratories, shell vial cultures are equal in sensitivity to traditional tube cultures, but others find them significantly less sensitive (10).

Viremia is being accepted with increasing frequency as the most meaningful measure of active infection in the immunocompromised host. Its increasing acceptance is based in large part on the application of two sensitive methods for detecting virus in blood, the antigenemia assay and PCR (47–49). For the antigenemia assay, leukocytes separated from whole blood are deposited on slides by cytocentrifugation. The cells are then fixed and stained with a CMV-specific monoclonal antibody. Viral antigen is found in neutrophils and mononuclear cells, and results are generally expressed as number of virus-infected cells/number examined (generally 200,000). Some investigators claim a direct relationship between the magnitude of the viremia and CMV disease, including pneumonia, but others have been unable to establish such a relationship. As well as providing same day diagnosis, antigenemia assays are more sensitive for detecting CMV in blood than traditional cell culture and shell vial assays in the hands of most investigators (48).

PCR is also gaining widespread acceptance as a tool for detecting CMV viremia. Extraction of viral DNA and treatment to remove inhibitors is the first step in the process. Amplifiable DNA can be extracted from serum, plasma, leukocyte preparations, and even whole blood. However, as yet neither specimen preparation nor PCR methods are standardized. Virtually all of the methods that are now used are investigator developed. Nevertheless, studies comparing PCR to culture invariably demonstrate approximately twofold greater sensitivity using PCR (49).

Serology is important for demonstrating titer rises and distinguishing between primary and recurrent infection; as already noted, pneumonia occurs more frequently among individuals experiencing primary infection. Serologically, primary infection is defined as conversion from seronegative to seropositive for CMV. A variety of serological assays, including latex agglutination, ELISA, and indirect fluorescent antibody assays, are used to measure antibody, and for the most part, similar results are obtained regardless of the assay used. However, to demonstrate seroconversion, it is necessary to have a serum specimen prior to the onset of illness. In many cases (transplantation, HIV$^+$

individuals), such sera are available in the laboratory. In the absence of a CMV-negative acute or preacute phase serum, IgM assays can be used to suggest primary infection. Unfortunately, IgM assays are not as reliable an indicator of primary CMV infection as seroconversion, because IgM antibody to CMV develops with some frequency during recurrent infection as well as primary infection. In addition, IgM assays vary more in sensitivity and specificity than do IgG assays. Interpreting serological findings is further complicated by the frequent use of fresh frozen plasma, transfusions, and immune globulin in the patients who most commonly experience difficulty with CMV infection (10).

XVI. Herpes Simplex

Herpes simplex virus is often isolated from the oropharynx and upper respiratory tract, but HSV is seldom implicated as a cause of lower respiratory tract disease. Although relatively uncommon, HSV pneumonia is a well-recognized complication of infection in newborns, immunocompromised hosts, burn patients, and rarely even in individuals with apparently intact immune function. In adults, infection of the lower respiratory tract appears to occur most often by direct spread of virus from the upper to the lower respiratory tract. Herpetic lesions are often observed in the oropharynx and in the tracheobronchial tree of patients with HSV pneumonia (50–52).

HSV is readily isolated in a variety of cell cultures, including human diploid fibroblasts, primary rabbit kidney cells, and primary African green monkey kidney cells. In most cases, HSV CPE is so distinctive that the experienced observer can identify the virus based solely on its growth characteristics with greater than 95% accuracy. Some laboratories issue final reports based on CPE alone, whereas others employ HSV 1- and HSV 2-specific monoclonal antibodies to identify and serotype isolates specifically. Cell culture isolation is both a sensitive and rapid means for detecting virus, and over 80% of isolates are detected within the first 2 days of incubation (52–53). Unfortunately, even if virus is isolated from bronchoscopically obtained specimens, the results may be difficult to interpret because virus is shed so commonly from the oropharynx, particularly during acute illnesses.

Cytological and histological examination of specimens from the lower respiratory tract is the best way to establish tracheobronchial and pulmonary involvement with HSV. Infection is established by demonstrating multinucleated giant cells and cells containing eosinophilic intranuclear inclusions. Although the cytological changes characteristic of HSV-infected cells are similar to those of VZV-infected cells, differentiation between HSV and VZV pneumonia is seldom a problem, since the latter rarely, if ever, occurs in the absence of typical cutaneous manifestations. Unfortunately, although finding the histological and cytological changes typical of HSV infections is specific for lower tract disease, it is relatively insensitive. Identification of typical cytopathology is often difficult, because HSV pneumonias and tracheobronchitis are frequently complicated by bacterial and fungal superinfections. Sensitivity and specificity can both be improved by the application of immunostains to the cells and tissues being examined.

XVII. Conclusion

A large and diverse group of viruses infect the respiratory tract, and many approaches can be used to detect them. To make effective use of laboratory facilities, clinicians should be familiar with the methods employed at the laboratory which they use and with the appropriate interpretations of the findings that are reported. It is likely that the use of viral diagnostic facilities will expand in the future, with further refinements in laboratory techniques and with the availability of additional therapeutic and preventive measures for respiratory viral infections.

References

1. Ahluwalia G, Embree J, McNicol P, Law B, and Hammond GW. Comparison of nasopharyngeal aspirate and nasopharyngeal swab specimens for respiratory syncytial virus diagnosis by cell culture, indirect immunofluorescence assay, and enzyme-linked immunosorbent assay. J Clin Microbiol 1987; 25:763–767.
2. Connolly MG Jr, Baughman RP, Dohn MN, Linnemann CC Jr. Recovery of viruses other than cytomegalovirus from bronchoalveolar lavage fluid. Chest 1994; 105:1775–1781.
3. Atmar RL, Englund JA. Laboratory methods for the diagnosis of viral diseases. In: Evans AS, Kaslow RA, eds. Viral Infections of Humans. 4th ed. New York: Plenum, 1997:59–88.
4. Gardner PS, McQuillan J. Rapid Viral Diagnosis: Application of Immunofluorescence. 2nd ed. London: Butterworth, 1980.
5. Khairulla NS, Lam SK. Evaluation of WHO monoclonal antibody kit for diagnosis of acute respiratory viral infections. Southeast Asian J Trop Med Public Health 1995; 26:263–267.
6. Ziegler T, Katz JM, Cox NJ, Regnery HL. Influenza viruses. In: Rose NR, Conway de Macario E, Folds JD, Lane HC, Nakamura RM, eds. Manual of Clinical Laboratory Immunology. 5th ed. Washington, DC: ASM Press, 1997:673–678.
7. Waner, JL. Parainfluenza viruses. In: Rose NR, Conway de Macario E, Folds JD, Lane HC, Nakamura RM, eds. Manual of Clinical Laboratory Immunology. 5th ed. Washington, DC: ASM Press, 1997:926–931.

8. Hierholzer JC. Adenoviruses. In: Rose NR, Conway de Macario E, Folds JD, Lane HC, Nakamura RM, eds. Manual of Clinical Laboratory Immunology. 5th ed. Washington, DC: ASM Press, 1997:947–955.
9. Tristram DA, Welliver RC. Respiratory syncytial virus. In: Rose NR, Conway de Macario E, Folds JD, Lane HC, Nakamura RM, eds. Manual of Clinical Laboratory Immunology. 5th ed. Washington, DC: ASM Press, 1997:932–939.
10. Gershon AA, Gold E, Nankervis GA. Cytomegalovirus. In: Evans AS, Kaslow RA, eds. Viral Infections of Humans. 4th ed. New York: Plenum, 1997:229–251.
11. Todd SJ, Minnich L, Waner JL. Comparison of rapid immunofluorescence procedure with TestPack RSV and Directigen Flu-A for diagnosis of respiratory syncytial virus and influenza A virus. J Clin Microbiol 1995; 33:1650–1651.
12. Tang Y, Procop GW, Persing DH. Molecular diagnostics of infectious diseases. Clin Chem 1997; 43:2021–2038.
13. Fan J, Hendrickson KJ. Rapid diagnosis of human parainfluenza virus type 1 infection by quantitative reverse transcription–PCR–enzyme hybridization assay. J Clin Microbiol 1996; 34:1914–1917.
14. Akhtar N, Ni J, Langston C, Demmler GJ, Towbin JA. PCR diagnosis of viral pneumonia from fixed-lung tissue in children. Biochem Mol Med 1996; 58:66–76.
15. Atmar RL, Baxter BD, Dominguez EA, Taber LH. Comparison of reverse transcription–PCR with tissue culture and other rapid diagnostic assays for detection of type A influenza virus. J Clin Microbiol 1996; 34:2604–2606.
16. Ireland DC, Kent J, Nicholson KG. Improved detection of rhinoviruses in nasal and throat swabs by seminested RT-PCR. J Med Virol 1993; 40:96–101.
17. Donofrio JC, Coonrod JD, Davidson JN, Betts RF. Detection of influenza A and B in respiratory secretions with the polymerase chain reaction. PCR Methods Appl 1992; 1:263–268.
18. Zhang WD, Evans DH. Detection and identification of human influenza viruses by the polymerase chain reaction. J Virol Methods 1991; 33:165–189.
19. Olive DM, Al-Mufti S, Khan MA, Pasca A, Stanway G, Al-Nakib W. Detection and differentiation of picornaviruses in clinical samples following genomic amplification. J Gen Virol 1990; 71:2141–2147.
20. Atmar RL, Baxter BD. Typing and subtyping clinical isolates of influenza virus using reverse transcription–polymerase chain reaction. Clin Diagn Virol 1996; 7: 77–84.
21. Wright KE, Wilson GA, Novosad D, Dimock C, Tan D, Weber JM. Typing and subtyping of influenza viruses in clinical samples by PCR. J Clin Microbiol 1995; 33:1180–1184.
22. Wald TG, Shult P, Krause P, Miller BA, Drinka P, Gravenstein S. A rhinovirus outbreak among residents of a long-term care facility. Ann Intern Med 1995; 123: 588–593.
23. Nicholson KG, Kent J, Hammersley V, Cancio E. Risk factors for lower rre complications of rhinovirus infections in elderly people living in the community: prospective cohort study. Br Med J 1996; 313:1119–1123.
24. Levandowski RA. Rhinoviruses. In: Belshe RB, ed. Textbook of Human Virology. 2nd ed. St. Louis: Mosby-Year Book, 1991:412–426.

25. Falsey AR, McCann RM, Hall WJ, Criddle MM, Formica MA, Wycoff D, Kolassa JE. The "common cold" in frail older persons: impact of rhinovirus and coronavirus in a senior daycare center. J Am Geriatr Soc 1997; 45(6):706–711.
26. Johnston SL, Sanderson G, Pattemore PK, Smith S, Vardin PG, Bruce CB, Lambden PR, Tyrrell DAJ, Holgate ST. Use of the polymerase chain reaction for picornavirus infection in subjects with and without respiratory symptoms. J Clin Microbiol 1993; 31:111–117.
27. McIntosh K. Respiratory Syncytial Virus. In: Evans AS, Kaslow RA, eds. Viral Infections of Humans. 4th ed. New York: Plenum, 1997:691–705.
28. Dowell SF, Anderson LJ, Gary HE Jr, Erdman DD, Plouffe JF, File TM Jr, Marston BJ, Breiman RF. Respiratory syncytial virus is an important cause of community-acquired lower respiratory infection among hospitalized adults. J Infect Dis 1996; 174:456–462.
29. Falsey AR, Cunningham CK, Barker WH, Kouides RW, Yuen JB, Menegus M, Weiner LB, Bonville CA, Betts RF. Respiratory syncytial virus and influenza A infections in the hospitalized elderly. J Infect Dis 1995; 172:389–394.
30. Englund JA, Sullivan CJ, Jordan MC, Dehner LP, Vercellotti GM, Balfuor HH Jr. Respiratory syncytial virus in immunocompromised adults. Ann Intern Med 1988; 109:203–208.
31. Harrington RD, Hooton RM, Hackman RC, Storch GA, Osborne B, Gelves CA, Benson A, Meyers JD. An outbreak of respiratory syncytial virus in a bone marrow transplant center. J Infect Dis 1992; 165:987–989.
32. Kellog JA. Culture vs. direct antigen assays for the detection of microbial pathogens from lower respiratory tract specimens suspected of containing the respiratory syncytial virus. Arch Pathol Lab Med 1991; 115:451–458.
33. Dominguez EA, Taber LH, Couch RB. Comparison of rapid diagnostic techniques for respiratory syncytial and influenza A virus respiratory infections in young children. J Clin Microbiol 1993; 31:2286–2290.
34. Falsey AR, McCann RM, Hall WJ, Criddle MM. Evaluation of four methods for the diagnosis of respiratory syncytial virus infection in older adults. J Am Geriatr Soc 1996; 44(1):71–73.
35. Glezen WP, Couch RB. Influenza Viruses. In: Evans AS, Kaslow RA, eds. Viral Infections of Humans. 4th ed. New York: Plenum, 1997:473–505.
36. Leonardi GP, Leib H, Birkhead GS, Smith C, Costello P, Conron W. Comparison of rapid detection methods for influenza A virus and their value in health-care management of institutionalized geriatric patients. J Clin Microbiol 1994; 32: 70–74.
37. Reina J, Munar M, Blanco I. Evaluation of a direct immunofluorescence assay, dot-blot enzyme immunoassay, and shell vial culture in the diagnosis of lower respiratory tract infections caused by influenza A virus. Diagn Microbiol Infect Dis 1996; 25:143–145.
38. Waner JL, Todd SJ, Shalaby H, Murphy P, Wall LV. Comparison of Directigen Flu-A with viral isolation and direct immunofluorescence for the rapid detection and identification of influenza A virus. J Clin Microbiol 1991; 29:479–482.
39. Glezen WP, Denny FW. Parainfluenza Viruses. In: Evans AS, Kaslow RA, eds. Viral Infections of Humans. 4th ed. New York: Plenum, 1997:551–567.

40. Wenzel RP, McCormick DP, Beam WE Jr. Parainfluenza pneumonia in adults. JAMA 1972; 221:294–295.
41. Wendt CH, Weisdorf DJ, Jordan MC, Balfor HH. Parainfluenza virus respiratory infection after bone marrow transplantation. N Engl J Med 1992; 326:921–926.
42. Grandien M, Petterson CA, Gardner PS, Linde A, Stanton A. Rapid viral diagnosis of acute respiratory infections: comparison of enzyme-linked immunosorbent assay and the immunofluorescent technique for detection of viral antigens in nasopharyngeal secretions. J Clin Microbiol 1985; 22:757–760.
43. Krisher KK, Menegus MA. Evaluation of three types of cell culture for recovery of adenovirus from clinical specimens. J Clin Microbiol 1987; 25:1323–1324.
44. Weiss LM, Movahed LA, Berry GJ, Billingham ME. In situ hybridization studies for viral nucleic acids in heart and lung allograft biopsies. Am J Clin Pathol 1990; 93:714–716.
45. Monto AS. Coronaviruses. In: Evans AS, Kaslow RA, eds. Viral Infections of Humans. 4th ed. New York: Plenum, 1997:211–227.
46. Hibberd PL, Snydman DR. Cytomegalovirus infection in organ transplant recipients. Infect Dis Clin North Am 1995; 9:863–877.
47. Abecassis MM, Koffron AJ, Kaplan B, Buckingham M, Muldoon JP, Cribbins AJ, Kaufman DB, Fryer JP, Stuart J, Stuart FP. Role of PCR in the diagnosis and management of CMV in solid organ recipients: what is the predictive value for the development of disease and should PCR be used to guide antiviral therapy? Transplant Proc 1996; 28:2–4.
48. The TH, van den Berg AP, Harmsen MC, van der Bij W, van Son WJ. The cytomegalovirus antigenemia assay: a plea for standardization. Scand J Infect Dis 1995; 99:25–29.
49. Gerna G, Baldanti F, Zella D, Furione M. Detection of human cytomegalovirus DNA: how, when, and where? Scand J Infect Dis 1995; 99(suppl):11–15.
50. Nash G. Necrotizing tracheobronchitis and bronchopneumonia consistent with herpetic infection. Hum Pathol 1972; 3:283.
51. Graham BS, Snell JD. Herpes simplex virus infection of the adult lower respiratory Ramsey PF, Fife KH, Hackman RC, Meyers JD, Corey L. Herpes simplex virus pneumonia. Ann Intern Med 1982; 97:813–820.
52. Stanberry LR, Jorgensen DM, Nahmias AJ. Herpes simplex viruses 1 and 2. In: Evans AS, Kaslow RA, eds. Viral Infections of Humans. 4th ed. New York: Plenum, 1997:419–446.
53. Stewart J. Herpes simplex virus. In: Rose NR, Conway de Macario E, Folds JD, Lane HC, Nakamura RM, eds. Manual of Clinical Laboratory Immunology. 5th ed. Washington, DC: ASM Press, 1997:625–630.

Part Four

TREATMENT

13

Therapy of Viral Respiratory Infections

ARNOLD S. MONTO

School of Public Health
University of Michigan
Ann Arbor, Michigan

I. Introduction

Although antimicrobial therapy has been widely used for bacterial respiratory infections over the last half century, antiviral therapy has been limited to a small number of drugs and types of infections. This situation reflects the difficulty encountered in developing effective and safe interventions to inhibit viral growth, yet not injure important cellular activities. This discussion of drugs and other methods to treat respiratory infections will focus on influenza, respiratory syncytial viral diseases, and the hantavirus pulmonary syndrome. These are the major respiratory viral infections for which specific antiviral therapies are available or are being evaluated. In some cases, drugs and other therapeutic approaches are useful in both prophylaxis and therapy, and both applications will be discussed in this chapter.

II. Amantadine and Rimantadine

A. Development and Introduction

These related compounds, amantadine and rimantadine, were both developed by the E.I. Dupont de Nemours Company (Wilmington, Delaware). Amantadine (1-aminoadamantane hydrochloride) was evaluated first, and it was found to prevent infection with type A influenza in the early 1960s (1). Early studies indicated that the in vivo effect of the compound was highly specific. There was in vitro activity against type B influenza, parainfluenza viruses types 2 and 3, respiratory syncytial virus, and rubella, as well as against influenza virus types A(H1N1) and A(H2N2). However, at concentrations achievable in humans, activity was restricted to type A influenza viruses and possibly rubella (2,3). Studies in humans of amantadine prophylaxis of type A(H2N2) influenza were at first limited to experimental challenge with attenuated strains, which quickly determined that the drug was efficacious and appeared to be safe (4–6). As a result, amantadine was approved for limited use in the prophylaxis of influenza type A(H2N2) in the fall of 1966. Thereafter, the drug's safety and efficacy was challenged by Albert B. Sabin in a "Special Communication" published in the *Journal of the American Medical Association* of June, 1967, which was answered in August 1967 by a statement by the American Medical Association's Council on Drugs (7,8). The main concerns were the potential of unacceptable side effects and the possibility of the emergence of strains resistant to the drug. Interestingly, it is these issues which have continued to raise concerns, and they have affected the broader use of amantadine (9). Sabin also raised the question of the lack of appropriate field trials to confirm the prophylactic efficacy of the drug, which was a deficiency that was shortly rectified (10,11). Finally, the potential for the inappropriate use was raised because of the difficulty in making a specific diagnosis of influenza based on clinical characteristics alone compared with the characteristic clinical picture of measles or polio myelitis, for example (12).

This earlier controversy regarding amantadine was compounded in 1968, 2 years after its licensure for type A(H2N2), when the type A(H3N2) influenza pandemic began. Based on the demonstration in cell culture that the new variant was as sensitive to amantadine as type A(H2N2), DuPont issued a press release suggesting the use of the drug in the pandemic. The U.S. Food and Drug Administration (FDA) objected because of the absence of any clinical studies, and the company was required to so notify all American physicians in a "Dear Doctor" letter. It was not until 1976 that the FDA accepted data indicating that amantadine would be effective against all type A subtypes. This meant that when type A(H1N1) viruses returned in 1977–1978, its use in that setting was an approved indication (13).

The hiatus in approved usage which followed the appearance of type A (H3N2) viruses in 1968 until 1976, when amantadine was approved for use against all influenza A strains, would ordinarily have resulted in its disappearance from the American commercial scene. However, it had been discovered, almost by chance, that amantadine controlled some symptoms of Parkinson's disease, and its use for this indication continued (14,15). During this period,

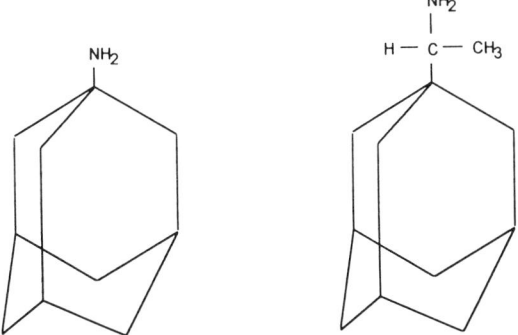

Figure 1 The chemical structures of amantadine (left) and rimantadine (right).

experimental studies on amantadine prophylaxis and therapy for type A influenza proceeded, especially in Europe (16,17). In addition, a related drug, rimantadine, was selected by the former Soviet Union in 1969 as the antiviral of choice after both amantadine and rimantadine had been extensively evaluated (18,19). This established a pattern which continued until 1993, in which rimantadine was used exclusively in the former Soviet Union and amantadine was used in certain other countries, especially the United States. From the start, the Russian investigators stressed their view that rimantadine was less likely to produce side effects than amantadine (19).

B. Structure and Activity

The amantadine compounds are stable, colorless, crystalline amines with an unusual symmetrical structure, as shown in Figure 1. Both have a large carbon ring (the adamantyl cage) and a primary amine. In amantadine, the amine is directly linked to the cage, but in rimantadine (α-methyl-1-adamantane methylamine hydrochloride), the amine is separated by a branched side chain which provides a center of asymmetry. In cell culture assays, both drugs inhibit type A strains at relatively low concentrations, with rimantadine being slightly more active on a weight basis. This difference is more pronounced in favor of rimantadine in organ culture (24,25).

Although the pharmacokinetics of these two drugs are very different, and result in different side effects, other characteristics are similar. Neither amantadine nor rimantadine prevent absorption of the virus to cells or viral penetration, as was originally thought. Rather the effects are complex and appear to take place at two points in viral replication (20). The early effect is still not fully defined, and it occurs prior to the onset of viral transcription through inhibition of viral uncoating. The late effect is of importance with only certain type A viruses, and it appears to be a direct consequence of specific changes in the structure of the viral hemagglutinin (21). Interaction of drug with the M2 protein is critical in terms of the antiviral action of both rimantadine and amantadine, and it appears to be related to both early and late effects. The best evidence for this comes from the association of M2 amino acid substitutions with the development of resistance to both drugs (22). The M2 protein forms a transmembrane channel across the membrane of normally acidic cellular vesicles (23). Amantadine and rimantadine block the normal acidic flux through this ion channel. The position of the amino acid substitutions which produce resistance is consistent with this explanation.

C. Pharmacokinetics

There are major differences in the metabolism of amantadine and rimantadine which may explain differences in side effects, such as those related to the central nervous system. Both drugs are administered orally as HCl salts and are well absorbed from the gastrointestinal tract, although the process can sometimes be slow (26). There is also experience with aerosol administration, but there is no preparation available for parenteral administration (27,28). After a single oral dose of amantadine, plasma peak levels are achieved in 2–4 hr. With rimantadine, peak levels are reached in 3–6 hr. The half-life of rimantadine is much longer (37 hr) than amantadine (17 hr). These differences are in part related to the volume of distribution of rimantadine, which is twice as large as that of amantadine. For the same dose, the peak levels of amantadine are nearly twice as high as those of rimantadine, but the concentration of rimantadine in nasal mucus is approximately 50% higher than that of amantadine. These differences have led to debates as to whether the two drugs should be compared at the same dosage, which has typically been the case (29–31).

The most profound difference between the drugs relates to metabolism and excretion. Amantadine is mainly excreted unchanged by renal tubular secretion. Rimantadine is extensively metabolized by the liver, with up to 90% excreted in the form of hydroxylated and conjugated metabolites, some of which possess antiviral activity. Only 2–20% of rimantadine is excreted unchanged. This has resulted in more concern about the use of amantadine in patients with decreased renal function, which likely accounts for the occurrence of side effects, especially in older individuals (31–34). For amantadine, the Advisory Committee on Immunization Practices (ACIP) of the U.S. Public

Table 1 Dosage for Prophylaxis and Treatment of Uncomplicated Influenza A in Those with Impaired Renal Function

Creatinine clearance (mL/min/1.73 m^2)	Amantadine dosage[a]
30–50	100 mg every day
15–29	100 mg every other day
<15	100 mg every 7 days

[a]After 200-mg loading dose.

Health Service has recommended that the dosage be reduced in patients with decreased kidney function. Table 1 shows the current recommendation for dosage reduction based on the level of creatinine clearance. It should only be employed as a guide, since results were based on small sample sizes (35). Reduction in rimantadine dosage for hepatic or renal disease is also recommended, but is not based on a specific schedule. The dosage of both compounds was empirically recommended to be reduced by half in all elderly patients in nursing homes, which was predicated on the decrease in creatinine clearance which is generally found in this population. In fact, the documented accumulation of rimantadine seen in the elderly would not have been predicted by single-dose pharmacokinetic studies, and thus it may be best correlated to the overall condition of the patients (36–38). Drug interactions have been more systematically evaluated with rimantadine than amantadine, partially because of its extensive metabolism (39). In a single dose study, plasma concentrations of rimantadine were consistently higher by 15–20% when cimetidine, a known inhibitor of hepatic oxidative drug-metabolizing enzymes, was coadministered. However, it was felt that these interactions were of little clinical significance, as was also the case with aspirin and acetaminophen.

D. Prophylaxis

Although the prophylactic efficacy of amantadine had been evaluated earlier in several small-scale studies, the pivotal investigation was conducted in University of Michigan students in the first outbreak of the reemergent type A (H1N1) viruses in 1978 (13). A similar pivotal study conducted in University of Vermont students in 1981 also compared rimantadine's prophylactic effect to that of amantadine or placebo (40). Both will be considered together, since the methodology and analytic design were similar. The Michigan study, lasting 6 weeks, was begun in the face of the influenza outbreak, which had begun

Table 2 Protective Efficacy of Antivirals Against Laboratory-Confirmed Clinical Influenza

Site and subtype	Efficacy (%)	Significance
Michigan[a]		
type A(H1N1)		
amantadine	71	$P < .001$
Vermont[b]		
types A(H3N2) and A(H1N1)		
amantadine	91	$P < .001$
rimantadine	85	

[a]*Source*: Ref. 13.
[b]*Source*: Ref. 40.

explosively, since type A(H1N1) virus possessed hemagglutinin and neuraminidase antigens which were new for this younger population. Amantadine was administered at 200 mg per day, and the first statistically significant difference in rates of illness between drug and placebo groups was seen 2 days after the onset of prophylaxis. As shown in Table 2, amantadine was 70% effective in preventing laboratory-confirmed clinical influenza (cough and two other respiratory symptoms). Laboratory confirmation of infection required a rise in antibody titer and/or viral isolation. When overall frequencies of rises in antibody titers were compared in individuals on drug with those on placebo, it was found that the drug efficacy was only 40%. This indicated that amantadine was more effective in preventing symptomatic compared with asymptomatic infection. If infection alone was used as an endpoint, as has sometimes been the case, the extent of the drug's effectiveness would be underestimated.

The Vermont study involved three groups of participants. Rimantadine and amantadine were both administered at doses of 200 mg per day, and the third arm was placebo. The major endpoint again was laboratory-confirmed clinical influenza, and the circulating viruses were A(H3N2) and A(H1N1). Type A(H1N1) predominated. As shown in Table 2, the efficacy of amantadine and rimantadine were similar—91 and 85%, respectively. The increased efficacy over the prior Michigan study may have been related to the fact that the Vermont population had some prior experience with the circulating strains, and it was thus not experiencing initial infection with a new subtype. The efficacies of the drugs in preventing symptomatic and asymptomatic infection were 74 and 66%, respectively, which again indicates that these drugs prevent clinical influenza more effectively than subclinical or inapparent infection. This is paradoxically an advantageous situation. With complete protection against infection, there would be no antibody that would persist after an outbreak to protect against subsequent infection.

Many other studies have confirmed the efficacy of both drugs in prophylaxis (41–44). Much of the similarity in results stems from the use of clear, well-defined endpoints: prevention of infection or disease. The investigations performed before the Michigan study are sometimes difficult to interpret, since many used experimental challenge, often with attenuated viruses. The number of subjects employed in several studies were too small for clear conclusions. In some studies, the illness rates were too low to provide firm estimates of efficacy, and only infection data were compared. Some studies addressed specific issues; for example, the use of amantadine to prevent nosocomial transmission of influenza during a community outbreak (45). Recent studies have addressed the issue of optimal dosage and evaluated the possibility of reducing the dosage from 200 to 100 mg per day. The reduction of dosage would have the advantage of reducing possible side effects, although it raises questions about the effect of missed doses in long-term use. These studies, some of which have suffered from low attack rates, have suggested that such a reduction in dosage does not reduce prophylactic efficacy (46,47).

Of particular interest are investigations which evaluated the use of antivirals in the family setting. The approach here had two objectives: (1) limitation of prophylaxis to a short period of exposure, unlike seasonal prophylaxis which might extend over an entire influenza outbreak; and (2) treatment of the first, or index, case in the family in addition to prophylaxis against disease in other family members. Two studies of Galbraith are among the earliest to employ this strategy (48,49). They have recently become the subject of renewed scrutiny, since the results differed. Amantadine was effective in prophylaxis during the first trial when the circulating virus was type A(H2N2), but it was not significantly protective in the second trial when A(H3N2) virus circulated. The investigators cited the absence of antibody against the novel H3N2 virus in the second trial as the explanation for apparent failure of the antiviral in prophylaxis, since relevant antibody was not present to provide additional protection. After recognition that antiviral resistance can occur quickly in therapy, it was appreciated that index cases were treated in the second study, whereas they were not treated in the first study. Thus a potential explanation for the failure of prophylaxis in the second study is that resistant virus was transmitted. Other examinations of the use of amantadine or rimantadine in the family setting have been more successful. Clover et al. used rimantadine in the prophylaxis of type A(H1N1) influenza in children with the aim of preventing both influenza in the recipients of drug and subsequent transmission to adults in the family (50). In the direct prophylaxis of infection in children, the drug was remarkably effective (90%), and there was also a trend toward indirect protection of the parents not on the drug. Similar, although less dramatic, results in a subsequent study confirmed the efficacy of rimantadine in the prophylaxis of children and also suggested that transmission to parents was reduced (51). A problem in approaches to the reduction of secondary transmission within families by administration of antivirals is that a substantial portion of new infections are introduced from contacts outside the family by infections in the community. Thus, even under the best of circumstances, indirect protection of other family members is not nearly as effective as direct protection (52).

E. Use in Treatment

Amantadine was demonstrated to affect symptoms of type A influenza illnesses at approximately the same time as it was recognized to be effective in prophylaxis (53–56). However, acceptance of the value of amantadine, and then rimantadine, as therapy for type A influenza took much longer than acceptance for prophylaxis. A large part of the problem relates to the endpoints which must be used in treatment studies. In prophylactic evaluations, infection or illness is either prevented or not; in treatment, the resolution of symptoms is more subjective, and this has been one of the reasons for an apparent inconsistency in therapeutic trials. Another issue involves characteristics of illness at time of recruitment into studies. The major sign of illness which can be evaluated is fever. However, it has often proven difficult to recruit individuals with high enough fever so that its decline can be used as an indicator of the efficacy of treatment. This, and the difficulty in controlling for differences in the severity of illness at the time of entry into the study likely contributed to the inconsistency in early results. Gradually data were produced which quantified the value of these drugs in therapy. One of the more definitive studies was conducted in 45 young adults infected in a type A(H1N1) outbreak in 1978 (56). Those on rimantadine and amantadine exhibited significantly faster resolution of fever. Symptom scores were reduced by 50% within 48 hr in treated individuals, whereas it took approximately 72 hr in individuals who received placebo. There was a reduction in viral shedding and a more rapid return to normal activity in those who received drug. Similar results were obtained comparing rimantadine to placebo in an A(H3N2) outbreak. There was also a statistically significant reduction in viral shedding by day 2 in that study (57).

Another important question was whether treatment with an antiviral offered greater relief than that provided by symptomatic therapy. This issue was resolved by another study in young adults with influenza A (H1N1) infection who were treated with the antiviral or with aspirin or placebo. As might be expected from the observation that it took 48 hr for amantadine to reduce symptoms by 50% in the above studies, aspirin was superior to amantadine in the first part of the illness, since its symptomatic effect was rapid. However, the antiviral was clearly superior in a more rapid resolution of the overall illness, demonstrating a difference between symptomatic and specific therapy

(58). An additional potential advantage of using an antiviral was demonstrated in a study involving the treatment of type A(H3N2) influenza with amantadine. This subtype of influenza has been found to cause transient abnormalities in small airway functions even in previously healthy adults. When delivered by aerosol, amantadine produced a more rapid resolution of such abnormalities (59). These observations indicate that the antiviral drug has a much more profound effect on the course of influenzal infection than simple reduction in bothersome symptoms. There are no data as to whether this beneficial effect will extend to cases of severe pulmonary complications of influenza, such as primary influenzal pneumonia. Studies to examine this question systematically have not been successful in the recruitment of adequate sample sizes. As a result, the clinical benefit, if any, of amantadine in the treatment of pulmonary complications of influenza is not established. Since these events generally occur late in the course of influenza, the value of an inhibitor of viral replication is open to question.

Children experience the highest frequency of influenzal infection and illness. Only a few studies have examined the question of whether antivirals have a role in the treatment of influenza in children. The most comprehensive investigation compared the use of rimantadine with acetaminophen in the treatment of influenza in children (60,61). As in adults, there was reduction in viral shedding, fever, and symptoms in children treated with rimantadine when compared not with placebo but with antipyretic analgesic therapy. In children, influenza generally lasts longer than in adults, and it is associated with longer viral shedding, so that the effect of an antiviral might be expected to be more profound. An unexpected finding, not associated with a return in symptoms, was a rebound in shedding of virus late in the illness in some of the rimantadine-treated children (60). The emergence of viruses resistant to the antiviral drug was subsequently recognized as the explanation for the return of viral shedding in some of the rimantadine-treated children (62).

F. Drug Resistance

The existence of drug-resistant viral variants of type A influenza has been recognized for many years (9). It has been estimated to occur naturally in a small proportion of both cell culture and egg-grown cultures. The resistant virus can be selected by passage in the presence of antiviral agents. Viruses resistant to either of the two drugs are resistant to the other. The fact that resistant viruses occur naturally and can be easily selected in vitro explains the rapid emergence of resistant viruses in some individuals during treatment. The genetic basis for resistance has been well defined and relates to the mechanism of action of the drugs. Reassortment studies have confirmed that changes in the M2 protein are responsible for amantadine and rimantadine resistance (63,64). These point mutations in the sequence of gene segment 7 result in substitutions of amino acids 26, 27, 30, 31, or 34 of the M2 protein. Different amino acid changes have been recognized at certain positions (20, 21). Because these changes can be tracked from one infected individual to another, it has become possible to follow the likely spread of resistant viruses. However, this tracking is not absolute, since some substitutions are more common than others and emergence of resistant variants rather than transmission can occur.

Resistant viruses usually emerge with treatment rather than with prophylaxis. They emerge with regularity, as would be predicted from in vitro observations. It is clear that, at least over the short term, resistant viruses can be transmitted and are pathogenic (65,66,67). In these properties, they do not appear to differ from sensitive strains. When surveillance of isolates is carried out, there is also no evidence that the proportion of resistant strains is increasing over time (68). This may indicate that these drugs have not been used sufficiently long or extensively for resistance to have reached a detectable level in surveillance of the general population. Alternatively, it may be that there is a competitive disadvantage to resistant virus in the absence of drug, since resistant variants exist naturally in a low proportion to sensitive ones. There is no evidence at present either to support or deny this hypothesis. There are ongoing surveillance programs in the United States to detect whether there is an increase in the frequency of naturally occurring resistant viruses. These programs use an enzyme-linked immunoassay (EIA) first to identify the isolates which are sensitive or resistant. The isolates are then genotyped, taking advantage of the point mutations in the M2 protein as the genotypic correlate of resistance.

G. Side Effects

Although the antiviral activities of the two drugs are similar, the pharmacokinetics are different, which probably accounts for major differences in reactogenicity (69). The differences are most apparent in prophylactic studies, in which healthy individuals take drug for long periods of time. In the 1978 study of seasonal prophylaxis, 8% of participants on amantadine withdrew, compared with 2% of placebo participants, for a reaction rate attributable to the drug of 6% (13). In the 1981 study, withdrawal rates for those on rimantadine were similar to those on placebo, whereas again amantadine produced an excess dropout rate in the study (41). Most of these withdrawals occurred early in the first week of prophylaxis. Various symptoms were reported, but they mainly involved central nervous system complaints such as jitteriness, insomnia, and difficulty in concentrating. Other studies have shown less difference between amantadine and placebo, although one small study showed a possible interaction between amantadine and the antihistamine chlorpheniramine during psychomotor testing (70).

The clearest and most dramatic occurrence of side effects has been reported in the elderly, and it is in that population in which the difference between the drugs may be most important. A study of seasonal prophylaxis in nursing home elderly did not demonstrate any difference between rimantadine and placebo in central nervous system reactions, but gastrointestinal symptoms were more frequent in patients taking the drug (71). In contrast, up to 33% of recipients of amantadine have reported adverse reactions, which were primarily a wide variety of neurological signs and symptoms, including hallucinations, visual disturbances, tremors, and convulsions (72–73). Precise estimates of rates of side effects are difficult to obtain, since many observations were not placebo-controlled but were based simply on the presence of an event at the time when amantadine was being taken. In addition, amantadine was used initially at a higher concentration than is now recommended for older individuals, since the effect of reduced renal clearance in this group was not appreciated. The use of rimantadine afforded a way to reduce the frequency and related concerns regarding central nervous system side effects, such as unsteadiness, and resultant falls in the elderly. Both gastrointestinal and central nervous system events have been described, but often not in sufficient frequency to be of statistical significance in small studies (74). Rarely, severe and even fatal events have been reported in patients on these drugs, but their causal relationship, potential interactions with other medications, and relationship to underlying disease has not been established (75).

H. Recommendations for Use

Because of the use of amantadine and rimantadine in both prophylaxis and therapy, and the issues of resistance and side effects, particular attention must be given to practical approaches to utilization. There is greatest consensus in managing illness in the institutionalized elderly (76). Outbreaks occur in spite of high vaccination rates, and antivirals are recommended for both therapy and prophylaxis in all nursing home residents. This means that the particular drug is in use simultaneously for both prophylaxis and therapy, a situation which has been documented sometimes to result in the emergence and transmission of resistant viruses (78). However, this phenomenon does not appear to have affected the ability of the drugs to terminate rapidly type A outbreaks in most cases. There has been discussion concerning the need for strict isolation of individuals who are ill and on drug. Standard practice for the control of outbreaks in institutions would encourage as much separation as possible of ill individuals from well individuals whether they are on antiviral drug or not. Since vaccine is not as protective in the frail elderly as in younger individuals, consideration can be given to the provision of chemoprophylaxis to nursing home residents before an outbreak occurs in an institution but after viral transmission has been documented in the community. This would be carried out in addition to standard vaccination programs (75). There is substantial evidence that amantadine and rimantadine provide significant added protection to the vaccinated elderly. Questions which need to be evaluated in terms of such prophylactic use would be the cost of such a program and the added likelihood of side effects when large numbers of older individuals are given another drug on a long-term basis and are already on many medications.

For younger individuals, there are fewer issues involving indications for use. Seasonal prophylaxis is an option for persons who decide not to be vaccinated. Vaccination is an absolute recommendation only for those younger persons with chronic conditions, although it may be taken by anyone wishing to prevent infection. Many individuals may wish to be vaccinated and to use the antiviral for 2 weeks thereafter while protective antibodies are developing. This strategy can be employed in the face of an outbreak when rapid protection is desired and is particularly appropriate for individuals in a "high-risk group." Antiviral treatment of adults and in some cases children can be considered whether or not there are preexisting conditions. As indicated above, specific therapy is better than symptomatic therapy, and it should not be restricted to the chronically ill. One area of concern is the use of combined prophylaxis and therapy in the family unit, where development of resistance has been shown to occur. If there is a high-risk person in the family, cases in other family members should probably not be treated because of the risk of transmission of resistant virus to the high-risk individual.

III. Ribavirin

A. Mechanism of Action

In contrast to amantadine and rimantadine, which have a narrow spectrum of antiviral activity, ribavirin has broad activity against some DNA and many RNA viruses, including influenza and respiratory syncytial virus. Unlike rimantadine and amantadine, ribavirin (L-beta-D-ribofuranosyl-1,2,4 triazole-3-carboxamide) inhibits several steps of viral replication. As shown in Figure 2, it is a nucleoside analogue which is related in structure to guanosine (79,80). Its activity in vitro can be abolished in some, but not all, cases by the addition of guanosine or related components to the medium. The mechanisms of action include inhibition of the function of RNA polymerases which are required for the formation of messenger RNA, inhibition of 5' capping of viral messenger RNA, and reduction of pools of cellular guanosine triphosphate

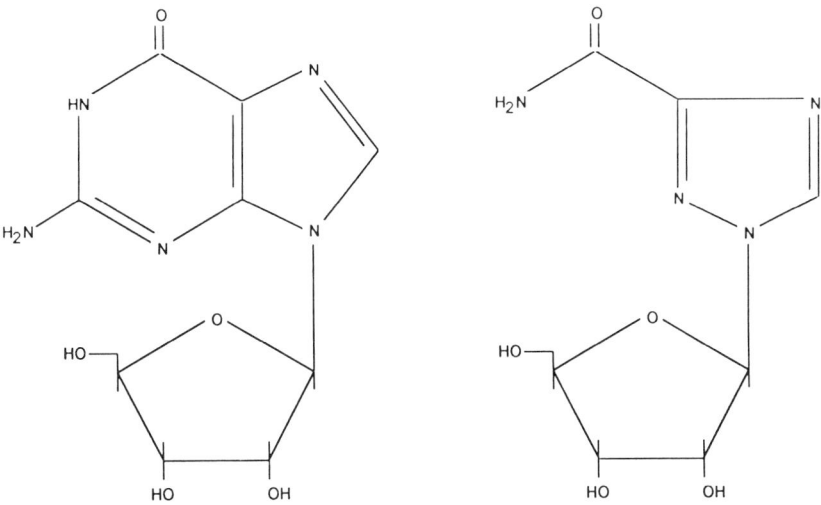

Figure 2 The structure of ribavirin (right) showing its relationship to that of guanosine (left).

(GTP) required for nucleic acid synthesis by competitive inhibition of inosine monophosphate dehydrogenase (81–83).

Ribavirin is water soluble and can be administered orally, intravenously, and, most importantly, directly into the respiratory tract through small-particle aerosol, which has become the major mode of use. About one third to 40% of the drug is excreted unchanged by the kidneys (84,85), and in its phosphorylated form, ribavirin accumulates in red cells, where it decays slowly, with a half-life of 40 days (86). Aerosol administration of ribavirin results in a peak concentration in respiratory secretions approximately 1000 times higher than that reached in plasma. However, at higher or longer applications of the drug, plasma concentrations can eventually approximate those reached by oral use. There is uncertainty about the precise site in the respiratory tract where the drug is deposited. However, methods have been developed to estimate the total amount of ribavirin delivered in the course of therapy (87).

The issue of the safety of ribavirin has been a prime consideration in determining its appropriate use. This, too, is related to its multiple mechanisms of action which may affect the host cell as well as the virus in certain circumstances. Early clinical investigations involving the oral administration of ribavirin suggested side effects, with reports of anemia, often not statistically significant in an individual study but reappearing at low levels from study to study. This effect was noted to be dose-related, was sometimes associated with duration of administration, and appeared to be reversible (88). In one field trial of oral ribavirin at a dosage of 1000 mg per day, reticulocytosis and elevated bilirubin levels were noted, with effects similar to those found in toxicological studies of the drug in certain laboratory animals (89). Central nervous system effects, including altered mood, irritability, and insomnia, have been reported in association with oral administration of high doses of ribavirin. In laboratory animals, such as rabbits and guinea pigs, the drug has been both teratogenic and embryolethal; these severe effects have not been reproduced in small studies in primates, but they remain a concern for hospital workers where ribavirin is administered by aerosol (90). Aerosol administration has also been reported to produce mild bronchospasm and to induce episodes of reversible dyspnea in asthmatic individuals (91). Skin rash has also been reported on rare occasions.

B. Treatment of Influenza

Ribavirin was of great interest clinically, since it was found to be effective in vitro against both types A and B influenza, unlike rimantadine and amantadine. The value of the drug in the prophylaxis and therapy of experimentally induced influenza was evaluated in early studies with inconsistent results (92, 93). Data suggested that the inconsistency might be related to different doses which were used. Therefore, a multicenter study was conducted to evaluate oral administration of a 1000-mg daily dose of ribavirin against naturally occurring influenza infection (89). These were outbreaks at only two study sites, both of which were caused by influenza type A(H1N1), the subtype which produces the mildest disease. In contrast to published studies with amantadine and rimantadine, no treatment effect could be detected in the 49 young adult males who received ribavirin as compared to the 48 who received placebo. Probably the most definitive finding in this study was elevated bilirubin, occurring mostly at one site, and thus prompting speculation that other factors might have been involved. Regardless of the interpretation, the results changed the approach of ribavirin therapy away from the oral route of administration to the use of aerosols.

A series of studies involving the generation of small-particle aerosols for administration of ribavirin then followed. For this purpose, a modified aerosol generator was developed, which has become the standard; the delivery characteristics of this device have been well described (94). However, there has been considerable variation in the design of clinical studies in which it has been employed. These have included differences in the method of administration, dependent to a large extent on the age and initial condition of the patient (this was typically a mask in adults, which in children might be modified to a tent or "oxyhood" or to a respirator), as well as duration of administration, amount of ribavirin in the reservoir, and, most importantly, the type of placebo employed. A number of studies were conducted in naturally acquired influenzal infection. Most showed a beneficial effect of the aerosol; however, the magnitude of that effect was variable, and it needed to be interpreted in light of the cost and discomfort of the lung duration of wearing the mask, which was up to 16–18 hr per day. In general, the therapy was deemed modestly successful against type A(H3N2) and type B infections, and antiviral resistance was not detected (87,95,96). Therapy against natural type A(H1N1) disease did not procure significant differences between the treated groups and those receiving placebo (96,97). These observations again produced speculation about the difficulty in the reduction of symptoms in this mildest form of influenza. Because of these modest and inconsistent results, the use of ribavirin against typical influenza has been largely abandoned. However, had its therapeutic effect been more consistent and profound, it might have been considered for evaluation against severe influenzal pneumonia. Unfortunately, the drug has not been systematically evaluated in older individuals, which is the population most likely to experience complications of influenza.

C. Treatment of Respiratory Syncytial Viral Infection

The most successful use of ribavirin has been in the therapy of respiratory syncytial viral (RSV) infection in very young children. Even here, the value of ribavirin has been questioned almost from the time of its approval, especially in terms of risk and cost benefits (98). Statements have periodically been published summarizing the published data, addressing various issues, and making recommendations for use (99). RSV produces bronchiolitis and pneumonia in otherwise healthy children, resulting in hospitalization at a very young age (mean of 5.7 months and median of 2.8 months) (see Chapter 7). When RSV infection occurs at a later age, the probability of severe disease is lower. In children with underlying diseases, especially cardiac, pulmonary, or immunosuppressive in nature, severe lower respiratory illnesses can occur throughout the first year of life and sometimes into the second (100). Antiviral therapy for RSV is attractive because of the severity of this disease, sometimes associated with respiratory failure, and especially since rapid diagnostic laboratory tests are available which facilitate specific use of the drug. Additionally, there is the suggestion that RSV illness early in life is followed at a later time by manifestations of chronic respiratory disease (101).

In the United States, the initial recommendation for the use of aerosolized ribavirin for infants and young children with RSV infection was based on the studies of Hall et al., and supported by the study of Taber and colleagues (102–104). A pilot study was carried out by Hall among adult volunteers who had been experimentally challenged with RSV, in which drug or water placebo was administered for 3 days (105). Reinfection in adults with RSV is known to result in frequent but relatively mild disease, so the purpose was mainly to evaluate safety and to detect any suggestion of beneficial effect (106). Adverse effects related to ribavirin were not detected. There were no significant differences in the occurrence of specific symptoms related to infection or viral shedding. Naturally infected infants were then studied with a treatment using a water placebo, which lasted for 3–6 days (102). The study was double blind, and a total of 33 infants, all with RSV pneumonia, were studied. The ribavirin-treated groups showed lower symptom severity scores by days 4 and 5 when the data were compared on a day-to-day basis. All infants were hypoxemic at the start of therapy, and by the end of treatment, they had all improved, although significantly more so in the treatment group. Duration of viral shedding was also reduced in the group receiving ribavirin, and no resistance to the drug was detected. The investigators did not report any significant side effects of the drug. In the Taber study, two designs were used; one used water as the placebo and the other was open label or observational (103). Again, there was a treatment benefit in improvement in symptoms on day 3, but this time no difference in viral shedding was seen. No further deterioration of status was noted in the treated groups, and no side effects were observed. Of particular interest to these investigators was the question of water absorption by infants receiving the aerosol, which they concluded was not excessive. They also reported the use of a device called an "oxyhood" for drug administration.

The use of ribavirin has continued to be evaluated after these pivotal studies both with randomized and, more recently, with observational designs (107–112). Surprisingly, appropriate use has become even more, rather than less, controversial over time, especially when costs are considered. Some intervention studies were blinded and placebo-controlled or others used an observed control. Investigators in some of the studies concluded that there was more rapid resolution of disease and less frequent adverse outcomes in children with underlying diseases. Others did not find significant differences. Critical reviews of these studies have suggested that there were deficiencies in some of the studies, including small sample sizes, the scoring system, which was felt to be unproven, and the entry criteria, which were not sufficiently specific. The question of whether the sterile water placebo could cause prolonged symptoms has also been raised. Some investigators have suggested the need for further evaluation, especially in those most likely to show benefit, namely, the very young and premature, as well as those children with serious preexisting conditions. The use of more precise endpoints has been recommended, such as the need for artificial ventilation, duration of hospital stay, and mortality.

These questions have been more recently addressed by observational studies, which have examined important endpoints such as duration of hospitalization. Of note are the timing of these studies, which were carried out after major improvements were made in the care of children with respiratory distress and after ribavirin was already being used in regular medical practice (110,111). Since they are observational, there is no placebo used, and thus the question of the effect that it might have on the outcome is not introduced. Decisions about use of ribavirin in these observational studies were made by the treating physicians. As a result, methods must be employed which adjust for selection differences in situations in which the drug is given. The adjustment is usually carried out by multivariate techniques such as logistic regression. An example of such a study is one conducted by Ohmit and colleagues over a 7-year period in children with RSV infections admitted to a single teaching hospital (112). Adjustment for factors which could have determined selection for antiviral treatment or which could have affected outcome, such as underlying conditions, were made using multivariate techniques. The investigators employed a single objective outcome, length of hospital stay, as an indicator of effect and found that ribavirin did not produce a reduction in hospitalization days. The average duration of stay in children without underlying conditions was 3.7 days, so it would have required a reduction in hospitalization by 27% to reduce stay by even 1 day. This and results from other similar studies probably reflect the advances made over the years in pediatric pulmonary intensive care, which has itself an improved outcome in both treated and untreated children. However, these studies may not indicate potential advantages of treatment which could occur in specific groups of children, such as the very young and those with certain underlying conditions. The studies also do not take into account any potential reduction in the chronic sequelae of RSV infection, which are now gaining increased recognition (101).

D. Use for Other Severe Lung Infections

Because of its broad spectrum, ribavirin was identified some years ago as being useful in treating severe infection by the Lassa virus (123). With a disease of this severity, the issue of side effects is muted. Both oral and intravenous administration have been evaluated, and the latter is preferred when there is more severe disease. The use of ribavirin has also been evaluated in the treatment of Korean hemorrhagic fever, now known to be caused by the Hantaan virus, a member of the hantavirus group (see Chap. 11). A prospective, placebo-controlled trial of hantaviral hemorrhagic fever with renal syndrome was conducted in cases occurring in China, with a significant reduction in mortality (124). Given this background, when the hantavirus pulmonary syndrome (HPS) was described in the western United States, it was natural to investigate the use of ribavirin in this disease.

The HSP is caused by an agent now termed sin nombre virus (SNV) and by at least three other related hantaviruses (see Chap. 11). It is considered an emergent infection that probably appears following a change in the regional ecology (125). It is clear from serological studies that the SNV or related agents are present in various parts of the United States, and they are not limited to the Southwest (126,127). Like some other bunyaviruses, HSP is a zoonosis that is mainly transmitted from animal to animal without necessarily involving humans. The animal hosts are typically rodents. In the American West, the host is the deer mouse, *Peromyscus maniculatus*, but other rodents may be involved in different parts of the United States and the rest of the world. Transmission to humans occurs principally through exposure to rodent urine or possibly feces. The ecological changes which resulted in the recognition of this infection have been hypothesized to involve an increase in the supply of pine nuts, a principal food of the rodents. This in turn would result in an increase in the rodent population, which would increase the likelihood of transmission of infection to humans who come in contact with rodents (128).

The outbreak in the southwestern United States was characterized by cases clustered in time and place, and because of the accompanying case fatality, there was interest in the utilization of specific antiviral therapy in addition to supportive therapy. Ribavirin was used to treat cases empirically at first, and then an open (uncontrolled) protocol was developed in an attempt to standardize its use. In the open protocol, nonpregnant adolescents and adults with a clinical diagnosis of the cardiopulmonary stage of the HPS were eligible for intravenous treatment with different doses of ribavirin. The protocol was in use from June 1993 to September 1994. In the period before ribavirin therapy was available, the case fatality was 63% of the 27 persons diagnosed, sometimes retrospectively, with the syndrome. Among those treated under the protocol, the case fatality was 47% (30 persons) compared with 50% of 34 individuals not treated. Because of the uncontrolled nature of the evaluation, it was not possible to conclude if antiviral treatment had any effect given the open selection of cases for drug administration and the improvement in the general level of care after the syndrome was recognized. In addition, there was clear toxicity associated with therapy, including reversible anemia in 75% of participants, some of whom required transfusions. Pancreatitis or hyperamylasemia was documented in 8% of those who were treated (129).

As a result, a formal placebo-controlled trial has been undertaken by the National Institutes of Allergy and Infectious Disease Collaborative Antiviral Study Group. Enrollment criteria were changed to allow inclusion of cases even during the febrile prodromal period. A problem with this trial will be the enrollment of sufficient participants for definitive conclusions to be drawn, since most cases occur largely in a limited geographical area of low population density. In other parts of the country where disease occurs more sporadically, it may be diagnosed too late for effective antiviral treatment.

IV. Other Antivirals for Treatment of Infections of the Lung

There have been a number of additional antivirals examined for use against lower respiratory infections, but most have failed because of low efficacy when evaluated in the experimental challenge model or in naturally occurring infection. Some have been unacceptably toxic, particularly when intended for use in infections that are, in general, self-limited. A number of neuraminidase inhibitors, active against both types A and B influenza, have recently entered evaluation. These compounds are examples of "engineered drugs," or drugs developed to complement the structure of the target macromolecule (130). The fact that compounds which affect influenza neuraminidase inhibit viral replication has been known for many years (131). Knowledge of the structure of the neuraminidase has allowed drug design to move broadly forward (132). One current candidate is the neuraminidase inhibitor 4-guanidino-Neu-5Ac2en (GG167). Clinical trials have not proceeded far enough to draw definitive conclusions about the value of this particular compound in prophylaxis or therapy. In a study of volunteers experimentally challenged with influenza A virus, it appeared highly efficacious in what would be the equivalent of prophylaxis and early therapy (133). This drug is administered topically while other neuraminidase inhibitors under development can be given orally (134). Considering the specificity of action, it is not likely that these compounds will be of use against viral infections other than influenza.

V. Conclusions

Given the many years since the identification of the principal viruses which cause pulmonary infection, the situation concerning antivirals available for treatment is disappointing. The number in use is not large, and the ones available are, in many cases, surrounded by controversy. This may reflect the problems associated with treating conditions which are mainly of relatively short duration, but it also reflects the lack of persistence by industry in developing new compounds. We can only hope that the situation is changing, as evidenced by the recent flurry of interest in neuraminidase inhibitors, resulting from new approaches in drug design, at least in part. Certainly most observers would agree that viral infections of the lung are frequent and severe enough to warrant more consistent attention than they have received in the past.

References

1. Davies WL, Grunert RR, Haff RF, McGahen JW, Neumayer EM, Paulshock M, et al. Antiviral activity of L-adamantanamine HCl. Science 1964; 144:862–863.
2. Maassab HF, Cochran KW. Rubella virus: inhibition in vitro by amantadine hydrochloride. Science 1964; 145:1443–1444.
3. Cochran KW, Maassab HF, Tsunoda A, et al. Studies on the antiviral activity of amantadine hydrochloride. Ann NY Acad Sci 1965; 130:432–439.
4. Jackson GG, Muldoon RL, Akers LW. Serological evidence for prevention of influenzal infection in volunteers by an antiinfluenzal drug amantadine hydrochloride. Antimicrob Agents Chemother 1963; 703–707.
5. Tyrrell DAJ, Bynoe ML, Hoorn B. Studies on the antiviral activity of 1-adamantanamine. Br J Exp Pathol 1965; 46:370–375.
6. Quilligan JJ Fr, Hirayama M, Baernstein HD Jr. The suppression of A2 influenza in children by the prophylactic use of amantadine. J Pediatr 1966; 69:572–575.
7. Sabin AB. Amantadine hydrochloride: analysis of data related to its proposed use for prevention of A2 influenza virus disease in human beings. JAMA 1967; 200:943–950.
8. Council on Drugs, American Medical Association. JAMA 1967; 201:372–373.
9. Oxford JS, Logan IS, Potter CW. In vivo selection of an influenza A2 strain resistant to amantadine. Nature 1970; 226:82–83.
10. Finklea JF, Hennessey AB, Davenport FM. A field trial of amantadine chemoprophylaxis in respiratory disease. Am J Epidemiol 1967; 85:403–412.
11. Muldoon RL, Stanley ED, Jackson GG. Use and withdrawal of amantadine chemoprophylaxis during epidemic influenza A. Am Rev Respir Dis 1967; 113:487–491.
12. Sabin AB. Mortality from pneumonia and risk conditions during influenza epidemics. High influenza morbidity during nonepidemic years. JAMA 1977; 237:2823–2828.
13. Monto AS, Gunn RA, Bandyk MG, et al. Prevention of Russian influenza by amantadine. JAMA 1979; 241:1003–1007.
14. Schwab RS, Poskanzer DC, England AC Jr, et al. Amantadine in Parkinson's disease. JAMA 1972; 222:792–795.
15. Parkes JD, Zilkha KJ, Marsden P, et al. Amantadine dosage in treatment of Parkinson's disease. Lancet 1970; 1:1130–1133.
16. Oker-Blom N, Hovi T, Leinikki P, et al. Protection of man from natural infection with influenza A2 Hong Kong virus by amantadine: a controlled field trial. Br Med J 1970; 3:676–678.
17. Nafia I, Turcanu AG, Braun I, et al. Administration of amantadine for the prevention of Hong Kong influenza. Bull WHO 1970; 42:423–427.
18. Smorodintsev AA, Karpuhin GI, Zlydnikov DM, et al. The prophylactic effectiveness of amanatdine hydrochloride in an epidemic of Hong Kong influenza in Leningrad in 1969. Bull WHO 1970; 42:865–872.
19. Zlydnikov DM, Kubar OI, Kovaleva TP, et al. Study of rimantadine in the USSR: a review of the literature. Rev Infect Dis 1981; 3:408–421.

20. Hay AJ, Zambon MC, Wolstenholme AJ, Skehel JJ, Smith MH. Molecular basis of resistance of influenza A viruses to amantadine. J Antimicrob Chemother 1986; 18:19–29.
21. Hay AJ. The mechanism of action of amantadine and rimantadine against influenza viruses. In: Notkins AL, Oldstone MBA, eds. Concepts in Viral Pathogenesis III. Berlin: Springer, 1989:561–567.
22. Hay AJ, Kennedy NTC, Skehel JJ, Appleyard G. The matrix protein gene determines amantadine-sensitivity of influenza viruses. J Gen Virol 1979; 42:189–191.
23. Sugrue RJ, Hay AJ. Structural characteristics of the M2 protein of influenza A viruses: evidence that it forms a tetrameric channel. Virology 1991; 180:617–624.
24. Browne MJ, Moss MY, Boyd MKR. Comparative activity of amantadine and ribavirin against influenza virus in vitro: possible clinical relevance. Antimicrob Agents Chemother 1983; 23:503–505.
25. Burlington DB, Meikeljohn G, Mostow SR. Anti-influenza A virus activity of amantadine hydrochloride and rimantadine hydrochloride in ferret tracheal ciliated epithelium. Antimicrob Agents Chemother 1982; 21:794–799.
26. Aoki FY, Sitar DS. Clinical pharmacokinetics of amantadine hydrochloride. Clin Pharmacokinet 1988; 14:35–51.
27. Atmar RL, Greenberg SB, Quarles JM, et al. Safety and pharmacokinetics of rimantadine small-particle aerosol. Antimicrob Agents Chemother 1990; 34:2228–2233.
28. Hayden FG, Hall WJ, Douglas RG Jr. Therapeutic effects of aerosolized amantadine in naturally acquired infection due to influenza A virus. J Infect Dis 1980; 141:535–542.
29. Aoki FY, Sitar DS, Olgilvie RI. Amantadine kinetics in healthy young subjects after long-term dosing. Clin Pharmacol Ther 1979; 26:729–736.
30. Tominack RL, Hayden FG. Rimantadine hydrochloride and amantadine hydrochloride use in influenza A virus infections. Infect Dis Clin North Am 1987; 1:459–478.
31. Hayden FG, Minocha A, Spyker DA, Hoffman HE. Comparative single-dose pharmacokinetics of amantadine hydrochloride and rimantadine hydrochloride in young and elderly adults. Antimicrob Agents Chemother 1985; 18:216–221.
32. Wu MJ, Ing TS, Soung LS, et al. Amantadine hydrochloride pharmacokinetics in patients with impaired renal function. Clin Nephrol 1982; 17:19–23.
33. Armbruster KFW, Rahn AC, Ing TS, et al. Amantadine toxicity in a patient with renal insufficiency. Nephron 1974; 13:183–186.
34. Borison RL. Amantadine-induced psychosis in a geriatric patient with renal disease. Am J Psychiatry 1979; 136:111–112.
35. Horadam VW, Sharp JG, Smilack JD, et al. Pharmacokinetics of amantadine hydrochloride in subjects with normal and impaired renal function. Ann Intern Med 1981; 94:454–458.
36. Capparelli EV, Stevens RC, Chow MS, Izard M, Wills RJ. Rimantadine pharmacokinetics in healthy subjects and patients with end-stage renal failure. Clin Pharmacol Ther 1988; 43:536–541.
37. Tominack RL, Wills RJ, Gustavson LE, Hayden FG. Multiple-dose pharmacokinetics of rimantadine in elderly adults. Antimicrob Agents Chemother 1988; 32:1813–1819.

38. Patriarca PA, Kater NA, Kendal AP, Bregman DJ, Smith JD, Sikes RK. Safety of prolonged administration of rimantadine hydrochloride in the prophylaxis of influenza A virus infections in nursing homes. Antimicrob Agents Chemother 1984; 26:101–103.
39. Wills RJ. Update on rimantadine's clinical pharmacokinetics. J Respir Dis 1989; 10(suppl):20–25.
40. Dolin R, Reichman RC, Madore HP, et al. A controlled trial of amantadine and rimantadine in the prophylaxis of influenza A infection. N Engl J Med 1982; 307: 580–584.
41. Togo Y, Hornick RB, Dawkis AT Jr. Studies on induced influenza in man. I. Double-blind studies designed to assess prophylactic efficacy of amantadine hydrochloride against A2/Rockville/I/65 strain. JAMA 1968; 203:1089–1094.
42. Likar M. Effectiveness of amantadine in protecting vaccinated volunteers from an attenuated strain of influenza A2/Hong Kong virus. Ann NY Acad Sci 1970; 173: 108–112.
43. Quarles JM, Couch RB, Cate TR, et al. Comparison of amantadine and rimantadine for prevention of type A (Russian) influenza. Antiviral Res 1981; 1:149–155.
44. Pettersson RF, Hellstrom PE, Penttinen K, et al. Evaluation of amantadine in the prophylazix of influenza A (H1N1) virus infection: A controlled field trial among young adults and high risk patients. J Infect Dis 1980; 142:377–383.
45. O'Donoghue JM, Ray CG, Terry DW Jr, Beaty HN. Prevention of nosocomial influenza with amantadine. Am J Epidemiol 1973; 97:276–282.
46. Brady MT, Sears SD, Pacini DL, et al. Safety and prophylactic efficacy of low-dose rimantadine in adults during an influenza A epidemic. Antimicrob Agents Chemother 1990; 34:1633–1636.
47. Reuman PD, Bernstein DI, Keefer MC, et al. Efficacy and safety of low dosage amantadine hydrochloride as prophylaxis for influenza A. Antiviral Res 1989; 11: 27–40.
48. Galbraith AW, Oxford JS, Schild GC, Watson GI. Protective effect of 1-adamantanamine hydrochloride on influenza A2 infections in the family environment. A controlled double-blind study. Lancet 1969; 2:1026–1028.
49. Galbraith AW, Oxford JS, Schild GC, Watson GI. Study of 1-adamantanamine hydrochloride used prophylactically during the Hong Kong influenza epidemic in the family environment. Bull WHO 1969; 41:677–682.
50. Clover RD, Crawford SA, Abell TD, et al. Effectiveness of rimantadine prophylaxis of children with families. Am J Dis Child 1986; 140:706–709.
51. Crawford SA, Clover RD, Abell TD, et al. Rimantadine prophylaxis in children: A follow-up study. Pediatr Infect Dis J 1988; 7:379–383.
52. Longini IM, Koopman JS, Monto AS, Fox JP. Estimating household and community transmission parameters for influenza. Am J Epidemiol 1982; 115:736–751.
53. Wingfield WL, Pollack D, Grunert RR. Therapeutic efficacy of amantadine HCl and rimantadine HCl in naturally occurring influenza A2 respiratory illness in man. N Engl J Med 1969; 281:579–584.
54. Togo Y, Hornick RB, Felliti VJ, et al. Evaluation of therapeutic efficacy of amantadine in patients with naturally occurring A2 influenza. JAMA 1970; 211: 1149–1156.

55. Knight V, Fedson D, Baldini J, et al. Amantadine therapy of epidemic influenza A2/Hong Kong. Infect Immun 1970; 1:200–204.
56. Van Voris LP, Betts RG, Hayden FG, et al. Successful treatment of naturally occurring iin A/USSR/77 H1N1. JAMA 1981; 245:1128–1131.
57. Hayden FG, Monto AS. Oral rimantadine hydrochloride therapy of influenza A virus H3N2 subtype infection in adults. Antimicrob Agents Chemother 1986; 29: 339–341.
58. Younkin SW, Betts RF, Roth FK, et al. Reduction in fever and symptoms in young adults with influenza A/Brazil/78 H1N1 infection after treatment with aspirin or amantadine. Antimicrob Agents Chemother 1983; 23:577–582.
59. Little JW, Hall WJ, Douglas RD Jr, et al. Amantadine effect on peripheral airways abnormalities in influenza. Ann Intern Med 1976; 85:177–182.
60. Hall CB, Dolin R, Gala CL, Markovitz DM, et al. Children with influenza A infection: treatment with rimantadine. Pediatrics 1987; 880:275–282.
61. Thompson J, Fleet LW, Lawrence E, Pierce E, Morris L, Wright P. A comparison of acetaminophen and rimantadine in the treatment of influenza A infection in children. J Med Virol 1987; 21:249–255.
62. Belshe RB, Hall-Smith M, Hall CB, Betts R, Hay AJ. Genetic basis of resistance to rimantadine emerging during treatment of influenza virus infection. J Virol 1988; 5:1508–1512.
63. Lubeck MD, Schulman JL, Palese P. Susceptibility of influenza A viruses to amantadine is influenced by the gene coding for M protein. J Virol 1978; 28:710–716.
64. Hay AJ, Wolstenholme AJ, Skehel JJ, Smith MH. The molecular basis of the specific antiinfluenza action of amantadine. EMBO J 1985; 4:3021–3024.
65. Hayden FG, Belshe RB, Clover RD, Hay AJ, Oakes MG, Soo W. Emergence and apparent transmission of rimantadine-resistant influenza A virus in families. N Engl J Med 1989; 321:1696–1702.
66. Hayden F, Sperber SJ, Belshe R, Clover R, Hay A, Pyke S. Recovery of drug-resistant influenza A virus during therapeutic use of rimantadine. Antimicrob Agents Chemother 1991; 35:1741–1747.
67. Sweet C, Hayden FG, Jakeman KJ, Grambas S, Hay AJ. Virulence of rimantadine-resistant human influenza A (H3N2) viruses in ferrets. J Infect Dis 1991; 164:969–972.
68. Belshe RB, Burk B, Newman F, Cerruti RL, Sim IS. Resistance of influenza A virus to amantadine and rimantadine: results of one decade of surveillance. J Infect Dis 1989; 159:430–435.
69. Hayden FG, Hoffman HE, Spyker DA. Differences in side effects of amantadine hydrochloride and rimantadine hydrochloride relate to differences in pharmacokinetics. Antimicrob Agents Chemother 1983; 23:458–464.
70. Millet VM, Dreisbach M, Bryson YJ. Double-blind controlled study of central nervous system side effects of amantadine, rimantadine, and chlorpheniramine. Antimicrob Agents Chemother 1982; 21:1–4.
71. Dolin R, Betts RF, Treanor JJ, et al. Rimantadine prophylaxis of influenza in the elderly, abstr. 691, p. 210. In: Program and abstracts of the 23rd Interscience Conference on Antimicrobial Agents and Chemotherapy. American Society for Microbiology, 1983, Washington, DC.

72. Postma JU, Van Tilburg W. Visual hallucinations and delirium during treatment with amantadine (Symmetrel). J Am Geriatr Soc 1975; 23:212–215.
73. Degelau J, Somani S, Cooper SL, Irvine PW. Occurrence of adverse effects and high amantadine concentrations with influenza prophylaxis in the nursing home. J Am Geriatr Soc 1990; 38:428–432.
74. Soo W. Adverse effects of rimantadine: summary from clinical trials. J Respir Dis 1989; 10(suppl):26–31.
75. Monto AS, Ohmit SE, Hornbuckle K, Pearce CL. Safety and efficacy of long-term use of rimantadine for prophylaxis of type A influenza in nursing homes. Antimicrob Agents Chemother 1995; 39:2224–2228.
76. Monto AS, Arden NH. Implications of viral resistance to amantadine in control of influenza A. Clin Infect Dis 1992; 15:362–367.
77. Centers for Disease Control and Prevention. Prevention and control of influenza. Part II. Antiviral agents—recommendations of the Advisory Committee on Immunization Practices (ACIP). MMWR 1994; 43:1–10.
78. Mast EE, Harmon MW, Gravenstein S, et al. Emergence and possible transmission of amantadine-resistant viruses during nursing home outbreaks of influenza A (H3N2). Am J Epidemiol 1991; 134:988–997.
79. Witkowski JT, Robins RK, Sidwell RW, et al. Design, synthesis, and broad spectrum antiviral activity of L-D-ribofuranosyl-1,2,4-triazole-3-carboxamide and related nucleosides. J Med Chem 1972; 15:1150–1154.
80. Sidwell RW, Hurrman JM, Khare GP, Allen LB, Witkowski JT, Robins RK. Broad spectrum antiviral activity of Virazole: 1-β-D-ribofuranosyl-1,2,4-triazole-3-carboxamide. Science 1972; 177:705–706.
81. Streeter DG, Witkowski JT, Khare GP, et al. Mechanism of action of 1-β-D-ribofuranosyl-1,2,4-triazole-3-carboxamide (Virazole), a new broad-spectrum antiviral agent. Proc Natl Acad Sci USA 1973; 70:1174–1178.
82. Goswami BB, Borek E, Sharma OK, Fujitaki J, Smith RA. The broad spectrum antiviral agent ribavirin inhibits capping of mRNA. Biochem Biophys Res Commun 1979; 89:830–836.
83. Patterson JL, Fernandez-Larsson. Molecular mechanisms of action ribavirin. Rev Infect Dis 1990; 12:1139–1146.
84. Connor JD, Hintz M, Van Dyke R, et al. Ribavirin pharmacokinetics in children and adults during therapeutic trials. In: Smith RA, Knight V, Smith JAD, eds. Clinical Applications of Ribavirin. New York: Academic Press, 1984:107–123.
85. Laskin OL, Longstreth JA, Hart CC, et al. Ribavirin disposition in high-risk patients for acquired immunodeficiency syndrome. Clin Pharmacol Ther 1987; 41:546–555.
86. Catlin DH, Smith RA, Samuels AI. C-ribavirin distribution and pharmacokinetics studies in rats, baboons and man. In: Smith RA, Kirkpatric W, eds. Ribavirin: A Broad Spectrum Antiviral Agent. New York: Academic Press, 1980:83–98.
87. McClung HW, Knight V, Gilbert BE, et al. Ribavirin aerosol treatment of influenza B virus infection. JAMA 1983; 249:2671–2674.
88. Shulman NR. Assessment of Hematologic effects of ribavirin in humans. In: Smith RA, Knight V, and Smith JAD, eds. In: Clinical Applications of Ribavirin. New York: Academic Press, 1984:79–96.

89. Smith CB, Charette RP, Fox JP, et al. Lack of effect of oral ribavirin in naturally occurring influenza A virus (H1N1) infection. J Infect Dis 1980; 141:548–554.
90. Rodriguez WJ, Dant Bui RH, Connor JD, et al. Environmental exposure of primary care personnel to ribavirin aerosol when supervising treatment of infants with respiratory syncytial virus infection. Antimicrob Agents Chemother 1987; 31:1143–1146.
91. Light B, Aoki FY, Serrette C. Tolerance of ribavirin aerosol inhaled by normal volunteers and patients with asthma and chronic obstructive airways disease. In: Smith RA, Knight V, and Smith JAD, eds. Clinical Applications of Ribavirin. New York: Academic Press, 1984:97–105.
92. Togo Y, McCraken EA. Chemoprophylaxis and therapy of respiratory viral infections: Double-blind clinical assessment of ribavirin (Virazole) in the prevention of induced infection with type B influenza virus. J Infect Dis 1976; 133:A109–A113.
93. Magnussen CR, Douglas RG Jr, Betts RF, et al. Double-blind evaluation of oral ribavirin (Virazole) in experimental influenza A virus infection in volunteers. Antimicrob Agents Chemother 1977; 12:498–502.
94. Young HW, Dominik JW, Walker JS, et al. Continuous aerosol therapy system using a modified Collison nebulizer. J Clin Microbiol 1977; 5:131–136.
95. Knight V, Wilson SZ, Quarles JM, et al. Ribavirin small-particle aerosol treatment of influenza. Lancet 1981; 2:945–949.
96. Gilbert BE, Wilson SZ, Knight V, et al. Ribavirin small-particle aerosol treatment of infections caused by influenza virus strains A/Victoria/7/83 (H1N1) and B/Texas/1/84. Antimicrob Agents Chemother 1985; 27:309–313.
97. Wilson SZ, Gilbert BE, Quarles JM, et al. Treatment of influenza A(H1N1) virus infection with ribavirin aerosol. Antimicrob Agents Chemother 1984; 26:200–203.
98. Wald ER, Dashefsky B, Green M. In re ribavirin: A case of premature adjudication? J Pediatr 1988; 112:154–158.
99. Committee on Infectious Diseases, American Academy of Pediatrics. Reassessment of the indications for ribavirin therapy in respiratory syncytial virus infections. Pediatrics 1996; 97:137–140.
100. McIntosh K. Respiratory syncytial virus infection in infants and children: diagnosis and treatment. Pediatr Rev 1987; 9:191–196.
101. Pullan CR, Hey EN. Wheezing, asthma, and pulmonary dysfunction 10 years after infection with respiratory syncytial virus in infancy. Br Med J 1982; 284:1665–1669.
102. Hall CB, McBride JT, Walsh EE, et al. Aerosolized ribavirin treatment of infants with respiratory syncytial viral infection: A randomized double-blind study. N Engl J Med 1983; 308:1443–1447.
103. Taber LH, Knight V, Gilbert BE, et al. Ribavirin aerosol treatment of bronchiolitis associated with respiratory syncytial virus infection in infants. Pediatrics 1983; 72:613–618.
104. Hall CB, McBride JT, Gala CL, et al. Ribavirin treatment of respiratory syncytial viral infection in infants with underlying cardiopulmonary disease. JAMA 1985; 254:3047–3051.

105. Hall CB, Walsh EE, Hruska JF, et al. Ribavirin treatment of experimental respiratory syncytial viral infection: A controlled double-blind study in young adults. JAMA 1983; 249:2666–2670.
106. Monto AS, Bryan ER, Rhodes LM. The Tecumseh study of respiratory illness. VII. Further observations on the occurrence of respiratory syncytial virus and mycoplasma pneumoniae infections. Am J Epidemiol 1975; 100:458–468.
107. Rodriguez WJ, Kim HW, Brand CD, et al. Aerosolized ribavirin in the treatment of patients with respiratory syncytial virus disease. Pediatr Infect Dis 1987; 6:159–163.
108. Smith DW, Frankel LR, Mathers LH, Tang ATS, Ariagno RL, Prober CG. A controlled trial of aerosolized ribavirin in infants receiving mechanical ventilation for severe respiratory syncytial virus infection. N Engl J Med 1991; 325:24–29.
109. Meert KL, Sarnaik AP, Gelmini MJ, Lieh-Lai MW. Aerosolized ribavirin in mechanically ventilated children with respiratory syncytial virus lower respiratory tract disease: a prospective, double-blind, randomized trial. Crit Care Med 1994; 22:566–572.
110. Wheeler JG, Wooford J, Turner RB. Historical cohort evaluation of ribavirin efficacy in respiratory syncytial virus infection. Pediatr Infect Dis J 1993; 12:209–213.
111. Law BJ, Wang EE, Stephens D. Ribavirin does not reduce hospital stay (LOS) in patients with respiratory syncytial virus (RSV) lower respiratory tract infection (LRTI). Pediatr Res 1995; 37:119A.
112. Ohmit SE, Moler FW, Monto AS, Khan AS. Ribavirin utilization and clinical effectiveness in children hospitalized with respiratory syncytial virus infection. J Clin Epidemiol 1996; 49:963–967.
113. Kapikian AZ, Mitchell RH, Chanock RM, Shevdoff RA, Stewart CE. An epidemiologic study of altered clinical reactivity to respiratory syncytial (RS) virus infection in children previously vaccinated with an inactivated RS virus vaccine. Am J Epidemiol 1969; 89:405–421.
114. Parrott RH, Kim HW, Arrobio JO, et al. Epidemiology of respiratory syncytial virus infection in Washington, DC. II. Infection and disease with respect to age, immunologic status, race and sex. Am J Epidemiol 1973; 98:289–300.
115. Lamprecht CL, Krause HE, Mufson MA. Role of maternal antibody in pneumonia and bronchiolitis due to respiratory syncytial virus. J Infect Dis 1976; 134:211–217.
116. Glezen WP, Paredes A, Allison JE, Taber LH, Frank AL. Risk of respiratory syncytial virus infection for infants from low-income families in relationship to age, sex, ethnic group, and maternal antibody level. J Pediatr 1981; 98:708–715.
117. Tristram DA, Welliver RC, Mohar CK, et al. Immunogenicity and safety of respiratory syncytial virus subunit vaccine in seropositive children 18-36 months old. J Infect Dis 1993; 167:191–195.
118. Hemming VG, Prince GA, Horswood RL, et al. Studies of passive immunotherapy for infections of respiratory syncytial virus in the respiratory tract of a primate model. J Infect Dis 1985; 152:1083–1087.
119. Siber GR, Leszczynski J, Pena-Cruz V, et al. Protective activity of a human respiratory syncytial virus immune globulin prepared from donors screened by microneutralization assay. J Infect Dis 1992; 165:456–463.

120. Hemming VG, Rodriguez W, Kim HW, et al. Intravenous immunoglobulin treatment of respiratory syncytial virus infections in infants and young children. Antimicrob Agents Chemother 1987; 31:1882–1886.
121. Groothuis JR, Simoes EA, Levin MJ, et al. Prophylactic administration of respiratory syncytial virus immune globulin to high-risk infants and young children. The Respiratory Syncytial Virus Immune Globulin Study. N Engl J Med 1993; 329:1524–1530.
122. Groothuis JR, Simoes EA, Hemming VG. Respiratory Syncytial Virus Immune Globulin Study Group. Pediatrics 1995; 95:463–467.
123. McCormick JB, King IJ, Webb PA, et al. Lassa fever: Effective therapy with ribavirin. N Engl J Med 1986; 314:20–26.
124. Huggins JW, Hsiang CM, Cosgriff TM, et al. Prospective, double-blind, concurrent, placebo-controlled clinical trial of intravenous ribavirin therapy of hemorrhagic fever with renal syndrome. J Infect Dis 1991; 164:1119–1127.
125. Elliot LH, Ksiazek TG, Rollin PE, et al. Isolation of the causative agent of hantavirus pulmonary syndrome. Am J Trop Med Hyg 1994; 51:102–108.
126. Tsai TF, Bauer SP, Sasso DR, et al. Serological and virological evidence of a Hantaan virus-related enzootic in the United States. J Infect Dis 1985; 152:126–136.
127. Childs JE, Glass GE, Korch GW, et al. Evidence of human infection with a rat-associated Hantavirus in Baltimore, Maryland. Am J Epidemiol 1988; 127:875–878.
128. Childs JE, Krebs JW, Ksiazek TG, et al. A household-based, case-control study of environmental factors associated with hantavirus pulmonary syndrome in the southwestern United States. Am J Trop Med Hyg 1995; 52:393–397.
129. Mertz B, Chapman L. Hantavirus infection in the United States: diagnosis and treatment. In: Mills J, Volberding PA, Corey I, eds. Antiviral Chemotherapy 4. New Directions for Clinical Application and Research. Advances in Experimental Medicine and Biology V. New York: Plenum Press, 1996:153.
130. von Itzstein M, Dyason JC, Oliver SW, et al. A study of the active site of influenza virus sialidase: an approach to the rational design of novel anti-influenza drugs. J Med Chemother 1996; 39:388–391.
131. Palese P, Schulman JL. Inhibition of influenza and parainfluenza virus replication in tissue culture by 2-deoxy-2,3-dehydro-N-trifluoroacetyl-neuraminic acid (FANA). Virology 1974; 59:490–498.
132. Air GM, Laver WG. The neuraminidase of influenza virus. Protein Struc Funct Genet 1989; 6:341–356.
133. Hayden FG, Treanor JJ, Betts RF, Lobo M, Esinhart JD, Hussey EK. Safety and efficacy of the neuraminidase inhibitor GG167 in experimental human influenza. JAMA 1996; 275:295–299.
134. Luo M, Air GM, Brouillette WJ. Design of aromatic inhibitors of influenza virus neuraminidase. In: Brown LE, Hampson AW, Webster RG, eds. Options for the Control of Influenza III. Amsterdam: Elsevier, 1996:702–712.

Part Five

PREVENTION

14

Prevention of Viral Respiratory Infections

PETER A. GROSS

New Jersey Medical School
Newark, New Jersey
and Hackensack University Medical Center
Hackensack, New Jersey

I. Influenza Virus Vaccines

A. History

Among viral infections of the lung, the influenza virus is responsible for more clinically significant morbidity and mortality than other respiratory viruses (1,2) (see Chap. 6). It therefore deserves our unwavering attention. The influenza virus was first isolated in 1933 by Smith, Andrewes, and Laidlaw, and within a few years, the first vaccine against influenza was tested by Chenoweth and colleagues (3,4). Subsequent years saw an improvement in the immunogenicity and a reduction in the reactogenicity of the vaccine.

Studies of influenza vaccine have yielded estimates of an approximately 55% reduction in the incidence of respiratory illness, pneumonia, hospitalization, and mortality during influenza outbreaks in the elderly. Yet the vaccine did not achieve widespread acceptance until recently. Perceptions of the lack of efficacy and the presence of side effects have impaired acceptance by patients and physicians alike. Periodic antigenic variability necessitates the need to change at least one of the three viral strains in the vaccine annually. The difference between antigenic drift and antigenic shift may confuse the average clinician or patient. Antigenic drift occurs frequently and represents a minor change in the viral surface proteins; that is, a <1% change in the nucleotide sequence of the hemagglutinin (H) or neuraminidase (N) genes (e.g., influenza A/Beijing/94 [H3N2] to A/Johannesburg/95 [H3N2]). Antigenic shift occurs infrequently and is a major change; that is, a >30% change in the nucleotide sequence of one or both genes and, hence, a new designation for the H or N component (e.g., influenza A/Aichi/57 [H2N2] to A/Hong Kong/68 [H3N2]). The short duration of vaccine-induced antibody requires the administration of vaccine annually even for vaccine strains that do not change (5).

With the complexity of interactive factors, let us look at the current status and future potential for protection against the influenza virus by vaccination. At present, the only licensed influenza vaccines are inactivated vaccines. Live virus vaccines are still investigational, and vaccines made with the new genetic technologies are being developed.

Currently, licensed influenza vaccines are either inactivated by formalin or split into their immunogenic parts by a detergent. Some are administered without further treatment; others undergo an additional purification step so that only the hemagglutinin and neuraminidase surface proteins remain. Although comparative efficacy studies have not been done, the licensed vaccines are assumed to be equally efficacious, because they are equally immunogenic.

B. Protective Efficacy Studies

The efficacy of influenza vaccine in the elderly has been recently summarized in a meta-analysis of 20 cohort studies (6). Along with three case-control, two cost-effectiveness studies, and one randomized, double-blind, placebo-controlled trial, it is apparent that influenza vaccine will reduce hospitalizations for pneumonia and influenza by 30–65% and will have a significant impact on reducing respiratory illness, pneumonia, and mortality from influenza (Table 1). The mortality calculations are based on almost 30,000 patients.

An unexpected finding in these studies is that hospitalization from all acute and chronic respiratory conditions was reduced by 27–39%, mortality from all respiratory conditions was reduced by 35–65%, and mortality from all causes was reduced by 27–54% (7,8).

In the meta-analysis of elderly vaccine recipients, the efficacy was the same whether the vaccine and the epidemic strain were similar or when the epidemic strain had drifted slightly from the vaccine strain. All the efficacy studies are confounded by several factors—the lack of a precise definition of pneumonia, the frequent lack of laboratory confirmation of influenza virus infection, confusion with other causes of pulmonary infiltrates such as the acute respiratory distress syndrome and congestive heart failure, the occurrence of other respiratory infectious microorganisms during the influenza season, and

Table 1 Summary of Influenza Vaccine Efficacy Studies in Elderly Persons: Reduction in Outcome Measured (Number or Range in Percentages [95% Confidence Interval])

Author (reference)	Type of study	Respiratory illness	Pneumonia	Hospitalization	Pneumonia & influenza mortality	All causes of mortality
Gross et al. (6)	Meta-analysis	56 (37–66)	53 (35–66)	50 (28–65)	68 (56–76)	—
Foster et al. (9)	Case-controlled	—	—	45 (14–64)	—	—
Fedson et al. (7)	Case-controlled	—	—	32–39	35–65	27–30
MIVDP (31)	Case-controlled	—	—	31–45	—	—
Nichol et al. (8)	Cost-effectiveness	—	—	48–57	—	39–54
Mullooy et al. (10)	Cost-effectiveness	—	—	30–40	—	—
Govaert et al. (11)	RDBPC	53	—	—	—	—

MIVDP, Medicare Influenza Vaccine Demonstration Project; RDBPC, Randomized, double-blind, placebo-controlled.

the causes of death. Yet, a comparison of the efficacy studies shows a remarkably similar range in outcomes (see Table 1) (9–11). Additionally, the estimates of vaccine efficacy are conservative and probably underestimated, whereas the case-mortality rates in vaccinated persons are overestimated (12).

In non–high-risk young adults, influenza vaccine also offers significant benefits. Nichol and colleagues reported that 25% fewer episodes of upper respiratory illness occurred in vaccinees versus placebo recipients, 43% fewer days of sick leave from work due to upper respiratory illness, and 44% fewer visits to physicians' offices for upper respiratory illness occurred in vaccine recipients. An estimated $46.85 per person vaccinated was saved (13).

The efficacy of vaccine in immunosuppressed patients has not been widely studied. Immunogenicity studies, however, have been done in patients on cancer chemotherapy and in acquired immunodeficiency syndrome (AIDS) patients and demonstrate that only 50% or less achieve presumed protective levels of serum antibody (14,15) (see Chap. 5).

A number of confounding issues need to be considered in assessing the results of the above studies. First, estimating reductions in upper respiratory illness from vaccination are difficult because of the common occurrence of other respiratory microorganisms during the winter influenza season. Without careful culture and serological studies, attribution of illness to influenza in vaccinated persons versus controls is difficult. A few studies have done this in the past, such as the one by Dowdle and colleagues in which they showed an 88% reduction in respiratory illness when serodiagnosis was one of the criteria (16).

Second, the issue of the efficacy of repeated annual vaccination is just beginning to be examined. Hoskins and associates found that repeated vaccination in adolescent boys in a boarding school may be detrimental when an antigenic drift variant is encountered during an influenza epidemic (17). More recent studies in young adults and the elderly indicated that repeated vaccination is not harmful and does not diminish the antibody response to vaccination (18,19).

Third, meta-analyses have been criticized for having a publication bias, in that, for example, negative studies on vaccination are usually not published, and if they are published, they might undo the weight of the findings in studies showing a positive vaccine effect. It is comforting to know that in the meta-analysis reported, it would have taken 952 unpublished null studies of respiratory illness, 153 unpublished null studies of pneumonia, 26 unpublished null studies of hospitalization, and 466 unpublished null studies of mortality to refute the results of the meta-analysis (6).

Finally, the positive findings in efficacy studies are also adversely affected by the fact that only outbreaks get studied. For example, in nursing homes where vaccination rates are high and no outbreaks develop because of herd immunity, the positive effect of vaccination would go unrecognized. Hence, underreporting of this positive vaccine effect would underestimate vaccine efficacy.

C. Role of Mucosal and Cellular Immunity

Mucosal immunity is an important part of our defenses against respiratory invaders. For influenza, a nasally administered, live-attenuated viral vaccine induces higher levels of secretory IgA levels than parenterally administered, inactivated vaccines. The secretory IgA produced is relatively short lived; that is, it is present less than 6 months (20). The protection against infection afforded by inactivated vaccine is correlated with adequate levels of serum antibody. On nasal challenge with live virus, mucosal IgA antibody correlates best with protection against infection. Nonetheless, serum hemagglutination inhibition antibody, which is much more readily measured than nasal antibody, remains the gold standard for predicting the likelihood of vaccine efficacy.

Cellular immunity may play a role in protection from infection or in the development and duration of clinical disease once infection occurs. In murine models, it conveys cross protection among strains. However, the precise role of cellular immunity in humans has not been clearly defined (21,22).

D. Side Effects

The perception of a high incidence of side effects from influenza vaccine has impaired the widespread acceptance of this effective public health measure. In a randomized, placebo-controlled study with a crossover design, Margolis et al. reported that the incidence of local and systemic side effects in adult males during the first 48 hr after vaccination was less than 5% (20). In a more recent study of healthy working adults, systemic symptoms of fever, fatigue, myalgias, malaise, and headaches were no more common in the vaccinated group than in a group receiving a placebo injection. The only difference was in a higher incidence of arm soreness at the injection site in the influenza vaccine recipients (24). Studies in children showed similar results.

It also is worthwhile to point out in randomized, placebo-controlled trials, the incidence of fever of ≥102°F was 3% in placebo vaccine recipients (25). The public needs to understand better that other respiratory and gastrointestinal infectious agents occur year round, including the time when a person is vaccinated, and that these infectious agents may cause fever and upper respiratory or gastrointestinal illnesses that are unrelated to the coincidental administration of a vaccine.

Allergic reactions can occur to some vaccine components. Therefore, the inactivated vaccine is contraindicated in persons with a history of anaphylaxis after eating eggs or with a history of allergy to the antibiotic, preservative, or detergent in the specific vaccine used.

The annual background incidence of Guillain-Barré syndrome (GBS) is one to two cases per 100,000 adult population. The incidence of GBS following the administration of the 1976 swine influenza vaccine exceeded the background rate by slightly less than one case per 100,000 vaccinations (1,39). Subsequent influenza vaccines have not been convincingly shown to increase the risk of GBS. Nevertheless, it is prudent to avoid giving influenza vaccine to persons who have developed GBS within 6 weeks of any previous influenza vaccination.

E. Pharmacoeconomic Analyses

Cost-effectiveness analysis evaluates the merits of reaching a desired health outcome by comparing the monetary cost of different courses of action. The desired outcome may be a reduction in morbidity and mortality by preventing the disease, as well as the reduction in productivity losses (26). Cost-benefit analyses evaluates health outcome in terms of the monetary value of medical resources saved, the avoidance of productivity losses, and the reductions in health status averted by vaccination.

The Office of Technology Assessment (OTA) performed an in-depth, cost-effectiveness study for the 7-year period between 1971 and 1972 and 1977 and 1978 (27). The study determined that during those years, 150 million influenza vaccinations resulted in approximately 13 million more years of healthy life at a cost of $63 per life gained for all ages. About $250 million in potential productivity losses were averted. The cost per life gained was lower among high-risk persons. For high-risk persons of all ages, it cost $10 per year of healthy life gained. Riddiough et al. (28) pointed out that the cost-effectiveness ratio in the OTA study rose (i.e., vaccination became less cost effective) with decreasing age. For example, the ratio increased from <0 (i.e., no net cost) for persons 65 years and older to $23 (in 1978 dollars) per year of healthy life gained for persons aged 45–64 years and peaked at $258 for those less than 3 years of age. However, and here is the rub in cost analyses, when you add in the cost of future medical care, the cost per year of healthy life gained increases significantly. For example, for all ages, without counting future medical care costs, the cost per year of healthy life gained is $63, but when you count future medical care costs, the cost per year of healthy life gained is $1956.

The cost-effectiveness studies also demonstrate that the lowest cost-effectiveness ratio (i.e., the greatest effectiveness for the least cost) was in elderly persons. In addition, vaccination of high-risk groups of any age was more cost effective than vaccinating the general population.

When performing cost-effectiveness studies, the reader should be aware of the importance of sensitivity analysis because of the imprecision of available data on the critical variables. Sensitivity analysis considers the effect of several factors on the study. The cost of vaccination will vary by whether the vaccine is administered in the private or public sector. An estimate of vaccine protective efficacy of 90% will decrease the cost compared with an estimate of 50% efficacy, and this effect is more significant for the elderly. The estimate of excess mortality during the influenza season also is important, especially in the elderly. The most profound impact on these studies was the cost produced when patients whose lives were saved by influenza vaccination lived longer, and therefore incurred expenses for additional medical care. The ethical concerns about including or excluding the additional medical costs for years of life saved have been hotly debated. The effects of herd immunity from vaccination and of antigenic variability in the epidemic strain versus the vaccine strain are usually not included in sensitivity analyses because of the paucity of data evaluating these factors (29).

Schoenbaum et al. (30) estimated the economic value of a mass immunization campaign when a new pandemic influenza strain appears. They determined that the cost benefit from the campaign would be greatest if the vaccine was restricted to adults 25 years of age and older and if the vaccine efficacy in that age group was 59% or better. If no vaccination was given, then the total cost would be $6 billion for the general population and $3 billion for the high-risk group alone in 1976 dollars.

In more recent cost analyses, Nichol et al. have shown that the cost of hospitalization was reduced for an average direct savings per year of $117 per person (8). And Mullooly and colleagues demonstrated that a net per person savings of $6.11 accrued to their health maintenance organization when vaccinating high-risk elderly persons.

How does an influenza vaccination program compare with other preventive medicine measures? A comparison of the cost effectiveness of influenza vaccination with that for the screening and treatment of hypertension and screening for cervical cancer with the Papanicolaou smear demonstrates that influenza vaccination is a relatively inexpensive disease-prevention program (26).

Standards for cost-effectiveness studies have recently been established (31,32). Until agreement is reached and uniformly applied, some authorities quip that "quantifying the value of nature is not ready for prime time and may never be" (33).

F. Acceptability of Vaccination

Until recently, influenza vaccine has not enjoyed widespread acceptability among the general public or the health-care profession. Individuals have tended to focus on the perceived low efficacy and high incidence of side effects even though both perceptions have recently been dispelled. In addition, individuals do not usually consider the total impact of the disease on society. With the newer efficacy information available, the public needs to be reminded that vaccination is cost effective and is a necessary part of preventive medicine. An annual influenza vaccination program will save billions of dollars and tens of thousands of lives, as well as substantially reduce productivity losses by preventing influenzal illness. Intensive health-education campaigns funded by the federal government have helped to make influenza vaccination more acceptable to the general public.

Vaccine acceptability has increased gradually over the past couple of decades. In the early 1980s, 20–23% of elderly persons were immunized. By the late 1980s, the percentage started to increase. During the 1993–1994 influenza season, 58% of elderly persons received influenza vaccine annually (34). Although this is still inadequate, the trend is encouraging. The fact that Medicare now reimburses for influenza vaccine has had a noticeable additional impact on increasing the number of elderly persons vaccinated.

G. Approaches to Encourage Vaccination

A number of approaches to improve vaccine usage have been recommended. In addition to the standard approaches of vaccination through private physicians' offices and public health clinics, vaccine can be administered to patients hospitalized for cardiorespiratory conditions just prior to discharge (35). It can be offered to health-care workers at their work sites. This approach can be used for non–health-care workers as well, since the vaccine is beneficial for all adults (10). Well-designed letters or postcards from authoritative sources, such as the physician or the Health Care Financing Administration (HCFA) administrator for Medicare, encourage usage. Checklists in the medical records of ambulatory care patients are helpful. Standing orders to administer vaccine in hospitals and clinics before the influenza season may help. Practice-based tracking systems that record the number and percentage of patients given vaccine serve as reminders and add a competitive spirit to the process. Public information campaigns reach a broad audience and should be an integral part of the effort (36).

Vaccine should be administered at least 2 weeks before influenza epidemics are expected to begin. In the United States, that would mean immunizations should be completed by early November.

H. Considerations for the Next Influenza Pandemic

Pandemics or worldwide epidemics of influenza periodically devastate the planet. In this century, pandemics have occurred in 1918, 1957, and 1968. They are associated with a major change in the hemagglutinin and often the neuraminidase surface proteins. In order to deal effectively with the next pandemic, we need to do the following (37):

1. Establish a surveillance network to detect the new strain.
2. Rapidly confirm that it is a new viral subtype.
3. Demonstrate that the new strain has epidemic potential in civilian populations.
4. Promptly prepare the new vaccine.
5. Identify and access the target groups for vaccination.
6. Define the role for antiviral drugs.

The first three items in the above list are in place or can be accomplished; the others are, to some degree, problematic. The World Health Organization has numerous laboratories in China and around the world to monitor the new influenzal strains isolated. The technology is available to confirm that a new strain is present. Confirmation of the epidemic potential is a straightforward epidemiological issue.

Problems occur, however, with the need for rapid vaccine production. Current manufacturing methods rely on embryonated eggs for vaccine production, and it takes approximately 6 months to produce a new vaccine. In that period of time, the first wave of the pandemic may have passed. The use of other tissue culture substrates or modern recombinant DNA technology for vaccine production may be more efficient but have not yet been fully developed (38). Determining the amount of vaccine to produce and for which segments of the population will require a Solomon-like decision, because we cannot make enough vaccine for our entire population. Although vaccination is the most effective method of disease prevention, antiviral drugs (i.e., amantadine and rimantadine) may be used for additional protection in high-risk persons or for prevention in nonvaccinated persons. Again, production capacity for the drugs would not be adequate, and the cost of long-term use of these drugs would be prohibitive.

Other issues have to be dealt with; for example, the number of doses required to provide adequate immunity. When a major antigenic shift occurs, it usually takes two doses of vaccine a month apart to provide adequate immunity (25). Also, legal liability may arise should adverse events occur, such as the Guillain-Barré syndrome (39). Finally, other nations depend on our vaccine production facilities.

Since most influenza pandemics appear to arise from human contact with certain animals, such as ducks and pigs, the potential for new strains is large. At least 15 hemagglutinins exist in the animal population, but only three of these (i.e., H1, H2, and H3) have infected humans (40).

In order to deal with this multifaceted problem, the National Institutes of Health (NIH), Centers for Disease Control and Prevention (CDC), and Food and Drug Administration (FDA) are developing pandemic and interpandemic plans. They are encouraging the development of influenza vaccines with enhanced immunity, improving methods for rapid vaccine manufacturing and administration, searching for a common epitope that would provide broad generic protection against a wide range of type A variant strains, developing a library of the remaining 12 animal hemagglutinin (HA) subtypes that have not infected humans yet, devising methods to reach the poorly immunized segments of our population, and adding more influenza surveillance sites around the world.

I. Experimental Influenza Vaccines

A number of different types of influenza vaccine are being investigated. For each vaccine, we will need to test whether the immunity induced by the new vaccines produces antibodies for all the immunoglobulin classes and whether they induce specific $CD4^+$, $CD8^+$ T-cell responses with no significant side effects. More importantly, we will need to demonstrate that the protection provided by the new vaccines is superior to that observed with the killed vaccines under both ideal study conditions (i.e., efficacy) as well as everyday use (i.e., effectiveness).

A number of vaccines have passed animal testing and are in at least phase I trials in humans. The different technologies include a cold-adapted live, attenuated virus; a purified viral HA subunit; a liposome containing viral HA; purified cytotoxic T-lymphocyte (CTL)–specific peptides; a microencapsulated inactivated virus; a purified, inactivated viral neuraminidase; a baculovirus-expressed recombinant HA subunit; a baculovirus-expressed nucleoprotein; and a transfected nucleic acid (DNA) plasmid expressing an HA subunit (41).

Distinct types of live-attenuated influenza vaccines have been investigated for the past few decades. The current live-attenuated vaccine being proposed for licensure is a cold-adapted vaccine. The term *cold-adapted* refers to the vaccine virus multiplying efficiently in the cooler upper respiratory passages of the nose and not in the warmer passageways of the lungs. Cold-adapted vaccines are administered by nasal drops or spray. They stimulate mucosal IgA immunity better than parenterally administered vaccine. Cold-adapted vaccines appear to have some advantages over inactivated vaccines, especially in children where they appear to be more acceptable than the injectable inactivated vaccines (41a). They promised to provide better protection for young children and broader, longer-lasting immunity against drift variants of the vaccine strains. Yet, the benefits of the cold-adapted strain have not been proven to be superior to the inactivated vaccine in influenza epidemics.

Advances in recombinant DNA technology have also been applied to making influenza vaccine production and are generating much excitement in the vaccine research world (38). The genome for the influenza HA has been cloned and inserted into a DNA plasmid, which is then injected intradermally with a gene gun. In response to the continuous transcription of the HA gene and translation into the H3 HA protein, antibody to the HA is produced for a period of time and then decays. There is no evidence of immunological tolerance induced by DNA immunization, although that is a theoretical consideration. Unexpectedly, cross-protective antibody to drift strains (e.g., various H3N2 strains) or to shifted or other subtypic strains (e.g., H1N1 strains) develop.

Vectors or carriers for recombinant-expressed influenza virus proteins, such as HA and matrix (M2) proteins, have been produced. The vectors may be avipox, vaccinia virus, baculovirus, or Venezuelan equine encephalitis virus. The gene for the influenza virus HA, for example, has been cloned and inserted into the baculovirus genome and then expressed in insect cells (42). The HA in this vaccine is in the form of the uncleaved HA (rHA0) that has epitopes distinct from the cleaved HA that is in the commercially available inactivated influenza vaccines. The rHA0 is glycosylated and hemagglutinates red blood cells (RBC). The vaccine is protective in young adults. The new vaccine may have the capacity to be more immunogenic, because a greater concentration of HA may be put into the vaccine than is possible with the current vaccines.

New presentation forms for influenza vaccines are being studied. Immunostimulating complexes (ISCOMS) are a novel antigen presentation form which may be more immunogenic in the elderly, since aged mice form a better immune response with Flu-ISCOMS than with the standard killed vaccine. Other new presentation forms for vaccines are unilaminar 150-nm spherical liposomes called immunopotentiating reconstituted influenza virosomes (IRIV) and chicken RBC ghosts.

II. Measles

Measles virus pneumonia is preventable by vaccination. It is more likely to occur in susceptible adults than in children. Although measles vaccine is most often administered as the trivalent measles, mumps, and rubella (MMR) vaccine, it also is available as a monovalent vaccine or a bivalent vaccine combined with rubella virus vaccine. The three-component MMR is usually preferred. A single dose of MMR provides protection in 95% of vaccine recipients. The second dose currently recommended is intended to provide protection to most of the rest of the subjects who do not respond to the initial dose and to boost immunity from the initial dose.

The first dose of MMR should be given at 15 months of age when maternal antibody against measles in the infant has ebbed. The second dose is given during the school-aged years. MMR is also recommended for adults (1) born after 1956 who do not have documentation of immunization with lives measles vaccine on or after their first birthday, (2) who have not had physician-diagnosed measles, or (3) with no laboratory evidence of measles immunity. In addition, persons should receive another dose of live measles vaccine who received live measles vaccine before their first birthday, or within several months after administration of immune globulin; those who received killed measles vaccine alone or killed measles vaccine followed within 3 months by live vaccine; or those who received a measles vaccine of unknown type between 1963 and 1967. Because knowledge of prior vaccination is often poor, a practical approach is to immunize all healthy adults born after 1956 with MMR (2,43). When two doses are administered, they should be separated by at least 1 month.

There is a caveat to the recommendation that persons born after 1956 should be revaccinated. Among health-care workers who developed measles during a study in the late 1980s, 29% were born before 1957. This dilemma may be avoided by serological screening of health-care workers for measles and rubella before reimmunizing all susceptibles regardless of age.

When exposed to a case of measles, susceptible persons should be vaccinated within 72 hr of exposure for protection. Alternatively, measles immune globulin, that is, normal immune globulin, should be given within 6 days of exposure to be effective. Immune globulin is particularly useful for persons who cannot take the live vaccine.

Adverse reactions to measles vaccine are not infrequent. Fever greater than 103°F (39.4°C) appears in 5–15% of vaccine recipients and occurs 5 to 12 days after vaccination. The fever lasts approximately 1–2 days. Febrile seizures can occur in children. Transient rashes also have been reported in 5% of vaccinated persons. Although encephalitis following measles vaccine has been reported, the incidence is not only less than the background incidence of encephalitis of unknown cause but is much less than encephalitis following naturally occurring measles.

Measles vaccine should not be given to pregnant women or to women considering becoming pregnant within 3 months of vaccination. It also should not be given to most immunocompromised persons whether the immunosuppression is from leukemia, lymphoma, or generalized malignancy or occurs as a result of large doses of corticosteroids, cancer chemotherapy, or radiation. There are a few exceptions. Persons with leukemia who are in remission and have not received chemotherapy within 3 months and adults infected with the human immunodeficiency virus (HIV) who have not progressed to AIDS may be vaccinated against measles. HIV-infected children <12 months old with

CD4$^+$ T-lymphocyte counts <750 or children aged 1–5 years with CD4$^+$ counts <500 should not receive MMR. Otherwise, children 6 years old or above may be vaccinated when their CD4$^+$ counts are >200 (44). Immune globulin can be used for exposure of susceptible immunocompromised patients to individuals with measles. The vaccine is also contraindicated in persons with anaphylaxis after ingesting eggs and receiving neomycin.

Only one severe adverse reaction has been reported in an HIV-infected person with AIDS and a CD4$^+$ count of 0. This individual developed pneumonia from a measles virus strain that resembled the vaccine strain, as documented by polymerase chain reaction (PCR) analysis. It was thought to have contributed to his death (44).

Transient increases in viral load occur in HIV-infected persons when they receive measles or influenza vaccine, but this is not considered clinically significant (45).

Other types of live, attenuated measles vaccines are currently being investigated as potential vaccine candidates. In addition, a high-titered live vaccine containing multiple strains of measles is being studied (41).

III. Varicella-Zoster Virus

Varicella-zoster virus (VZV) pneumonia is one of the many complications of varicella-zoster virus infection. It is most common in adults who have not had chickenpox in childhood (46,47). Most patients who develop this complication have cough and dyspnea within 1–6 days after the onset of rash. Pneumonia diagnosed by chest radiograph actually appears in up to 10–20% of adults, but it may be mild and transient and clear without acyclovir therapy in 48 hr. In others, it may progress to bilateral infiltrates, severe hypoxemia, and fulminant respiratory failure.

A live-attenuated VZV vaccine was recently licensed (48,49). Universal childhood immunization is recommended and thought to be cost beneficial (50). In adolescents and adults, vaccine is indicated when they are shown to be susceptible by serological testing. The vaccine provides protection from mild disease in 77% and from severe disease in 98% of vaccinated persons (51).

The vaccine elicits humoral as well as T-lymphocyte responses. The T-lymphocyte responses are comparable to that elicited by natural infection. In children, the T-lymphocyte response is superior to that seen in adults. Consequently, one dose is recommended for ages 12 months to 13 years when susceptible by history, and two doses given 4–8 weeks apart are recommended for ages 13 years and above when susceptible by serological testing.

The vaccine is contraindicated in immunodeficiencies whether they are congenital or acquired except for acute lymphocytic leukemia where children in remission for 1 year or more may be immunized under a research protocol. (Contact the Varivax Coordinating Center by telephone at 215/283-0891.) The vaccine is also contraindicated for symptomatic HIV infection, pregnancy, high-dose corticosteroid use (i.e., ≥2 mg of prednisone per kg per day for children or ≥20 mg of prednisone for ≥1 month), allergy to neomycin, or intercurrent illness. The use of immune globulin or other blood products within 5 months will interfere with vaccination. Salicylates given within 6 weeks pose the possible risk of Reye's syndrome.

A number of mild adverse reactions to the VZV vaccine may occur. Fever ≥102°F occurs in 15% of vaccinees and local pain in 19%. A localized rash at the injection site appears in 3% of vaccinees, with a median of two lesions which occur at 8–19 days after vaccination. A generalized rash occurs in 4% vaccinees, with a mean of five lesions that appear 5–26 days after vaccine is administered. When a healthy vaccinee develops a rash, transmission to susceptible persons has been reported (52). Although VZV has been detected by PCR in the oropharynx of 7% of healthy children, infectious virus has not been recovered.

Passive immunity may be provided with varicella-zoster immune globulin (VZIG), which is distributed by the American Red Cross Blood Services. VZIG is indicated when the following groups of individuals have significant exposure to chickenpox: immunocompromised children with no history of varicella; pregnant women with no history of varicella and no laboratory evidence of prior infection; infants born to mothers with varicella beginning within 5 days before or two days after delivery; hospitalized premature infants with no maternal history of varicella and/or no antibodies to VZV; and premature infants <28 weeks of gestation or weighing <1000 g regardless of maternal history. Isolation of hospitalized patients with varicella can reduce the risk of spread to at-risk patients.

A close exposure to varicella is defined as a household contact; close indoor contact (i.e., face-to-face exposure) for greater than 1 hr; hospital contact with an index case in the same room, ward, or nursery; hospital contact by face-to-face exposure to an infected person; or newborn exposure to maternal varicella.

When the decision is made to give VZIG, it must be given within 96 hr, preferably within 48 hr (53). VZIG lowers the risk of varicella pneumonia, but breakthrough cases have been reported in 11% in one series (54).

IV. Respiratory Syncytial Virus

The respiratory syncytial virus (RSV) is one of the most common causes of pneumonia in infants and children and is being increasingly recognized as a cause of pneumonia in high-risk adults. RSV presents distinct problems. First, although the level of human neutralizing, F, and G antibodies correlate directly with resistance to reinfection, the protection is by no means complete. Reinfection occurs in 25% of individuals with the highest levels of antibody (55). Second, potentiation of natural RSV infection occurs when a killed, whole virus RSV vaccine has been given to children previously. So new methods of vaccine production are being tested.

A purified fusion (F) surface glycoprotein of RSV was tested in children without ill effect. Further studies are necessary to be certain that the vaccine does not potentiate illness when the vaccine recipient is exposed to naturally occurring RSV. In addition, live, attenuated temperature-sensitive and/or cold-adapted strains are being tested as vaccines (41). Eventually, an RSV vaccine may be studied in certain high-risk adults, as RSV is associated with pneumonia and death in adult bone marrow transplant recipients (56) (see Chap. 5).

RSV immunoglobulin (RSVIG) is given to high-risk infants and children, because it is effective in preventing serious lower respiratory tract infection caused by RSV (57). Target groups for administration are children less than 24 months of age with a history of bronchopulmonary dysplasia or premature birth (i.e., ≤ 35 weeks' gestation). It is given 1 month prior to the start of the RSV season and continued monthly throughout the season.

V. Parainfluenza Virus

Parainfluenza viruses commonly cause pneumonia in infants and children and are an occasional cause in high-risk adults. Parainfluenza virus type 3 (PIV-3) cold-adapted and temperature-sensitive mutant human vaccine strains are safe and immunogenic when tested in infants and children as well as being phenotypically stable (58). In addition to the human PIV-3, a bovine PIV-3 strain antigenically related to human strains and a purified HN and F protein subunit vaccine are being investigated (41).

VI. Summary

The world of respiratory virus vaccine development is moving rapidly forward. Influenza vaccine has been shown significantly to reduce the morbidity and mortality from frequent epidemics of influenza virus infection. Broader usage promises to have a large impact on the prevention of disease. Molecular virology techniques are being applied to further improve influenza vaccine.

Vaccines against other common causes of viral pneumonia, such as parainfluenza virus and respiratory syncytial virus, are being studied. Vaccines against less common causes of viral pneumonia, such as measles virus and varicella-zoster virus, are already available.

References

1. Centers for Disease Control and Prevention. Prevention and control of influenza: recommendations of the Advisory Committee on Immunization Practices (ACIP). MMWR 1996; 45:1–4.
2. Gardner P, Eickhoff T, Griffin M, Gross P, LaForce FM, Schaffner W, Strikas R, eds. Guide for Adult Immunization. Philadelphia: American College of Physicians, 1994:143–151.
3. Smith W, Andrewes CH, Laidlaw PP. A virus obtained from influenza patients. Lancet 1933; 2:66–68.
4. Chenoweth A, Waltz AD, Stokes J Jr, Gladen RG. Active immunization with the viruses of human and swine influenza. Am J Dis Child 1936; 52:757–758.
5. Kilbourne ED. Influenza. New York: Plenum Press, 1987.
6. Gross PA, Hermogenes AW, Sacks HS, Lau J, Levandowski RA. The efficacy of influenza vaccine in elderly persons. A meta-analysis and review of the literature. Ann Intern Med 1995; 123:518–527.
7. Fedson DS, Wajda A, Nicol P, Hammond GW, Kaiser DL, Roos LL. Clinical effectiveness of influenza vaccination in Manitoba. JAMA 1993; 270:1956–1961.
8. Nichol KL, Margolis KL, Wuorenma J, Von Sternberg T. The efficacy and cost effectiveness of vaccination against influenza among elderly persons living in the community. N Engl J Med 1994; 331:778–784.
9. Foster DA, Talsma A, Furomoto-Dawson A, Ohmit SE, Margulies JR, Arden NH, Monto AS. Influenza vaccine effectiveness in preventing hospitalization for pneumonia in the elderly. Am J Epidemiol 1992; 136:296–307.
10. Mullooy JP, Bennett MD, Hornbrook MC, Barker WH, Williams WW, Patriarca PA, Rhodes PH. Influenza vaccination programs for elderly persons: cost-effectiveness in a health maintenance organization. Ann Intern Med 1994; 121:947–952.
11. Govaert TM, Thijs CT, Masurel N, Sprenger MJ, Dinant GJ, Knottnerus JA. The efficacy of influenza vaccination in elderly individuals. A randomized double-blind placebo-controlled trial. JAMA 1994; 272:1661–1665.
12. Strassburg MA, Greenland S, Sorvillo FJ, Lieb LE, Habel LA. Influenza in the elderly: report of an outbreak and a review of vaccine effectiveness reports. Vaccine 1986; 4:38–44.
13. Nichol KL, Lind A, Margolis KL, Murdoch M, McFadden R, Hauge M, Magnan S, Drake M. The effectiveness of vaccination against influenza in healthy, working adults. N Engl J Med 1995; 333:889–893.
14. Gross PA, Gould AL, Brown AE. Effect of cancer chemotherapy on the immune response to influenza virus vaccine: review of published studies. Rev Infect Dis 1985; 7:613–618.

15. Ortbals DW, Liebhaber H, Presant CA, Van Amburg AL III, Lee JY. Influenza immunization of adult patients with malignant diseases. Ann Intern Med 1977; 87:522–527.
16. Dowdle WR, Moslow SR, Coleman MT, Kaye HS, Schoenbaum SC. Inactivated influenza vaccines. 2. Laboratory indices of protection. Postgrad Med J 1973; 49: 159–163.
17. Hoskins TW, Davies JR, Smith AJ, Miller CL, Allchin A. Assessment of inactivated influenza-A vaccine after three outbreaks of influenza at Christ's Hospital. Lancet 1979; 1:33–35.
18. Gross PA, Denning CR, Gaerlan PF, Bonelli J, Bernius M, Dran S, Munk G, Vassallo M, Quinnan GV, Levandowski R, Cataruozolo PE, Wallenstein S. Annual influenza vaccination: immune response in patients over 10 years. Vaccine 1996; 14:1280–1284.
19. Keitel WA, Case TR, Couch RB. Efficacy of sequential annual vaccination with inactivated influenza virus vaccine. Am J Epidemiol 1988; 12:353–364.
20. Clements ML, Murphy BR. Development and persistence of local and systemic antibody responses in adults given live-attenuated or inactivated influenza a virus vaccine. J Clin Microbiol 1986; 23:66–72.
21. Bender BS, Johnson MP, Small PA. Influenza in senescent mice: impaired cytotoxic T-lymphocyte activity is correlated with prolonged infection. Immunology 1991; 72:514–519.
22. Kutza J, Gross P, Kaye D, Murasko DM. Natural killer cell cytotoxicity in elderly humans after influenza immunization. Clin Diag Lab Immunol 1996; 3:105–108.
23. Margolis KL, Nichol KL, Poland GA, Pluhar RE. Frequency of adverse reactions to influenza vaccine in the elderly. A randomized, placebo-controlled trial. JAMA 1990; 264:1139–1141.
24. Nichol KL, Margolis KL, Lind A, Murdoch M, McFadden R, Hauge M, Magnan S, Drake M. Side effects associated with influenza vaccination in healthy working adults. Arch Intern Med 1996; 156:1546–1550.
25. Gross PA. Reactogenicity and immunogenicity of bivalent influenza vaccine in one- and two-dose trials in children: a summary. J Infect Dis 1977; 136:s616–s623.
26. Perez-Tirse J, Gross PA. Review of cost-benefit analyses of influenza vaccine. PharmacoEconomics 1992; 2:198–206.
27. Office of Technology Assessment, US Congress. Cost Effectiveness of Influenza Vaccination. Washington, DC: Government Printing Office, 1982.
28. Riddiough MA, Slak JE, Bell JC. Influenza vaccination: cost-effectiveness and public policy. JAMA 1983; 249:3189–3195.
29. Glezen WP. Emerging infections: pandemic influenza. Epidemiol Rev 1996; 18: 1–13.
30. Schoenbaum SC. Economic impact of influenza, individual's perspective. Am J Med 1987; 19:(suppl 6A):26–30.
31. Weinstein MC, Siegel JE, Gold MR, Kamlet MS, Russell LB. Recommendations of the panel on cost-effectiveness in health and medicine. JAMA 1996; 276:1253–1258.
32. Naylor D. Editorial: Cost-effectiveness analysis: are the outputs worth the inputs? ACP Journal Club 1996; Jan/Feb:A12–A14.

33. Stevens WK. But cost-benefit analysis is problematic. New York Times 1995; April 25:C4.
34. Schmitz R. Influenza vaccination in the first year of the Medicare influenza vaccine benefit. Cambridge, MA: Abt Associates, 1994.
35. Fedson DS. Influenza vaccination of medical residents at the University of Virginia: 1986 to 1994. Infect Control Hosp Epidemiol 1996; 17:431–433.
36. GAO Report to congressional requesters. Immunization: HHS could do more to increase vaccination among older adults. United States General Accounting Office. GAO/PEMD-95-14.
37. Gross PA. Preparing for the next influenza pandemic: a reemerging infection. Ann Intern Med 1996; 124:682–685.
38. Donnelly JJ, Ulmer JB, Liu MA. Immunization with DNA. J Immunol Methods 1994; 176:145–152.
39. Hurwitz ES, Schonberger LB, Nelson DB, Holman RC. Guillain-Barré syndrome and the 1978–1979 influenza vaccine. N Engl J Med 1981; 304:1557–1561.
40. Webster RG, Schafer JR, Suss J, Bean WJ, Kawaoka Y. Evolution and ecology of influenza viruses. In: Hannoun C, Kendal AP, Klenk HD, Ruben FL, eds. Options for the Control of Influenza II: Proceedings of the International Conference on Options for the Control of Influenza, Courchevel, September 27–October 2, 1992. New York: Excerpta Medica, 1993:177–185.
41. Baker PJ, ed. The Jordan Report: accelerated development of vaccines 1996. Division of Microbiology and Infectious Diseases, National Institutes of Health, Bethesda, MD, 1996.
41a. Belshe RB, Mendelman PM, Treanor J, King J, Gruber WC, Piedra P, Bernstein DI, Hayden FG, Kotloff K, Zangwill K, Iacuzio D, Wolff M. The efficacy of live attenuated, cold-adapted, trivalent, intranasal influenzavirus vaccine in children. N Engl J Med 1998; 338(20):1405–1412.
42. Lakey DL, Treanor JJ, Betts RF, Smith GE, Thompson J, Sannella E, Reed G, Wilkinson BE, Wright PF. Recombinant baculovirus influenza A hemagglutinin vaccines are well tolerated and immunogenic in healthy adults. J Infect Dis 1996; 174:838–841.
43. Peter G, Halsey NA, Marcuse EK, Pickering LK, eds. Report of the Committee on Infectious Diseases. 23nd ed. Elk Grove Village, IL: American Academy of Pediatrics, 1994.
44. Mealses pneumonitis following measles-mumps-rubella vaccination of a patient with HIV infection, 1993. MMWR 1996; 45:603–606.
45. Stanley SK, Ostrowski MA, Justement BS, Gantt K, Hedayati S, Mannix M, Roche K, Schwartzentruber DJ. Effect of immunization with a common recall antigen on viral expression in patients infected with human immunodeficiency virus type 1. N Engl J Med 1996; 334:1222–1230.
46. Gogos CA, Bassaris HP, Vagenakis AG. Varicella pneumonia in adults. A review of pulmonary manifestations, risk factors and treatment. Respiration 1992; 59:339–343.
47. Krugman S, Goodrich CH, Ward R. Primary varicella pneumonia. N Engl J Med 1957; 257:843–847.
48. Gershon AA. Varicella-zoster virus: prospects for control. Adv Pediatr Infect Dis 1995; 10:93–124.

49. Arvin AM. Varicella-zoster virus. Clin Microbiol Rev 1996; 9:361–381.
50. Lieu TA, Cochi SL, Black SB, Halloran ME, Shinefield HR, Holmes SJ, Wharton M. Cost-effectiveness of a routine varicella vaccination program for US children. JAMA 1994; 271:375–381.
51. American Academy of Pediatrics Committee on Infectious Diseases. Recommendations for the use of live-attenuated varicella vaccine. Pediatrics 1995; 95:791–796.
52. Hughes P, LaRussa P, Pearce JM, Lepow M, Steinberg S, Gershon A. Transmission of varicella-zoster virus from a vaccinee with leukemia, demonstrated by polymerase chain reaction. J Pediatr 1994; 124:932–935.
53. Centers for Disease Control. Varicella-zoster immune globulin for the prevention of chickenpox: recommendations of the Immunizations Practices Advisory Committee. Ann Intern Med 1984; 100:859–865.
54. Feldman S, Lott L. Varicella in children with cancer: impact of antiviral therapy and prophylaxis. Pediatrics 1987; 80:465–472.
55. Hall CB, Walsh EE, Long CE, Schnabel KC. Immunity to and frequency of reinfection with respiratory syncytial virus. J Infect Dis 1991; 163:693–698.
56. Whimbey E, Couch RB, Englund JA, Andreeff M, Goodrich JM, Raad II, Lewis V, Mirza N, Luna MA, Baxter B, Tarrand JJ, Bodey GP. Respiratory syncytial virus pneumonia in hospitalized adult patients with leukemia. Clin Infect Dis 1995; 21:376–379.
57. Groothuis JR. Role of antibody and use of respiratory syncytial virus (RSV) immune globulin to prevent severe RSV disease in high-risk children. J Pediatrics 1994; 124:S28–S32.
58. Karron RA, Wright PF, Newman FK, Makhene M, Thompson J, Samorodin R, Wilson MH, Anderson EL, Clements ML, Murphy BR, Belshe RB. A live human parainfluenza type 3 virus vaccine is attenuated and immunogenic in healthy infants and children. J Infect Dis 1995; 172:1445–1450.

AUTHOR INDEX

Italic numbers give the page on which the complete reference is listed.

A

Abbas, J, 92, 93, *101*
Abbott, RD, 265, *277*
Abdallah, PS, 32, *48*
Abe, K, 113, *141*
Abecassis, MM, 320, *324*
Abell, TD, 333, 334, *348*
Abina, MA, 242, *250*
Abramson, JS, 111, 113, *140, 141*
Abzug, MJ, 239, *248*
Achiwa, K, 137, *159*
Acsadi, G, 132, *156*
Ada, GL, 117, *145*
Adams, EG, 163, *187*
Adams, JM, 30, *44*
Adelson, L, 111, *140*
Adler, JL, 29, *42*, 124, *147*
Adler, WH, 56, *74*
Adrian, T, 224, 226, 235, *244*
Agius, G, 30, *45*, 63, 65, 66, *78*, 177, *199*
Aherne, W, 26, *40*, 171, *196*
Ahle, ET, 31, *46*
Ahluwalia, G, 308, *322*
Ahn, Y, 65, *79*

Ailing, DW, 180, *200*
Air, GM, 345, *353*
Aj, NW, 264, *277*
Akaike, T, 113, *141*
Aker, M, 93, *101*
Akerlind, B, 166, *191*
Akerlund, A, 268, 269, *279*
Akers, LW, 328, *346*
Akhtar, N, 311, *323*
Akizuki, S, 29, *43*, 68, *80*
al-Mazron, A, 128, *152*
Al-Mufti, S, 311, 313, *323*
Al-Nakib, W, 311, 313, *323*
Alam, A, 27, *41*
Albano, C, 93, *101*
Albrecht, JK, 264, *277*
Albritton, W, 240, *249*
Alexandrova, GI, 130, *154*
Alexson, C, 165, 176, *190*
Alford, RH, 111, *140*
Alix, D, 270, 271, *280*
Alkner, U, 268, *279*
Allan, I, 55, 58, *74*
Allan, ID, 63, *79*, 270, *279*
Allan, JE, 210, *218*
Allan, W, 116, 117, *144, 145*

Allard, JP, 59, 75
Allchin, A, 128, *152*, 358, *371*
Allen, ID, 29, *41*
Allen, JR, 129, *153*
Allen, LB, 338, *350*
Allen, SE, 292, *305*
Allen, U, 180, *200*
Alling, DW, 163, *187*
Allison, AC, 115, *143*
Allison, JE, 127, *149*, 342, *352*
Almond, JW, 255, *274*
Alonso-Caplan, FB, 108, *139*
Altman, DG, 16, *22*
Alwan, W, 171, 173, *196, 197*
Ambrose, MW, 180, *200, 201*
An, S, 173, *197*
Anapol, H, 284, *301*
Anas, NG, 175, *198*
Anderson, B, 287, 293, *303, 305*
Anderson, CW, 232, *244*
Anderson, DC, 296, *305*
Anderson, DJ, 27, *41*
Anderson, E, 131, *155*
Anderson, EL, 130, 131, *153, 155*, 183, *203*, 369, *373*
Anderson, G, 31, *46*
Anderson, J, 168, 170, *192*
Anderson, K, 163, 170, 183, *187, 188, 195, 202*, 284, *301*
Anderson, KG, 29, *41*, 86, *98*
Anderson, LJ, 30, *44*, 92, *100*, 161, 163, 166, 167, 177, *184, 186, 190, 191*, 224, 226, 235, 239, *244, 248*, 314, *324*
Anderson, MS, 31, *46*, 96, *102*
Anderson, R, 181, 182, *201*
Andersson, E, 269, *279*
Andersson, J, 89, *99*
Andersson, M, 268, 269, *279*
Andiman, WA, 33, *49*
Ando, M, 113, *141*
Andreef, M, 91, *100*
Andreeff, M, 369, *373*
Andreis, K, 264, *277*
Andrewes, CH, 355, *370*
Andrews, RI, 31, *46*

Angelillo, VA, 33, *49*
Angliker, H, 113, *142*
Ansari, SA, 216, *221*
Antipa, C, 25, 29, *39*
Antkowiak, JG, 31, *46*
Anzueta, A, 96, *102*
Aoki, FY, 330, 340, *347, 351*
Aoudjhane, M, 30, *43*, 86, 87, *98*, 177, *199*
Aoyagi, T, 298, *306*
Apalsch, AM, 213, *219*
Apkom, CA, 16, *22*
Appleyard, G, 115, *143*, 273, *280*, 330, *347*
Apuzzio, JJ, 31, *46*
Aquilina, AT, 113, *141*
Araki, S, 113, *141*
Arbiza, JR, 27, *40*
Arden, NH, 60, 61, 62, 69, *76, 77*, 92, *100*, 128, 134, *151, 157, 158*, 337, 350, 358, *370*
Ariagno, RL, 65, *79*, 342, *352*
Arikawa, J, 284, 286, *302*
Arisumi, D, 25, *39*
Armbruster, KFW, 330, *347*
Armstron, JA, 127, *151*
Armstrong, LR, 34, *51*, 284, *301*
Arnold, E, 255, *274*
Arnold, R, 167, *191*
Arrobio, J, 92, 94, *101*
Arrobio, JO, 123, *147*, 161, 165, 170, 172, 182, 183, *184, 189, 195, 202*, 224, 237, 238, *244*, 342, *352*
Arroyo, JC, 54, 63, 67, *73*, 128, *152*
Arruda, E, 257, *275*
Artenstein, BC, 236, *247*
Artenstein, MS, 240, *249*
Arvin, AM, 366, *372*
Aschan, J, 89, *99*
Ascher, M, 284, *301*
Ash, RC, 235, 237, *246, 248*
Ashley, R, 33, *50*
Ashmun, RA, 266, 268, *278*
Askonas, BA, 117, *144, 145*, 163, 169, 170, 172, *187, 188, 194, 195*
Asperilla, MO, 32, 35, *47*

Atkinson, WL, 134, *157*
Atmar, RL, 34, *51,* 94, *101,* 126, *149,* 209, 270, 272, *280,* 308, 310, 311, 313, 314, 315, 316, 317, *322, 323,* 330, *347*
Atsuhiro, K, 33, *50*
August, MJ, 239, *248*
Avery, RK, 27, *41*
Avila, M, 27, *40, 41*
Avsi-Zupanc, T, 284, *301*
Aylward, RB, 30, *45,* 65, *79*
Aymard, M, 128, *152*
Azimi, PH, 91, *100*

B

Babbitt, J, 235, 237, *246, 248*
Babish, JD, 57, *74*
Babiuk, LA, 26, *40,* 113, *141*
Bachi, T, 162, *185*
Bacik, I, 163, *188*
Bacum, RJ, 127, *149*
Bader, I, 29, *43*
Baek, LJ, 287, *303*
Baernstein, HD, 328, *346*
Baes, L, 27, *41*
Bagdzhadhzyan, A, 266, 267, *278*
Baguet, JC, 30, *43,* 88, *99*
Baker, CJ, 240, *249*
Baker, DJ, 61, 63, 71, *76,* 128, *152,* 270, *280*
Baker, PJ, 364, 366, 369, *372*
Baker, VV, 29, *42*
Baldanti, F, 320, *324*
Baldini, J, 334, *349*
Balfour, HH, 27, 29, 30, 32, *41, 43, 44, 49,* 86, 87, 88, 96, *98, 102,* 161, 166, 167, 180, *185,* 213, *219,* 314, 316, *324*
Baljet, M, 61, *76*
Balk, RA, 290, 292, *304*
Ball, LA, 162, 163, 169, 170, 183, *186, 187, 194, 195, 202*
Balliigand, Jl, 298, *306*
Balser, CF, 230, *247*

Baltiev, A, 25, 29, *39*
Balzano, GJ, 58, *75,* 128, *152*
Ban Amburg, AL, 358, *371*
Bandyk, MG, 328, 331, 336, *346*
Bangham, CRM, 163, 169, 170, *187, 194, 195*
Bar-Yishay, E, 180, *200*
Baradaran, K, 162, 163, *185*
Barbas, CF, 181, *201*
Barbone, F, 113, *142*
Barclay, WS, 131, *156*
Bardin, PG, 258, 261, *275, 276*
Barigazzi, G, 121, *146*
Barker, DJP, 161, *185*
Barker, WH, 29, 38, *42, 43, 51,* 55, 56, 58, 62, 63, 64, *73, 74, 77,* 118, 127, *145, 149,* 161, 180, *185,* 270, *280,* 314, *324,* 358, *370*
Barnaure, F, 25, 29, *39*
Barnes, MW, 111, *140*
Barnes, ND, 88, *98*
Baron, P, 169, 181, *194, 201*
Barrett, FF, 30, *45*
Barrett, MJ, 125, *147*
Barry, DW, 115, *143*
Barton, R, 255, *274*
Bartoni, K, 96, *102*
Bass, DA, 113, *141*
Bassallo, M, 358, *371*
Bassaris, HP, 31, *47,* 366, *372*
Bauer, SP, 34, *51,* 344, *353*
Baughman, RP, 32, *49,* 308, *322*
Baum, SG, 241, *249*
Baumann, PC, 33, *50*
Baumgarth, N, 116, 117, *144*
Baxter, B, 91, *100,* 126, 131, *148, 149, 155,* 369, *373*
Baxter, BB, 64, *79,* 165, 169, *189, 193*
Baxter, BD, 128, 131, *151, 155, 156,* 214, *219,* 270, 272, *280,* 311, 313, *323*
Bayley, P, 106, *138*
Baylor, N, 108, *138*
Beal, R, 238, *248*
Beale, AJ, 205, *216*
Beale, J, 115, *143*

Beall, AC, 31, *46*, 96, *102*
Beam, WE, 29, *43*, 316, *324*
Beam, WEJ, 66, *80*
Bean, WJ, 119, 121, 122, 135, *146, 147, 158*, 363, *372*
Beard, CW, 135, *158*
Beare, PAS, 117, *145*
Beasley, P, 261, *276*
Beasley, PP, 265, *277*
Beatie, BL, 128, *152*
Beaton, AR, 108, *138*
Beattie, BL, 56, 62, *74*, 77
Beaty, HN, 333, *348*
Bebear, C, 25, 29, *39*
Bechard, DE, 34, *50*
Becht, H, 117, *144*
Bechtereva, T, 126, *148*
Becker, S, 164, 167, *189, 191*
Becroft, DM, 238, *248*
Beeler, JA, 163, *187*
Beem, M, 168, 169, 172, *192*
Beier, P, 168, *192*
Belchis, D, 91, *100*
Beljaev, AL, 130, *154*
Bell, DM, 65, *79*, 180, *200*
Bell, JA, 205, *217*, 223, *244*
Bell, LM, 175, *198*
Bell, PR, 88, *99*
Bellanti, JA, 210, *218*, 236, *247*
Belshe, R, 336, *349*
Belshe, RB, 60, *76*, 128, 130, 131, 134, 135, *152, 153, 155, 157, 158*, 166, 171, 172, 182, 183, *191, 196, 202, 203*, 214, 215, *220*, 335, 336, *349*, 369, *373*
Bende, M, 269, *279*
Bender, BS, 26, *40*, 128, *151*, 359, *371*
Bender, CA, 120, *146*
Benham, C, 109, *139*
Bennett, MD, 38, *51*, 62, *77*, 358, *370*
Bennink, JR, 163, *188*
Benson, A, 30, *43, 44*, 86, 87, *98*, 314, *324*
Bentley, D, 133, *157*
Bentley, DW, 29, *43*, 58, 61, 62, 63, 64, *75, 76, 78*, 166, *190*

Bentur, L, 180, *200*
Berbari, N, 88, *99*
Bereiter-Hahn, J, 298, *306*
Berencsi, K, 236, *247*
Bergert, SM, 229, *245*
Bergin, J, 93, *101*
Bergin, M, 240, *249*
Berlin, BS, 127, *150*
Berman, S, 17, *23*
Bernhardt, LL, 272, *280*
Bernius, M, 358, *371*
Bernstein, DI, 136, *159*, 333, *348*
Bernstein, JM, 163, *188*
Berntsson, E, 25, 29, *39*
Berry, GJ, 318, *324*
Beschorner, WE, 95, *102*
Beshe, RB, 130, *153*
Bethell, R, 137, *159*
Bethell, RC, 136, *159*
Betts, R, 55, 57, 58, 59, 60, *73*, 128, 132, *152, 157*, 335, *349*
Betts, RF, 29, *43*, 55, 56, 61, 62, 63, 64, 65, 66, 67, 69, 70, 71, *73, 77, 78, 82*, 93, *101*, 115, 116, 125, 127, 130, 131, 133, 134, 136, 137, *143, 147, 150, 153, 154, 157, 158, 159*, 161, 166, 177, 180, *185*, 265, *277*, 311, 313, 314, *323, 324*, 334, 335, 337, 340, 345, *349, 351, 353*, 365, 372
Bew, M, 169, *194*
Beyer, B, 31, *47*
Beyer, WE, 127, *151*
Beyer, WEP, 56, 61, *74, 76*, 93, *101*
Beytout, D, 30, *43*, 88, *99*
Bharadwaj, M, 284, *301*
Bhat, BM, 183, *202*, 242, *250*
Bhat, R, 242, *250*
Bhat, RA, 183, *202*
Bice, DE, 297, *305*
Biddison, WE, 116, *144*
Bienvenu, J, 128, *152*
Biggar, R, 164, 165, *189*
Biggar, RJ, 30, *45*, 63, 65, 66, *78*, 177, *199*
Bigl, S, 128, *152*

Billaudel, S, 178, *199*
Billeter, MA, 216, *221*
Billingham, ME, 318, *324*
Billups, LC, 115, *143*
Binder, C, 261, *276*
Bird, T, 26, *40,* 171, *196*
Birgenheier, R, 128, *152*
Birkhead, GS, 29, *42,* 59, *75,* 315, 316, *324*
Birnbaumer, DM, 34, *50*
Bitterman, PB, 30, *44,* 86, 87, *97,* 166, 171, 177, *190*
Bjarnason, R, 173, 174, *197, 198*
Bjorksten, B, 173, 174, *197*
Bjornson, G, 128, *152*
Blac-Payne, CA, 30, *45*
Black, RA, 115, *142*
Black, SB, 366, *372*
Black, SH, 232, *246*
Blackwelder, W, 127, 128, *150*
Blackwelder, WC, 126, *148*
Blaine, WG, 117, *145*
Blainey, AD, 25, *38*
Blair, G, 68, *80*
Blanche, S, 91, *100*
Blanco, I, 316, *324*
Blass, D, 108, *138,* 255, *274*
Blatnik, B, 60, 61, *76*
Blau, DM, 208, *217*
Bleackley, CR, 62, *77*
Bleackley, RC, 128, *152*
Bleakley, RC, 56, *74*
Blisel, P, 131, *156*
Block, MJ, 165, 166, 177, *189*
Blomberg, J, 25, 29, *39*
Bloom, H, 169, *193*
Bloom, HH, 63, *78*
Blossom, P, 164, *189*
Blount, RE, 161, *184*
Blumberg, EA, 93, *101*
Blumefield, HL, 29, *42*
Blumenfeld, HL, 58, *75,* 113, 124, *141*
Bobo, L, 59, *75,* 214, *220*
Bocchini, JA, 30, *45,* 165, *189*
Bock, MJ, 87, *98*

Bodey, GP, 32, *48,* 87, 88, *98,* 117, 123, *145,* 369, *373*
Boggs, JM, 34, *50*
Bohte, R, 25, 29, *40*
Boland, FJ, 131, *156*
Bona, C, 131, *156*
Bona, CA, 115, 126, *142, 148*
Bone, RC, 290, 292, *304*
Bonelli, J, 358, *371*
Bonville, CA, 29, *43,* 314, *324*
Bootman, JS, 129, *153*
Borek, E, 339, 350
Borison, RL, 330, *347*
Borkowsky, W, 90, *100,* 176, *199*
Bornstein, N, 25, 29, *39*
Borst, RJA, 126, 128, *149*
Borysiewicz, LK, 26, 32, *40, 48*
Bosher, J, 229, *245*
Bosshard, S, 32, *48*
Bot, A, 115, *142*
Bovbjerg, DH, 263, *277*
Boven, K, 240, *249*
Bowden, RA, 32, 33, 35, *48, 49, 50,* 86, 87, 88, 95, *98*
Boyd, K, 32, *47*
Boyd, MKR, 329, *347*
Boyel, TR, 257, *275*
Boyer, KM, 127, *149*
Bozeman, FM, 126, *148*
Braam, J, 108, *138*
Braciale, TJ, 116, *144*
Braciale, VL, 116, *144*
Bradshaw, GL, 113, *142*
Brady, HA, 231, *247*
Brady, MT, 333, *348*
Bragina, VE, 130, *154*
Brain, EA, 261, *276*
Braine, HG, 95, *102*
Braman, P, 133, *157*
Bramson, JL, 242, *250*
Brand, CD, 342, *352*
Brand, CM, 115, *143*
Brandenburg, AH, 179, *200*
Brandriss, M, 62, *77,* 162, 163, 169, *186, 187, 194*
Brandriss, MW, 163, *187*

Brandt, BS, 236, *247*
Brandt, CD, 91, *100,* 123, *147,* 161, 162, 165, 170, 172, 181, *184, 185, 189, 195, 201,* 224, 237, 238, *244*
Brasier, A, 167, *192*
Brassard, DL, 107, 109, *138, 139*
Bratton, S, 89, *99*
Braun, I, 329, *346*
Bregman, DJ, 127, *150,* 331, *348*
Breiman, RF, 30, 34, *44, 51,* 92, *100,* 289, 292, 297, *304, 305,* 314, *324*
Breinig, MK, 88, 89, *98*
Breyer, RH, 31, *46*
Bribskov, CL, 256, *274*
Bricourt, F, 30, *43,* 86, 87, *98*
Brideau, RJ, 216, *220*
Briggs, DD, 33, *49*
Briggs, KD, 88, *99*
Brillman, JC, 290, 292, *304*
Briselli, M, 163, *187*
Broadbent, DA, 113, *141*
Brochstein, JA, 32, *48*
Brodine, S, 55, *73*
Brodman, R, 127, *151*
Brody, SL, 242, *250*
Broker, TR, 229, *245*
Brondel, L, 66, *80*
Brooks, JG, 175, *198*
Bross, P, 127, 128, *150*
Brossmer, R, 109, *139*
Brouard, J, 179, *200*
Brouilette, WJ, 345, *353*
Broussard, RC, 32, *47*
Brown, A, 128, *152*
Brown, AE, 358, *370*
Brown, CS, 62, *78*
Brown, E, 106, *138*
Brown, EG, 113, *142*
Brown, L, 116, *144*
Brown, PK, 263, *277*
Brown, R, 181, *201*
Brown, RB, 25, *38*
Brown, VA, 216, *221*
Browne, MJ, 329, *347*
Bruce, CB, 313, *324*
Brugh, M, 135, *158*

Bruhn, F, 173, *197*
Bruner, JM, 32, *48*
Brunet, F, 292, *304*
Brunner, AH, 268, 270, *278*
Bryan, ER, 69, *81,* 342, *352*
Bryan, RT, 34, *51*
Bryant, CL, 96, *102*
Bryant, J, 32, *48*
Bryant, RE, 30, 31, *45, 47*
Bryer, A, 32, *47*
Bryson, YJ, 337, *349*
Brytting, M, 32, *49*
Bucens, MR, 89, *99*
Buchanan, MR, 31, *46*
Buckingham, M, 320, *324*
Buckler-White, AJ, 130, *154*
Budahazi, G, 256, *274*
Buescher, EL, 236, 238, *247, 248*
Buffone, GJ, 32, *48*
Buhles, WC, 96, *102*
Bui, M, 107, 109, *138, 139*
Bui, PT, 169, 174, 183, *194, 198, 202*
Bukrinskaya, AG, 132, *157*
Bunin, N, 235, 237, *246, 248*
Bunting, D, 183, *203*
Bunton, L, 169, 170, 171, *194*
Burakoff, SJ, 116, *144*
Burch, B, 181, *201*
Burch, C, 291, 292, *304*
Burch, GE, 111, *140*
Burchak, E, 240, *249*
Burda, J, 243, *250*
Burdge, DR, 30, *45,* 65, *79*
Burgert, EO, 84, *97*
Burgert, HG, 230, *247*
Burgess, BG, 127, *149*
Burk, B, 135, *158,* 336, *349*
Burke, A, 171, *196*
Burke, PJ, 95, *102*
Burkreyev, AA, 163, 183, *188*
Burlington, DB, 329, *347*
Burnette, TC, 96, *102*
Burns, BA, 130, *154,* 215, *220*
Burns, WH, 95, *102,* 115, *143*
Burtseva, EP, 130, *154*
Buscho, RO, 58, *74*

Author Index

Busse, WW, 260, 261, 262, *276*
Bustamante, EA, 293, *305*
Butler, JC, 34, *51,* 92, *100,* 284, *302*
Butler, T, 27, *41*
Butsumyo, A, 30, *44,* 63, 64, 66, *78,* 166, 177, *190*
Bynoe, ML, 328, *346*
Byrd, RW, 131, *156*

C

Caba, D, 181, *201*
Cabera, B, 178, *199*
Cade, JF, 31, *46*
Cagle, PT, 32, *48*
Calder, MA, 30, *44,* 63, 64, *78*
Caldwell, J, 25, 29, *39*
Calhoun, NH, 96, *102*
Calhoun, WJ, 262, *276*
Callahan, PL, 255, 264, *273, 277*
Callow, KA, 268, 269, *279*
Calne, RY, 88, *98*
Calvin, JE, 292, *304*
Camargo, E, 163, 182, 183, *188, 202*
Camazine, B, 31, *46*
Camerson, JM, 136, *159*
Camitta, B, 237, *248*
Camner, P, 113, *141*
Campbell, RJ, 84, *97*
Canchola, JG, 162, 172, *185*
Cancio, E, 313, *323*
Candor, OS, 30, *44*
Cane, PA, 166, *191*
Canepa, E, 27, *40*
Caniglia, M, 91, *100*
Cannon, MJ, 163, 170, 172, *187, 195*
Canny, G, 180, *200*
Capote, PF, 25, *38*
Capparelli, EV, 331, *347*
Carballal, G, 27, *40, 41*
Carcelen, R, 111, *140*
Cardellichio, CB, 266, 268, *278*
Carding, SR, 116, *144*
Carey, RW, 33, *49*
Carilla, A, 177, *199*

Carilli, AD, 30, *45*
Carins, CB, 34, *50*
Carlisle, JT, 91, *100*
Carmack, MA, 180, *201*
Carnitta, B, 235, *246*
Carpenter, RJ, 29, *43*
Carr, MN, 33, *49*
Carre, P, 88, *99*
Carrigan, DR, 33, *50,* 95, *102,* 235, 237, *246, 248*
Carrion, ME, 228, *245*
Carson, JL, 9, 20, *21*
Carter, ML, 128, *151*
Case, TR, 358, *371*
Casey, WM, 231, *247*
Cash, P, 169, *193*
Caskey, CT, 243, *250*
Casola, A, 167, *192*
Casper, JT, 235, *246*
Cassidy, LF, 111, 113, *140, 141*
Castets, M, 30, *45*
Castrucci, MR, 109, 121, 122, 131, *139, 146, 147, 156*
Catalano, M, 27, *41*
Cataruozolo, PE, 358, *371*
Cate, TR, 29, *42,* 55, 58, *73,* 126, 128, 131, *148, 149, 153, 155,* 232, 241, *246, 249,* 257, *275,* 333, *348*
Catena, R, 298, *306*
Catlin, DH, 339, 350
Cauvin, JM, 270, 271, *280*
Cavallaro, JJ, 7, *21,* 54, 71, *73, 81*
Cays, M, 96, *102*
Cederberg, DM, 96, *102*
Cefalo, RC, 29, *42*
Cengiz, M, 292, *304*
Centers for Disease Control and Prevention, 38, *51,* 53, 58, 63, *73,* 75, *78,* 287, 300, *303, 306,* 337, 350, 355, 360, 368, *370, 373*
Cerami, A, 231, *247*
Cerqueiro, MC, 27, *40, 41*
Cerruti, RL, 336, *349*
Chabanon, G, 25, 29, *39*
Chace, BA, 96, *102*
Chaeffer, CI, 161, 165, *184*

Chakraverty, P, 128, *152*
Chalmers, A, 127, *151*
Chambers, GW, 62, *77*
Chambers, TM, 119, *146*
Champlin, E, 166, 177, 181, *190*
Champlin, R, 25, 29, *40*, 86, 87, 88, *98*
Champlin, RE, 91, 94, 96, *100, 101, 102*, 117, 123, *145*, 181, *201*
Chan, S, 243, *250*
Chanda, PK, 242, *250*
Chandrasekar, PH, 30, *45*
Chandwani, S, 90, *100, 176, 199*
Chang, V, 66, *80*
Chanock, R, 161, 165, *184*
Chanock, RM, 63, 66, 71, *78, 80, 81*, 115, 123, 130, *142, 143, 147, 154*, 162, 163, 169, 170, 172, 180, 181, 182, 183, *185, 188, 193, 194, 195, 200, 201, 202*, 205, 210, *216, 217, 218*, 224, 227, 230, 232, 233, 237, 238, 241, *244, 245, 246, 247, 248, 249*, 270, *279*, 342, *352*
Chantarojanasiri, T, 27, *41*
Chao, RK, 71, *81*
Chapman, L, 344, *353*
Chapman, LE, 34, *51*
Chapnick, EK, 34, *50*
Charette, RP, 340, *351*
Chastel, C, 270, 271, *280*
Chastre, J, 66, *80*, 177, *199*
Chatten, J, 91, *100*
Chavez-Giles, F, 287, *303*
Cheigh, JS, 29, *43*
Chen, AY, 131, *156*
Chen, DYH, 95, *102*
Chen, HH, 243, *250*
Chen, SJ, 243, *250*
Chengalvala, M, 242, *250*
Chengalvala, MV, 242, *250*
Chenoweth, A, 355, *370*
Cheresh, DA, 227, 232, *245*
Cherian, T, 59, *75*
Chernick, V, 240, *249*
Cherrie, AH, 163, 170, *187*
Cherry, JD, 30, *46*, 126, 127, *148, 149*
Cheung, H, 291, 292, *304*

Chiba, S, 166, 170, *191, 195*
Chiba, Y, 166, 169, 171, *191, 194*
Childs, J, 286, *303*
Childs, JE, 284, 286, *301, 303*, 344, *353*
Chin, J, 162, *185*, 215, *220*
Chin, TD, 127, *150*
Chinnock, BJ, 96, *102*
Chiparelli, H, 27, *40*
Chitkara, R, 32, 35, *47*
Choi, H, 243, *250*
Chomel, CC, 59, *75*
Chomel, JJ, 32, *48*
Chong, W, 132, *156*
Chonmaitree, T, 123, *147*, 168, 174, 175, 176, *192, 198, 199*
Choosakul, S, 212, *219*
Choppin, P, 171, *196*
Choppin, PW, 107, *138*, 211, *218*
Chow, LT, 229, *245*
Chow, MS, 331, *347*
Christiansen, G, 216, *221*
Christmas, WA, 134, *158*
Chu, CS, 242, *250*
Chu, YK, 300, *306*
Church, MK, 259, *276*
Church, NR, 175, *198*
Chytil, F, 173, *197*
Ciborowski, P, 26, *40*
Circo, R, 61, 69, *76*, 134, *158*
Cirino, N, 168, *192, 193*
Cisse, MF, 30, *45*
Claas, ECJ, 179, *200*
Clark, GPM, 31, *46*, 96, *103*
Clark, JG, 32, *49*
Clark, M, 170, *195*
Clark, RJ, 31, *46*
Clark, S, 132, *157*
Clarke, JR, 71, *81*, 268, 270, 271, *278*
Clarke, S, 171, 173, *196*
Clarke, SD, 25, *38*
Clarke, SKR, 165, *189*
Class, ECJ, 126, *148*
Clay, SJ, 89, *99*
Clemenets, ML, 115, 116, 130, *142, 143, 154*, 369, *373*
Clemens, J, 171, *196*

Clemens, PR, 243, *250*
Clement, J, 284, *301*
Clements, ML, 56, 74, 93, *101*, 115, 126, 127, 130, 131, 133, *143, 149, 151, 154, 155, 157*, 359, *371*
Clemmer, TP, 290, 292, *304*
Clover, R, 336, *349*
Clover, RC, 118, *145*
Clover, RD, 60, *76*, 134, 135, *157, 158*, 333, 334, 336, *348, 349*
Clover, RS, 60, *76*
Clyde, WA, 7, 9, 10, 13, 15, *21*, 27, *40*, 123, *147*, 161, 165, 169, 174, 176, 180, *184, 190, 198, 200*, 205, 212, *217, 219*, 232, 246
Clyde, WAJ, 238, *248*
Clyde, WE, 17, *23*
Coates, JAV, 136, *159*
Coch, RB, 85, 86, 87, *97*
Cochi, SL, 366, *372*
Cochran, KW, 328, *346*
Coelingh, KLVW, 207, 212, 215, *217, 219, 220*
Coffield, LM, 292, 293, 294, 295, 296, *305*
Coffman, RL, 117, *144*
Cogliano, RC, 111, *140*
Cohen, HJ, 84, *97*
Cohen, JI, 32, *48*
Cohen, S, 263, 268, 271, *277, 279*
Cohen-Abbo, A, 90, *100*
Cohn, S, 93, *101*, 127, *151*
Colby, TV, 29, *43*, 113, *141*, 238, 248
Coleclough, C, 216, *220*
Coleman, MT, 71, *82*, 126, *149*, 358, *371*
Coles, FB, 58, *75*, 128, *152*
Collett, MS, 285, *302*
Colley, D, 171, 173, *196*
Collier, AM, 7, 10, 15, *21, 22*, 27, *40*, 123, *147*, 165, 169, 174, 176, *190*, *198*, 205, *217*, 238, *248*
Collins, A, 169, *194*
Collins, AR, 273, *280*
Collins, P, 162, 163, *185*

Collins, PL, 162, 163, 166, 169, 183, *186, 187, 188, 194, 202*, 210, 216, *218, 220*
Colman, PM, 121, 136, *146, 159*, 207, *217*
Colonno, RJ, 255, 264, 265, *273, 277*
Colson, P, 284, *301*
Colville, A, 25, 29, *40*
Compans, RM, 208, *217*
Compton, SR, 266, 268, *278*
Condon, B, 256, *274*
Cone, R, 33, *50*
Conley, WG, 161, 165, *184*
Conner, EM, 265, *277*
Conney, MK, 63, *79*
Connolly, MG, 32, *49*, 308, *322*
Connor, JD, 94, *102*, 238, *248*, 339, 340, 350, *351*
Connors, M, 117, *145*, 163, 171, 183, *188, 196, 202*
Conron, W, 29, *42*, 59, *75*, 315, 316, *324*
Cook, K, 205, *216*
Cook, MK, 205, *216*
Cooke, J, 233, *246*
Cookson, JB, 69, 71, *81*
Cooley, MH, 30, *45*
Cooney, MK, 7, *21*, 29, *41*, 55, 58, *74*, 224, *244*, 257, 263, 270, *275, 277, 279*
Coonrod, JD, 125, *147*, 311, 313, *323*
Cooper, JA, 111, *140*
Cooper, JD, 298, *306*
Cooper, SL, 61, *76*, 134, *158*, 337, *350*
Copeland, JG, 94, *102*, 136, *159*
Cordell, AR, 31, *46*
Cordier, L, 242, *250*
Corey, GR, 32, *48*
Corey, L, 30, 33, *44, 45, 50*, 237, *248*
Cormier, D, 33, *49*
Cosgriff, TM, 342, 343, *353*
Costello, P, 29, *42*, 59, *75*, 315, 316, *324*
Cote, PJ, 163, 169, *187, 194*
Cotten, M, 242, *250*
Cottey, R, 128, *151*
Couch, R, 87, 88, *98*

Couch, RB, 55, 58, *74,* 91, *100,* 117, 123, 126, 128, 131, 136, *145, 148, 149, 153, 155, 158, 159,* 166, 177, 181, *190,* 214, *219,* 232, 241, *246, 249,* 253, 254, 256, 257, 263, 264, 270, 272, *273, 275, 277, 280,* 314, 315, *324,* 333, *348,* 358, 369, *371, 373*
Couch, RBG, 118, *145*
Couch, RG, 115, *142*
Couchonnal, G, 30, *45*
Court, S, 171, *196*
Court, SD, 26, *40*
Courtieu, A, 178, *199*
Couture, LA, 227, 233, 242, *245, 250*
Cowan, J, 127, *150*
Cox, GB, 107, *138*
Cox, H, 263, *277*
Cox, N, 61, *76,* 94, *101,* 130, *154*
Cox, NJ, 120, 129, *146, 153,* 310, 313, *322*
Cox, SM, 31, *46*
Coxon, R, 298, *305*
Craft, AW, 84, *97*
Craighead, JF, 30, *45*
Cram, DL, 30, *44*
Crawford, GE, 34, *50*
Crawford, SA, 333, 334, *348*
Crawford, SW, 32, *49*
Crawford-Miksza, L, 235, *246*
Cribbins, AJ, 320, *324*
Criddle, MM, 55, 61, 63, 64, 69, *73, 79,* 179, *200,* 270, *280,* 313, 314, *324*
Crocker, RJ, 161, *185*
Crompton, J, 236, *247*
Cross, AS, 113, *141*
Cross, KW, 63, *78,* 166, 177, *190*
Crossley, KB, 61, *76,* 134, *158*
Crowe, JE, 169, 181, 183, *194, 201, 202,* 215, *220*
Crowe, JHE, 163, *188*
Crowell, RE, 289, 290, 291, 292, 293, *304*
Crowell, RL, 227, *245*
Crump, C, 93, *101*
Crystal, RG, 233, 242, *246, 250*

Cryz, SJ, 62, *77*
Cuello, JA, 25, *38*
Culbreth, R, 111, *140*
Cullison, JP, 88, *99*
Cummings, JE, 127, *150*
Cunha, BA, 88, *99*
Cunningham, CK, 29, *43,* 58, 63, 64, *74,* 161, 180, *185,* 314, *324*
Cunningham, DG, 291, 292, *304*
Cunningham, FG, 31, *46*
Cunningham, I, 32, *48*
Cunningham, JA, 227, *245*
Curiel, DT, 228, 243, *245, 251*
Curlin, GT, 126, *148*
Currier, PF, 267, *273, 278*
Curruri, RL, 135, *158*

D

D'Alessio, DJ, 256, *275*
d'Arthis, P, 66, *80*
Dab, I, 167, *192*
Daisy, JA, 125, *147*
Dallabetta, GA, 93, *101*
Dalrymple, JM, 284, 285, *302*
Dalton, MJ, 297, *305*
Dandliker, PS, 32, 35, *48,* 96, *102*
Danel, C, 91, *100,* 242, *250*
Daniels, RD, 129, *153*
Dant Bui, RH, 340, *351*
Daroca, DJ, 91, *100*
Dashefsky, B, 341, *351*
Dauber, JH, 32, *48*
Dave, VP, 210, *218*
Davenport, FM, 328, *346*
David, DS, 29, *43*
Davidson, JN, 311, 313, *323*
Davies, JR, 128, *152,* 358, *371*
Davies, WL, 328, *346*
Daview, JA, 268, 270, *278*
Daview, R, 128, *151*
Davis, AR, 183, *202,* 242, *250*
Davis, C, 125, *147*
Davis, JP, 134, *158*
Davis, R, 96, *102,* 284, *301*

Davis, T, 169, *194*
Dawkis, AT, 333, 336, *348*
Dawson, A, 229, *245*
Dawson, FW, 27, *41*
de Blic, J, 91, *100*
de Diego, A, 31, *46*
De Graff-Meeder, B, 240, *249*
De La Luna, S, 110, *139*
de Leon, LE, 27, *41*
de Miranda, P, 96, *102*
de oliveira, CB, 240, *249*
De Silva, LM, 240, *249*
Dearden, C, 264, *277*
DeArmond, B, 96, *102*
Debbas, M, 228, 230, *245*
DeBorde, D, 131, *154*
DeBorde, DC, 130, *154*
DeCarvalho, V, 165, *190*
DeCastro, G, 172, *197*
Deck, RR, 132, *156*
Decker, JL, 127, *151*
Decker, M, 56, *74*, 117, *145*
DeCorato, D, 110, *139*
DeFarbritus, AM, 29, *43*
Defayolle, M, 128, *152*
Degclau, J, 134, *158*
Degelau, J, 61, *76*, 337, *350*
Dehner, LP, 30, *44*, 87, *98*, 161, 166, 167, 180, *185*, 314, *324*
Deitzschold, B, 115, *143*
Delgado, T, 163, 170, *188*
DeMeules, JE, 298, *306*
Demmler, GJ, 32, *48*, 311, *323*
Dempsey, MH, 136, *159*
Denison, MR, 267, 273, *278*
Dennehy, JJ, 240, *249*
Denning, C, 29, *43*, 62, *77*, 127, *150*
Denning, CR, 358, *371*
Denny, FW, 7, 9, 10, 12, 13, 15, 17, 20, *21, 22, 23*, 27, *40*, 123, *147*, 165, 169, 176, *190*, 205, *217*, 238, *248*, 316, 317, *324*
Derish, MT, 178, *199*
Dermody, TS, 29, *41*, 86, *98*
Descamps, V, 242, *250*
Deteix, P, 30, *43*

Detjen, BM, 108, *138*
Detreix, P, 88, *99*
Devine, R, 56, *74*
Devlin, R, 167, *192*
DeWitt, CM, 132, *156*
Dhainault, JF, 292, *304*
Dhar, S, 53, *73*
Dick, CR, 256, *275*
Dick, EC, 256, 260, 261, 262, *274, 275, 276*
Dicker, RC, 30, *44*
Didier, A, 88, *99*
Didier, JP, 66, *80*
Dietlein, LF, 111, *140*
Dietzman, DE, 125, *147*
Dimock, C, 311, 313, *323*
Dinant, GJ, 62, *77*, 127, 128, *150*, 358, *370*
Dinarello, CA, 259, *275*
Dindinaud, G, 30, *45*, 63, 65, 66, *78*, 177, *199*
Dingle, J, 223, 226, *244*
Dingle, JH, 223, *244*
Disney, FA, 134, *158*
Dixon, A, 30, *45*
Dloin, R, 131, *155*
Doan, R, 30, *44*
Dobretsova, A, 126, *148*
Dobson, PM, 31, *46*, 96, *103*
Doherty, PC, 116, 117, *144, 145*, 209, 210, *217, 218*
Dohn, MN, 32, *49*, 308, *322*
Dolin, R, 25, 35, *38, 51*, 60, *76*, 83, *97*, 126, 127, 128, 131, 132, 133, 134, 137, *148, 150, 151, 154, 156, 157, 158, 159*, 331, 335, 337, *348, 349*
Doller, G, 59, *75*, 125, *148*
Dolph, PJ, 229, *245*
Dominguez, EA, 270, 272, *280*, 311, 314, *323, 324*
Dominik, JW, 340, *351*
Donatelli, I, 121, *146*
Donnelly, JJ, 132, *156*, 363, *372*
Donofrio, JC, 311, 313, *323*
Dorff, GJ, 25, 29, *39*
Dorinsky, PM, 292, *304*

Dorward, M, 261, *276*
Dotsch, C, 216, *221*
Douay, L, 30, *43*, 86, 87, *98*
Doud, JR, 88, *99*
Douglas, AR, 119, *146*
Douglas, GC, 232, *246*
Douglas, JT, 228, 243, *245*, *251*
Douglas, RD, 335, *349*
Douglas, RG, 27, 30, 31, *41*, *45*, *46*, 58, 60, 62, 66, *75*, *77*, *80*, 93, 96, *101*, *102*, 113, 127, 128, 132, 134, 135, *141*, *150*, *152*, *157*, *158*, 164, 165, 166, 168, 175, 176, *189*, *190*, *192*, *199*, 263, *277*, 330, 340, *347*, *351*
Douglas, RGB, 168, *192*
Douglas, RGJ, 113, *141*, 257, *275*
Douglas, RM, 17, *22*
Dowda, H, 128, *152*
Dowdle, WR, 25, 29, *39*, 84, *97*, 126, *149*, 358, *371*
Dowell, SF, 30, *44*, 166, *190*, 314, *324*
Downham, MAPS, 171, *196*
Downing, A, 30, *44*
Downs, TD, 56, *74*
Doyle, HK, 238, *248*
Doyle, WJ, 259, 262, 264, 265, *275*, *276*, *277*
Drabkin, PD, 58, *75*
Drake, M, 127, *150*, 358, 359, *370*, *371*
Dran, S, 358, *371*
Drasar, BS, 113, *141*
Dreisbach, M, 337, *349*
Driedger, AA, 291, 292, *304*
Drinka, P, 60, 61, 62, 63, 64, 69, 70, 71, *76*, *78*, *81*, 313, *323*
Drinkwater, DC, 93, *101*
Drobyski, WR, 33, *50*, 235, 237, *246*, *248*
Droguett, G, 227, *245*
Dubovi, EJ, 180, *200*, 232, *246*
Duchin, JS, 34, *51*, 289, 292, *303*
Dudding, BA, 30, *45*, 238, *248*
Duffour, MT, 242, *250*
Duffy, L, 174, *198*
Duhamel, JF, 179, *200*
Duhaut, SD, 109, *139*

Dulberg, CS, 84, *97*
Dull, SM, 290, 292, *304*
Dummer, JS, 32, *48*, 83, 95, *97*
DuMond, C, 96, *102*
Dumyati, G, 62, *77*, *78*, 128, 131, *152*, *155*
Duncan, AJ, 32, *48*
Duncan, SJ, 232, *244*
Dungworth, D, 174, *198*
Dunin, CM, 29, *42*
Dunleavy, U, 129, *153*
Dunn, DL, 27, *41*
Duong, CM, 31, *46*
Dupont, WD, 131, *155*
Durante, W, 298, *305*
Dure, L, 136, *158*
Duthie, EH, 62, *78*
Dwarki, VJ, 132, *156*
Dyason, JC, 136, *159*, 345, *353*
Dybdahl-Sissoko, N, 110, *140*

E

Eadie, MB, 69, 71, *81*
Eastman, R, 33, *49*
Eaton, OM, 33, *49*
Ebekian, B, 27, *40*
Ebeling, DF, 96, *102*
Eckels, DD, 115, *143*
Edelstein, A, 287, *303*
Eder, SE, 31, *46*
Edwards, EA, 237, 241, *247*, *249*
Edwards, KM, 131, *155*, 211, *219*, 237, *248*
Efrat, S, 230, *247*
Eggleston, PA, 261, *276*
Eichelberger, M, 117, *145*
Eickhoff, CS, 62, *77*
Eickhoff, T, 355, *370*
Eickhoff, TC, 127, *149*, *151*
Eillehay, DL, 231, *247*
Einarsson, O, 167, *191*, 255, 259, 264, *274*
Eissa, NT, 242, *250*
Eith, JD, 235, *246*

Elango, N, 162, 183, *186, 202*
Elfenbein, GJ, 32, *48*
Elias, JA, 167, *191,* 255, 259, 264, *274*
Eling, LS, 117, 123, *145*
Elis, JT, 58, *75*
Elkins, WR, 169, 183, *194, 202*
Ell, JC, 360, *371*
Eller, JJ, 71, *81,* 162, *185,* 215, *220*
Elliott, LH, 284, 286, *301, 302,* 344, *353*
Elliott, WM, 235, *246*
Ellis, DS, 285, *302*
Ellis, EF, 71, *81*
Ellis, JT, 113, 124, *141*
Ellis, ME, 31, *46*
Elliver, R, 94, *101*
Elmore, LW, 231, *247*
Elsea, W, 171, *196*
Elting, L, 32, *48*
Elting, LS, 87, *98*
Emanuel, D, 32, 35, *48, 51*
Embree, J, 308, *322*
Embrey, RP, 29, *42*
Enami, M, 109, 131, *139, 156*
Enders, JF, 223, *244*
Enelow, TJ, 91, *100*
Engelhard, D, 93, *101*
England, AC, 328, *346*
Englehardt, OG, 131, *156*
Englund, J, 87, 88, *98*
Englund, JA, 30, 34, *44, 51,* 64, 65, *79,* 85, 86, 87, 91, 94, 95, *97, 98, 100, 101, 102,* 161, 165, 166, 171, 177, 180, 181, 183, *185, 189, 190, 201, 203,* 209, 308, 310, 313, 314, 315, 316, 317, *322, 324,* 369, *373*
Ennis, FA, 117, 126, 128, *145, 148*
Enria, D, 287, *303*
Epstein, SL, 117, *145*
Erb, S, 62, *77, 78,* 127, 128, 131, 137, *150, 152, 155, 159*
Erdman, DD, 30, *44,* 166, *190,* 314, *324*
Erice, A, 27, *41,* 96, *102*
Erickson, JW, 255, *274*
Eriksson, BM, 32, *49*
Erscoiu, S, 25, 29, *39*
Esinhart, JD, 136, *159,* 345, *353*

Eskola, J, 174, 176, *198*
Esmonde, TF, 31, *46*
Espy, MJ, 35, *51,* 125, *147*
Estani, SS, 287, *303*
Eugene, C, 179, *200*
Evans, D, 110, *140*
Evans, DH, 311, 313, *323*
Evans, KD, 90, *100*
Everitt, E, 227, *245*
Ewart, G, 107, *138*

F

Fagon, J, 66, *80,* 177, *199*
Fairclough, DL, 123, *147,* 238, *248*
Falsey, AR, 29, *43,* 55, 58, 61, 63, 64, 65, 66, 67, 69, 70, 71, *73, 74, 78, 79, 80, 82,* 161, 166, 177, 179, 180, 183, *185, 200, 203,* 270, *280,* 313, 314, *324*
Fan, J, 311, *323*
Fan, LL, 131, *156*
Fang, GD, 25, *39*
Fannin, SL, 30, *44,* 63, 64, 66, *78,* 166, 177, *190*
Farley, J, 171, *196*
Farmer, SG, 25, 29, *39*
Faro, S, 29, *43*
Farquhar, A, 61, 63, 71, *76,* 270, *280*
Farr, B, 258, *275*
Farr, BM, 259, 265, *275, 277*
Farzadagan, H, 93, *101*
Fasano, MB, 134, *157*
Fauci, AS, 90, *99*
Feddersen, RM, 292, 293, 294, 295, 296, 297, *304, 305*
Fedlmann, H, 287, 288, *303*
Fedson, D, 334, *349*
Fedson, DS, 127, *150,* 356, 362, *370, 372*
Fehrenbach, FJ, 25, 29, *40*
Fein, A, 290, 292, *304*
Fejer, G, 230, *247*
Fekety, FR, 25, 29, *39*
Feldman, H, 296, *305*

Feldman, ME, 215, *220*
Feldman, S, 31, *47,* 84, *97,* 128, *152,* 368, *373*
Feldmann, H, 284, 286, *301, 302, 303*
Felgner, PL, 132, *156*
Felliti, VJ, 334, *348*
Fels, A, 32, *48*
Felton, A, 269, 272, *279*
Felton, AL, 30, *46*
Ferbas-Grovit, K, 127, *151*
Ferguson, R, 32, *49*
Ferko, B, 131, *156*
Fermaglich, DR, 33, *49*
Fernandez, N, 242, *250*
Fernandez-Larsson, 339, 350
Fernandez-Sesma, A, 117, 137, *144, 159*
Fernie, BF, 163, 166, 169, *186, 187, 190, 191, 194*
Ferre, RA, 256, *274*
Ferren-Garnder, C, 181, 182, *201*
Ferris, JAJ, 171, *196*
Fibbe, WE, 30, *43*
Fife, KH, 30, 31, *45, 46,* 237, *248*
File, TM, 30, *44,* 314, *324*
File, TMJ, 166, *190*
Finberg, R, 209, *217*
Finberg, RW, 227, *245*
Finch, E, 58, *74*
Finch, RG, 25, 29, *39*
Finck, ES, 29, *43*
Fine, M, 25, *39*
Finer, MH, 243, *250*
Finger, R, 30, *44*
Finkel, B, 62, *77*
Finkel, MS, 298, *306*
Finklea, JF, 328, *346*
Finland, M, 111, *140*
Fiorentino, D, 168, *193*
Fireman, P, 262, *276*
Firestone, C, 163, 171, 183, *188, 196, 202*
Fischschweiger, W, 113, *141*
Fishaut, M, 171, *196*
Fisher, CJ, 290, 292, *304*
Fisher, KJ, 243, *250*

Fitch, WM, 120, *146*
FitzGibbon, PA, 54, *73*
Fitzharris, P, 268, *279*
Fitzmaurice, J, 33, *50*
Fitzpatrick, J, 93, *101*
Flamholc, L, 31, *46*
Flanagan, TD, 163, *187*
Flavell, RA, 243, *251*
Fleet, LW, 335, *349*
Fleet, W, 134, *158,* 182, 183, *202*
Fleischer, B, 117, *144*
Fleisher, GR, 33, *49*
Fleming, DM, 63, *78,* 166, 177, *190*
Fleming, E, 285, *302*
Fleming, K, 173, *197*
Fletcher, C, 96, *102*
Fleurette, J, 25, 29, *39*
Flomenberg, P, 235, 237, *246,* 248
Flor, SM, 178, *199*
Florey, CV, 16, *22*
Flowers, D, 71, *81,* 268, 270, 271, 272, *278, 279*
Fogy, I, 255, *274*
Folland, DS, 126, 127, *148*
Fontillas, G, 32, *48*
Ford, AB, 54, *73*
Forder, AA, 25, 29, *39*
Forman, SJ, 83, 96, *97*
Formica, MA, 55, 61, 63, 64, 69, *73,* 270, *280,* 313, *324*
Forni, AL, 34, *50*
Forsgren, M, 66, *80,* 89, *99*
Forsyth, B, 177, *199*
Forsyth, BR, 69, *81*
Forte, CP, 265, *277*
Foster, DA, 62, *77,* 126, *149,* 358, *370*
Foucar, K, 292, 293, 294, 295, 296, 297, *304, 305*
Fouillard, L, 30, *43,* 86, 87, *98,* 177, *199*
Fox, JM, 213, *219*
Fox, JMK, 88, *99*
Fox, JP, 55, 58, *74,* 224, *244,* 257, 263, 270, *275, 277, 279,* 334, 340, *348, 351*
Foy, HH, 55, 58, *74*

Foy, HM, 7, *21,* 29, *41,* 55, 58, 63, *74, 79,* 126, 127, *148,* 263, 270, *277, 279*
Foye, HR, 84, *97*
Fraenkel, DJ, 258, 261, *275, 276*
Fraisse, A, 33, *49*
France-Fernandez, MT, 284, *301*
Francis, AB, 134, *158*
Frank, A, 169, *193*
Frank, AL, 16, 17, *22,* 113, 128, *142, 151,* 209, 210, 214, *217, 218, 219,* 342, *352*
Frank, PF, 237, *247*
Frankel, LR, 65, *79,* 178, *199,* 342, *352*
Frankenberger, EA, 255, *274*
Fransen, H, 25, 30, *38, 44,* 63, 66, *79, 80*
Franze-Fernandez, MT, 287, *303*
Frases, VJ, 31, *46,* 96, *103*
Fraundorfer, F, 255, *274*
Freda Pietrobon, PJ, 62, *77*
Freeman, RB, 93, *101,* 127, *150*
Freemont, AJ, 33, *50*
Freihorst, J, 174, *198*
French, GR, 30, *45*
Freundlich, CB, 55, 56, *73*
Freymuth, F, 179, *200*
Friday, WW, 71, *82*
Friebertshauser, K, 174, *198*
Friedman, A, 132, *156*
Friedman, HW, 125, *147*
Fries, LF, 56, *74,* 130, 131, *154, 155*
Froehlich, JL, 216, *221*
Froelich, Jl, 214, *220*
Frogel, M, 91, *100*
Frost, A, 32, *48*
Fry, J, 58, 63, 64, *74*
Fryd, DS, 32, *49*
Fudutomi, A, 113, *142*
Fujimura, M, 34, *51*
Fujitaki, J, 339, 350
Fukayama, M, 242, *250*
Fukuchi, Y, 240, *249*
Fukuda, R, 110, 111, *140,* 296, *305*
Fukuda, T, 136, *159*
Fukutomi, A, 211, *218*
Fulginiti, VA, 71, *81,* 162, *185,* 215, *220*

Fuller, DJ, 95, *102*
Fulton, DR, 92, *101*
Funari, P, 208, *217*
Furione, M, 320, *324*
Furomoto-Dawson, A, 358, *370*
Furth, EE, 236, *247*
Furumoto-Dawson, A, 62, *77*
Furze, J, 170, 171, *195*
Fusco, JJ, 29, *42*

G

Gaerlan, P, 29, *43,* 127, *150*
Gaerlan, PF, 62, *77,* 358, *371*
Gage, K, 284, *301*
Gage, PW, 107, *138*
Gajdusek, DC, 287, *303*
Gala, CL, 9, *22,* 65, *79,* 84, *97,* 161, 164, 165, 176, 180, *185, 189, 199, 200, 201,* 335, 342, *349, 351*
Gala, GL, 134, *158*
Galbraith, AW, 134, *157,* 333, *348*
Galinski, MS, 163, *188,* 210, *218*
Gallaher, MM, 34, *51,* 289, 292, *303*
Gallati, H, 167, *191*
Gallichan, WS, 242, *250*
Gamellie, RL, 298, *306*
Gandhi, VC, 127, *150*
Gantt, K, 366, *372*
Gantz, NM, 235, *246*
Garafalo, R, 167, 174, *192, 198*
Garb, JL, 25, *38*
Garb, JR, 25, *38*
Garbe, L, 33, *49*
Garcia, J, 163, *188,* 230, *247*
Garcia-Barreno, B, 162, 163, 170, *186, 188*
Garcia-Prats, JA, 240, *249*
Garcia-Sastre, A, 109, 131, *139, 156*
Gardner, G, 17, *22*
Gardner, P, 171, *196,* 355, *370*
Gardner, PS, 26, *40,* 84, *97,* 165, *189,* 209, *217,* 310, 317, *322, 324*
Garibaldi, RA, 53, 55, *73*
Garnacho, J, 25, *38*

Garner, JS, 92, *100*
Garrard, CS, 113, *141*
Garrity, ER, 88, *99*
Garten, W, 113, *142*
Garvie, DG, 30, *44*, 63, 64, *78*
Gary, HE, 30, *44*, 166, *190*, 314, *324*
Gaudet, M, 66, *80*
Gauldie, J, 242, *250*
Gavaert, TME, 62, *77*
Gaviria, M, 284, *301*
Gavrilovskaya, I, 284, 287, *301, 303*
Gaynor, R, 230, *247*
Gazuy, N, 30, *43*, 88, *99*
Geelan, S, 240, *249*
Geever, EF, 31, *47*
Gegory, DW, 232, *244*
Geiman, JM, 164, 165, 166, 168, 175, 176, *189, 190, 192, 199*
Geis, WP, 127, *150*
Geist, LJ, 29, *42*
Gelfand, EW, 214, *219*
Gelinas, RE, 229, *245*
Gelman, JM, 66, *80*
Gelmini, MJ, 181, *201*, 342, *352*
Gelves, CA, 314, *324*
Gennetay, E, 179, *200*
Gentry, SR, 89, *99*
George, R, 32, *47*
George, RB, 30, *45*
George, RC, 113, *141*
Geradts, J, 31, *46*
Geratz, JD, 180, *200*
Gergelson, JM, 227, *245*
Gerhard, H, 31, *46*
Gerhard, W, 115, 117, 119, *143, 145, 146*
Germillion, DH, 34, *50*
Gern, JE, 260, 261, *276*
Gerna, G, 320, *324*
Gerone, JP, 257, *275*
Gerone, PJ, 111, *140*, 232, *246*
Gerrity, TR, 113, *141*
Gershon, A, 368, *373*
Gershon, AA, 310, 313, 319, 320, 321, *323*, 366, *372*
Gershwin, L, 174, *198*

Gerth, HJ, 59, *75*, 125, *148*
Gertzen, J, 30, *45*
Ghadge, GD, 229, *246*
Ghendon, YZ, 130, *154*
Giangreco, B, 267, *278*
Gibb, FR, 113, *141*
Gilardi, P, 242, *250*
Gilbert, BE, 29, *42*, 65, *79*, 136, *158, 159*, 180, *200, 201*, 339, 341, 342, *350, 351*
Gilbert, F, 233, *246*
Gilbert, I, 168, *192*
Gilbert, R, 32, *48*
Gilfillan, R, 127, *151*
Gill, EP, 270, 272, *280*
Gill, V, 66, *80*
Gilles, P, 33, *49*
Gillessen, D, 115, *143*
Gillis, S, 259, *275*
Gillmore, LK, 223, *244*
Gimenez, H, 169, *193*
Gingsberg, HS, 230, *247*
Ginsberg, HS, 227, 230, 232, 233, *245, 246*
Giroux, JD, 270, 271, *280*
Gladen, RG, 355, *370*
Glasgow, KW, 68, *80*
Glass, D, 127, *151*
Glassroth, J, 90, *99*
Glathe, H, 128, *152*
Gleaves, CA, 30, 32, *43, 44, 49*, 65, *79*, 86, 87, 96, *98, 102*, 166, 177, 181, *190*
Glezen, WO, 210, *218*, 361, 364, *371*
Glezen, WP, 7, 9, 12, 15, 16, *21, 22*, 25, *39*, 55, 56, 58, *74*, 117, 118, 126, 127, 131, *145, 148, 149, 155, 156*, 161, 165, 169, *184, 193*, 209, 212, *217, 219*, 315, 316, 317, *324*, 342, *352*
Gloster, E, 91, *100*
Gluck, R, 62, *77*
Gmelich, JT, 30, *45*
Goddard, CM, 298, *305*
Godfrey, E, 166, *191*
Goergakopoulos, K, 181, *201*

Goetz, MB, 35, *51*
Gogos, CA, 31, *47,* 366, *372*
Gohd, R, 134, *157,* 177, *199*
Gohd, RS, 91, *100*
Gold, E, 310, 313, 319, 320, 321, *323*
Gold, JW, 224, 226, 235, *244*
Gold, MR, 361, *371*
Gold, RS, 30, *45*
Golden, CA, 29, *42,* 69, *81,* 113, *141*
Golden, JA, 34, *50*
Goldman, MJ, 227, 232, *245*
Goldsmith, CS, 284, 286, 292, 293, 294, 295, 296, *301, 302, 305*
Goldstein, AL, 260, *276*
Gomolin, IH, 60, *76*
Gonczol, E, 236, *247*
Gonzelez-Rothi, RJ, 128, *151*
Goodenberger, DM, 31, *46,* 96, *103*
Gooding, LR, 229, 231, *245, 247*
Goodman, RA, 29, *42,* 58, *75*
Goodrich, CH, 366, *372*
Goodrich, HM, 96, *102*
Goodrich, JM, 32, *48,* 87, 88, 91, *98, 100,* 166, 177, 181, *190, 201,* 369, *373*
Gorbalenya, A, 267, *278*
Gorbalenya, AE, 266, 267, *278*
Gordon, FCA, 232, *244*
Gordon, HR, 32, *47*
Gordon, R, 32, 35, *47*
Gordon, W, 30, *45,* 177, *199*
Gordon, YJ, 240, *249*
Gorman, O, 121, *146*
Gorman, OT, 119, *146*
Gorodkova, N, 115, *142*
Gorse, GJ, 62, *77,* 131, *155*
Gorsgren, M, 30, *44,* 63, *79*
Goswami, BB, 339, *350*
Gotch, FM, 117, *145*
Gottlieb, LS, 29, *42,* 111, *140*
Gottschalk, J, 163, 166, *186*
Gouin, F, 33, *49*
Gould, AL, 358, *370*
Gould, S, 173, *197*
Govaert, TM, 127, 128, *150,* 358, *370*
Govorkova, EA, 129, *153*

Graber, J, 34, *51*
Grace, S, 183, *203*
Gradon, JD, 34, *50*
Graham, BS, 167, 169, 170, 171, 173, 180, *192, 193, 194, 196, 197, 200,* 321, *324*
Graham, FL, 242, *250*
Graham, MB, 116, *144*
Graham, ML, 95, *102*
Graham, NMH, 8, 17, *21, 22*
Graham, SM, 227, 233, 242, *245, 250*
Grajower, B, 115, *143*
Graman, PS, 27, *41,* 66, 69, *80*
Grambas, S, 135, *158,* 336, *349*
Grandien, M, 30, *44,* 63, 65, *79,* 317, *324*
Grandt, CD, 182, 183, *202*
Grant, JP, 17, 18, *23*
Grassauer, A, 131, *156*
Gravenstein, S, 60, 61, 62, 63, 64, 69, 70, 71, *76, 78, 81,* 134, *158,* 313, *323,* 337, 350
Graves, P, 127, *149, 151*
Gray, FD, 113, *141*
Gray, J, 30, *44,* 63, 64, *78*
Gray, JJ, 32, *48*
Gray, M, 173, *197*
Grayston, JT, 7, *21,* 25, *39,* 236, *247*
Green, I, 262, *276*
Green, JL, 134, *158*
Green, M, 88, 89, *99,* 176, *199,* 213, *219,* 341, *351*
Green, RW, 240, *249*
Greenberg, SB, 25, 31, 35, *39, 46, 51,* 113, *141,* 264, 270, 272, *277, 280,* 330, *347*
Greenland, S, 62, *77,* 358, *370*
Greenman, R, 284, *301*
Greenspoon, JS, 34, *50*
Greer, PW, 292, 293, 294, 295, 296, *305*
Gregg, I, 261, *276*
Gregory, RJ, 227, 233, 242, *245, 250*
Greiff, L, 268, 269, *279*
Greve, JM, 265, *277*
Grewal, IS, 243, *251*
Griffin, M, 355, *370*

Griffis, CA, 214, *219*
Griffith, BP, 32, *48*
Griffith, JP, 255, *274*
Grigorieva, EP, 130, *154*
Grillner, L, 25, 29, *40*
Grist, NR, 69, 71, *81,* 257, *275*
Grogaard, J, 173, *197*
Grogan, TM, 94, *102,* 136, *159*
Grogard, J, 173, *197*
Gromkowski, SH, 132, *156*
Groothuis, JR, 92, 94, *101,* 127, *149,* 165, 176, 182, *190, 199, 201, 202,* 342, 343, *353,* 369, *373*
Grosche, A, 128, *152*
Groschel, DH, 261, *276*
Grosfeld, H, 163, *188,* 216, *220*
Gross, P, 126, 128, *148,* 355, 359, *370, 371*
Gross, PA, 29, *43,* 61, 62, 63, 67, *76, 77,* 93, *101,* 127, *149, 150,* 356, 358, 359, 360, 361, 363, *370, 371, 372*
Grossman, RF, 290, 292, *304*
Grover, FL, 96, *102*
Grubb, A, 273, *280*
Gruber, C, 162, 172, *186, 197*
Gruber, W, 169, 181, *194*
Gruber, WC, 95, *102,* 131, *155, 156,* 173, *197,* 226, 240, *244, 249*
Gruenberger, M, 255, *274*
Gruendler, P, 255, *274*
Grunert, RR, 328, 334, *346, 348*
Grynoch, R, 56, *74*
Guay, DRP, 60, 61, *76,* 134, *158*
Gubareva, LV, 129, 137, *153, 159*
Guidry, GG, 30, *45*
Guinea, R, 131, *156*
Guion, A, 25, 29, *40*
Gujihashi, D, 116, *144*
Gullace, M, 84, *97*
Gump, D, 25, 29, *39,* 177, *199*
Gump, DW, 69, *81*
Gundelfinger, BF, 236, *247*
Gunn, RA, 328, 331, 336, *346*
Gupta, CK, 164, *189*
Gupta, KK, 164, *189*
Gurney, TJ, 106, *138*

Gustafson, E, 163, *188*
Gustafson, LM, 265, *278*
Gustavson, LE, 331, *347*
Gutierrez, KM, 176, *199*
Gwaltney, JJ, 255, 256, 257, 258, 259, 261, 263, 264, 265, 268, 270, *274, 275, 276, 277, 278*
Gwaltney, JM, 35, *51,* 61, 69, 71, *76, 80, 81,* 126, 128, *148, 149,* 257, 258, 262, 268, *275, 276*
Gyory, I, 230, *247*

H

Haahtela, T, 128, *151*
Habel, LA, 62, *77,* 358, *370*
Hackett, CJ, 115, 117, *143, 144*
Hackett, CS, 130, *153*
Hackman, CR, 32, *49*
Hackman, RC, 30, 31, 33, *43, 44, 45, 46, 50,* 65, *79,* 86, 87, *98,* 166, 177, 181, *190,* 237, *248,* 314, *324*
Haddada, H, 242, *250*
Hadley, WK, 34, *50*
Haff, RF, 328, *346*
Haghighat, A, 255, *274*
Haidl, S, 31, *46*
Hall, CB, 9, *22,* 27, 29, 30, 34, *41, 43, 45, 50,* 55, 56, 58, 63, 64, 65, 66, 67, 68, 69, 71, *73, 75, 78, 79,* 80, *82,* 84, 92, 94, *97, 101,* 126, 127, 132, *148, 149, 157,* 161, 163, 164, 165, 166, 167, 168, 169, 170, 175, 176, 177, 178, 180, 182, *185, 187, 189, 190, 191, 192, 195, 198, 199, 200, 201,* 212, *219,* 335, 342, *349, 351, 352,* 369, *373*
Hall, CE, 55, 58, *74,* 224, *244,* 257, 263, *275, 277*
Hall, EH, 129, *153*
Hall, SL, 215, *220*
Hall, W, 134, *158*
Hall, WJ, 30, 34, *45, 50,* 55, 61, 63, 64, 69, *73, 78, 79,* 113, *141,* 161, 164, 175, 177, 179, *185, 189, 198, 200,*

Author Index

[Hall, WJ]
  270, *280,* 313, 314, *324,* 330, 335, 347, *349*
Hall, WN, 29, *42,* 58, *75,* 127, *150*
Hall-Smith, M, 335, *349*
Haller, A, 33, *50*
Hallin, GW, 289, 290, 291, 292, 293, *304*
Halloran, ME, 366, *372*
Halonen, P, 17, *22*
Halonen, PE, 125, *147,* 239, *248*
Halperin, SA, 261, *276*
Halsey, NA, 130, *154,* 365, *372*
Hamilton, JD, 32, *48*
Hammar, SP, 29, *42*
Hammersley, V, 313, *323*
Hammill, H, 34, *51*
Hammond, GW, 127, *150,* 308, *322,* 356, *370*
Hammond, M, 88, *99*
Hamory, BH, 232, *246*
Hamparian, V, 261, *276*
Hamre, D, 263, *277*
Handy, J, 167, *192*
Handzel, ZT, 261, *276*
Hano, JE, 127, *150*
Hanscome, PJ, 62, *77*
Hardan, I, 93, *101*
Harisiadi, J, 27, *41*
Harman, MW, 134, *158*
Harmon, MW, 61, 69, *76,* 125, 134, *147, 157,* 264, *277,* 337, *350*
Harmsen, MC, 320, *324*
Harn, N, 170, *195*
Harnett, GB, 89, *99*
Harper, J, 130, *154*
Harrich, D, 230, *247*
Harrington, RD, 30, *43, 44,* 65, *79,* 86, 87, *98,* 166, 177, 181, *190,* 314, *324*
Harris, DO, 215, *220*
Harris, PJ, 165, 176, *190*
Harris, RE, 31, *47*
Harrison, AK, 286, *302*
Harrison, B, 30, *44*
Harrison, FJ, 284, *301*
Harrison, K, 128, *152*

Harrison, KJ, 25, *38*
Hart, CC, 339, 350
Hart, GJ, 137, *159*
Hart, RJC, 30, *44,* 63, 64, 66, *78*
Harter, DH, 29, *42*
Hartley, JW, 71, *81,* 270, *279*
Hartzman, RJ, 115, *143*
Harvey, BG, 233, *246*
Hashimoto, G, 117, *144*
Hashimoto, Y, 33, *49*
Hasony, HJ, 270, *279*
Hasty, SE, 286, *302*
Hattler, BG, 298, *306*
Hauge, M, 127, *150,* 358, 359, *370, 371*
Hawe, LA, 132, *156*
Hay, AJ, 60, *76,* 132, 134, 135, *157, 158,* 330, 335, 336, *347, 349*
Hay, J, 285, *302*
Hay, JG, 242, *250*
Hay, RT, 229, 236, *245, 247*
Hayani, K, 173, *197*
Hayashi, S, 231, 235, *246*
Hayden, F, 93, *101*
Hayden, FG, 60, *76,* 86, 94, *98, 101, 102,* 123, 134, 135, 136, *147, 157, 158, 159,* 257, 259, 260, 263, 264, 265, 272, *275, 276, 277, 278, 280,* 330, 331, 334, 336, 345, *347, 349, 353*
Hayes, N, 136, *158*
Hayle, A, 170, *195*
Hazarika, P, 298, *305*
He, B, 167, *192*
He, S, 121, *146*
He, SQ, 121, *146*
Healy, N, 136, *159*
Hebert, PC, 298, *306*
Hecht, HH, 255, *274*
Hedayati, S, 366, *372*
Hedberg, CW, 125, *147*
Hedgpeth, D, 174, 176, *198*
Hedlund, J, 25, 29, *40*
Hegele, RG, 33, *50*
Heidrich, B, 25, 29, *40*
Heigl, Z, 30, *44,* 63, 66, *79,* 80
Heinrich, W, 236, *247*

Heinz, F, 66, *80*
Heinzer, I, 163, 166, *186*
Heister, A, 266, 268, *278*
Helenius, A, 107, 109, *138, 139,* 285, *302*
Helgerson, SD, 128, *151*
Hellstrom, PE, 333, *348*
Hemingway, BR, 163, *188*
Hemming, VG, 169, 171, 181, 182, *194, 196, 201, 202,* 342, *352, 353*
Hemphill, M, 61, *76*
Henderson, FW, 10, 15, *22,* 27, 30, *40, 44,* 123, *147,* 165, 167, 169, 174, 176, *190, 192, 193, 198,* 205, *217,* 238, *248*
Henderson, G, 171, 173, *196*
Hendley, J, 71, *81*
Hendley, JO, 61, 69, 71, *76, 80, 81,* 126, *149,* 256, 257, 258, 259, 261, 265, 268, 270, *274, 275, 276, 277, 278*
Hendricks, DA, 162, 163, *185*
Hendrickson, KJ, 311, *323*
Hendry, RM, 163, 166, 167, *186, 190, 191*
Hengartner, H, 170, *195*
Henke, D, 167, *191*
Henle, W, 33, *49*
Henneman, PL, 34, *50*
Hennessey, AB, 328, *346*
Hennessy, T, 297, *305*
Henrickson, KJ, 213, *219*
Henry, K, 90, *99*
Henry, S, 88, *99*
Henschke, C, 233, *246*
Hensley, M, 62, *78*
Henttonen, H, 284, *301*
Her, C, 292, *304*
Herata, Y, 298, *306*
Herbert, FA, 240, *249*
Herbertson, MJ, 298, *305*
Herdman, G, 31, *46*
Herena, J, 233, *246*
Hermiston, TW, 231, *247*
Hermogenes, AW, 62, *77,* 356, 358, *370*
Hernandez, M, 31, *46*

Herold, J, 266, 267, *278*
Herrier, G, 109, *139*
Herrington, D, 131, *154*
Hers, JFP, 111, *140*
Hertz, MI, 29, 30, *43, 44,* 86, 87, 88, *97, 98, 99,* 166, 168, 171, 177, *190, 193,* 213, *219*
Herva, E, 25, 29, *40*
Herz, C, 106, *138*
Hess, KR, 126, *149*
Heussner, RC, 27, *41*
Hey, EN, 341, 343, *351*
Heyduk, J, 286, *302*
Heyman, P, 174, *198,* 284, *301*
Hiatt, P, 65, *79*
Hibbard, PL, 83, 96, *97,* 319, *324*
Hicks, BN, 284, *301*
Hierholzer, JC, 25, 29, *39,* 71, *82,* 126, *149,* 163, 166, *186,* 224, 226, 235, 238, 239, *244, 246, 248,* 310, 313, 317, 318, *323*
Higashidate, Y, 170, *195*
Higenbottam, TW, 32, *48*
Higgins, AM, 261, *276*
Higgins, PG, 272, *280*
Higuchi, Y, 29, *43,* 68, *80,* 110, *140,* 296, *305*
Hildebrandt, HM, 125, *147*
Hildreth, S, 65, *79*
Hildreth, SW, 164, 166, 167, 180, 183, *189, 191, 200, 202*
Hill, MG, 163, 169, *188, 194,* 216, *220*
Hilleman, MR, 223, 236, *244*
Hiller, FC, 34, *50*
Hillerdal, G, 32, *49*
Hillman, BC, 127, *149*
Himes, S, 174, *198*
Hinkamp, T, 88, *99*
Hinshaw, VS, 110, 130, *140, 154*
Hintz, M, 339, 350
Hirayama, M, 328, *346*
Hirokawa, M, 240, *249*
Hirsch, M, 261, *276*
Hirschhorn, LR, 29, *41,* 86, *98*
Hirschtick, RE, 90, *99*
Hirsh, D, 61, *76*

Hirst, EMA, 132, *157*
Hiscox, SA, 136, *159*
Hishino, Y, 211, *219*
Hisson, FK, 215, *220*
Hitchcock, W, 29, *43*
Hjelle, B, 284, 286, 287, 288, 293, *301, 302, 303, 305*
Hjort, L, 66, *80*
Hlady, WG, 284, *301*
Ho, M, 83, 88, 89, 95, *97, 98,* 127, *151*
Ho, WG, 96, *102*
Hoble, GR, 29, *42*
Hockberger, RS, 31, *47*
Hockenbery, D, 228, 230, *245*
Hodder, SL, 54, *73*
Hodes, DS, 161, 165, *184*
Hodges, GR, 30, 34, *45, 50*
Hoestetler, KY, 132, *157*
Hofer, F, 255, *274*
Hoffken, G, 25, 29, *40*
Hoffman, HE, 330, 336, *347, 349*
Hoffman, LS, 71, *81*
Hoffman, S, 168, *193*
Hofling, K, 109, *139*
Hogan, PM, 164, 165, *189*
Hogerman, D, 183, *203*
Hogerman, DA, 183, *202*
Hogg, JC, 33, *50,* 231, 235, *246*
Hoglund, S, 233, *246*
Hogue, BG, 270, 272, *280*
Holgate, ST, 161, *185,* 258, 259, 261, 271, 272, *275, 276, 280,* 313, *324*
Hollander, H, 34, *50*
Holman, RC, 34, *51,* 363, *372*
Holmber, H, 25, 29, *39*
Holmes, K, 171, *196*
Holmes, KV, 253, 254, 264, 265, 266, 268, *273, 278*
Holmes, SJ, 366, *372*
Holsinger, LJ, 107, *138*
Holt, DA, 88, *99*
Homa, FL, 216, *220*
Hong, JS, 227, *245*
Honickey, RE, 16, *22*
Honjo, K, 170, *195*
Honjo, T, 166, *191*

Hoorn, B, 328, *346*
Hooton, RD, 86, 87, *98*
Hooton, RM, 30, *43,* 166, 177, 181, *190,* 314, *324*
Hooton, TM, 30, *44,* 65, *79*
Hoover, G, 174, *198*
Hoover, LH, 265, *277*
Hopewell, PC, 90, *99*
Horadam, VW, 331, *347*
Horimoto, T, 113, *142*
Horlick, D, 174, 176, *198*
Horn, ME, 261, 272, *276*
Hornbrook, MC, 38, *51, 62, 77,* 358, *370*
Hornbuckle, K, 337, 338, *350*
Horner, GJ, 113, *141*
Hornick, RB, 333, 334, 336, *348*
Hornsleth, A, 66, *80*
Horowitz, MM, 235, 237, *246, 248*
Horstmann, DM, 33, *49*
Horswood, RL, 169, 171, 183, *194, 196, 202,* 227, 230, 233, *245, 246, 247,* 342, *352*
Hortal, M, 27, *40*
Horvath, CM, 107, *138*
Horwitz, MS, 224, 227, *244, 245*
Hoskalski, PB, 71, *81*
Hoskins, TW, 128, *152,* 358, *371*
Hossain, SU, 256, *274*
Hotham, VJ, 136, *159*
Hotrakitya, S, 27, *41*
Hou, S, 209, 210, *217, 218*
Houck, P, 61, *76*
Hous, S, 210, *218*
Houston, J, 210, *218*
Housworth, J, 84, *97*
Hovi, T, 32, *48,* 329, *346*
Howard, C, 170, 171, *195*
Howard, JB, 123, *147*
Howard, M, 168, *193*
Howie, V, 123, *147*
Hoyne, PA, 207, *217*
Hruska, J, 163, *187*
Hruska, JF, 342, *352*
Hsia, J, 260, *276*
Hsiang, CM, 342, 343, *353*

Hsu, KL, 183, *202*
Hsu, MT, 233, *246*
Hsu, SA, 181, *201*
Hu, Y, 233, *246*
Huang, J, 229, *245*
Huang, KL, 127, *151*
Huang, MW, 33, *50*
Huang, Y, 162, *186*
Huang, YT, 162, 163, *186, 187,* 209, *217*
Huber, M, 216, *221*
Hudson, I, 240, *249*
Huebner, RJ, 205, *216, 217,* 223, 241, 244, *249*
Huettinger, M, 255, *274*
Huggins, JW, 342, 343, *353*
Hughes, P, 368, *373*
Hughes, PJ, 255, *274*
Hughes, SA, 267, *278*
Huhtala, L, 240, *249*
Huie, SF, 30, *44,* 63, 64, 66, *78,* 166, 177, *190*
Humbert, B, 167, *191*
Humphrey, CD, 284, *301*
Humphries, JE, 210, *218*
Hung, PP, 183, *202,* 237, 242, *248, 250*
Hunninghake, G, 167, *192*
Hunt, LA, 132, *156*
Huq, F, 27, *41*
Hurd, D, 61, 63, 71, *76,* 128, *152,* 270, *280*
Hurrman, JM, 338, *350*
Hurwitz, ES, 125, *147,* 363, *372*
Hurwitz, JL, 210, 216, *218, 220*
Hus, LC, 125, *147*
Husak, P, 113, *142*
Hussey, EK, 136, *159,* 345, *353*
Hutchins, G, 171, *196*
Hutchins, GM, 95, *102*
Huttunen, JK, 128, *151*
Hyde, RW, 113, *141*

I

Iacobescu, V, 25, 29, *39*
Icart, J, 88, *99*

Icenogle, TB, 94, *102,* 136, *159*
Ijaz, MK, 268, 270, *278*
Ikeda, A, 137, *159*
Ikeda, RM, 58, *75*
Ikeda, S, 208, *217*
Illarramendi, A, 27, *40*
Imagawa, DT, 30, *44*
Ing, TS, 127, *150,* 330, *347*
Inglis, JM, 30, *44,* 63, 64, *78,* 261, *276*
Ingram, J, 174, *198*
Ingram, RH, 71, *82*
Inhorn, SL, 256, *274*
Inoue, S, 240, *249*
Iorio, AM, 128, *152*
Ireland, DC, 261, 272, *276,* 311, 313, *323*
Irvine, CS, 270, *280*
Irvine, PW, 337, *350*
Irving, WR, 238, *248*
Irwin, W, 284, *301*
Isaacs, D, 27, *40,* 71, *81,* 170, *195,* 268, 270, 271, 272, *278, 279*
Isaacs, R, 93, *101*
Isacson, P, 171, *196*
Ishard, F, 86, 87, *98*
Ishikawa, K, 167, *192*
Isnard, F, 30, *43*
Isnard, LF, 177, *199*
Isobe, H, 115, 117, 131, *142, 144, 156*
Issekutz, TB, 296, *305*
Itabashi, S, 235, *246*
Itamura, S, 113, *142*
Ito, E, 167, *192*
Iwamoto, I, 33, *49*
Izard, M, 331, *347*

J

Jackson, D, 116, *144*
Jackson, E, 84, *97*
Jackson, GG, 127, *150,* 241, *249,* 260, *276,* 328, *346*
Jacob, TD, 298, *306*
Jacobson, JA, 25, *38*
Jaenisch, R, 117, *145,* 210, *218*

Jaffe, HA, 242, *250*
Jaffe, R, 30, *45,* 235, *246*
Jahn, CL, 30, *46*
Jakab, GJ, 26, *40*
Jakeman, KJ, 135, *158,* 336, *349*
Jallat, S, 242, *250*
Jalonen, E, 25, 29, *40*
Jamaluddin, M, 167, *192*
James, DS, 289, 290, 291, 292, 293, *304*
Jamison, RM, 30, *45,* 127, *149,* 165, *189*
Jani, A, 132, *156*
Janner, D, 91, *100*
Janson, CA, 256, *274*
Jarstrand, C, 113, *141*
Jarvis, WR, 214, *219*
Javato, MC, 27, *41*
Jay, M, 284, *301*
Jefferson, LS, 180, *201*
Jeffries, BC, 161, 165, *184, 189,* 224, 237, 238, *244*
Jeffries, WA, 231, *246*
Jekel, JF, 128, *151*
Jenison, S, 284, 286, 287, 293, *302, 303, 305*
Jenkins, DE, 31, *46,* 96, *102*
Jennings, G, 285, *302*
Jennings, GB, 300, *306*
Jennings, LC, 256, *274*
Jensen, K, 162, 172, *185*
Jenson, A, 171, *196*
Jenson, AB, 233, *246*
Jentzen, JM, 125, *147*
Jewell, A, 64, *79,* 165, 183, *189, 203*
Jewett, PH, 212, *219*
Jin, B, 136, *159*
Jindal, P, 128, *151*
Jing, L, 173, *197*
Joglekar, VM, 63, 64, 66, *78*
Johanson, WGJ, 113, *141*
Johansson, BE, 115, 126, *143, 148*
Johansson, KH, 125, *147,* 239, *248*
Johansson, M, 65, *79*
Johnson, BL, 93, *101*
Johnson, DH, 88, *99*
Johnson, G, 94, *101*
Johnson, HN, 31, *47*

Johnson, JE, 25, 29, *39,* 255, *274*
Johnson, K, 169, *193*
Johnson, KM, 63, *78,* 205, *216,* 284, *300, 301*
Johnson, LC, 268, 270, *278*
Johnson, MP, 359, *371*
Johnson, PB, 236, *247*
Johnson, PE, 264, *277*
Johnson, PR, 128, *152,* 163, 166, *186, 187*
Johnson, RW, 30, *44*
Johnston, F, 58, *75,* 127, 128, *149*
Johnston, S, 272, *280*
Johnston, SL, 258, 259, 261, 271, 272, *275, 276, 280,* 313, *324*
Johnston, SLG, 178, *200*
Jokela, P, 128, *151*
Jones, JG, 290, 292, *304*
Jones, PK, 54, *73*
Jones, TM, 181, *201*
Jordan, C, 87, *98*
Jordan, CJ, 87, *98*
Jordan, MC, 29, 30, *43, 44,* 86, 87, 88, 90, 96, *98, 99, 102,* 127, *150,* 161, 166, 167, 180, *185,* 213, *219,* 314, 316, *324*
Jordan, W, 54, 63, 67, *73*
Jordan, WS, 69, *80, 81*
Jordon, MC, 27, *41*
Jorgensen, DM, 321, *324*
Jorgensen, ED, 207, *217*
Josephs, L, 271, 272, *280*
Josephs, S, 91, *100*
Joyner, JW, 215, *220*
Joyner, MW, 162, *185*
Jukkara, A, 128, *151*
Jules-Elysee, K, 32, *48*
Jullaney, D, 136, *158*
Justement, BS, 366, *372*

K

Kaelin, K, 216, *221*
Kaempf, L, 163, 166, *186*
Kagey, SA, 258, *275*

Kagey-Sobotka, A, 258, *275*
Kairys, SW, 215, *220*
Kaiser, DL, 264, *277,* 356, *370*
Kaiser, H, 95, *102*
Kaji, M, 111, *140*
Kakinuma, K, 111, *140*
Kalin, M, 25, 29, *40*
Kallings, I, 25, 29, *40*
Kalser, DL, 127, *150*
Kamer, G, 255, *274*
Kamlet, MS, 361, *371*
Kanegae, Y, 242, *250*
Kanetake, H, 89, *99*
Kang, EY, 32, *48*
Kanner, RE, 29, *42,* 69, *81,* 113, *141*
Kantakamalakul, W, 27, *41*
Kantawateera, P, 27, *41*
Kantor, OS, 63, *79*
Kapadia, S, 298, *305*
Kapikian, AZ, 71, *81,* 162, *185,* 205, *217,* 270, *279,* 342, *352*
Kaplan, B, 320, *324*
Kaplan, M, 91, *100*
Kapoor, W, 25, *39*
Karakorpi, T, 128, *151*
Karalakulasingam, R, 29, *42*
Kardatzke, DR, 262, *276*
Karkowitz, N, 90, *99*
Karpel, JP, 63, *79*
Karpuhin, GI, 329, *346*
Karron, RA, 59, *75,* 214, 215, 216, *220, 221,* 369, *373*
Karzon, DT, 113, 117, 126, 127, 130, *142, 144, 148, 154,* 169, 170, 171, 182, 183, *193, 194, 195, 196, 202*
Kasal, JA, 115, *142*
Kasel, GL, 16, *22*
Kasel, J, 169, *193*
Kasel, JA, 111, 115, *140, 143,* 210, *218,* 240, *249*
Kashtan, CE, 89, *99*
Kashyap, GH, 30, *44,* 63, *79*
Kaslow, R, 127, 128, *150*
Kaslow, RA, 29, *43,* 61, 63, 67, *76,* 127, *150*
Kataja, M, 128, *151*

Kater, N, 61, *76*
Kater, NA, 331, *348*
Katinger, H, 131, *156*
Katsuda, S, 33, *50*
Katunoma, N, 113, *142*
Katunuma, N, 211, *218*
Katz, J, 16, *22,* 121, *146*
Katz, JM, 125, 126, 129, *148, 153,* 310, 313, *322*
Katze, M, 109, 110, *139*
Katze, MG, 108, *138,* 229, *246*
Katzenstein, AL, 33, *49*
Kauffman, RS, 25, *39*
Kauffman, J, 29, *42*
Kaul, A, 169, 171, *194, 195*
Kaul, T, 174, *198*
Kauppinen, MT, 25, 29, *40*
Kava, T, 128, *151*
Kaverin, NV, 129, *153*
Kavet, J, 119, *146*
Kawaguchi, Y, 211, *218*
Kawahara, EK, 33, *50*
Kawana, R, 270, *279*
Kawaoka, Y, 109, 117, 119, 121, 122, 125, 131, 135, *139, 145, 146, 147, 148, 156, 158,* 363, *372*
Kawaoko, Y, 113, *142*
Kawata, N, 93, *101*
Kay, AB, 268, *279*
Kaye, D, 359, *371*
Kaye, HS, 126, *149,* 358, *371*
Keefer, MC, 333, *348*
Keegan, JM, 32, *47*
Keeling, J, 173, *197*
Keicho, N, 235, *246*
Keil, K, 63, *79*
Keir, H, 169, *193*
Keitel, WA, 118, 126, 128, 131, *145, 149, 153, 155,* 358, *371*
Keller, E, 261, *276*
Keller, N, 293, *305*
Kellner, G, 261, *276*
Kellog, JA, 314, *324*
Kellogg, JA, 178, *199*
Kelly, EA, 260, 261, *276*
Kelly, RA, 298, *306*

Kelsey, DK, 269, 272, *279*
Kelso, A, 116, 117, *144*
Kempe, A, 84, *97*
Kempson, RL, 29, *42*
Kendal, AP, 29, *42,* 58, *75,* 115, 119, 125, 127, 130, 134, *142, 143, 146, 147, 150, 154, 157, 158,* 331, *348*
Kendal, SP, 128, *151*
Kennedy, DJ, 130, *153*
Kennedy, NTC, 330, *347*
Kenny, GE, 55, 58, *74*
Kent, J, 61, 63, 69, 71, *76, 81,* 128, *152,* 261, 270, 272, *276, 280,* 311, 313, *323*
Kenyon, K, 33, *49*
Kerem, E, 180, *200*
Kernahan, J, 84, *97*
Kernan, NA, 32, *48*
Kerns, FT, 30, *45*
Kerttula, Y, 25, 29, *39*
Ketai, LH, 292, *305*
Keunecke, H, 231, *246*
Keyes, LD, 227, 233, *245*
Khabbaz, RF, 34, *51,* 284, *301*
Khairulla, NS, 310, *322*
Khan, AS, 34, *51,* 63, 64, 66, *78,* 284, 292, 293, 294, 295, 296, *301, 305,* 342, 343, *352*
Khan, MA, 311, 313, *323*
Khare, GP, 338, 339, *350*
Khen, F, 32, 35, *47*
Kido, H, 113, *142,* 211, *218, 219*
Kilbourne, ED, 29, *42,* 58, *75,* 113, 115, 119, 124, 126, *141, 143, 146, 148,* 356, *370*
Kilian, PL, 227, 232, 233, *245*
Kim, H, 91, *100*
Kim, HW, 123, 130, *147, 154,* 161, 162, 165, 170, 171, 172, 180, 181, 182, 183, *184, 185, 189, 195, 196, 200, 201, 202,* 224, 237, 238, *244,* 342, *352, 353*
Kim, JC, 267, 273, *278*
Kimball, AM, 29, *41,* 63, *79*
Kimpen, J, 174, *198*
Kimura, Y, 111, *140*

Kinchington, PR, 240, *249*
Kind, P, 115, *143*
King, AMQ, 163, 169, 170, *187, 194, 195*
King, IJ, 342, 343, *353*
King, J, 130, *154,* 171, *196*
King, JC, 90, *100,* 131, *155*
King, T, 233, *246*
Kinner, J, 170, *195*
Kirchweger, R, 255, *274*
Kirk, LE, 96, *102*

Kirkpatrick, CJ, 127, *149*
Kirshon, B, 29, *43*
Kishino, Y, 113, *142,* 211, *218*
Kisselev, O, 126, *148*
Kitabayashi, A, 240, *249*
Kitayama, T, 89, *99*
Kitchen, LW, 30, *45*
Kiyono, H, 116, *144*
Kjellman, B, 173, 174, *197*
Klainer, AS, 31, *46*
Klassen, LW, 127, *151*
Klassen, TP, 215, *220*
Klauber, MR, 113, *141*
Klemola, E, 32, *48*
Klenk, H, 109, *139*
Klenk, HD, 26, *40,* 113, 115, *142,* 211, 212, *218, 219*
Klessig, DF, 232, *244*
Kleter, GEM, 126, *148*
Klima, A, 131, *156*
Klimov, A, 94, *101*
Kline, MW, 90, *100*
Klocke, RA, 240, *249*
Klotman, ME, 32, *48*
Klutinis, BS, 236, *247*
Knight, V, 29, 31, *42, 46,* 96, *102,* 111, 136, *140, 158, 159,* 169, 180, *193, 201,* 232, 241, *246, 249,* 334, 339, 341, 342, *349, 350, 351*
Knorr, R, 115, *143*
Knott, AM, 212, *219*
Knottnerus, JA, 62, *77,* 127, 128, *150,* 358, *370*
Knox, KK, 33, *50*

Kobashigawa, JA, 93, *101*
Kobzik, L, 298, *306*
Kochanek, S, 243, *250*
Kodinka, RL, 91, *100*
Koffron, AJ, 320, *324*
Kohler, R, 25, *39*
Kohmoto, O, 298, *306*
Kohn, MA, 284, *301*
Kok, GB, 136, *159*
Kolassa, JE, 270, *280,* 313, *324*
Kolb, AF, 266, 268, *278*
Kolber, M, 284, *301*
Kolls, J, 167, *192*
Komatsu, T, 111, *140*
Komishan, SV, 30, *45*
Kondo, S, 113, *141*
Konig, W, 167, *191*
Koonin, E, 267, *278*
Koonin, EV, 266, 267, *278*
Koopman, JS, 334, *348*
Kopelman, AE, 176, *199*
Kopriva, S, 233, *246*
Koren, H, 167, *191, 192*
Kormos, RL, 32, *48*
Kornfeld, SJ, 209, *217*
Kornilayeva, GV, 132, *157*
Korsmeyer, S, 228, 230, *245*
Kort, BA, 29, *42*
Kosak, K, 269, 272, *279*
Kositanont, U, 27, *41*
Koskela, M, 25, 29, *39*
Kostek, B, 183, *202*
Koster, FT, 34, *51,* 284, 289, 290, 291, 292, 293, 294, 295, 296, 297, *301, 303, 304, 305*
Kotok, DI, 164, 165, *189*
Kouides, RW, 29, *43,* 58, 63, 64, *74,* 161, 180, *185,* 314, *324*
Kovaleva, TP, 329, *346*
Koven, NL, 33, *49*
Kovesdi, I, 228, *245*
Kowalski, H, 255, *274*
Kowalski, RP, 240, *249*
Kozlowska, W, 173, *197*
Krane, E, 89, *99*
Krasinski, K, 90, *100,* 176, *199*

Krasnykh, VN, 228, 243, *245, 251*
Krause, HE, 27, *41,* 71, *81,* 161, 165, *184,* 342, *352*
Krause, M, 33, *50*
Krause, P, 69, 70, 71, *81,* 313, *323*
Krauss, S, 121, *146*
Kravetz, H, 169, *193*
Krebs, JW, 284, 286, *301, 303,* 344, *353*
Kremer, E, 242, *250*
Kretzschmar, E, 109, *139*
Krieger, M, 162, *186*
Krilov, L, 261, *276*
Krilov, LR, 35, *51,* 91, *100*
Krisher, KK, 317, *324*
Krithivas, A, 227, *245*
Kroes, ACM, 30, *43*
Krolikowski, J, 287, *303*
Kronberg, R, 32, *49*
Krosl, P, 298, *306*
Krug, R, 109, 110, *139*
Krug, RM, 106, 108, *138, 139*
Krugman, S, 366, *372*
Krystal, M, 120, 131, 136, *146, 156, 158*
Krystofik, D, 172, *197*
Ksiazek, TG, 34, *51,* 284, 286, 287, 288, 289, 292, 297, *301, 303, 305,* 344, *353*
Kubar, OI, 329, *346*
Kubiet, MA, 128, *151*
Kudo, K, 167, *192*
Kuechler, E, 108, *138,* 255, *274*
Kuhn, MS, 213, *219*
Kuip, LVD, 111, *140*
Kuis, W, 240, *249*
Kujala, P, 25, 29, *40*
Kulhanjian, JA, 178, *199*
Kulkarni, AB, 163, 171, *188, 196,* 215, *220*
Kumar, ML, 54, *73*
Kumar, SS, 93, *101,* 127, *151*
Kundi, M, 261, *276*
Kunigawa, K, 298, *306*
Kunin, CM, 29, *42,* 111, *140*
Kunkel, SL, 298, *306*
Kunz, C, 261, *276*
Kuosma, E, 240, *249*

Kurasawa, K, 33, *49*
Kurita, T, 111, *140*
Kuroki, J, 240, *249*
Kurt-Jones, EA, 227, *245*
Kurtz, S, 136, *158*
Kusaba, Y, 89, *99*
Kussisto, P, 128, *151*
Kutza, J, 359, *371*
Kuwano, K, 231, *246*
Kvale, PA, 90, *99*
Kvist, S, 230, *247*

L

La Montagne, JR, 127, 128, *150*
LaBree, L, 240, *249*
Lacarpa, S, 258, *275*
Lacroix, S, 61, 66, *76, 80*
LaForce, FM, 355, *370*
Lagergard, T, 25, 29, *39*
Lahdensuo, A, 128, *151*
Lai, MMC, 253, 254, 264, 265, 266, 267, *273, 278*
Laidlaw, PP, 355, *370*
Laitinen, LA, 240, *249*
Lakey, DL, 130, *153*, 365, *372*
Laks, H, 93, *101*
Lam, SK, 310, *322*
Lamb, JR, 115, *143*
Lamb, RA, 107, 109, 115, 136, *138, 139, 143, 158*, 208, *217*
Lambden, P, 169, *193*
Lambden, PR, 313, *324*
Lambert, DM, 162, *186*
Lamborn, KR, 69, *81*
Lamm, ME, 209, *217*
LaMonica, N, 266, 267, *278*
LaMontagne, JR, 29, *43*, 61, 63, 67, *76*, 126, 127, *148, 150*
Lampe, F, 258, 271, 272, *275, 280*
Lamphear, BJ, 255, *274*
Lamprecht, CL, 342, *352*
Lamson, TH, 238, *248*
Landau, LI, 240, *249*
Landry, M, 167, *191*

Landry, ML, 255, 259, 264, *274*
Lane, J, 94, *102*
Lang, DJ, 241, *249*
Langedijk, JPM, 162, *186*
Langer, L, 63, 64, *78*
Langmuir, AD, 84, *97*, 223, 226, *244*
Langston, C, 311, *323*
Lansing, RM, 29, *42*
Lant, AF, 25, 29, *39*
Lanteri, CJ, 180, *200*
Lanzi, R, 287, *303*
Lapied, R, 178, *199*
Laporte, JP, 30, *43*, 86, 87, *98*
Laposata, E, 287, *303*
Larsen, JW, 29, *42*
Larsen, RA, 25, *38*
Larson, HE, 71, *81*, 111, *140*, 270, 279
LaRussa, P, 368, *373*
Laskin, OL, 339, 350
Laster, S, 231, *247*
Latz, JM, 210, *218*
Lau, J, 62, *77*, 356, 358, *370*
Lau, LC, 261, *276*
Lauer, BA, 127, *149*, 165, 176, *190, 199*
Lavandowski, RA, 260, *276*
Laver, J, 32, *48*
Laver, WG, 115, 136, *143, 159*, 345, *353*
Law, B, 308, *322*
Law, BJ, 342, 343, *352*
Lawrence, E, 134, *158*, 335, *349*
Lawrence, EC, 32, *48*
Lawrence, LA, 162, *186*
Lawrence, MC, 207, *217*
Lawrence, R, 90, *100*, 176, *199*
Lawson, CM, 117, 131, *145, 156*
Lazaro, ME, 284, 287, *301, 303*
Lazicki, ME, 93, *101*
Lazzarini, R, 108, *138*
Leader, I, 63, 65, *79*
Leander, KR, 132, *156*
LeBourgeois, M, 91, *100*
Lechelt, KE, 62, *77*, 128, *152*
Lecocq, LP, 242, *250*
Leddy, JP, 161, *185*

Ledesma-Medina, J, 88, 89, *99,* 176, *199,* 213, *219*
LeDuk, JW, 287, *303*
Lee, H, 93, *101*
Lee, HJ, 266, 267, *278*
Lee, HW, 286, *302*
Lee, JY, 358, *371*
Lee, PW, 286, *302*
Lee, SG, 237, 242, *248, 250*
Lee, SW, 284, *301*
Lee, WM, 261, *276*
Lees, DE, 292, *304*
Legrand, MC, 270, 271, *280*
Lehman, DJ, 216, *220*
Lehot, JJ, 32, *48*
Lehtomaki, K, 240, *249*
Leib, H, 29, *42,* 59, *75,* 315, 316, *324*
Leib, HB, 60, *76*
Leibovitz, A, 238, *248*
Leibovitz, E, 174, *198*
Leigh, MW, 9, 20, *21*
Leikin, S, 170, 172, *195*
Leinikki, P, 329, *346*
Leiononen, M, 25, 29, *39, 40*
Leland, DS, 35, *51*
Lennette, EH, 162, *185,* 215, *220*
Lennon, R, 171, *196*
Lenora, RAK, 53, *73*
Leonard, SA, 125, *147*
Leonardi, GP, 29, *42,* 59, *75,* 315, 316, *324*
Leophante, P, 88, *99*
Leowski, J, 8, 18, *21*
Lepow, M, 368, *373*
Lerch, RA, 163, *187*
Lerman, SJ, 127, *149*
Leser, GP, 107, *138*
Leslie, N, 134, *157*
Leszczynski, J, 164, 181, 182, *189, 201,* 342, *352*
Levandowski, R, 358, *371*
Levandowski, RA, 62, *77,* 113, 127, *141, 149,* 260, *276,* 313, 314, *323,* 356, 358, *370*
Levely, ME, 163, 170, *187, 188, 195*
Levenson, RM, 30, *44,* 63, *79*

Levin, MJ, 92, *101,* 127, *149,* 182, *201,* 235, 239, *246, 248,* 342, 343, *353*
Levin, S, 172, *197*
Levine, DP, 30, *45*
Levine, HD, 161, 165, *184*
Levine, PA, 272, *280*
Levine, S, 162, *186*
Levine, SM, 96, *102*
Levis, R, 266, 268, *278*
Levy, H, 289, 290, 291, 292, 293, 299, *304, 305, 306*
Lewensohn-Fuchs, S, 89, *99*
Lewis, ED, 84, *97*
Lewis, JK, 131, *156*
Lewis, V, 86, 87, 88, 91, *98, 100,* 369, *373*
Li, D, 284, *301*
Li, S, 113, 131, *142, 156*
Lichtenstein, D, 162, 163, *186*
Lichtenstein, LM, 258, *275*
Lieb, LE, 62, *77,* 358, *370*
Lieb, T, 181, *201*
LIebhaber, H, 358, *371*
Lief, FS, 125, *147*
Lieh-Lai, MW, 342, *352*
Liepins, A, 33, *50*
Lieu, TA, 366, *372*
Liew, FY, 115, *143*
Light, B, 340, *351*
Ligthart, GJ, 126, 128, *149*
Likar, M, 333, *348*
Lilleby, KE, 32, 35, *48*
Lillington, GA, 29, *42*
Lin, J, 173, *197*
Lin, YL, 117, *144*
Lind, A, 127, *150,* 358, *370*
Linde, A, 32, *49,* 317, *324*
Linden, M, 269, *279*
Lindgren, C, 173, *197*
Lindgren, KM, 263, *277*
Lindholm, K, 31, *46*
Linnemann, CC, 32, *49,* 125, *147,* 308, *322*
Linton, PN, 35, *51,* 60, *76,* 133, *157*
Lipman, BJ, 31, *46*
Lipson, SM, 91, *100*

Lipton, SD, 32, *48*
Little, DW, 60, 61, *76*
Little, J, 134, *158*
Little, JW, 113, *141, 335, 349*
Little, PF, 33, *49*
Littman, M, 31, *47*
Litton, PA, 128, *152*
Liu, C, 111, *140,* 238, *248*
Liu, KJ, 134, *157*
Liu, MA, 132, *156,* 363, *372*
Liu-Yin, JA, 33, *50*
Ljungman, P, 32, *48,* 87, 88, 89, *98, 99*
Lo, W, 117, 123, *145*
Lobo, M, 136, *159,* 345, *353*
Loda, FA, 7, 9, 15, 17, *21, 22,* 161, 165, *184*
Loda, FSA, 212, *219*
Lode, H, 25, 29, *40*
Logan, IS, 328, 335, *346*
London, WT, 130, 131, *154, 155,* 169, 181, 183, *194, 201, 202*
Long, CE, 55, 56, *73,* 92, *101,* 164, 165, 166, 167, 169, 182, *189, 191, 201,* 212, *219*
Long, Ce, 369, *373*
Long, WJ, 264, *277*
Longini, IM, 334, *348*
Longson, M, 30, *44*
Longstreth, JA, 339, *350*
Longworth, DL, 27, *41*
Look, AT, 266, 268, *278*
Loosli, Cg, 236, *247*
Lopaschuk, Gd, 298, *306*
Lopez, N, 284, 287, *301, 303*
Lotshaw, RR, 32, *47*
Lott, L, 368, *373*
Louria, DB, 29, *42,* 113, 124, *141*
Louria, DE, 58, *75*
Low, FN, 111, *140*
Low-Friedrich, I, 298, *306*
Lowenstein, CJ, 298, *306*
Lu, X, 171, 173, *196,* 267, 273, *278*
Lu, Y, 108, *139,* 267, *278*
Lubeck, MD, 132, *157,* 183, *202,* 242, *250,* 336, *349*
Luby, J, 31, *46*

Luby, JP, 117, *145*
Lucas, SJ, 115, *143*
Lucero, MG, 27, *41*
Lucet, JC, 30, *43,* 86, 87, *98,* 177, *199*
Luckey, A, 205, *216*
Ludwig, WR, 29, *42*
Luft, BJ, 287, *303*
Luijt, DS, 59, *75*
Lukacher, AE, 117, *144*
Lukason, MJ, 227, 233, *245*
Lum, CT, 96, *102*
Luna, M, 87, 88, *98*
Luna, MA, 32, *48,* 91, *100,* 369, *373*
Lundholm-Beuchamp, U, 230, *247*
Lundkvist, A, 284, *301*
Luo, G, 136, *158*
Luo, M, 255, *274,* 345, *353*
Luytjes, W, 131, *156*
Lybass, TG, 71, *81*
Lyles, DS, 111, 113, *140, 141*
Lyn, D, 209, *217*
Lyons, MJ, 286, *302*

M

Ma, Y, 229, *246*
Maassab, HF, 130, 131, *154, 155,* 328, *346*
MacDonald, KL, 125, *147*
MacDonald, NE, 84, *97,* 164, 165, 176, *189, 190*
Macek, V, 233, *246*
Macfarlane, JT, 25, 29, *39, 40*
Macfarlane, RM, 25, 29, *40*
Machat, H, 255, *274*
MacInnes, K, 284, 286, *302*
Maciu, H, 93, *101*
Mackenzi, J, 121, *146*
MacKenzie, CD, 117, *145*
MacKenzie, JS, 128, *152*
Macknight, K, 261, *276*
Mackow, ER, 284, 287, *301, 303*
Macnaughton, MR, 71, *81,* 268, 270, 271, 272, *278, 279*
Macrae, AD, 25, 29, *39*

Madar, D, 292, 293, 294, 295, 296, 297, 304
Madore, HP, 35, *51,* 60, *76,* 133, *157,* 331, *348*
Madore, PH, 134, *158*
Maeda, H, 113, *141*
Maehara, N, 167, 168, *192*
Magdangal, DM, 27, *41*
MaGill, FB, 161, *185*
Magnan, S, 127, *150,* 358, 359, *370, 371*
Magnussen, CR, 340, *351*
Magoffin, RL, 162, *185,* 215, *220*
Mahan, K, 261, *276*
Mahmoo, W, 35, *51*
Mahoney, JD, 128, *152*
Maile, J, 266, 268, *278*
Maj, H, 175, 180, *198, 200*
Major, D, 129, *153*
Makela, PH, 25, 29, *39*
Makene, M, 215, *220,* 369, *373*
Makino, S, 167, 168, *192*
Malefyt, R, 168, *193*
Maletzky, AJ, 7, *21*
Mallick, NP, 30, *44*
Malone, RW, 132, *156*
Mandal, SK, 63, 64, 66, *78*
Mandema, JM, 59, *75*
Manguara, BT, 90, *99*
Mangubat, NV, 27, *41*
Mann, DL, 298, *305*
Mann, T, 168, *193*
Mann, TN, 111, *140*
Manning, JA, 165, 176, *190*
Mannix, M, 366, *372*
Mansury, L, 128, *151*
Manzanec, MB, 209, *217*
Mao, SH, 127, *151*
Mapel, V, 297, *305*
Marakami, M, 137, *159*
Marcuse, EK, 365, *372*
Margolick, J, 93, *101*
Margolis, KL, 62, *77,* 127, *150,* 356, 358, 359, 361, *370, 371*
Margulies, JR, 62, *77,* 358, *370*
Mariguchi, JD, 93, *101*
Marine, WM, 25, 29, *39, 42,* 124, *147*

Mark, EJ, 33, *49*
Mark, JBD, 32, *48*
Markovitz, DM, 134, *158,* 335, *349*
Markowitz, RI, 33, *49*
Marks, MI, 25, 29, *40*
Markwell, MAk, 208, *217*
Marlin, SD, 255, 265, *274, 277*
Marlor, CW, 265, *277*
Marsden, P, 328, *346*
Marsh, M, 285, *302*
Marshall, WF, 35, *51*
Marston, BJ, 30, *44,* 314, *324*
Martin, CM, 29, *42,* 111, *140*
Martin, J, 119, *146,* 233, *246*
Martin, K, 107, 109, *138, 139*
Martin, MA, 87, *98,* 165, 166, 177, *189*
Martin, SM, 117, 128, *145, 151*
Martinez, A, 31, *47*
Martinez, D, 132, *156*
Martinez, E, 31, *46*
Martinez, FD, 161, *185*
Massab, HF, 125, *147*
Massicot, JG, 130, *154*
Massion, PP, 208, *217*
Mast, EE, 61, 69, *76,* 134, *158,* 337, 350
Mastrangcli, A, 233, *246*
Mastrangeli, A, 242, *250*
Mastronarde, J, 167, *192*
Mastrota, FM, 205, *217*
Masurel, N, 56, 61, 62, *74, 76, 77,* 93, *101,* 111, 126, 127, 128, *140, 148, 149, 150, 151,* 179, *200,* 358, *370*
Mather, U, 58, *75*
Mathers, LH, 342, *352*
Mathews, MB, 229, *246*
Mathias, P, 227, 232, *245*
Mathisen, G, 35, *51*
Mathur, U, 29, *43,* 62, 63, 64, *77, 78,* 166, *190*
Mathurs, LH, 65, *79*
Matlock, M, 29, *41,* 63, *79*
Matsuda, T, 34, *51*
Matsui, H, 240, *249*
Matsukawa, S, 296, *305*
Matsumiya, S, 55, *73*
Matsumoto, I, 270, *279*

Matsumotot, K, 136, *159*
Matsusc, T, 231, *246*
Matsuse, T, 240, *249*
Matsushima, K, 167, *192*
Matsuya, F, 89, *99*
Matthay, RA, 292, *304*
Matthews, DA, 166, *191,* 256, *274*
Matthews, J, 25, 29, *39*
Matthieu, MC, 242, *250*
Mattison, HR, 62, *77,* 131, *155*
Mauch, H, 25, 29, *40*
Mauch, TJ, 89, *99*
Maupin, G, 284, *301*
Maxson, W, 25, 29, *39*
Mayer, L, 233, *246*
Maynard, R, 35, *51,* 60, *76,* 133, *157*
Mazanec, MB, 209, *217*
Mbawuike, I, 131, *156*
McAuliffe, T, 235, 237, *246, 248*
McBean, AM, 57, *74*
McBride, JT, 65, *79,* 180, *200, 201,* 342, *351*
McBride, T, 259, 265, *275*
McBride, TP, 264, *277*
McCann, RM, 55, 61, 63, 64, 69, *73, 79,* 179, *200,* 270, *280,* 313, 314, *324*
McCarthy, AJ, 240, *249*
McCarthy, CA, 165, 170, 175, 180, *190, 195*
McCarthy, N, 209, *218*
McCarthy, P, 33, *49*
McCauley, JW, 109, *139*
McClelland, A, 265, *277*
McClung, HW, 136, *159,* 339, 341, *350*
McConnochie, KM, 161, 166, 167, *185, 191*
McCormick, DP, 29, *43,* 66, *80,* 316, *324*
McCormick, JB, 284, *301,* 342, 343, *353*
McCracken, JS, 25, 29, *39*
McCraken, EA, 340, *351*
McDonald, DM, 208, *217*
McDonald, MI, 31, *46*
McDonnell, PJ, 240, *249*
McElhancy, JE, 128, *152*
McElhaney, JE, 56, 62, *74,* 77

McElroy, HE, 256, *274*
McElvaney, NG, 242, *250*
McFadden, J, 168, *192*
McFadden, R, 127, *150,* 358, 359, *370, 371*
McFarland, L, 284, *301*
McGahen, JW, 328, *346*
McGann, K, 91, *100*
McGhee, JR, 116, *144*
McGlave, P, 166, 171, 177, *190*
McGlave, PB, 30, *44,* 86, 87, *97*
McIntosh, K, 16, 17, *22, 23,* 29, *41,* 69, 71, *81,* 86, 90, 91, *98, 99,* 126, 127, *148, 149,* 161, 162, 163, 166, 167, 168, 171, 173, *184, 185, 190, 191, 192, 196, 197,* 209, *217,* 253, 254, 261, 264, 265, 270, *273, 276, 279,* 314, *324,* 341, *351*
McKee, KT, 287, *303*
McKenna, BA, 93, *101,* 127, *150*
McKenna, P, 284, *301*
McKenzie, IFC, 117, *145*
McKinlay, MA, 255, *274*
McKinney, WP, 29, *42*
McLeod, DL, 205, *216*
McMichael, A, 170, *195*
McMichael, AJ, 117, *145*
McMickle, A, 116, *144,* 210, *218*
McMillan, JA, 176, *199,* 261, 276
McNabb, WR, 25, 29, *39*
McNamara, MJ, 69, *81*
McNeil, MM, 92, *100*
McNicol, P, 308, *322*
McPhie, JL, 232, *244*
McQuillan, J, 310, 317, *322*
McQuillin, J, 26, *40,* 84, *97,* 171, *195, 196,* 209, *217*
Meade, R, 31, *47*
Meagher, MP, 166, 176, *190, 199*
Meert, KL, 181, *201,* 342, *352*
Mei, YF, 224, 232, *244, 247*
Meier, M, 30, *45*
Meignier, B, 129, *153*
Meiklejohn, G, 127, *149, 151,* 162, *185,* 215, *220,* 329, *347*

Meissner, HC, 92, *101*
Melchers, F, 115, *143*
Melero, JA, 162, 163, 170, *186, 188*
Melia, RJW, 16, *22*
Meloen, RH, 162, *186*
Menegus, M, 29, *43,* 58, 63, 64, *74,* 161, 180, *185,* 314, *324*
Menegus, MA, 27, 30, *41, 45,* 55, 56, *73,* 317, *324*
Menegus, ME, 164, 165, 176, *189*
Meneilly, GS, 62, *77,* 128, *152*
Mera, JR, 32, *48*
Merigan, TC, 32, *48*
Merlin, TL, 292, 293, 294, 295, 296, 297, *304*
Merluzzi, VJ, 255, 265, *274, 277*
Merolla, R, 167, 168, *192, 193*
Mertz, B, 344, *353*
Mertz, GJ, 289, 290, 291, 292, 293, *304*
Meruman, O, 174, 176, *198*
Meryers, JD, 96, *102*
Merz, D, 171, *196*
Meschievitz, CK, 256, 269, 272, *274, 275, 279*
Messner, MK, 166, 175, 176, *190*
Metcalf, M, 33, *50*
Metz, CG, 290, 292, *304*
Meurman, O, 169, *193*
Meyer, AL, 163, *188*
Meyer, AM, 265, *277*
Meyer, HL, 180, *200*
Meyer, K, 261, *276*
Meyers, DR, 95, *102*
Meyers, JD, 30, 32, 33, 35, *43, 44, 45, 48, 49, 50,* 86, 87, 96, *98, 102,* 237, *248,* 314, *324*
Meyerson, LR, 180, *201*
Meziere, A, 178, *199*
Michaels, MG, 30, *45,* 235, *246*
Middleton, E, 209, *218*
Middleton, PJ, 214, *219*
Midulla, F, 167, 168, *192*
Miettinen, AK, 240, *249*
Mignot, P, 30, *43,* 88, *99*
Mikata, A, 33, *49*
Mikheeva, GV, 228, 243, *245, 251*

Miller, BA, 60, 61, 62, 63, 64, 69, 70, 71, *76, 78, 81,* 313, *323*
Miller, CL, 128, *152,* 358, *371*
Miller, G, 33, 34, *49, 51*
Miller, GL, 292, 293, 294, 295, 296, *305*
Miller, NT, 130, *154*
Miller, R, 117, 121, *145*
Miller, RA, 53, *73*
Miller, RD, 257, *275*
Miller, RW, 176, *199*
Millet, VM, 337, *349*
Milligan, L, 54, 63, 67, *73*
Mills, J, 90, *99,* 118, 123, *146,* 169, *194*
Mills, JN, 287, *303*
Mills, SA, 31, *46*
Milner, M, 171, *196*
Milner, RA, 175, 180, *198, 200*
Minamitani, M, 162, *185,* 215, *220*
Minguez, JA, 31, *47*
Mink, KA, 256, *274*
Minnefor, A, 265, *277*
Minnefore, AB, 93, *101*
Minnich, L, 311, 314, *323*
Minnich, LL, 94, *102,* 136, *159*
Minocha, A, 330, *347*
Minor, PD, 255, *274*
Miotti, P, 127, *151*
Miotti, PG, 93, *101*
Mirza, MQ, 87, 88, *98*
Mirza, N, 91, *100,* 181, *201,* 369, *373*
Mirza, NQ, 91, *100*
Mischler, R, 62, *77*
Misplon, JA, 117, *145*
Mitani, K, 243, *250*
Mitchell, D, 87, *98*
Mitchell, M, 170, *195*
Mitchell, RH, 162, *185,* 342, *352*
Mitnaul, LJ, 109, *139*
Mittler, S, 181, *201*
Mitzutani, S, 255, *273*
Miura, AB, 240, *249*
Miyasaka, M, 296, *305*
Miyawaki, T, 111, *140*
Mizutani, S, 242, *250,* 255, *273*
Mocega, HE, 27, *41*
Mocega-Gonzalez, HE, 161, 165, *184*

Modlin, JF, 127, *149*
Moffet, HL, 238, *248*
Mogabgab, WJ, 30, *45,* 111, *140*
Mohar, CK, 183, *202,* 342, *352*
Mokrohisky, S, 173, *197*
Moldawer, LL, 227, 232, 233, *245*
Moler, Fw, 342, 343, *352*
Molla, A, 113, *141*
Mollat, C, 178, *199*
Momomura, S, 298, *306*
Monath, TP, 181, *201*
Moncada, S, 298, *306*
Monick, M, 167, *192*
Monroe, M, 284, *301*
Monte, S, 171, *196*
Montgomery, DL, 132, *156*
Monto, A, 69, *81*
Monto, AS, 7, *21,* 54, 56, 60, 61, 66, 71, *73, 74, 76, 80, 81,* 115, 126, 127, 130, 134, *143, 148, 149, 154, 157, 158,* 318, *324,* 328, 331, 334, 336, 337, 338, 342, 343, *346, 348, 349,* 350, *350, 352,* 358, *370*
Montoya, J, 297, *305*
Moodie, J, 32, *47*
Moodie, JW, 25, 29, *39*
Moolenaar, RL, 34, *51,* 289, 292, *303*
Moore, C, 229, *245*
Moore, GM, 284, *301*
Moore, K, 168, *193*
Moore, M, 235, *246*
Moore, RV, 136, *159*
Morag, A, 93, *101*
Morales, F, 30, *44,* 63, 64, *78*
Moran, T, 131, *156*
Moran, TM, 117, 126, 137, *144, 148, 159*
Morel-Barbey, CL, 211, *219*
Morens, D, 125, *147*
Morgan, WJ, 161, *185*
Morgante, O, 240, *249*
Mori, I, 111, *140*
Mori, M, 96, *102*
Mori, S, 240, *249*
Morice, RC, 91, *100*
Morrell, RE, 25, 29, *40*

Morris, AH, 292, *304*
Morris, C, 287, 293, *303, 305*
Morris, DJ, 33, *50*
Morris, JA, 161, 169, *184, 193*
Morris, L, 134, *158,* 335, *349*
Morrow, PE, 113, *141*
Morse, DL, 58, *75,* 128, *152*
Morse, IH, 171, *196*
Mortimer, EAJ, 54, *73*
Morzunov, S, 284, 286, 293, *301, 302, 303, 305*
Morzunov, SP, 287, 288, *303*
Moscona, A, 208, 210, *217, 218*
Mosega, HE, 71, *81*
Moslow, SR, 358, *371*
Mosmann, T, 168, *193*
Moss, B, 162, 183, *186, 202*
Moss, MY, 329, *347*
Mosser, AG, 255, *274*
Mostow, RA, 126, *149*
Mostow, Sr, 329, *347*
Mottet, G, 162, *186*
Motzel, SL, 132, *156*
Mountford, RC, 255, *274*
Mouthaon, L, 177, *199*
Mouthon, L, 30, *43,* 86, 87, *98*
Movahed, LA, 318, *324*
Muchmore, HG, 210, *218*
Muder, RR, 25, *39*
Mudholkar, GS, 113, *141*
Mueller, M, 298, *306*
Mueller, RE, 241, *249*
Mufson, M, 171, 172, 182, 183, *196*
Mufson, MA, 27, *41,* 58, 63, 66, 71, *74, 78, 80, 81,* 163, 166, 167, 169, *186, 191, 193,* 342, *352*
Mukaika, N, 167, *192*
Mulder, J, 111, *140*
Mulder, PGH, 56, *74*
Muldoon, JP, 320, *324*
Muldoon, Rl, 241, *249,* 328, *346*
Muller, NL, 32, *48*
Mulligan, MS, 296, *305*
Mullinix, MG, 130, *154*
Mullooly, JP, 29, 38, *42, 51,* 56, 62, *74, 77,* 118, 127, *145, 149,* 358, *370*

Multz, AS, 63, *79*
Munar, M, 316, *324*
Mundy, GR, 33, *49*
Munk, G, 358, *371*
Munn, NJ, 131, *155*
Munns, RE, 31, *46*
Munoz, J, 170, *195*
Munro, TF, 58, *75*
Murasko, DM, 359, *371*
Murdoch, M, 127, *150,* 358, 359, *370, 371*
Murdoch, PS, 30, *44,* 63, 64, *78*
Murphy, B, 123, *147*
Murphy, BR, 56, *74,* 115, 116, 117, 121, 122, 126, 130, 131, *142, 143, 145, 149, 154, 156,* 161, 162, 163, 165, 169, 171, 180, 181, 183, *184, 186, 187, 188, 193, 194, 196, 200, 201, 202,* 207, 210, 212, 215, *217, 218, 219, 220,* 359, 369, *371, 373*
Murphy, D, 91, *100*
Murphy, FA, 286, *302*
Murphy, M, 125, *148*
Murphy, P, 59, *75,* 316, *324*
Murphy, TF, 27, *40,* 205, *217*
Murray, JF, 290, 292, *304*
Murray, S, 261, *276*
Murrin-Espin, M, 88, *99*
Murtagh, P, 27, *41*
Murthy, KK, 242, *250*
Murthy, S, 242, *250*
Murti, KG, 109, 137, *139, 159*
Muster, T, 131, *156*
Muth, RG, 127, *150*
Mutson, MA, 161, 165, *184*
Myasaka, M, 296, *305*
Myerowitz,RL, 235, *246*
Myers, G, 284, 286, *302*
Myers, JL, 33, *49,* 238, *248*
Myers, ML, 292, *304*
Myers, R, 161, *184*
Myers, T, 89, *99*
Mygind, N, 258, *275*
Myint, S, 272, *280*
Myint, SH, 271, 272, *280*
Myou, S, 34, *51*

N

Naclerio, RM, 258, 259, 265, *275*
Nadel, JA, 208, *217*
Nadel, S, 91, *100*
Naeve, C, 121, *146*
Nafia, I, 329, *346*
Nagase, T, 240, *249*
Nagelkerken, L, 126, 128, *149*
Nagler, A, 93, *101*
Nahar, N, 27, *41*
Nahmias, AJ, 321, *324*
Nair, P, 171, *196*
Nair, RC, 268, 270, *278*
Nakada, S, 108, *139*
Nakagawa, Y, 108, *139*
Nakakuki, K, 111, *140*
Nakamura, S, 110, *140,* 296, *305*
Nakanishi, I, 33, *50*
Nakanishi, Y, 110, 111, *140,* 296, *305*
Nakayama, T, 167, 168, *192*
Namazi, A, 127, *151*
Nankevis, GA, 310, 313, 319, 320, 321, *323*
Naparstek, E, 93, *101*
Napoli, A, 263, *277*
Narmanbetova, RA, 132, *157*
Nash, G, 31, *46,* 321, *324*
Nasu, N, 29, *43,* 68, *80*
Nathanson, C, 291, 292, *304*
Nathanson, N, 119, *146*
Natuk, RJ, 242, *250*
Nava, MER, 31, *46*
Navas, L, 165, 175, *190, 198*
Nawas, SR, 284, *301*
Nawata, Y, 33, *49*
Naylor, D, 361, *371*
Neal, KR, 31, *46*
Neale, JM, 263, *277*
Nedrud, JG, 209, *217*
Neill, SU, 284, *301*
Nelson, DB, 125, *147,* 363, *372*
Nelson, DL, 115, *142,* 169, *193*
Nelson, KE, 93, *101,* 127, *151*
Nemerow, GR, 227, 232, *245*
Neri, M, 128, *152*

Nerome, K, 136, *159*
Neuberger, K, 31, *47*
Neufeld, R, 29, *43,* 127, 128, *150*
Neumann, JL, 91, *100*
Neumayer, EM, 328, *346*
Neuzil, K, 167, 171, 173, *192, 196, 197*
Nevins, JR, 228, *245*
Newman, F, 131, 135, *155, 158,* 336, *349*
Newman, FK, 62, *77,* 131, *155,* 215, *220,* 369, *373*
Newman, R, 129, *153*
Newman, RW, 129, *153*
Newton-John, H, 240, *249*
Ng, VL, 34, *50*
Nguyen, A, 284, *301*
Nguyen, MLT, 27, *41*
Ni, J, 311, *323*
Ni, K, 91, *100*
Nichol, KL, 62, *77,* 127, *150,* 356, 358, 359, 361, *370, 371*
Nichol, S, 34, *51,* 289, 292, *303*
Nichol, ST, 34, *51,* 284, 286, 287, 288, 293, *301, 302, 303, 305*
Nicholas, JA, 163, *187, 188*
Nichols, JA, 170, *195*
Nichols, L, 96, *102*
Nicholson, KG, 61, 63, 69, 71, *76, 79, 81,* 128, *152,* 166, *190,* 261, 270, 272, *276, 280,* 311, 313, *323*
Nicol, JP, 127, *150*
Nicol, P, 356, *370*
Nicolson, C, 129, *153*
Niederman, MS, 31, *47*
Niemisto, M, 128, *151*
Nieto, A, 110, *139*
Niitsu, H, 240, *249*
Nishinari, T, 240, *249*
Noah, T, 167, *191, 192*
Noble, GR, 58, *75,* 84, *97,* 115, 117, 126, 127, *142, 145, 148, 150*
Noble, RL, 29, *42*
Noble, TC, 84, *97*
Nolte, K, 284, 286, *302*
Nolte, KB, 34, *51,* 289, 292, 293, 294, 295, 296, 297, *303, 304, 305*

Norden, J, 168, 170, *192*
Norman, D, 29, *43,* 63, *78*
Norrby, E, 166, *191*
Norton, HJ, 240, *249*
Notkins, AL, 115, *143*
Nour, B, 213, *219*
Novoa, I, 255, *274*
Novosad, D, 311, 313, *323*
Nubojewski, RA, 93, *101*
Numasaki, Y, 136, *159*
Nunes, FA, 236, *247*

O

O'Brien, D, 62, *77, 78,* 127, 128, 131, *150, 152, 155*
O'Brien, J, 178, *199*
O'Brien, KL, 216, *221*
O'Brien, WA, 127, *151*
O'Connor, FT, 215, *220*
O'Donoghue, JM, 333, *348*
O'Donohue, WJ, 33, *49*
O'Garra, A, 168, *193*
O'Neill, RE, 137, *160*
O'Toole, S, 271, 272, *280*
Oakes, MG, 60, *76,* 134, *157,* 336, *349*
Oda, K, 33, *49,* 108, *139*
Oda, Y, 33, *50*
Oddis, CV, 298, *306*
Odelin, MF, 128, *152*
Oeltmann, TN, 211, *219*
Offit, PA, 33, *49*
Ogilvie, M, 169, *193*
Ogra, PL, 163, 167, 169, 170, 171, 172, 174, *187, 192, 193, 194, 195, 197, 198,* 209, *218*
Oguri, K, 136, *159*
Ohashi, K, 111, *140*
Ohmit, S, 69, *81*
Ohmit, SE, 62, *77,* 337, 338, 342, 343, *350, 352,* 358, *370*
Ohori, NP, 30, *45,* 235, *246*
Okada, I, 298, *306*
Okada, Y, 33, *50*
Okamoto, Y, 167, 174, *192, 198*

Oker-Blom, N, 286, *302,* 329, *346*
Olcen, P, 30, *44,* 63, *79*
Olding-Stenkvist, E, 32, *49*
Oleske, J, 265, *277*
Olgilvie, Ri, 330, *347*
Olive, DM, 311, 313, *323*
Oliver, SW, 136, *159,* 345, *353*
Olley, PM, 298, *306*
Olmstead, EM, 215, *220*
Olmsted, RA, 162, 163, 166, *186, 187,* 210, 216, *218, 220*
Olsen, CW, 110, *140*
Olsen, MA, 178, 179, *199, 200*
Olson, AL, 267, *278*
Olson, RW, 34, *50*
Onuma, M, 166, *191*
Ooi, A, 33, *50*
Openshaw, P, 169, 170, 171, 172, 173, *194, 195, 196, 197*
Openshaw, PJM, 163, 170, *187,* 188
Orenstein, WA, 58, *75,* 127, *150*
Orimo, H, 240, *249*
Orloff, J, 25, *39*
Ortbals, DW, 358, *371*
Ortin, J, 110, *139*
Ortqvist, A, 25, 29, *40*
Orvell, C, 166, *191*
Osanloo, EO, 127, *150*
Osborne, B, 30, *43, 44,* 65, *79,* 86, 87, *98,* 166, 177, 181, *190*
Osborne, G, 314, *324*
Osborne, JS, 16, *22*
Oseasohn, R, 111, *140*
Osterholm, MT, 125, *147*
Osterweil, D, 29, *43,* 63, *78*
Ostrowski, MA, 366, *372*
Otto, EE, 62, *77*
Ou, DW, 260, *276*
Ovcak-Derzic, S, 127, *151*
Ovcharenko, AV, 215, *220*
Overland, E, 290, 292, *304*
Owen, MJ, 174, 176, *198*
Oxford, JS, 129, 134, *153, 157,* 328, 333, 335, *346, 348*
Oxman, MN, 235, *246*

P

Paakko, PK, 242, *250*
Pabico, RC, 93, *101,* 127, *150*
Pachon, J, 25, *38*
Pachucki, CT, 260, *276*
Pacini, DL, 232, *246,* 333, *348*
Padula, P, 284, 287, *301, 303*
Page, Y, 32, *48*
Pagtakhan, RD, 240, *249*
Pain, MC, 31, *46*
Palache, AM, 61, *76,* 126, 128, *149*
Paladin, JF, 27, *41*
Palencia, R, 31, *47*
Palese, P, 109, 113, 120, 131, 132, 137, *139, 142, 146, 156, 157, 160,* 336, 345, *349, 353*
Palladino, G, 117, *145*
Palmer, JM, 264, *277*
Palmer, PS, 131, *155*
Palomo, C, 162, *186*
Panas, DL, 298, *306*
Panuskas, J, 167, 168, *192, 193*
Paolini, J, 237, *248*
Papazian, L, 33, *49*
Paradis, A, 31, *46*
Paradis, IL, 32, *48*
Paradiso, P, 183, *202*
Parag, G, 93, *101*
Parce, JW, 113, *141*
Pardon, D, 59, *75*
Paredes, A, 16, *22,* 127, *149,* 209, *217,* 342, *352*
Parfrott, RH, 224, 237, 238, *244*
Park, CL, 128, *151*
Park, EJ, 131, *156*
Park, J, 127, *151*
Parker, D, 126, *148*
Parker, MD, 285, *302*
Parker, MM, 291, 292, *304*
Parker, RA, 127, *150,* 161, 173, *184, 197*
Parker, SE, 132, *156*
Parkes, JD, 328, *346*
Parkinson, AJ, 210, *218*
Parks, LW, 231, *247*

Parquhar, A, 128, *152*
Parrillo, JE, 291, 292, *304*
Parrott, RH, 71, *81,* 91, *100,* 123, 126, 127, 130, *147, 148, 154,* 161, 165, 170, 171, 172, 181, *184, 195, 196, 201,* 205, *216,* 223, *244,* 270, *279,* 342, *352*
Parry, HF, 269, 272, *279*
Parry, RP, 111, *140*
Partiarca, PA, 331, *348*
Parvin, JD, 131, *156*
Parvirani, A, 242, *250*
Parvu, C, 25, 29, *39*
Pasca, A, 311, 313, *323*
Pascal, W, 233, *246*
Pastoor, DW, 59, *75*
Patel, JA, 174, 176, *198*
Patel, K, 113, *141*
Paton, AM, 88, *99*
Paton, MC, 88, *99*
Patriarca, P, 61, *76*
Patriarca, PA, 38, *51,* 62, *77,* 127, 128, 134, *150, 151, 157,* 358, *370*
Pattemore, PK, 271, 272, *280,* 313, *324*
Patterson, C, 127, *151*
Patterson, JL, 162, 163, *185,* 284, 285, *302,* 339, 350
Patterson, S, 268, *279*
Patz, EF, 32, *48*
Patzelt, E, 108, *138*
Paul, WS, 127, *150*
Paulshock, M, 328, *346*
Paun, L, 25, 29, *39*
Pawlik, KM, 125, *147*
Payne, AA, 56, *74*
Payne, DK, 30, 32, *45, 47*
Peallen, MA, 165, 166, 177, *189*
Pearce, CL, 337, 338, *350*
Pearce, JM, 368, *373*
Pearson, BA, 136, *159*
Pearson, L, 230, *247*
Pearson, RD, 30, *45*
Peckinpaugh, RO, 241, *249*
Pedra, PA, 91, *100*
Peeples, ME, 163, *188*
Pegg, MS, 136, *159*

Peigue-Lafeuille, H, 30, *43,* 88, *99*
Peiper, SC, 33, *49*
Pellegrini, J, 235, *246*
Pellicchia, JA, 31, *46,* 96, *103*
Peluso, RW, 208, *217*
Pemberton, RM, 163, *187*
Pena-Cruz, V, 181, 182, *201,* 342, *352*
Penas, C, 162, *186*
Penn, CC, 238, *248*
Penn, CR, 136, 137, *159*
Penttinen, K, 333, *348*
Pepys, J, 128, *151*
Perez-Tirse, J, 360, 361, *371*
Perkins, M, 131, *154*
Perkis, V, 130, *154*
Perlman, S, 267, *278*
Pernis, B, 230, *247*
Perricaudet, M, 242, *250*
Perrine, KG, 163, *188*
Perrotta, DM, 56, *74,* 117, *145*
Perry, HC, 132, *156*
Persing, DH, 311, *323*
Persson, CG, 268, 269, *279*
Peter, G, 365, *372*
Peters, CJ, 34, *51,* 284, 286, 287, 288, 289, 292, 293, 296, 297, *300, 301, 302, 303, 305*
Petersdorf, RG, 29, *42*
Petersen, DM, 227, 233, *245*
Peterson, GF, 125, *147*
Peterson, JA, 256, *275*
Peterson, PJ, 54, *73*
Peterson, PK, 32, *49,* 66, *80*
Petijean, J, 179, *200*
Petric, M, 180, *200*
Petru, AM, 91, *100*
Petterson, CA, 317, *324*
Pettersson, C, 65, *79*
Pettersson, RF, 333, *348*
Pettersson, U, 233, *246*
Pevear, DC, 257, *275*
Peyre, R, 30, *45,* 63, 65, 66, *78,* 177, *199*
Pfaller, MA, 87, *98*
Pfitzenmeyer, P, 66, *80*
Phan, TV, 136, *159*
Phelan, MA, 115, *142*

Philipson, K, 113, *141*
Philipson, L, 223, 226, *244*
Phillips, C, 177, *199*
Phillips, CA, 69, *81*
Phillips, CD, 257, *275*
Phillips, IA, 69, *81*
Phillpotts, RJ, 272, *280*
Pianigiani, G, 119, *146*
Pichichero, ME, 134, *158*
Pichuantes, S, 284, *301*
Pickens, D, 173, *197*
Pickering, LK, 365, *372*
Piedra, P, 165, 174, 180, 181, 183, *189, 198, 201, 203*
Piedra, PA, 29, *42,* 64, 65, *79,* 94, 95, *102,* 118, 131, *145, 155, 156,* 240, *249*
Pieler, C, 255, *274*
Pierce, AK, 113, *141*
Pierce, E, 134, *158,* 335, *349*
Pierce, WE, 236, 241, *247, 249*
Pierik, L, 261, *276*
Pierik, LT, 166, 167, *191*
Pigula, FA, 298, *306*
Pimplikar, SW, 209, *217*
Pincus, PH, 9, *22,* 164, 176, *189, 199*
Pingleton, SK, 30, *45*
Pingleton, W, 34, *50*
Pingleton, WW, 30, *45*
Pini, N, 287, *303*
Pinto, LH, 107, 109, 136, *138, 139, 158*
Pinus, PH, 27, *41*
Pio, A, 8, 18, *21*
Pisareva, M, 126, *148*
Pitalion, AK, 33, *50*
Pitts, L, 290, 292, *304*
Plastts-Mills, T, 174, *198*
Plaut, AG, 209, *217*
Plorde, JJ, 29, *41,* 63, *79*
Plotch, SJ, 108, *139*
Plotkin, SA, 33, *49*
Plouffe, JF, 30, *44,* 166, *190,* 314, *324*
Pluhar, RE, 359, *371*
Plummer, WDJ, 131, *155*
Plyusnin, A, 126, *148,* 284, *301*
Pohl, C, 88, 89, *99,* 176, *199*
Pohl, KA, 272, *280*
Poland, GA, 359, *371*
Polk, BF, 93, *101,* 127, *151*
Pollack, D, 334, *348*
Polly, SM, 33, *49*
Polonis, V, 131, *156*
Polsky, B, 32, *48*
Poole, PM, 165, *189*
Pope, J, 168, *192*
Popli, S, 127, *150*
Popow, KT, 261, *276*
Porter, DA, 233, *246*
Porter, DD, 209, *218*
Portner, A, 209, 210, *217, 218*
Poskanzer, DC, 328, *346*
Postic, B, 128, *152*
Postlethwaite, R, 232, *244*
Postma, JU, 337, *350*
Potgieter, P, 32, *47*
Potgieter, PD, 25, 29, *39*
Potter, CW, 328, 335, *346*
Poupet, JY, 30, *45*
Powell, KR, 9, *22,* 164, 165, 176, *189, 199*
Power, UF, 210, *218*
Powers, DC, 56, 62, *74, 77,* 128, 130, 131, *152, 153, 155*
Pozzetto, B, 128, *152*
Prados, MD, 25, *38*
Preblud, SR, 31, *47*
Prellner, T, 31, *46*
Premkumar, A, 107, *138*
Premkumar, LS, 107, *138*
Presant, CA, 358, *371*
Preston, F, 168, *192*
Preti, A, 32, *48*
Pretorius, J, 298, *306*
Prill, A, 168, *193*
Prill, AH, 111, *140*
Prince, GA, 163, 169, 171, 180, 181, 183, *187, 193, 194, 196, 200, 201, 202,* 209, 210, *218,* 227, 230, 232, 233, *245, 245, 246, 247,* 342, *352*
Pringle, CR, 166, *191*
Prober, CG, 65, *79,* 180, *201,* 342, *352*
Procop, GW, 311, *323*

Protnoy, B, 126, 127, *148*
Proud, D, 258, 259, 265, *275, 278*
Prout, S, 25, 29, *39*
Pruett, T, 93, *101*
Przepiorka, D, 87, 88, 91, *98, 100*
Public Health Laboratory Service Communicable Disease Surveillance Centre, 66, *80*
Public Health Laboratory Service Communicable Diseases Surveillance Centre, 63, 64, 66, *78*
Puga, AP, 227, 233, *245*
Pugh, S, 87, *98*
Puhakka, H, 174, 176, *198*
Pullan, CR, 161, 171, *185, 195,* 341, 343, *351*
Pulverer, G, 26, *40*
Purcell, RH, 210, *218*
Purtshcer, M, 131, *156*
Puthavathana, P, 27, *41*
Pyhala, R, 128, *151*
Pyke, S, 60, *76,* 135, *158,* 336, *349*
Pyles, G, 162, 165, 172, 182, 183, *185, 189, 202*

Q

Quarles, JM, 126, 131, 136, *149, 155, 158,* 330, 333, 341, *347, 348, 351*
Quay, J, 167, *191*
Que, JU, 62, *77*
Qui, Y, 108, *139*
Quian, XY, 108, *139*
Quilligan, JJ, 328, *346*
Quinlan, K, 173, *197*
Quinnan, G, 127, 128, *150*
Quinnan, GV, 29, *43,* 126, 127, 128, *148, 150, 152,* 358, *371*
Quinnan, GVJ, 62, *77*
Quint, WGV, 126, *148*

R

Raabe, T, 266, 267, 272, *278, 280*
Raad, I, 91, 92, 93, *100, 101,* 166, 177, 181, *190,* 369, *373*

Rabalais, GP, 127, *149*
Radecke, F, 216, *221*
Raff, JM, 29, *42*
Raftery, AT, 30, *44*
Rahman, M, 27, *41,* 216, *221*
Rahn, AC, 330, *347*
Raider, L, 32, *48*
Rakes, G, 174, *198*
Ramphal, R, 111, 113, *140, 141*
Ramsey, PG, 31, *46*
Rand, KH, 32, *48*
Randrianarison-Jewtoukoff, 242, *250*
Ranger, S, 30, *45,* 63, 65, 66, *78,* 177, *199*
Rao, L, 228, 230, *245*
Rasmussen, L, 286, *302*
Raven, JM, 180, *200*
Ravid, Z, 93, *101*
Ravkov, E, 284, *301*
Rawlings, JA, 284, *301*
Ray, A, 255, 259, 264, *274*
Ray, CG, 94, *102,* 125, 136, *147, 159,* 333, *348*
Raymond, SJ, 298, *306*
Raynor, WJ, 256, *274*
Reay, PA, 115, *143*
Rebert, N, 168, *193*
Rebert, NA, 167, *191*
Reck, LJ, 130, *154*
Record, F, 171, 173, *196, 197*
Redington, M, 227, 232, 233, *245*
Redl, H, 298, *306*
Reed, EC, 32, 35, *48*
Reed, G, 130, *153,* 212, *219,* 365, *372*
Reed, GW, 131, *155*
Reed, ME, 125, *147*
Reed, MH, 240, *249*
Reed, SE, 71, *81,* 269, 270, 271, *279*
Reef, S, 34, *51*
Reef, SE, 34, *51,* 289, 292, *303*
Regnery, H, 94, *101*
Regnery, HL, 120, 127, 129, *146, 149, 153,* 310, 313, *322*
Reichlin, A, 115, *142*
Reichman, RC, 25, 35, *38, 51,* 60, *76,* 133, 137, *157, 159,* 331, *348*

Reid, JL, 165, *189*
Reid, MM, 84, *97*
Reimer, CB, 169, 180, *193, 200*
Reina, J, 316, *324*
Reinacher, M, 8, *21,* 58, *75,* 113, *142,* 211, *219*
Reinertsen, JL, 127, *151*
Reisman, JJ, 180, *200*
Reiss, CS, 116, 117, *144, 145*
Reithmann, C, 298, *306*
Rekstin, AR, 130, *154*
Remarque, EJ, 126, 128, *149*
Renegar, KB, 115, *143*
Renzetti, AD, 29, *42,* 69, *81,* 113, *141*
Renzulio, PO, 128, *151*
Resenbaum, MJ, 237, *247*
Reucker, RR, 253, 254, 255, 256, 257, 264, 265, *273*
Reuman, PD, 136, *159,* 333, *348*
Reynolds, CJ, 258, *275*
Rhame, FS, 27, *41,* 166, 177, *190*
Rhoades, AJ, 205, *216*
Rhoades, ER, 30, 31, *45, 47*
Rhoads, RE, 255, *274*
Rhodes, GH, 132, *156*
Rhodes, LJ, 131, *156*
Rhodes, LM, 342, *352*
Rhodes, PH, 38, *51,* 358, *370*
Richert, JH, 240, *249*
Richman, DD, 132, *157*
Riddiough, MA, 360, *371*
Rifkind, D, 169, *193*
Riggio, RR, 29, *43*
Riggs, N, 216, *221*
Riker, DK, 257, 259, 264, 265, 272, *275, 277, 280*
Riley, G, 62, *78,* 128, *152*
Riley, MA, 62, *78,* 128, *152*
Rimland, D, 134, *157*
Rindge, B, 224, 237, 238, *244*
Ringden, O, 89, *99*
Riva, C, 287, *303*
Rivard, S, 216, *221*
Road, JD, 298, *306*
Roberts, C, 113, *142*
Roberts, N, 168, *192, 193*

Roberts, NJ, 111, *140*
Roberts, RB, 34, *50*
Roberts, RJ, 229, *245*
Roberts, SR, 162, 163, *186*
Robertson, J, 108, *138*
Robertson, JS, 129, *153*
Robins, RK, 338, *350*
Robinson, J, 165, *190*
Robonson, HL, 132, *156*
Rocha, EP, 129, *153*
Roche, K, 366, *372*
Rodrigues, J, 31, *47*
Rodriguez, W, 342, *353*
Rodriguez, WH, 94, *101*
Rodriguez, WJ, 92, *101,* 181, 182, *201,* 340, 342, *351, 352*
Rodstein, M, 29, 33, *43, 49,* 61, 63, 67, *76,* 127, 128, *150*
Rogers, DE, 58, *75,* 113, 124, *141*
Rogers, MF, 125, *147*
Roghmann, KJ, 161, 166, 167, *185, 191*
Rohm, C, 121, *146*
Rolfs, A, 25, 29, *40*
Rollin, PE, 34, *51,* 284, 286, 287, 288, 289, 292, 296, 297, *301, 303, 305,* 344, *353*
Rolston, K, 87, 88, *98*
Romansky, MJ, 66, *80*
Roos, LL, 127, *150,* 356, *370*
Root, RK, 30, *44*
Rorke, LB, 237, *248*
Rosales, T, 171, *196*
Rose, DH, 25, 29, *39, 40*
Rose, JK, 109, *139*
Rose, RC, 91, *100*
Rosen, MJ, 90, *99*
Rosenbaum, MJ, 241, *249*
Rosenfeld, MA, 242, *250*
Rosenkranz, MA, 93, *101*
Rosenthal, KL, 242, *250*
Rosenthal, KU, 180, *200*
Ross, LA, 29, *43*
Rossen, RD, 298, *305*
Rossi, C, 284, 287, *301, 303*
Rossman, MG, 255, *274*
Rota, PA, 115, *142*

Roth, F, 137, *159*
Roth, FK, 58, *75,* 113, 127, 134, *141, 150, 158,* 335, *349*
Rothbarth, PH, 179, *200*
Rothlein, R, 255, *274*
Rott, R, 8, *21, 26, 40,* 58, *75,* 113, 117, *142, 144,* 211, 212, *218, 219*
Rott, RR, 211, *218*
Rousseau, WE, 127, *150*
Rowe, MJ, 113, *141*
Rowe, PC, 215, *220*
Rowe, WP, 223, 241, *244, 249*
Roziman, B, 161, *184*
Ruangkanchanasetr, S, 27, *41*
Ruben, EL, 58, *75*
Ruben, F, 262, *276*
Ruben, FL, 25, 27, 29, *39, 41, 42,* 127, 128, *149*
Rubenis, M, 260, *276*
Rubin, BK, 25, *39*
Rubin, DH, 209, *217*
Rubin, LG, 91, *100*
Rubin, RA, 237, *248*
Rubin, RH, 33, *49*
Rubino, KL, 163, 170, *187, 188, 195*
Rubio, S, 270, 271, *280*
Ruckdeschel, G, 25, 29, *40*
Rudenko, LG, 130, *154*
Ruigrok, RWH, 132, *157*
Rupp, ME, 34, *50*
Rusche, JR, 296, *305*
Rush, JD, 90, *99,* 118, 123, *146*
Russel, JA, 298, *305*
Russell, DJ, 226, *244*
Russell, LB, 361, *371*
Russell, NH, 87, *98*
Russell, SM, 115, *143*
Russi, JC, 27, *40*
Russler, SK, 33, *50*
Rutstein, R, 91, *100*
Ruuskanen, O, 17, *22,* 174, 176, *198*
Ruutu, P, 32, *48*
Ruutu, T, 32, *48*
Ryan, DM, 136, *159*
Ryan, KW, 210, *218*
Ryan, ME, 94, *101*
Ryan, P, 17, *22*
Ryan-Pourier, KA, 125, *148*
Ryerse, JS, 231, *247*
Rytel, MW, 25, 29, *39,* 93, *101*

S

Saah, AJ, 29, *43,* 61, 63, 67, *76,* 127, 128, *150*
Sabbarao, EK, 131, *156*
Sabbatini, P, 228, 230, *245*
Sabin, AB, 328, *346*
Sable, CA, 86, 94, *98, 102,* 123, *147*
Sabry, M, 167, *192*
Sach, DA, 27, *41*
Sacks, HS, 62, *77,* 356, 358, *370*
Sacks, SL, 35, *51*
Saed, F, 32, *48*
Safrin, S, 90, *99,* 118, 123, *146*
Saikku, P, 25, 29, *40,* 286, *302*
Saito, I, 167, *192,* 242, *250*
Saito, Y, 89, *99*
Sakai, K, 113, *142,* 211, *218, 219*
Saker, BM, 89, *99*
Salbenblatt, CK, 165, 176, *190*
Salomon, H, 27, *40, 41*
Salt, A, 88, 89, *98*
Sambol, AR, 178, 179, *199, 200*
Samo, T, 32, *48*
Samo, TC, 29, *43,* 264, *277*
Samorodin, R, 369, *373*
Samorodin, RK, 130, *154*
Samuels, AI, 339, 350
Sanchez, A, 284, 286, *301, 302, 303*
Sande, MA, 61, *76,* 126, *149*
Sanders, A, 233, *246*
Sanderson, G, 258, 261, 271, 272, *275, 276, 280,* 313, *324*
Sanford, JP, 113, *141*
Sangster, M, 117, *144,* 216, *220*
Sangster, MY, 116, *144*
Sannella, E, 130, *153,* 365, *372*
Santos, GW, 95, *102*
Sanyal, MA, 123, *147,* 174, 176, *198,* 238, *248*

Sanz-Esquerro, JJ, 110, *139*
Saral, R, 95, *102*
Sarawar, SR, 116, 117, *144*
Sargaison, M, 88, *98*
Sarkkinen, H, 169, 174, 176, *193, 198*
Sarnaik, AP, 181, *201*, 342, *352*
Saski, K, 167, 168, *192*
Sasso, DR, 344, *353*
Satlzman, RL, 66, *80*
Sattar, SA, 216, *221*, 268, 270, *278*
Saunders, D, 168, 170, *192*
Saux, P, 33, *49*
Savage, RE, 161, *184*
Savatski, LL, 213, *219*
Saxtan, D, 58, *74*
Scanga, CA, 266, 268, *278*
Scanlon, G, 25, 29, *39*
Scaria, A, 231, *247*
Scarpa, B, 62, *77*
Scarpace, PJ, 26, *40*
Schaaper, WMM, 162, *186*
Schacht, RA, 29, *42*
Schafer, G, 224, *244*
Schafer, JR, 122, *147*, 363, *372*
Schaffer, FL, 119, *146*
Schaffer, RL, 30, *45*
Schaffner, W, 355, *370*
Schaller, JG, 125, *147*
Schecker, WE, 54, *73*
Schefft, G, 173, *197*
Scheiblauer, H, 8, *21*, 58, *75*, 211, *219*
Scheid, A, 171, *196*, 211, *218*
Scheifele, D, 127, *151*
Scheifiele, DW, 128, *152*
Scheinmann, P, 91, *100*
Schell, M, 121, *146*
Schelle, PB, 266, 267, *278*
Scherle, PA, 117, *145*
Schieble, JH, 162, *185*
Schiff, GM, 136, *159*
Schild, GC, 129, 134, *153, 157*, 333, *348*
Schilz, R, 243, *251*
Schirm, J, 59, *75*
Schlag, G, 298, *306*
Schlarb, JE, 268, 271, *279*
Schleimer, RP, 259, *275*

Schlesinger, JJ, 162, 163, 169, *186, 187, 194*
Schlesinger, RW, 113, *142*
Schlievert, PM, 125, *147*
Schlossberg, D, 31, *47*
Schluger, NW, 34, *50*
Schmaljohn, AL, 284, 285, *301, 302*
Schmaljohn, CS, 284, 285, 300, *301, 302, 306*
Schmidt, OW, 270, *279*
Schmitz, H, 236, *247*
Schmitz, R, 362, *372*
Schnabel, KC, 9, *22*, 164, 165, 166, 167, 169, 176, 180, *189, 191, 199, 201*, 369, *373*
Schneider, RJ, 229, *245*
Schnurr, DP, 235, *246*
Schoenbaum, SC, 57, *74*, 119, 126, *146, 149*, 358, 361, *371*
Schoeppe, W, 298, *306*
Schonberger, LB, 127, *150*, 363, *372*
Schonberger, LN, 125, *147*
Schooley, R, 126, 128, *148*
Schooley, Rt, 33, *49*
Schrock, CG, 125, *147*
Schroder, FP, 59, *75*
Schroter, G, 127, *151*
Schubert, M, 108, *138*
Schuck, KM, 178, 179, *199, 200*
Schuckett, R, 127, *151*
Schuette, W, 291, 292, *304*
Schuh, S, 180, *200*
Schuller, D, 31, *46*, 96, *103*
Schulman, J, 113, 115, *142*
Schulman, JL, 117, 137, *145, 159*, 336, 345, *349, 353*
Schultz, SB, 256, *274*
Schulz, P, 131, *156*
Schulz, R, 298, *306*
Schur, PH, 127, *151*
Schuy, W, 59, *75*, 125, *148*
Schwab, RS, 328, *346*
Schwartz, LB, 262, *276*
Schwartz, ML, 34, *50*
Schwartzentruber, DJ, 366, *372*
Schwarzmann, SW, 29, *42*, 124, *147*

Scott, EJ, 69, 71, *81*
Scott, EN, 210, *218*
Scott, GM, 272, *280*
Scott, JP, 32, *48*
Scott, LV, 210, *218*
Scott, M, 169, 171, *194*
Scott, R, 168, 169, 170, 171, *192, 194, 195*
Sears, SD, 131, 133, *154, 155, 157,* 333, *348*
Sedmak, G, 93, *101*
Sedmak, GV, 235, 237, *246, 248*
Seeds, M, 113, *141*
Segura, EL, 287, *303*
Sehgal, PB, 227, 232, 233, *245*
Seita, U, 62, *77*
Sell, SH, 182, 183, *202*
Sell, SHW, 126, 127, *148*
Selling, BH, 183, *202*
Selwyn, BJ, 17, *23*
Semenova, VA, 287, 288, *303*
Sempel, DA, 13, *22*
Senior, RJ, 7, *21,* 161, 165, *184*
Senne, D, 122, *147*
Senterfit, LB, 29, *43*
Sergeant, M, 269, 272, *279*
Serizawa, T, 298, *306*
Seroky, JT, 262, *276*
Serrette, C, 340, *351*
Setia, U, 128, *152*
Seto, JT, 211, 212, *218, 219*
Setoguchi, M, 29, *43,* 68, *80*
Sewell, CM, 297, *305*
Sfakianaki, ED, 284, *301*
Shaheen, SO, 161, *185*
Shalaby, H, 59, *75,* 125, *148,* 316, *324*
Shandera, WX, 30, *44,* 63, 64, 66, *78,* 166, 177, *190*
Shands, JWJ, 111, 113, *140, 141*
Shanley, JD, 26, 27, *40, 41*
Shanson, DC, 25, 29, *39*
Shapiro, LH, 266, 268, *278*
Sharma, G, 109, *139*
Sharma, OK, 339, 350
Sharp, GB, 121, *146*
Sharp, JG, 331, *347*

Sharp, PA, 229, *245*
Sharrow, SO, 116, *144*
Shastri, SR, 53, *73*
Shaughnessy, MA, 136, *158*
Shaw, E, 113, *142*
Shaw, KN, 175, *198*
Shaw, MW, 107, 120, *138, 146*
Shaw, RJ, 268, *279*
Sheaffer, CI, 7, *21*
Shearer, GM, 116, *144*
Shearer, LA, 162, *185,* 215, *220*
Shelhamer, JH, 291, 292, *304*
Shenk, T, 227, 229, *244*
Shepp, DH, 96, *102*
Sherman, FT, 60, *76*
Sherman, NH, 175, *198*
Sherry, MK, 31, *46*
Sherwood, JR, 136, *159*
Shevdoff, RA, 342, *352*
Shieble, JH, 215, *220*
Shieh, CK, 266, 267, *278*
Shields, AF, 30, *45,* 237, *248*
Shiell, A, 161, *185*
Shigeru, M, 110, *140*
Shild, GC, 115, *143*
Shindo, K, 89, *99,* 109, *139*
Shinefield, HR, 366, *372*
Shinozaki, T, 182, 183, *202*
Shirodaria, PV, 285, *302*
Shiver, JW, 132, *156*
Short, AIK, 292, *304*
Shortridge, KF, 122, *147*
Shrples, LD, 32, *48*
Shu, CY, 240, *249*
Shu, L, 121, *146*
Shu, LL, 121, *146*
Shulman, JL, 117, 132, *144, 157*
Shulman, NR, 340, *350*
Shult, P, 63, 64, 69, 70, 71, *78, 81,* 313, *323*
Shultz, PS, 58, *74*
Shute, JK, 259, *276*
Shvedoff, RA, 162, *185*
Sibbald, WJ, 291, 292, *304*
Siber, GR, 164, 181, 182, *189, 201,* 342, *352*

Sibert, GR, 169, 183, *194*
Siddell, S, 272, *280*
Siddell, SG, 266, 267, 268, 272, *278, 280*
Siddiqui, T, 32, *48*
Sidoli, I, 121, *146*
Sidwell, RW, 338, *350*
Sieber, OF, 162, *185*, 215, *220*
Siegel, AC, 238, *248*
Siegel, CS, 178, *200*
Siegel, JE, 361, *371*
Siegfried, W, 242, *250*
Siggaard-Anderson, J, 66, *80*
Sigurbergsson, F, 173, 174, *197*
Sigurs, N, 173, 174, *197, 198*
Sikes, K, 58, *75*
Sikes, RK, 331, *348*
Silver, HM, 33, *49*
Sim, I, 135, *158*
Sim, IS, 336, *349*
Simmons, RL, 32, *49*, 83, 95, *97*, 298, *306*
Simmons, WW, 298, *306*
Simoes, EA, 94, *101*, 342, 343, *353*
Simoes, EAF, 182, *201, 202*
Simon, G, 69, *80, 81*
Simon, GL, 260, *276*
Simons, R, 168, *192*
Simonsen, L, 297, *305*
Simose, EAF, 92, *101*
Simpson, DIH, 285, *302*
Simpson, GL, 34, *51*, 289, 292, *303*
Simpson, H, 165, *189*, 272, *280*
Simpson, SQ, 289, 290, 291, 292, 293, 297, 299, *304, 305, 306*
Singh-Naz, N, 216, *221*
Sinnott, JT, 88, *99*
Sirinovin, S, 27, *41*
Sisson, W, 256, *274*
Sissons, JGP, 26, *40*
Sitar, DS, 330, *347*
Six, HR, 131, *155*
Sizun, J, 270, 271, *280*
Skeggs, DBL, 84, *97*
Skehel, JJ, 119, 132, *146, 157*, 330, 336, *347, 349*

Skern, T, 255, *274*
Sklar, DP, 290, 292, *304*
Skoner, DP, 262, *276*
Slak, JE, 360, *371*
Slepushkin, AN, 130, *154*
Slotman, GJ, 290, 292, *304*
Sly, PD, 180, *200*, 240, *249*
Small, PA, 113, *141*, 359, *371*
Small, PAJ, 111, 115, *140, 143*
Smeg, RA, 32, 35, *47*
Smilack, JD, 331, *347*
Smith, AE, 227, 233, 242, *245, 250*
Smith, AJ, 128, *152*, 358, *371*
Smith, AP, 263, *277*
Smith, C, 29, *42*, 59, *75*, 315, 316, *324*
Smith, CB, 29, *42*, 69, *81*, 113, *141*, 210, *218*, 340, *351*
Smith, CW, 296, *305*
Smith, DW, 65, *79*, 178, *199*, 342, *352*
Smith, FS, 210, 216, *218*, 220
Smith, GE, 130, *153*, 365, *372*
Smith, JD, 331, *348*
Smith, JF, 285, *302*
Smith, JI, 126, *148*
Smith, MH, 132, *157*, 330, 336, *347, 349*
Smith, RA, 339, 350
Smith, S, 271, 272, *280*, 313, *324*
Smith, SC, 58, *75*
Smith, SH, 61, 63, 71, *76*, 128, *152*, 270, *280*
Smith, TF, 35, *51*, 84, *97*, 125, *147*
Smith, TW, 298, *306*
Smith, W, 355, *370*
Smith, WW, 256, *274*
Smith,RA, 339, 350
Smorodintsev, AA, 329, *346*
Smyth, RL, 32, *48*
Smythe, ML, 136, *159*
Snell, JD, 321, *324*
Snider, MT, 287, 292, *303*
Snover, D, 30, *44*, 86, 87, *97*, 166, 171, 177, *190*
Snyder, DN, 56, *74*
Snyder, MH, 131, *154, 155*, 180, *200*
Snydman, DR, 83, 96, *97*, 319, *324*

Sobod, KS, 210, *218*
Sobonya, RE, 30, 34, *45, 50*
Soergel, ME, 119, *146*
Solomon, LR, 30, *44*
Somani, S, 337, *350*
Somani, SK, 61, *76,* 134, *158*
Sommer, A, 16, *22*
Sommergruber, W, 255, 265, *274, 277*
Sommerville, RG, 30, *45*
Sonenberg, N, 255, *274*
Song, JW, 284, 287, *301, 303*
Song, W, 284, *301*
Sonoda, S, 167, 168, *192*
Soo, W, 60, *76,* 134, *157,* 336, 337, *349, 350*
Soong, T, 128, *152*
Sopp, P, 170, 171, *195*
Sorli, J, 233, *246*
Sorrentino, J, 258, *275*
Sorrentino, JV, 259, 264, 265, 272, *275, 277, 280*
Sorvillo, FJ, 30, *44,* 62, 63, 64, 66, *77, 78,* 166, 177, *190,* 358, *370*
Sotnikov, A, 171, *196*
Soto-Quiros, ME, 240, *249*
Soukup, J, 164, 167, *189, 191*
Soukup, JM, 180, *200*
Soung, LS, 330, *347*
Soupre, D, 270, 271, *280*
Sparer, TE, 231, *247*
Speer, ME, 30, *45*
Speers, DM, 30, *45,* 63, *78,* 113, 134, *141, 158,* 164, 175, 177, *189, 198*
Speilhofer, P, 216, *221*
Spelman, DW, 30, *45,* 63, *79*
Spence, L, 25, 29, *40*
Spence, RA, 267, 273, *278*
Sperber, K, 233, *246*
Sperber, SJ, 60, *76,* 135, *158,* 264, 272, *277, 280,* 336, *349*
Spessert, C, 31, *46,* 96, *103*
Spinelli, S, 183, *203*
Spiropoulou, CF, 284, 286, 287, 288, 293, *301, 302, 303, 305*
Sprenger, MJ, 56, *74,* 127, 128, *150,* 358, *370*

Sprenger, MJW, 62, *77,* 126, 128, *148, 149,* 179, *200*
Spriggs, MK, 163, 166, *186,* 210, *218*
Spring, SB, 130, *154*
Springer, C, 180, *200*
Springer, TA, 255, 265, *274, 277*
Springthorpe, VS, 216, *221*
Spyker, DA, 330, 336, *347, 349*
Srinivasakumar, N, 163, *187*
St George, JA, 227, 233, *245*
St. Angelo, C, 108, *138*
Stachowiak, J, 30, *43,* 86, 87, *98*
Stackiw, W, 205, *216*
Stahlman, M, 173, *197*
Stalder, H, 31, *47,* 235, *246*
Stanberry, LR, 321, *324*
Stanek, J, 66, *80*
Stange, K, 60, 61, *76*
Stanley, ED, 328, *346*
Stanley, PA, 30, *45,* 63, *79*
Stanley, SK, 90, *99,* 366, *372*
Stanton, A, 317, *324*
Stanway, G, 255, *274,* 311, 313, *323*
Starzl, TE, 88, 89, *98*
Staton, E, 127, *149*
Staub, NC, 290, 292, *304*
Staunton, DE, 255, 265, *274, 277*
Stavnezer, E, 106, *138*
Steece, RS, 29, *42,* 58, *75*
Steigbigel, RT, 111, *140*
Steihoff, D, 25, 29, *40*
Stein, SJ, 34, *50*
Steinberg, AD, 127, *151*
Steinberg, S, 368, *373*
Steinhoff, MC, 59, *75,* 130, 131, *154, 155,* 215, *220*
Steinus-Aarniala, B, 128, *151*
Stekeler, B, 59, *75,* 125, *148*
Stenstrom, R, 32, *48*
Stenzel, KH, 29, *43*
Stephens, D, 342, 343, *352*
Sterner, G, 30, *44,* 63, *79*
Stevens, DJ, 119, *146*
Stevens, M, 240, *249*
Stevens, RC, 331, *347*
Stevens, WK, 361, *372*

Stevenson, D, 240, *249*
Stewart, CE, 162, *185,* 342, *352*
Stewart, J, 321, *324*
Stewart, S, 32, *48*
Stieneke-Grober, A, 113, *142*
Stier, LE, 242, *250*
Stiver, HG, 127, *151*
Stokes, DC, 31, *47*
Stokes, J, 355, *370*
Stone, AA, 263, *277*
Stone, Y, 163, 166, *186*
Storch, GA, 30, *43, 44,* 65, *79,* 86, 87, *98,* 166, 173, 177, 181, *190, 197,* 314, *324*
Stott, EJ, 169, 170, 183, *194, 195, 202*
Stouch, WH, 69, *81*
Stover, D, 32, *48*
Strachowiak, J, 177, *199*
Strangert, K, 7, *21*
Strassburg, MA, 30, *44,* 62, 63, 64, 66, *77, 78,* 166, 177, *190,* 358, *370*
Stratford-Perricaudet, L, 242, *250*
Stratowa, C, 265, *277*
Straube, DC, 119, *146*
Straus, SE, 224, *244*
Strauss, N, 93, *101*
Streeter, DG, 339, 350
Streiff, EJ, 58, *75,* 127, 128, *149*
Strikas, R, 355, *370*
Strikas, RL, 161, *184*
Strine, T, 34, *51*
Strope, GL, 13, *22*
Stuart-Harris, CH, 29, *42*
Stutman, H, 94, *101*
Su, Q, 242, 243, *250, 251*
Subbarao, EK, 117, 131, *145, 154, 156*
Sudo, M, 111, *140*
Suffin, SC, 164, 165, 176, *189, 190*
Suga, K, 166, 170, *191, 195*
Sugg, M, 84, *97*
Sugrue, Rj, 330, *347*
Sullender, WM, 163, 166, *186*
Sullivan, BJ, 180, *200*
Sullivan, CJ, 30, *44,* 87, *98,* 161, 166, 167, 180, *185,* 314, *324*
Sullivan, KM, 66, *80,* 126, *149*

Sullivan, M, 128, *151*
Sullivan, RFJ, 124, *147*
Sullivan, RJ, 25, 29, *39, 42*
Sun, M, 209, *218*
Sundell, H, 173, *197*
Sunico, ME, 27, *41*
Sunstrom, NA, 107, *138*
Suratt, P, 261, *276*
Suss, J, 121, 122, *146, 147,* 363, *372*
Sutcliffe, T, 215, *220*
Sutehall, G, 88, *98*
Suwanjutha, S, 27, *41*
Suzich, JQ, 285, *302*
Suzuki, H, 111, *140*
Svedmyr, A, 30, *44,* 63, 66, *79, 80*
Svensson, C, 268, 269, *279*
Svitkin, Y, 255, *274*
Swan, AV, 16, *22*
Swarminathan, S, 229, *246*
Sweeney, MS, 88, *99*
Sweet, C, 135, *158,* 336, *349*
Swischuk, LE, 175, *199*
Syrjala, H, 25, 29, *40*
Sztein, M, 260, *276*

T

Taber, LH, 16, *22,* 113, 118, 126, 127, 131, *142, 145, 148, 149, 156,* 169, 180, *193, 201,* 209, 210, *217, 218,* 311, 314, *323, 324,* 342, *351, 352*
Tablan, OC, 92, *100*
Tabor, LH, 17, *22*
Taivianen, A, 128, *151*
Takabayashi, K, 33, *49*
Takahashi, K, 270, *279*
Takahashi, T, 298, *306*
Takeuchi, K, 109, 111, *139, 140*
Takimoti, T, 210, *218*
Takimoto, CH, 30, *44*
Takita, H, 31, *46*
Takizawa, T, 110, 111, *140,* 296, *305*
Talis, AL, 166, *191*
Talpey, WB, 134, *158*
Talsma, A, 62, *77,* 358, *370*

Tamatani, T, 296, *305*
Tamblyn, SE, 68, *80*
Tan, D, 311, 313, *323*
Tan, WD, 32, *47*
Tang, ATS, 65, *79*, 342, *352*
Tang, W, 255, 259, 264, *274*
Tang, Y, 167, 169, 171, 173, *192, 194, 196, 197*, 311, *323*
Tanner, MA, 55, 61, 63, 64, 69, *73*, 270, *280*
Tapper, MA, 33, *50*
Tappero, J, 34, *51*
Taraf, H, 168, *193*
Tardy, JC, 32, *48*
Tarrand, JJ, 369, *373*
Tarwatjo, I, 16, *22*
Tashiro, M, 8, *21, 26, 40, 58, 75*, 113, *142*, 211, 212, *218, 219*
Taylor, G, 169, 170, 171, *194, 195*, 224, *244*
Taylor, P, 170, 172, *195*, 261, *276*
Taylor, PM, 117, *145*
Taylor-Robinson, D, 263, *277*
Tegtmeier, GE, 127, *150*
Telepak, RJ, 292, *305*
Tempest, B, 34, *51*, 289, 292, *303*
ten Dam, HG, 8, 18, *21*
Teran, LM, 259, *276*
Terry, Dw, 333, *348*
Teufel, A, 127, *151*
Thach, B, 173, *197*
Thickett, A, 31, *46*, 96, *103*
Thierney, EL, 215, *220*
Thijs, CT, 127, 128, *150*, 358, *370*
Thijs, CTMCN, 62, *77*
Thimmapaya, B, 229, *246*
Thomas, G, 113, *142*
Thomas, L, 170, 171, *195*
Thomas, P, 33, *49*
Thompson, J, 32, *47*, 126, 127, 130, 131, 134, *148, 153, 155, 158*, 182, 183, *202*, 212, 215, *219*, 220, 237, *248*, 335, *349*, 365, 369, *372, 373*
Thompson, JM, 128, *152*
Thomsen, DR, 216, *220*

Thongcharoen, P, 27, *41*
Thorne, TE, 231, *247*
Threlkeld, SC, 135, *158*
Throop, B, 169, 181, *194*
Throop, BJ, 95, *102*
Thumar, JB, 131, *155*
Thurn, JR, 90, *99*
Tibbetts, C, 226, *244*
Ticehurst, J, 136, *159*
Tidwell, RR, 180, *200*
Tierney, EL, 115, 116, 130, 131, *142, 143, 154*
Tilling, J, 136, *159*
Timbury, MC, 88, *99*
Tisdale, M, 273, *280*
Tjhen, KY, 59, *75*, 125, *148*
Tobin, JO, 165, *189*
Tobita, K, 211, 212, *218, 219*
Todd, RF, 296, *305*
Todd, SJ, 59, *75*, 125, *148*, 311, 314, 316, *323, 324*
Togawa, K, 167, *192*
Togo, Y, 333, 334, 336, 340, *348, 351*
Tollefson, AE, 231, *247*
Tollefson, S, 212, 215, *219, 220*
Tolpin, MD, 130, *154*
Tominack, RL, 330, 331, *347*
Toms, G, 168, 170, *192*
Toogood, CI, 236, *247*
Top, FHJ, 238, *248*
Topham, DJ, 116, *144*
Torre-Amione, G, 298, *305*
Torres, CU, 27, *41*
Torrez-Martinez, N, 284, 286, 287, 288, 293, *301, 302, 303, 305*
Toth, EL, 56, *74*
Towbin, JA, 311, *323*
Toyoda, Y, 242, *250*
Tracey, KJ, 231, *247*
Treanor, J, 117, 121, 122, 128, 137, *145, 152, 159*
Treanor, JJ, 55, 61, 62, 63, 64, 66, 67, 68, 69, 70, 71, *73, 77, 78, 80, 82*, 115, 127, 130, 131, 133, 136, *143, 150, 153, 154, 155, 157, 159*, 161,

[Treanor, JJ]
  166, 177, 180, *185,* 270, *280,* 337, 345, *349, 353,* 365, *372*
Trentin, JT, 224, *244*
Tresnan, DB, 266, 268, *278*
Treuhaft, MW, 180, *200*
Triebwasser, JH, 31, *47*
Trinkle, JK, 96, *102*
Tripp, RA, 116, *144,* 210, *218,* 231, *247*
Tristram, DA, 176, 183, *199, 202,* 310, 313, 314, *323,* 342, *352*
Trkola, A, 131, *156*
Trousdale, MD, 240, *249*
Trow, T, 167, *191*
Truant, A, 123, *147*
Tsai, Tf, 344, *353*
Tsivitse, P, 168, *193*
Tsou, C, 163, 166, 167, *186, 191*
Tsou, CJ, 239, *248*
Tsukui, T, 242, *250*
Tsunoda, A, 328, *346*
Tsutsumi, H, 166, 170, *191, 195*
Tu, Q, 136, *158*
Tubergen, D, 171, *196*
Tucehurst, J, 136, *159*
Tufariello, J, 230, *247*
Tukiainen, P, 32, *48*
Tuler, J, 266, 267, *278*
Tunevall, G, 30, *44*
Tupasi, TE, 27, *41*
Turcanu, AG, 329, *346*
Turner, HC, 71, *81,* 270, *279*
Turner, NM, 96, *103*
Turner, RB, 181, *201,* 257, 258, 269, 272, *275, 279,* 342, 343, *352*
Turse, SE, 240, *249*
Tuthill, RW, 25, *38*
Tutschka, PJ, 95, *102*
Tuxen, DV, 31, *46*
Tyrrell, D, 272, *280*
Tyrrell, DA, 253, 254, 263, 264, 268, 269, 270, 271, 272, *273, 277, 279, 280*
Tyrrell, DAJ, 71, *81,* 111, *140,* 313, *324,* 328, *346*
Tyska, G, 134, *158*

U

Ueki, I, 208, *217*
Ueno, T, 34, *51*
Ukkonen, P, 32, *48*
Ullman, BM, 54, *73*
Ulmanen, I, 108, *138*
Ulmer, JB, 132, *156,* 363, *372*
Ultman, BM, 7, *21*
Umland, ET, 34, *51,* 289, 292, 297, *303, 305*
Ungureanu-Longrois, B, 298, *306*
Ura, T, 89, *99*
Urano, T, 167, 168, *192*
Urquhart, GE, 257, *275*
Utell, MJ, 113, *141*
Uwayyed, K, 180, *200*

V

Vaara, S, 128, *151*
Vaca, L, 298, *305*
Vagenakis, AG, 31, *47,* 366, *372*
Vaheri, A, 284, *301*
Valainis, GT, 91, *100*
Valenti, WM, 27, *41*
Valliant, V, 30, *45, 63,* 65, 66, *78,* 177, *199*
Valman, HB, 71, *81,* 268, 270, 271, *278*
van Beek, R, 126, *148*
van Beek, WC, 126, 128, *149*
van den Berg, AP, 320, *324*
van den Broek, PJ, 25, 29, *40*
van der Bij, W, 320, *324*
Van der Meer, JWM, 32, *47*
van Dijken, P, 240, *249*
Van Dissel, JT, 30, *43*
Van Dyke, R, 94, *101,* 339, 350
van Furth, R, 25, 29, *40*
Van Kirk, J, 169, *194*
Van Niewstadt, AI, 164, *189*
van Oirschot, JT, 162, *186*
Van Scoy, RE, 84, *97*
van Son, WJ, 320, *324*
Van Strik, R, 56, *74*

Van Tilburg, W, 337, *350*
Van Voris, JP, 134, *158*
Van Voris, LP, 334, *349*
van Wyke Coelingh, K, 163, *187*
Vander Ban, M, 164, *189*
Vander, JB, 33, *49*
VanderWerf, B, 127, *151*
Vanduwex, B, 93, *101*
vanMilaan, AJ, 179, *200*
Vanner, C, 287, *303*
VanVoris, LP, 171, 172, 182, 183, *196, 202*
Vapalahti, O, 284, *301*
Vaporciyan, AA, 296, *305*
Vardin, PG, 313, *324*
Varga, MJ, 227, *245*
Varghese, JN, 136, *159*
Vargosko, A, 205, *216*
Vargosko, AJ, 224, 237, 238, *244*
Varini, J, 296, *305*
Vartivarian, SE, 87, *98*
Vaughn, WT, 126, 127, *148*
Vazauez, F, 31, *47*
Veal, CF, 33, *49*
Venkatesan, S, 183, *202*
Ventura, AK, 93, *101,* 127, *151*
Vercellotti, GM, 30, *44,* 87, *98,* 161, 166, 167, 180, *185,* 314, *324*
Verhoff, J, 164, *189*
Versluis, DJ, 93, *101,* 127, *151*
Versteeg, J, 32, *47*
Vesterinen, E, 128, *151*
Vey, M, 113, *142*
Vianiopaa, R, 169, *193*
Vieira, P, 168, *193*
Vikerfors, T, 30, *44,* 63, 65, *79*
Villafranca, JE, 256, *274*
Villani, A, 167, 168, *192, 193*
Vink, P, 171, *196*
Virelizier, JL, 115, *142, 143*
Virolainen, E, 174, 176, *198*
Vitalis, TZ, 235, *246*
Vivo, A, 163, *188*
Vladimarsdottir, H, 263, *277*
Voelkel-Johnson, C, 231, *247*

Volin, L, 32, *48*
Volkert, P, 29, *42*
Volovitz, B, 172, *197*
Volvovitz, F, 130, *153*
von Bonsdorff, CH, 286, *302*
von Essen, R, 32, *48*
von Itzstein, M, 136, *159,* 345, *353*
von Segesser, L, 33, *50*
Von Sternberg, T, 62, *77,* 127, *150,* 356, 361, *370*
Vorkunova, NK, 132, *157*
Voss, TG, 296, *305*
Vrtis, R, 260, 261, *276*

W

Wade, MS, 242, *250*
Wadell, G, 224, 232, *244, 247*
Wagner, DK, 169, 180, *193, 200*
Wagner, J, 25, 29, *40*
Wagner, R, 108, *138*
Wagner, SC, 30, *45*
Wajda, A, 127, *150,* 356, *370*
Wakabayashi, T, 240, *249*
Wakai, Y, 298, *306*
Walcott, SM, 136, *159*
Wald, ER, 88, 89, *99,* 176, *199,* 213, *219,* 341, *351*
Wald, TG, 63, 64, 69, 70, 71, *78, 81,* 313, *323*
Walker, E, 32, *47*
Walker, JS, 340, *351*
Walker, W, 84, *97*
Wall, LV, 59, *75,* 125, *148,* 316, *324*
Wallace, J, 272, *280*
Wallace, JM, 90, *99*
Wallenstein, S, 29, *43,* 61, 63, 67, *76,* 127, *150,* 358, *371*
Walley, KR, 298, *305, 306*
Walls, HH, 125, *147*
Wallwork, J, 32, *48*
Walsh, EE, 55, 61, 63, 64, 65, 66, 67, 69, 70, 71, *73, 78, 79, 80,* 161, 162, 163, 164, 165, 166, 167, 169, 171, 177, 180, 183, *185, 186, 187, 188,*

[Walsh, EE]
189, 191, 193, 194, 196, 200, 203,
342, *351, 352,* 369, *373*
Walsh, JJ, 111, *140*
Waltz, AD, 355, *370*
Wandell, G, 223, 237, *244*
Waner, JL, 59, *75,* 125, *148,* 310, 313, 316, 317, *322, 324*
Waner, Jl, 311, 314, *323*
Wang, E, 165, *190*
Wang, EE, 342, 343, *352*
Wang, EEL, 175, 180, *198, 200*
Wang, M, 126, 129, *148, 153*
Wang, Q, 243, *250*
Wang, SP, 25, *39*
Ward, CW, 121, *146*
Ward, K, 169, *193*
Ward, MJ, 25, 29, *39*
Ward, PA, 296, *305*
Ward, R, 366, *372*
Ward, TG, 223, *244*
Wardlaw, AJ, 268, *279*
Warford, AL, 239, *248*
Wargow, CD, 256, *274*
Waring, JJ, 31, *47*
Waris, M, 166, *191*
Warner, GS, 35, *51*
Warner-Stevenson, L, 93, *101*
Warnock, M, 31, *46*
Warren, JL, 57, *74*
Washburne, JF, 165, *189*
Wasi, C, 27, *41*
Wasil, R, 71, *81*
Wasil, RE, 161, 165, *184*
Watanabe, I, 34, *50*
Wathen, MSW, 216, *220*
Watkins, JM, 123, *147,* 174, 176, *198,* 238, *248*
Watkins, SC, 298, *306*
Watson, D, 261, *276*
Watson, GI, 333, *348*
Watt, P, 169, *193*
Watters, LK, 215, *220*
Watthana-Kasetr, S, 27, *41*
Webb, AK, 31, *46*
Webb, PA, 342, 343, *353*

Webber-Jones, J, 35, *51,* 60, *76,* 133, *157*
Weber, DM, 31, *46,* 96, *103*
Weber, J, 127, *151*
Weber, JA, 127, *150*
Weber, JM, 311, 313, *323*
Webster, RG, 84, *97,* 113, 115, 117, 119, 121, 122, 125, 126, 127, 129, 132, 135, 137, *142, 143, 145, 146, 147, 148,* 149, *153, 156, 158, 159,* 363, *372*
Weg, JG, 31, *46,* 96, *102*
Wegmann, W, 31, *47*
Weibull, C, 227, *245*
Weimar, W, 93, *101,* 127, *151*
Weiner, LB, 29, *43,* 176, *199,* 261, *276,* 314, *324*
Weinstein, L, 31, *47*
Weinstein, MC, 361, *371*
Weis, W, 106, *138*
Weisdorf, DJ, 86, 87, 88, *98,* 213, *219,* 316, *324*
Weisdorf, FJ, 29, *43*
Weisensee, D, 298, *306*
Weiss, G, 31, *46*
Weiss, LM, 318, *324*
Weissenbacher, M, 27, *40, 41*
Weissenbacher, MC, 287, *303*
Weksler, ME, 62, *77,* 128, *152*
Welliver, R, 90, *100,* 172, 176, 183, *197, 199, 202*
Welliver, RC, 92, *101,* 171, 174, *195, 198,* 209, *218,* 310, 313, 314, *323,* 342, *352*
Wells, CR, 16, *22,* 209, *217*
Wells, GA, 292, *304*
Wells, JM, 113, *142,* 209, *217*
Wells, RM, 287, *303*
Welsh, MJ, 242, *250*
Weltzin, R, 181, *201*
Wendt, CH, 29, 30, *43,* 86, 87, 88, 89, *98, 99,* 213, *219,* 316, *324*
Wenman, WM, 240, *249*
Wenting, GJ, 93, *101,* 127, *151*
Wentworth, BB, 30, *44,* 63, *79*
Wenzel, RP, 29, *43,* 61, 66, 71, *76, 80, 81,* 87, *98,* 126, *149,* 165, 166, 177, *189,* 268, 270, *278,* 316, 317, *325*

Author Index

Werchau, H, 167, *191*
Werdan, K, 298, *306*
Werner, HA, 298, *305*
Wertz, GW, 162, 163, 166, 169, 170, 183, *186, 187, 188, 194, 202*
Westrich, MK, 131, *155*
Wharton, J, 106, *138*
Wharton, M, 366, *372*
Wheeler, A, 298, *305*
Wheeler, EO, 33, *49*
Wheeler, JC, 181, *201*
Wheeler, JG, 113, *141,* 342, 343, *352*
Whimbey, E, 32, *48,* 64, *79,* 85, 86, 87, 88, 91, 92, 93, 94, 95, *97, 98, 100, 101, 102,* 117, 123, *145,* 165, 166, 177, 181, *189, 190, 201,* 369, *373*
Whitcomb, ME, 292, *304*
White, DA, 32, *48*
White, E, 228, 230, *245*
White, HF, 136, *159*
White, R, 232, *244*
White, RG, 31, *47*
White, RJ, 25, *38*
Whitehead, S, 183, *202*
Whitfield, SG, 286, *302*
Whitney, SE, 131, *156*
Whittaker, G, 107, *138*
Wickham, TJ, 227, 228, 232, *245*
Wiedemann, HP, 292, *304*
Wield, G, 161, *185*
Wigand, R, 224, 226, 235, 236, *244, 247*
Wilcosky, TC, 90, *99*
Wilcox, HNA, 232, *244*
Wildin, SR, 175, *199*
Wiley, D, 106, *138*
Wiley, DC, 119, *146*
Wilkinson, BE, 130, *153,* 365, *372*
Wilkinson, D, 240, *249*
Williams, AJ, 297, *305*
Williams, D, 127, *151*
Williams, GW, 127, *151*
Williams, JL, 230, *247*
Williams, L, 117, 123, *145*
Williams, MA, 107, *138*
Williams, MS, 127, *149*
Williams, OB, 69, *81*
Williams, P, 30, *45,* 132, *156,* 235, *246*
Williams, RK, 266, 268, *278*
Williams, T, 31, 32, *46, 48,* 96, *102*
Williams, TD, 25, 29, *39*
Williams, WW, 38, *51,* 62, *77,* 358, *370*
Williamson, J, 30, *44,* 63, 64, *78*
Williamson, MR, 292, *305*
Willis, G, 136, *158*
Willis, PWI, 125, *147*
Wills, RJ, 331, *347, 348*
Willy, M, 216, *221*
Wilson, GA, 311, 313, *323*
Wilson, GP, 296, *305*
Wilson, JM, 227, 232, 236, 242, 243, *245, 247, 250, 251*
Wilson, MH, 130, *154,* 215, *220,* 369, *373*
Wilson, S, 169, 181, *194*
Wilson, SZ, 95, *102,* 136, *158, 159,* 180, *201,* 341, *351*
Wingard, JR, 95, *102*
Wingfield, WL, 334, *348*
Winkelstein, W, 171, *196*
Winn, N, 87, *98*
Winston, DJ, 96, *102*
Winter, CC, 207, 212, 215, *217,* 219, 220
Winter, PE, 238, *248*
Winterbauer, RH, 29, *42*
Winther, B, 257, 258, 268, *275*
Wiselka, M, 59, *75*
Wiselka, MJ, 69, 71, *81*
Witkowski, JT, 338, 339, 350, *350*
Wkehel, J, 106, *138*
Wnag, HJ, 127, *151*
Woestenborghs, R, 264, *277*
Wofford, J, 181, *201*
Wold, AD, 35, *51*
Wold, LJ, 231, *247*
Wold, WM, 229, 231, *245, 247*
Wold, WSM, 230, 231, *247*
Wolf, JL, 209, *217*
Wolf, M, 30, *43,* 86, 87, *98*
Wolff, JA, 93, *101,* 132, *156*
Wolff, M, 31, *46*
Wolff, T, 137, *160*

Wollmer, P, 268, *279*
Wolontis, S, 30, *44,* 63, 66, *79, 80*
Wolstenholme, AJ, 132, *157,* 330, 336, *347, 349*
Wong, D, 169, *193*
Wong, DC, 205, *217*
Wong, DT, 209, *218*
Wong, RD, 35, *51*
Wood, FT, 130, *154*
Wood, JM, 129, *153*
Wood, SC, 66, *80,* 161, 165, *184*
Woodhead, MA, 25, 29, *39*
Woodin, KA, 84, *97*
Woods, JM, 136, *159*
Woodward, C, 88, *98*
Woody, JN, 115, *143*
Wooford, J, 342, 343, *352*
Woolridge, RL, 236, *247*
Wortman, I, 167, *192*
Woyskovsky, N, 27, *40*
Wreghitt, TG, 32, *48,* 88, *98*
Wright, J, 30, *45*
Wright, KE, 311, 313, *323*
Wright, P, 134, *158,* 335, *349*
Wright, PF, 90, *100,* 113, 115, 117, 126, 127, 128, 130, 131, *142, 144, 148, 152, 153, 154, 155,* 169, 170, 171, 180, 182, 183, *194, 200, 202,* 211, 212, 215, *219, 220,* 237, *248,* 365, 369, *372, 373*
Wright, SM, 122, *147*
Wu, F, 230, *247*
Wu, MJ, 330, *347*
Wu, SP, 61, 69, *76*
Wu, WP, 134, *158*
Wu, WY, 136, *159*
Wu, Y, 255, 259, 264, *274*
Wuarles, JM, 136, *159*
Wulffraat, N, 240, *249*
Wunderlich, D, 265, *277*
Wuorenma, J, 62, *77,* 127, *150,* 356, 361, *370*
Wycoff, D, 313, *324*
Wyde, P, 169, 181, *194*
Wyde, PR, 94, 95, *101, 102,* 180, *200, 201*
Wyld, S, 170, 171, *195*

X

Xu, X, 120, 129, *146, 153*
Xuan, BB, 32, *48*

Y

Yadon, ZE, 287, *303*
Yamada, T, 284, 286, 287, 293, *302, 303, 305*
Yamakawa, M, 211, 212, *218, 219*
Yamamoto, S, 29, *43,* 68, *80*
Yamashita, M, 120, *146*
Yanagihara, R, 284, 287, *301, 303*
Yang, E, 25, *39*
Yang, Y, 236, 242, 243, *247, 250, 251*
Yankaskas, JR, 164, *189*
Yao, A, 298, *306*
Yap, KL, 117, *145*
Yasui, M, 34, *51*
Yazaki, P, 132, *157*
Ye, Z, 108, *138*
Yeager, AM, 95, *102*
Yeager, CL, 266, 268, *278*
Yealland, SJ, 261, *276*
Yelandi, AV, 29, *43,* 113, *141*
Yen, TSB, 31, *46*
Yermian, C, 127, *151*
Yewdell, JW, 117, *144,* 163, *188*
Yinnon, A, 62, *77,* 131, *155*
Yokogoshi, Y, 113, *142,* 211, *218*
Yokoyama, T, 298, *305*
Yokoyama, WM, 115, *142*
Yolken, RH, 59, *75,* 214, *220*
Yoneyama, K, 242, *250*
Yong-doo, K, 34, *50*
York, MK, 34, *50*
Yorke, MA, 119, *146*
Yoshida, S, 29, *43,* 68, *80,* 270, *279*
Yoshimura, K, 242, *250*
Yoshiro, Y, 224, *244*
Young, EC, 136, *159*
Young, HW, 340, *351*
Young, KKY, 170, 183, *195, 202*
Younkin, SW, 134, *158*

Younkin, Sw, 335, *349*
Yousem, SA, 30, 32, *45, 48,* 235, *246*
Yousuf, H, 94, *101*
Yousuf, HM, 87, 88, *98*
Yu, R, 167, *192*
Yu, VL, 25, *39*
Yu, Y, 163, *188*
Yuen, JB, 29, *43,* 58, 63, 64, *74,* 161, 180, *185,* 314, *324*

Z

Zabner, J, 227, 233, 242, *245, 250*
Zack, JA, 127, *151*
Zaghouani, H, 131, *156*
Zahradnik, JM, 30, *45*
Zaia, JA, 83, 96, *97*
Zaki, S, 286, 296, *303, 305*
Zaki, SR, 34, *51,* 284, 286, 287, 289, 292, 293, 294, 295, 296, 297, *301, 302, 303, 304, 305*
Zambon, MC, 330, 336, *347*
Zambrano, MAR, 31, *47*
Zamora, CA, 96, *102*
Zandotti, C, 33, *49*
Zapol, WM, 287, 292, *303*
Zardiz, M, 169, *193*
Zaroukian, MH, 30, *44,* 63, 65, *79*
Zarraga, AL, 30, *45*
Zbinden, R, 163, 166, *186*
Zebedee, SL, 115, *143,* 181, *201*

Zeh, J, 33, *50*
Zei, T, 128, *152*
Zella, D, 320, *324*
Zellar, JA, 30, *45*
Zenati, MA, 32, *48*
Zhang, T, 121, *146*
Zhang, TJ, 121, *146*
Zhang, WD, 311, 313, *323*
Zhang, YQ, 134, *158*
Zheng, T, 167, *191*
Zhirnov, OP, 215, *220*
Zhou, N, 121, *146*
Zhou, NN, 121, *146*
Zhu, Z, 255, 259, 264, *274*
Ziebuhr, J, 267, *278*
Ziegler, T, 310, 313, *322*
Ziglmans, JMJM, 30, *43*
Zijlstra, M, 117, *145,* 210, *218*
Zike, K, 30, *44*
Zilkha, KJ, 328, *346*
Ziment, I, 69, 70, 71, *81*
Zimmerman, GA, 292, *304*
Zinkernagel, R, 170, *195*
Zitelli, B, 88, 89, *98*
Zlotnik, A, 168, *193*
Zlydnikov, DM, 329, *346*
Zoltick, PW, 267, *278*
Zumwalt, R, 284, 286, *302*
Zumwalt, RE, 292, 293, 294, 295, 296, *305*
Zurawin, RK, 29, *43*
Zweygberg-Wirgart, B, 32, *49*

SUBJECT INDEX

A

Adenovirus
  and conjunctivitis, 238
  and immunocompromised hosts, 237
  and pharyngitis, 238
  classification, 224
  early genes, 229–230
  epidemiology, 236
  fiber protein, 231
  gene expressions, 228
  history, 223
  morphology, 226
  persistence, 233
  pneumonia, 30
  serotypes and organ specificity, 225
  vaccines, 240–241
Amantadine
  history, 327–329
  mechanism of action, 329–330
  pharmacokinetics, 330–331
  prophylaxis, 331–334
  resistance, 335–336
  therapy, 132–136, 334–335
  toxicity, 336–337
Apnea
  and respiratory syncytial virus, 175

Asthma
  and coronavirus, 271
  and respiratory syncytial virus, 173
  and rhinovirus, 260

B

Bronchiolitis
  and respiratory syncytial virus, 171, 175

C

Conjunctivitis
  and adenovirus, 238
Coronavirus
  and asthma, 271
  diagnosis, 272
  in elderly, 71–72
  epidemiology, 270
  experimental infection, 269
  microbiology, 266
  receptor, 266
  upper respiratory infections, 271
Croup
  and steroid therapy, 215

Cytokines
  in rhinovirus infection, 258–260
Cytomegalovirus, 31–33, 95–96

D

Diagnosis
  adenovirus, 317–318
  antigen detection, 309
  cell cultures, 309
  coronavirus, 272, 318–319
  cytomegalovirus, 319–321
  enzyme-linked immunosorbent
    assays, 310–311
  hantaviruses, 293–294
  herpes simplex virus, 321–322
  immunofluorescence, 210
  influenza viruses, 125–126, 314–316
  parainfluenza virus, 214, 316
  polymerase chain reaction, 311–312
  respiratory syncytial virus, 178–180, 314
  rhinovirus, 313–314
  serology, 312–313
  specimen collection, 308

E

Epidemiology
  adenovirus, 236
  coronavirus, 270
  parainfluenza virus, 212
  respiratory syncytial virus, 164
  rhinovirus, 263
Epstein-Barr virus, 11

H

Hantavirus
  animal reservoir, 286
  classification, 282–284
  clinical manifestations, 288–291
  diagnosis, 293–294
  epidemiology, 285–286

[Hantavirus]
  histopathology, 294–295
  laboratory findings, 292–293
  pathogenesis, 295–298
  prevention, 300
  radiographic findings, 293
  replication, 284–285
  structure, 285
  therapy, 298–300, 343–344
History
  adenovirus, 223
  parainfluenza virus, 205
  respiratory syncytial virus, 161

I

IgA immunity
  and parainfluenza virus, 209
Immunocompromised hosts
  and adenovirus infections, 85, 89, 91, 237
  and cytomegalovirus infections, 95–96
  and herpes simplex virus infections, 31, 95
  and influenza virus infections, 84–91, 123
  and parainfluenza virus infections, 85–91, 213
  prevention of respiratory virus infections, 91–93
  and respiratory syncytial virus infections, 85–91, 166
  respiratory virus infections
    in bone marrow transplants, 85–88
    in cancer, 84–85
    in HIV infections, 89–91
    in solid organ transplants, 88–89
  treatment of respiratory virus infections, 94–95
  and varicella-zoster virus infections, 31, 96
Immunoglobulin prophylaxis
  in respiratory syncytial virus, 182

Immunoglobulin therapy
  in respiratory syncytial virus, 181
Influenza A and B viruses
  antigenic variation, 119–122
  chemoprophylaxis, 132–136
  clinical manifestations, 29, 123–125
  complications, 124–125
  diagnosis, 125–126
  in elderly, 55–62
  epidemiology, 117–119
  genetics, 106
  histopathology, 111–113
  immune responses, 114–117
  and immunocompromised hosts, 123
  pathogenesis, 109–111
  replication, 106–109
  treatment
    amantadine, 132–136
    neuroaminidase inhibitors, 136–137, 345
    rimantadine, 132–136
  vaccines
    inactivated, 126–130
    live, 130–131

L

Lower respiratory infections
  causes in adults, 27–29
  causes in children, 7
  in developing countries, 17–20
  etiology by age, 10–11, 14
  etiology by syndrome, 12
  susceptibility in children, 15

M

Measles
  pneumonia, 33–34
  vaccines, 365
Microbiology
  coronavirus, 266
  parainfluenza virus, 206

[Microbiology]
  respiratory syncytial virus, 162–164
  rhinovirus, 254

P

Pharyngitis
  and adenovirus, 238
Parainfluenza virus
  and immunocompromised hosts, 213
  comparison with influenza, 207
  comparison with respiratory syncytial virus, 207
  diagnosis, 214
  in elderly, 67–69
  epidemiology, 212
  history, 205
  IgA immunity, 209
  microbiology, 206
  pneumonia, 29–30
  receptor, 208
  vaccine, 215

R

Receptor
  coronavirus, 266
  parainfluenza virus, 208
  rhinovirus, 255
Respiratory syncytial virus
  and apnea, 175
  and asthma, 173
  and bronchiolitis, 171, 175
  diagnosis, 178–180
  disease due to inactivated vaccine
  disease in infancy, 175
  in elderly, 62–67, 177
  epidemiology, 164
  and epithelial cells,
  history, 161
  immunocompromised hosts, 166
  immunoglobin prophylaxis, 182
  immunoglobin therapy, 181

[Respiratory syncytial virus]
   microbiology, 162–164
   in organ transplant patients, 177
   pneumonia, 30
   ribavirin, 180
   role of antibody in protection, 169
   role of t-lymphocytes in protection, 170
   strain, 166
   vaccines
      live, 183
      subunit, 183
Rhinovirus
   cytokines, 258–260
   in elderly, 67–71
   epidemiology, 263
   microbiology, 254
   pneumonia, 30
   receptor, 255
   sinusitis, 257
   transmission, 256
   treatment, 264
   upper respiratory infections, 263
Ribavirin
   aerosol administration, 339
   in hantavirus infections, 299, 343–344
   in influenza virus infections, 136, 340–341
   mechanism of action, 338–339
   pharmacokinetics, 339
   in respiratory syncytial virus infection, 180, 341–343
Rimantadine
   mechanism of action, 329–330
   pharmacokinetics, 330–331
   prophylaxis, 331–334

[Rimantadine]
   resistance, 335–336
   therapy, 132–136, 334–335
   toxicity, 336–337

S

Sinusitis
   rhinovirus as a cause, 257
Surface protein cleavage
   in parainfluenza virus, 211

U

Upper respiratory infections
   and coronaviruses, 271
   and rhinoviruses, 263

V

Vaccines
   adenovirus, 240–241
   influenza
      cost effectiveness, 361
      in elderly, 356–358
      history, 355
      side effects, 359
   live
      respiratory syncytial virus, 183
   measles, 365
   parainfluenza virus, 215
   subunit
      respiratory syncytial virus, 183
Varicella-zoster virus, 31, 96
Viral–bacterial interactions, 8